History of Modern Clinical Toxicology

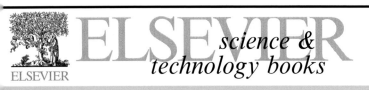

Companion Web Site:

https://www.elsevier.com/books-and-journals/book-companion/978012822218

History of Modern Clinical Toxicology
Alan Woolf, Philip Wexler, Editors

This site provides the following resources:

- The History of Modern Clinical Toxicology Study Guide

- The History of Modern Clinical Toxicology Study Guide ANSWER KEY

ELSEVIER

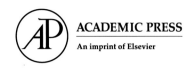
ACADEMIC PRESS
An imprint of Elsevier

History of Toxicology and Environmental Health Series

History of Modern Clinical Toxicology

Editor
Alan D. Woolf
Boston Children's Hospital & Harvard Medical School, Boston, Massachusetts, United States

Series Editor
Philip Wexler

Section Editors
Nicholas Bateman
Jeffrey Brent
Jou-Fang Deng
Susan Smolinske
Chen-Chang Yang

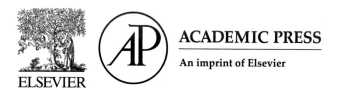

ELSEVIER

ACADEMIC PRESS
An imprint of Elsevier

Academic Press is an imprint of Elsevier
125 London Wall, London EC2Y 5AS, United Kingdom
525 B Street, Suite 1650, San Diego, CA 92101, United States
50 Hampshire Street, 5th Floor, Cambridge, MA 02139, United States
The Boulevard, Langford Lane, Kidlington, Oxford OX5 1GB, United Kingdom

Notices
Knowledge and best practice in this field are constantly changing. As new research and experience broaden our understanding, changes in research methods, professional practices, or medical treatment may become necessary.

Practitioners and researchers must always rely on their own experience and knowledge in evaluating and using any information, methods, compounds, or experiments described herein. In using such information or methods they should be mindful of their own safety and the safety of others, including parties for whom they have a professional responsibility.

To the fullest extent of the law, neither the Publisher nor the authors, contributors, or editors, assume any liability for any injury and/or damage to persons or property as a matter of products liability, negligence or otherwise, or from any use or operation of any methods, products, instructions, or ideas contained in the material herein.

Library of Congress Cataloging-in-Publication Data
A catalog record for this book is available from the Library of Congress

British Library Cataloguing-in-Publication Data
A catalogue record for this book is available from the British Library

ISBN: 978-0-12-822218-8

For information on all Academic Press publications
visit our website at https://www.elsevier.com/books-and-journals

Publisher: Stacy Masucci
Acquisitions Editor: Kattie Washington
Editorial Project Manager: Tracy Tufaga
Production Project Manager: Swapna Srinivasan
Cover Designer: Matthew Limbert

Typeset by STRAIVE, India

Working together
to grow libraries in
developing countries

www.elsevier.com • www.bookaid.org

Dedication

I dedicate this book to my family: my wife Linda, daughter Kristina (who helped with the research and editing), and son Nicholas. Their love, encouragement, and support have been invaluable. Dr. Frederick H. Lovejoy, Jr., has been my preceptor, my mentor, an inspiration, and my role model since I first arrived in Boston more than 35 years ago. I also acknowledge an important debt to my dear friend and colleague, Dr. Michael W. Shannon, who taught me so much before his untimely death in 2009. Finally, I dedicate this book to all the hardworking colleagues in clinical and medical toxicology and the staffs of poison control centers worldwide, whose dedication to their work helps others and saves lives.

Contents

Section 1
Disasters: Examples of toxic calamities in modern times

Alan D. Woolf

1.1 Triortho cresyl phosphate "Ginger Jake" disaster—United States, 1930s

Alan D. Woolf

1.2 Three methylmercury poisoning disasters

Alan D. Woolf

1.2.1 Minamata Bay, Japan

1.3   Community dioxin disaster—Seveso Italy, 1976

Alan D. Woolf

1.4   Arsenic in tube well water—Bangladesh, 1970s–1990s

Alan D. Woolf

1.5   Toxic oil syndrome—Spain, 1981

Alan D. Woolf

1.6   Eosinophilia-myalgia syndrome—United States, 1989

Alan D. Woolf

1.10 Japan "Yusho" poisoning, 1968 and Taiwan "Yucheng" poisoning, 1979

Alan D. Woolf

Section 2
Notable pharmaceutical poisoning incidents and poisoned people

Alan D. Woolf

2.1 Sulfanilamide (diethylene glycol) disaster— United States, 1937

Alan D. Woolf

2.6 Yushchenko (dioxin), 2004 and Markov (ricin), 1978: Two political poisonings

Alan D. Woolf

2.6.1 Viktor Yushchenko

2.6.2 Markov incident—Ricin—London, 1978

Section 3
Discovery of selected modern antidotes

Alan D. Woolf and Jeffrey Brent

3.1 *N*-Acetylcysteine

John Rague

3.2 Fomepizole

Kenneth E. McMartin

3.3 Methylene blue

Mary Ann Howland

3.4 British anti-lewisite (dimercaprol)

Marissa Hauptman and Alan D. Woolf

3.5 Pralidoxime and oximes

Alexander F. Barbuto and Michele M. Burns

3.6 Naloxone

David Toomey and Edward W. Boyer

3.7 Physostigmine

Nathan Kunzler and Timothy B. Erickson

Section 4
Clinical toxicology and poison control in the United States
Alan D. Woolf

Section 5
Clinical toxicology and poison information in Europe, Scandinavia, and Israel

D. Nicholas Bateman

5.1   United Kingdom and Ireland

D. Nicholas Bateman and Alex Proudfoot

5.2   Czech Republic and other Central European and Eastern European countries

Daniela Pelclova

5.5 The Netherlands

Irma de Vries and Antoinette van Riel

5.6 Belgium

Anne-Marie Descamps and Dominique Vandijck

Section 6
Clinical toxicology and poison control in Asia and Australia
Alan D. Woolf, Jou-Fang Deng, and Chen-Chang Yang

6.1 Australia
Andrew Dawson, Nicole Wright, and Ian Whyte

6.2 The Chinese mainland
Xiangdong Jian and Mei Zeng

6.3 Taiwan
Chen-Chang Yang and Jou-Fang Deng

6.4 The Philippines

Irma Reyes Makalinao and Lynn Crisanta del Rosario Panganiban

6.5 Vietnam

Nguyen Trung Nguyen

6.6 Thailand

Winai Wananukul and Charuwan Sriapha

6.7 South Korea

Hyung-Keun Roh

Contributors

Numbers in parenthesis indicate the pages on which the authors' contributions begin.

Alexander F. Barbuto (255), Department of Emergency Medicine, Carl R. Darnall Army Medical Center, Ft. Hood, TX, United States

D. Nicholas Bateman (369, 371, 505), Honorary Professor of Clinical Toxicology, University of Edinburgh, Edinburgh, United Kingdom

Vikhyat S. Bebarta (279), Center for Combat Medicine and Battlefield (COMBAT) Research, Aurora, CO; Translational Research, Innovation, and Antidote Development (TRIAD) Research, Aurora, CO; Department of Emergency Medicine, Anschutz Medical Campus, University of Colorado, Aurora, CO; Rocky Mountain Poison and Drug Safety, Denver Health and Hospital Authority, Denver, CO; Office of the Chief Scientist, 59th Medical Wing/Science and Technology, Joint Base San Antonio, San Antonio, TX, United States

Yedidia Bentur (481), Israel Poison Information Center, Rambam Health Care Campus, The Rappaport Faculty of Medicine, Technion-Israel Institute of Technology, Haifa, Israel

Edward W. Boyer (265), Department of Emergency Medicine, Brigham and Women's Hospital, Harvard Medical School, Boston, MA, United States

Jeffrey Brent (199), Distinguished Clinical Professor of Medicine and Emergency Medicine, University of Colorado School of Medicine, Aurora, CO, United States

Mary Jean Brown (97), Department of Social and Behavioral Sciences, Harvard T. H. Chan School of Public Health, Boston, MA, United States

Michele M. Burns (255), Harvard Medical Toxicology Fellowship/Division of Emergency Medicine, Boston Children's Hospital, Boston, MA, United States

Andrew Dawson (515), Clinical Toxicology and Drug Health, Royal Prince Alfred Hospital; New South Wales Poisons Information Centre, Children's Hospital Westmead, Sydney, NSW, Australia

Jou-Fang Deng (511, 527), Division of Clinical Toxicology & Occupational Medicine, Department of Medicine, Taipei Veterans General Hospital, Taipei, Taiwan

Anne-Marie Descamps (421), Belgian Poison Center, Brussels; Faculty of Medicine and Health Sciences, Ghent University, Ghent, Belgium

Herbert Desel (403), German Federal Institute for Risk Assessment, Berlin, Germany

Ana Ferrer Dufol (441), Unit of Clinical Toxicology, Clinic University Hospital, Zaragoza; Spanish Foundation of Clinical Toxicology, Barcelona, Spain

Timothy B. Erickson (271), Chief, Division of Medical Toxicology, Department of Emergency Medicine, Mass General Brigham, Harvard Medical School, Harvard Humanitarian Initiative, Boston, MA, United States

Robert Garnier (431), Paris Poison Control Centre, Federation of Toxicology, Fernand-Widal Hospital, University of Paris, Paris, France

Gabriel C. Gaviola (85), Resident Physician, Harvard T.H. Chan School of Public Health, Boston, MA, United States

Yu. S. Goldfarb (395), N.V. Sklifosovsky Research Institute for Emergency Medicine (RIA) of the Moscow Health Department; Federal State Budgetary Educational Institution of Additional Professional Education "Russian Medical Academy of Continuous Professional Education" of the Ministry of Healthcare of the Russian Federation, Moscow, Russia

Rose Goldman (85), Associate Professor of Medicine, Harvard Medical School, Boston; Associate Professor in the Department of Environmental Health, Harvard T.H. Chan School of Public Health, Boston; Department of Medicine, Cambridge Health Alliance, Cambridge, MA, United States

John Haines (493), Formerly International Programme on Chemical Safety, World Health Organization, Geneva, Switzerland

Marissa Hauptman (243), Boston Children's Hospital & Harvard Medical School, Boston, Massachusetts, United States

Lotte C.G. Hoegberg (471), Department of Anesthesiology and The Danish Poisons Information Centre, Copenhagen University Hospital Bispebjerg, Copenhagen, Denmark

Mary Ann Howland (231), Clinical Professor of Pharmacy, St. John's University College of Pharmacy and Health Sciences Adjunct Professor of Emergency Medicine, New York University School of Medicine Bellevue Hospital Emergency Department Senior Consultant in Residence, New York City Poison Center New York, NY, United States

Xiangdong Jian (519), Department of Poisoning and Occupational Diseases, Emergency, Qilu Hospital, Cheeloo College of Medicine, Shandong University, Jinan, Shandong, China

Nathan Kunzler (271), Department of Emergency Medicine, Medical Toxicology Fellowship Program, Regions Hospital, St. Paul, MN, United States

Hugo Kupferschmidt (465), Poisons Centre, Charité-Universitätsmedizin Berlin, Berlin, Germany

Carlo Alessandro Locatelli (451), Toxicology Unit, Pavia Poison Centre and National Toxicology Information Centre, Laboratory of Clinical and Experimental Toxicology, IRCCS Hospital of Pavia, Istituti Clinici Scientifici Maugeri, Pavia, Italy

Joseph K. Maddry (279) Department of Emergency Medicine, Brooke Army Medical Center, San Antonio, TX; Emergency Medicine, Uniformed Services University of the Health Sciences, Bethesda, MD; United States Army Institute of Surgical Research, San Antonio, TX, United States

Irma Reyes Makalinao (537), Department of Pharmacology and Toxicology, College of Medicine, University of the Philippines; University of the Philippines National Poison Management and Control Center, Philippine General Hospital, Manila, Philippines

Kenneth E. McMartin (213), Department of Pharmacology, Toxicology & Neuroscience, Louisiana State University Health Sciences Center, Shreveport, LA, United States

Bruno Mégarbane (431), Department of Medical and Toxicological Critical Care, Federation of Toxicology, Lariboisière Hospital, University of Paris, Paris, France

Patrick C. Ng (279), Department of Emergency Medicine, Brooke Army Medical Center, San Antonio, TX; Emergency Medicine, Uniformed Services University of the Health Sciences, Bethesda, MD; Emergency Medicine, University of Colorado Anschutz Medical Campus, Aurora, CO; En Route Care Research Center, 59th Medical Wing/Science and Technology, Joint Base San Antonio, San Antonio, TX, United States

Nguyen Trung Nguyen (547), Poison Control Center of Bach Mai Hospital, Hanoi, Vietnam

Yu. N. Ostapenko (395), N.V. Sklifosovsky Research Institute for Emergency Medicine (RIA) of the Moscow Health Department; Federal State Budgetary Educational Institution of Additional Professional Education "Russian Medical Academy of Continuous Professional Education" of the Ministry of Healthcare of the Russian Federation; Research and Applied Toxicological Center of the Russian Federal Medical and Biological Agency, Moscow, Russia

Lynn Crisanta del Rosario Panganiban (537), Department of Pharmacology and Toxicology, College of Medicine, University of the Philippines; University of the Philippines National Poison Management and Control Center, Philippine General Hospital, Manila, Philippines

Daniela Pelclova (383), Toxicological Information Centre, Department of Occupational Medicine, First Faculty of Medicine, Charles University in Prague and General University Hospital Prague, Czech Republic

Alex Proudfoot (371), Former Physician Royal Infirmary of Edinburgh and Director Scottish Poisons Information Bureau, Edinburgh, United Kingdom

John Rague (201), Rocky Mountain Poison and Drug Safety; Department of Emergency Medicine, Denver Health and Hospital Authority, Denver, CO, United States

Antoinette van Riel (413), Dutch Poisons Information Center, University Medical Center Utrecht, Utrecht University, Utrecht, The Netherlands

Hyung-Keun Roh (563), Past President, The Korean Society of Clinical Toxicology

Susan Smolinske New Mexico Poison & Drug Information Center; Pharmacy Practice and Administration, University of New Mexico, Albuquerque, NM, United States

Charuwan Sriapha (555), Ramathibodi Poison Center, Faculty of Medicine Ramathibodi Hospital, Mahidol University, Bangkok, Thailand

Andreas Stürer (403), Mainz Poison Centre, University Medical Center of the Johannes Gutenberg University Mainz [JGIU], Mainz, Germany

Joanna Tempowski (493), Formerly International Programme on Chemical Safety, World Health Organization, Geneva, Switzerland

David Toomey (265), Department of Emergency Medicine, Brigham and Women's Hospital, Harvard Medical School, Boston, MA, United States

Dominique Vandijck (421), Belgian Poison Center, Brussels; Faculty of Medicine and Health Sciences, Ghent University, Ghent, Belgium

Irma de Vries (413), Dutch Poisons Information Center, University Medical Center Utrecht, Utrecht University, Utrecht, The Netherlands

Winai Wananukul (555), Ramathibodi Poison Center; Department of Medicine, Faculty of Medicine Ramathibodi Hospital, Mahidol University, Bangkok, Thailand

Ian Whyte (515), Department of Clinical Toxicology and Pharmacology, Calvary Mater Newcastle, Waratah, NSW, Australia

Alan D. Woolf (1, 5, 15, 35, 45, 61, 71, 97, 109, 121, 137, 139, 149, 155, 165, 177, 183, 199, 243, 287, 297, 311, 329, 341, 357, 511), Boston Children's Hospital & Harvard Medical School, Boston, Massachusetts, United States

Nicole Wright (515), New South Wales Poisons Information Centre, Children's Hospital Westmead, Sydney, NSW, Australia

Santiago Nogué Xarau (441), Spanish Foundation of Clinical Toxicology, Barcelona, Spain

Chen-Chang Yang (511, 527), Institute of Environmental & Occupational Health Sciences, School of Medicine, National Yang Ming Chiao Tung University; Division of Clinical Toxicology & Occupational Medicine, Department of Medicine, Taipei Veterans General Hospital, Taipei, Taiwan

Mei Zeng (519), Department of Poisoning and Occupational Diseases, Emergency, Qilu Hospital, Cheeloo College of Medicine, Shandong University, Jinan, Shandong, China

Foreword

Poisons have been a part of human history passed down verbally for millennia and written through recorded history. Paracelsus (1493–1541) almost 600 years ago stated (translated from the original German), "All substances are poisons: there is none which is not a poison. The right dose differentiates a poison from a remedy." This knowledge has permitted medicine to advance treatment of disease states with appropriate dosing and at the same time has resulted in everything from mass murder to accidental death. The use of raw materials from plants as medications resulted in a wide variety of effects, some of which were helpful and some of which were not. Physicians had gardens from which they collected treatments such as digitalis but with erratic dosing. It was the development of the United States Pharmacopeia in the early 1800s and eventually the Food and Drug Administration by Harvey Wiley in the early 20th century that led to the safer use of medications. The last 200–250 years have been defined as the Industrial Revolution resulting in an explosive growth of the use of chemicals in just about every aspect of life. In addition to industrial accidents, well described in this book, the poisoning of our air, water, and land with a myriad of substances coupled with climate change has certainly created challenges for the future of every living thing on earth.

There have been numerous cases of accidental poisonings such as the accidental substitution of arsenic for "daft" in the making of candy in Yorkshire in 1858. Arsenic remained a common poison agent memorialized in the play, "Arsenic and Old Lace." Arsenic was responsible for a wave of poisonings in the middle 1800s as it became well known. Eleven Blue Men is a classic report of the substitution of sodium nitrite for sodium chloride in breakfast oatmeal as one of 12 epidemiologic medical detective stories from the New Yorker published in the book by Berton Roueche. The television series "Breaking Bad" had several instances of poison use including ricin and *Convallaria majalis* known as Lily of the Valley in addition to the main issue which was methamphetamine and a classic implementation of hydrofluoric acid. Accidental poisoning in farm animals from sweet clover, described in the 1920s, led to the medically important anticoagulant WARFARIN (chemically discovered and named at the *W*isconsin *A*lumni *R*esearch *F*oundation *In*corporated).

Examples of industrial accidents primarily due to questionable practices continue to be an ongoing concern. Methyl isocyanate released at a Union Carbide plant in Bhopal killed up to 10,000 people with many more injured. Slower actions such as 2,3,7,8-tetrachlorodibenzo-*p*-dioxin (TCDD) from the Seveso disaster in 1976 with thousands exposed led to an unknown number of illnesses and deaths. The Minamata Bay disaster from release of methylmercury led to thousands of patients over time and a striking book by photographers Eugene and Aileen Smith published in 1975. And the 1937 sulfanilamide-diethylene glycol disaster, which caused 365 poisonings and 105 deaths, led to a much more robust Food and Drug Administration. While each accident has led to our knowledge, it has been a difficult way to develop safer practices.

Deliberate poisonings such as cyanide-laced Tylenol killed 7 in 1982; the perpetrator has never been found and the motivation for doing this remains unknown. Physicians, pharmacists, and nurses have certainly provided their share of murder by poisons. Dr. Hawley Crippen utilized hyoscine to murder Cora Turner and was the first to be caught by radio as told by Erick Larson in the book: *"Thunderstruck"*. Michael Swango, MD, killed with medications repeatedly (perhaps 60 times) and even after a conviction in 1985 was allowed back into a residency and to work at other hospitals until he was finally sent to the supermax prison in Colorado for life in 2000. H. H. Holmes, MD, of Chicago, known as America's first serial killer, was responsible for as many as 200 deaths in a chamber outfitted with carbon monoxide. His misdeeds were well described in the book, *"Devil in the White City"* by Erik Larson. The pharmacist, Mitesh Patel, killed his wife with insulin followed by asphyxiation. The fourth season of the television series Fargo has an apparently psychopathic nurse who causes illness in a family with syrup of ipecac and poisons others with a variety of poisons. An illness, "Munchausen syndrome by proxy" due to intentional poisoning by care-givers, must be considered as part of the differential diagnosis especially in young children with repetitive, difficult to explain illnesses.

Caustics have been well recognized as a health hazard resulting in the Federal Caustic Poison Act passed in 1927. However, the use of lye, originally sold to make soap, has progressed to its use in drain cleaners and is still sold today, albeit with child-resistant packaging. Liquid caustics for household use were introduced in 1967 and created extreme injury since it coated all mucosal surfaces when ingested. In 1971, surgeon Lucian Leape, MD, and colleagues used Liquid-Plumr, which was 30.5% sodium hydroxide, to demonstrate experimentally that a 3-s exposure to 1 mL of this solution produced a severe injury. This product and other similar liquid caustic products were eventually reformulated to be safer. Acids such as sulfuric are still sold and along with solid caustics are readily available. In 2019, the American Association of Poison Control Centers reported 3496 exposures to these agents with 412 moderate or major injuries and 4 deaths despite compliance with the Poison Prevention Packaging Act of 1970. Clearly, prevention has fallen short.

Reye's syndrome was a well-recognized entity in the 1960s and 1970s. The cause of the syndrome was unknown, and many theories were presented. In the

1970s, there were several conferences examining research on the syndrome. The battle between companies marketing aspirin and acetaminophen resulted at one point in the aspirin industry accusing the acetaminophen industry of causing the syndrome. Acetaminophen had been shown to produce hepatic necrosis as well as elevated intracranial pressure in severe cases. One of us (BHR) presented data that showed the pathology, course of events, and laboratory data associated with Reye's syndrome was not consistent with acetaminophen. He was attacked at a conference for that position. The other of us (FHL) rose in response and presented clear and convincing data that Reye's syndrome and acetaminophen toxicity were clearly different entities. In 1979, a statistical link with a case–control series implicated aspirin as a causative agent. The CDC issued warnings for the use of aspirin in 1980 and labeling was added to aspirin products by the FDA in 1986 for children under the age of 12. However, the number of cases of Reye's syndrome decreased dramatically prior to FDA warning labels and it is not entirely clear whether indeed aspirin was truly the causative agent.

While development of antidotes has saved countless lives, it is critical to remember that most poisons do not have a specific treatment and are primarily addressed in patients with supportive and intensive care. The pioneering work by Henry Matthew, MD, at the Poisons Unit of the Royal Infirmary of Edinburgh led to the current practice of modern toxicology. His treatment of barbiturate overdoses in the 1960s with ventilator support until the drug was metabolized rather than the use of analeptic agents changed toxicology forever. The statement, "treat the patient, not the poison" has been attributed to many over the years. Regardless, it is a wise concept as we are faced with many patients having unknown or multiple ingestions. The "salad bowl" parties of the 1970s and 1980s have been replaced with "pharm parties" of more recent vintage where groups gather and mix tablets and capsules in a bowl and consume them. Patients are confusing clinicians at best, and should be treated conservatively with supportive care until a specific diagnosis can be made and the patient's physical findings warrant intervention.

Poison centers and professionalism in the field of medical toxicology have developed world-wide since the first poison center in Chicago in 1953. Development of the current National Poison Data System in the United States with about 2.5 million cases per year and similar systems in many other countries have benefitted public health and other organizations by providing specific and in some cases real time information to deal with common as well as emerging hazards at every level.

The authors of this Foreword have seen the approach to treatment of exposures to many entities change dramatically during their 50-year careers in this field. What was accepted as treatment in the 1970s is in many cases no longer accepted. Antidote charts were widespread with erroneous or false information in the middle of the last century but no longer are required to be posted in emergency departments. A few things that have changed over the past 50 years:

- Potassium permanganate was encouraged for heroin and strychnine toxicity, despite its toxicity when administered orally due to its strong oxidation. Just how taken orally it could help an intravenous injection has never been clear.
- Syrup of ipecac was encouraged to be placed in every home and utilized for many ingestions since it induced vomiting even though it produced little benefit in removing substances and has now been abandoned.
- Gastric lavage, especially with a large bore tube, was considered an appropriate first treatment for any medication ingestion until it was shown to produce only a small amount of recovery in most cases.
- Vinegar and lemon juice were on the labels of caustics to be administered in case of ingestion, despite the exothermic reaction that occurred, aggravating burns in the esophagus.
- Corn starch was recommended for iodine ingestion primarily because it changed color.
- Physostigmine, while helpful in some circumstances, was overused and misused resulting in its decrease in application.
- Acid diuresis was recommended for meprobamate ingestion due to its ability to ionize, despite the small amount recovered in this way and the hazards of acidifying a patient.

While there are many other examples, most of these early approaches were not based on pharmacologic principles as in many cases the mechanisms were not understood. Those approaches were based on the knowledge at the time and have been largely abandoned over time. Of course, the "retrospect-o-scope" is the sharpest instrument in our bags, so looking back we can easily deride many of the previous approaches. It is best to learn from those who came before us and change our treatments as knowledge progresses. That is certainly true for the future as our knowledge of genetics, metabolomics, and other new areas provide evidence for specific approaches.

But, just as treatments listed earlier have been abandoned, it is intriguing to wonder what things we are doing today will be abandoned in the next 50 years as we come to a greater understanding of basic mechanisms of action. This book also provides the history of many effective treatments for overdoses or the toxicity of beneficial and lifesaving medications and treatments.

FAB fragments are an early example of a very specific approach to neutralizing the toxic effects of digoxin overdose and snakebites. Acetylcysteine was developed following a series of outstanding papers by Mitchell et al. determining the exact mechanism of toxicity and an understanding of the molecular basis by which it could be treated. Fomepizole is a very specific treatment for methanol and ethylene glycol poisoning based on understanding the mechanism of action. Fomepizole is in the early stages of research for acetaminophen overdose again, based on an understanding of specific mechanisms. Fomepizole may become an adjunct to acetylcysteine for this purpose and may eventually replace it.

Today, there is substantially greater understanding of the precise pharmacologic mechanisms of many substances which can produce toxicity at certain dose levels. For example, ricin, obtained from castor beans contains an enzymic polypeptide that catalyzes the *N*-glycosidic cleavage of a specific adenine residue from 28S ribosomal RNA joined by a single disulfide bond to a galactose (cell)-binding lectin. The enzymatic activity renders ribosomes containing depurinated 28S RNA incapable of protein synthesis causing cell death. Even with this detailed knowledge, there is still no specific treatment or antidote. There is hope that by determining such mechanisms research will eventually produce the ability to treat such poisonings just as this kind of understanding has produced treatment for other poisonings and diseases.

Clinical toxicology is progressing from the time of the mythical Merlin and dark arts to the time of a basic science understanding and an approach to specific targeted treatments for exposures and overdoses.

Dr. Alan Woolf and chapter authors of this book have assembled a detailed critical review with examples of many of the most important incidents and agents. The lesson is clear that whether deliberate, accidental, or due to negligence, poisonings with a large variety of substances are and will continue to be a constant feature of public health.

It is incumbent on all levels of medicine and public health to maintain a high index of suspicion. It is also critical to maintain a skeptical view of both diagnoses and treatments. Evidence-based decisions must be the gold standard. When sufficient data are not available, it must be made clear what degree of speculation has been incorporated in any conclusions that have been drawn. One of us (FHL) provided the following statement in the 1970s, "Make your science last." The clear challenge with this statement is for all involved in clinical toxicology to not go beyond the evidence and data on what we publish and teach.

The context provided in this book is the basis for the future of clinical toxicology. Starting from the materials in each of these chapters, young investigators (and occasionally old investigators) can find where careful methodical research can lead to the future approaches for successful treatment and alleviation of associated suffering and illness. Prevention should always be the goal but needs to occur at every level, from poison-proofing a home with young children to examination of risks in industrial products and processes. We look forward to the next book 50 years from now and the advancements that will occur from the knowledge in this current publication.

Frederick H. Lovejoy, Jr., M.D.
Associate Physician-in-Chief and Deputy Chairman,
Department of Pediatrics, Boston Children's Hospital, Boston, MA,
United States.
William Berenberg Distinguished Professor of Pediatrics,
Department of Pediatrics, Harvard Medical School, Boston, MA,
United States.
frederick.lovejoy@childrens.harvard.edu

Barry H. Rumack, M.D.
Professor Emeritus of Emergency Medicine and Pediatrics,
Departments of Emergency Medicine and Pediatrics,
University of Colorado School of Medicine, Aurora, CO, United States.
barry.rumack@cuanschutz.edu

Disclaimer

This is a history book. It is not intended to be used by clinicians in the course of clinical decision-making for the care of patients or as a guide to their medical management. Please refer to other appropriate resources for such purposes.

Acknowledgments

Other texts in this Elsevier series explore ancient contributions to the art and science of modern clinical toxicology. I thank Dr. Phillip Wexler, a friend and colleague who gave me the opportunity to participate in this project. For their editorial advice, encouragement, and support, I thank the staff at Elsevier, especially Tracy Tufaga, Swapna Srinivasan, S. Praveen Anand, and Kattie Washington. Kristina Woolf served as a second copyeditor for this book.

I thank the chapter contributors who donated their considerable time and effort to this project. Without their dedication, interest, and invaluable perspective, this undertaking would not have been possible.

I thank the Section Editors: Nicholas Bateman, Jeffrey Brent, Chen-Chang Yang, Jou-Fang Deng, and Susan Smolinske for their encouragement and invaluable help with editing and in some cases, the translation.

I thank Frederick H. Lovejoy Jr., Barry Rumack, and Toby Litovitz for their help as readers and peer reviewers of the chapters as well as for their renowned roles as champions of clinical toxicology.

Finally, I acknowledge John Trestrail, the founder of the AACT's Toxicological History Society and Mark Thoman, the AACT's unofficial (or official?) historian, for their passion for all aspects of the history of clinical toxicology and their inspirational teaching of us all.

Abbreviations

Agencies

ATSDR	Agency for Toxic Substances and Disease Registry (United States)
BPC	Belgian Poison Center
CDC	Centers for Disease Control and Prevention (United States)
CIAV	Portuguese Poison Control Center
CPSC	Consumer Product Safety Commission (United States)
DPIC	Dutch Poisons Information Center
DPIC	Danish Poisons Information Center
EMS	Emergency Medical Services
EPA	United States Environmental Protection Agency
EU	European Union
FDA	United States Food and Drug Administration
FPIC	Finnish Poison Information Center
GfKT	Gesellschaft fur klinische Toxikologie (Germany)
HAZMAT	Hazardous Materials Teams
HRSA	Health Resources Service Administration (United States)
IARC	International Agency for Research on Cancer (part of WHO)
ILO	International Labor Organization
IOM	Institute of Medicine (now known as National Academy of Medicine) (United States)
IPCS	International Programme on Chemical Safety (WHO)
IPIC	Israel Poison Information Center
NAPC	Nordic Association of Poisons Centers (Scandinavia)
NAS	National Academies of Science, Health and Medicine Division (United States)
NEMC	National Emergency Medical Center (South Korea)
NHS	National Health Service (United Kingdom)
NHSO	Ministry of Public Health (Thailand)
NIDA	National Institute on Drug Abuse (United States)
NIEHS	National Institute for Environmental Health Sciences (United States)
NIH	National Institutes of Health (United States)
NIOSH	National Institute of Occupational Safety and Hygiene (United States)
NITFS	National Institute of Toxicology and Forensic Sciences (Spain)
NLM	National Library of Medicine (United States)
NPIC	Norwegian Poisons Information Centre
NPIS	National Poisons Information Service (United Kingdom)
OCHP	Office of Child Health Protection (within the US EPA)
OSHA	Occupational Safety and Health Administration (United States)

PCC-Taiwan	Poison Control Center-Taiwan
RCPT	Royal College of Physicians of Thailand
RIA	N.V. Sklifosovsky Emergency Medicine Research Institute (Russia)
RIVM	National Institute for Public Health and the Environment (Netherlands)
RPC	Ramathibodi Poison Center (Thailand)
RTIAC	Federal Medical Biological Agency of Russia
SAMHSA	Substance Abuse Mental Health Services Administration (United States)
TVGH	Taipei Veterans General Hospital
UNEP	United Nations Environment Program
UP	University of the Philippines
UPNPMCC	University of the Philippines National Poison Management and Control Center
USP	United States Pharmacopoeia
WHO	World Health Organization

Societies

AAPCC	American Association of Poison Control Centers
AACT	American Academy of Clinical Toxicology
ABAT	American Board of Applied Toxicology
ABMS	American Board of Medical Subspecialties
ABMT	American Board of Medical Toxicology
ACMT	American College of Medical Toxicology
AETOX	The Spanish Association of Toxicology
AOEC	Association of Occupational and Environmental Clinics
APAMT	Asian-Pacific Association of Medical Toxicology
APT	Portuguese Toxicology Association
CST	Chinese Society of Toxicology
EAPCCT	European Association of Poisons Centres and Clinical Toxicologists
FETOC	The Spanish Foundation of Clinical Toxicology
IUTOX	International Union of Toxicology
KSCT	Korean Society of Clinical Toxicology
MENATOX	Middle East and North Africa Clinical Toxicology Association
PSCOT	Philippine Society of Clinical and Occupational Toxicology, Inc.
SITOX	Italian Society of Toxicology
SOT	Society of Toxicology
SOFT	Society of Forensic Toxicologists, Inc.
TEOMA	Taiwan Environmental and Occupational Medical Association
TNAP	Toxicology Nurses Association of the Philippines
TSTA	Toxicology Society of Taiwan

Other

ADR	adverse drug reaction
ADSL	asymmetric digital subscriber line
ASHT	alerting system for chemical health threats
CSPI	certified specialist in poison information
CTU	clinical toxicology units

DEG	diethylene glycol
ED	emergency department
ELISA	enzyme-linked immunosorbent assay
EU	European Union
EXTRIP	EXtracorporeal TReatments In Poisoning
GC/MS	gas chromatography/mass spectrometry
GPS	global positioning system
HPLC	high performance liquid chromatography
ICP/MS	inductively coupled plasma mass spectrometry
ICU	intensive care unit
IRT	IUTOX recognized toxicologist
IV	intravenous
LAN	local area network
LC/MS-MS	liquid chromatography/tandem mass spectrometry
LD50	lethal dose (chemical that kills 50% of the animals of the species under investigation)
MSDS	material safety data sheets
NCHPCC	National Clearinghouse for Poison Control Centers
NPDS	National Poison Data System
PC	poison center
PCCs	poison control centers
PEHSU	pediatric environmental health specialty unit (https://www.pehsu.net)
PICs	poisons information centers
PIMs	poisons information monographs
PIP	poison information provider
Q-TOF/MS	quadrupole-time of flight
RCT	randomized controlled trial
RTECS	Registry of Toxic Effects of Chemical Substances (https://www.cdc.gov/niosh/rtecs/default.html)
SPI	specialist in poison information
SMS	short messaging service (text messaging)
TC	toxicology centers
TESS	toxic exposure surveillance system
THC	tetrahydrocannabinol
TIC	Toxicological Information Centers
TIK	Toxicological Information and Knowledge Bank (Netherlands)
TIS	Toxicological Information Service (Spain)
TLC	thin-layer chromatography
ToxIC	Toxicology Investigators Consortium (https://www.toxicregistry.org)
wte	whole time equivalents

Preface to the series

In the realm of communicating any science, history, though critical to its progress, is typically a neglected backwater. This is unfortunate, as it can easily be the most fascinating, revealing, and accessible aspect of a subject which might otherwise hold appeal for only a highly specialized technical audience. Toxicology, the science concerned with the potentially hazardous effects of chemical, biological, and certain physical agents, has yet to be the subject of a full-scale historical treatment. Overlapping with many other sciences, it both draws from, and contributes to, them. Chemistry, biology, and pharmacology all intersect with toxicology. While there have been chapters devoted to history in toxicology textbooks, and journal articles have filled in bits and pieces of the historical record, this new monographic series aims to further remedy the gap, by offering an extensive and systematic look at the subject from antiquity to the present.

Since ancient times, men and women have sought security of all kinds. This includes identifying and making use of beneficial substances, while avoiding the harmful ones, or mitigating harm already caused. Thus, food and other natural products, independently or in combination, which promoted well-being, or were found to have druglike properties and effected cures, were readily consumed, applied or otherwise self-administered, or made available to friends and family. On the other hand, agents found to cause injury or damage—what we might call *poisons* today—were personally avoided, although sometimes used to wreak havoc on one's enemies.

While natural substances are still of toxicological concern, synthetic, and industrial chemicals now predominate as the emphasis of research. Through the years, the instinctive human need to seek safety and avoid hazard, has served as an unchanging foundation for toxicology, and will be explored from many angles in this series. Although largely examining the scientific underpinnings of the field, chapters will also delve into the fascinating history of toxicology and poisons in mythology, arts, society, and culture more broadly. It is a subject that has captured our collective consciousness.

The series is intentionally broad, thus the title *History of Toxicology and Environmental Health*. Clinical and research toxicology, environmental and occupational health, risk assessment and epidemiology, to name but a few examples, are all fair game subjects for inclusion. The opening volume of the series focuses on toxicology in antiquity, taken roughly to be the period up to the fall of the Roman empire and stopping short of the Middle Ages, with which period future volumes will continue. These opening volumes explore toxicology from the perspective of some of the great civilizations of the past, including Egypt, Greece, Rome, Mesoamerica, and China. Particular substances, such as harmful botanicals, lead, cosmetics, kohl, and hallucinogens, serve as the focus of other chapters. The role of certain individuals as either victims or practitioners of toxicity (e.g., Cleopatra, Mithridates, Alexander the Great, Socrates, and Shen Nung) serves as another thrust of these volumes.

History proves that no science is static. As Nikola Tesla said, "The history of science shows that theories are perishable. With every new truth that is revealed we get a better understanding of Nature and our conceptions and views are modified."

Great research derives from great researchers who do not, and cannot, operate in a vacuum, but rely on the findings of their scientific forebears. To quote Sir Isaac Newton, "If I have seen further it is by standing on the shoulders of giants." Welcome to this toxicological journey through time. You will surely see further and deeper and more insightfully by wafting through the waters of toxicology's history.

Phil Wexler

Other published books

Wexler, *History of Toxicology and Environmental Health: Toxicology in Antiquity, Volume I,* May 2014, *978-0-12-800045-8.*

Wexler, *History of Toxicology and Environmental Health: Toxicology in Antiquity, Volume II,* September 2014, *978-0-12-801506-3.*

Wexler, *Toxicology in the Middle Ages and Renaissance,* March 2017, 978-0-12-809554-6.

Bobst, *History of Risk Assessment in Toxicology,* October 2017, 978-0-12-809532-4.

Balls, Combes, and Worth, *The History of Alternative Test Methods in Toxicology,* October 2018, 9780128136973.

Wexler, *Toxicology in Antiquity,* Second Edition, October 2018, 9780128153390.

Preface

Clinical Toxicology can be defined as the study of the adverse effects that substances such as chemicals, drugs, botanicals, venoms, radionuclides, and naturally occurring substances and other xenobiotics have when they come into contact with the human body. In the United States, a distinction is sometimes made between clinical toxicologists, whose expertise represents a range of professions including those primarily trained as physicians, nurses, pharmacists, veterinarians and others, and medical toxicologists, referring to physicians who specialize in this field. Other fields within the broad scope of toxicology, such as analytical (laboratory) toxicology, occupational toxicology, forensic toxicology, experimental (bench research) toxicology, and environmental toxicology certainly overlap and inform clinical and medical toxicologists.

Clinical and medical toxicologists work in a variety of capacities: as health policy makers, as teachers in academic centers, as educators in toxicology and poisoning prevention, as managers or directors of poison control centers, as specialists and educators working in poison control centers, as members and leaders of regional, national or international professional societies, and as members of the health care team working in the care of patients. They may be involved with epidemiology and public health, occupational toxicology, forensic and legal consultation, pharmaceutical or chemical industries, environmental or analytical toxicology, private toxicology practice, forensic evaluations, and conducting scientific research in pharmacology and toxicology. They may be involved with diverse activities, such as the review of industry practices, the study of venomous animals (toxinology), drug development, national emergency preparedness, food and drug safety, warfare toxicology, and media consultation.

The use of plants and potions for treating humans—as well as the history of known and discovered poisons—goes back into antiquity. While this book will focus on the growth of modern clinical toxicology since the 1950s, the current advanced state of toxicological science was built on the discoveries of our forerunners in earlier ages. There is a heritage of innovative pioneers in medicine and toxicology, such as Paracelsus (full name: Philippus Aureolus Theophrastus Bombastus von Hohenheim, 1493–1541), Percival Potts (1714–1788), Francois Magendie (1783–1855), Mathieu Orfila (1787–1853), Oswald Schmiedeberg (1838–1921), Louis Lewin (1850–1929), Claude Bernard (1813–1878), and many others in the 18th, 19th, and early 20th centuries. They were foundational to all of the tremendous advances in the science and practice of clinical toxicology and poison control we have witnessed in recent times.

This book includes a compendium of recent historical events in clinical toxicology: poisoning disasters, infamous poisonings, and the incredible stories of the discovery of important antidotes that changed the practice of medicine. Every student with a love of clinical toxicology, whether in training or in practice or in retirement, already knows or should know some of these stories and how these disasters and poisoning events shaped the world in which we live. For example, they changed how consumer products are packaged, how laboratories are regulated, and how chemical industries are regulated and sited. The stories of antidote discoveries show examples of how innovative thinking is instrumental in the development of an antidote. And sometimes the discovery of an effective antidote depends on that rare combination of methodical science, intuition, and blind luck.

This is the first book to bring together stories of the founding and growth of the poison control movement in countries around the world. It is a timely recounting because, in many cases, a country's history was recent enough so that recollections could be captured from the original scientists and founders who were there at the beginning. These authors and consultants lend to their chapters an authenticity that adds so much to memorializing that country's journey. I hope that you will find these histories as fascinating as I have. In reading their individual accounts, it is striking to me how all countries share certain commonalities: visionary scientists, persistent founding champions, struggles with limited funding and few trained personnel, and the slow recognition and acceptance of clinical toxicology by government officials and academics as its own science and its own medical subspecialty. The professionalization of our discipline is still early and still unfolding in many countries. But eventually all countries will come to recognize their clinical and medical toxicologists and poison control specialists as valued experts. Eventually, all countries will recognize their poison control systems as indispensable facets of a country's health services for its people and a key component of public health preparedness for disasters, terrorist attacks, chemical emergencies, and pandemics.

My apologies in advance for not including all of the countries in the world and their advances in clinical toxicology. We could only tell the stories of a sampling. There were limitations of space and the availability of volunteer authors for this project; but there was no intention to overlook the ongoing efforts of any country to make progress both in clinical toxicology and poison control. Each country has its individual history of initiatives to better address the poisonings and toxic exposures affecting their own population.

Finally, it is my sincere hope that this book brings those of us working in clinical toxicology and related fields around the world a little closer. We know so well the enormous value of connecting with each other.

Alan D. Woolf
Boston, Massachusetts
December 2020

Section 1

Disasters: Examples of toxic calamities in modern times

Alan D. Woolf

Boston Children's Hospital & Harvard Medical School, Boston, Massachusetts, United States

Introduction

There have been many notable chemical toxic events in the recent history of clinical toxicology, affecting whole communities and large numbers of people. Often children are disproportionately more affected as victims in such catastrophes, due to their small size and larger dose per weight and their inability to escape without the help of adults. Hindsight is the great teacher. Chemical toxic disasters often are the motivators for changes in governmental infrastructure and regulatory policy, changes in industrial practices and oversight to improve safety, production changes affecting commercial products and foodstuffs, and other measures designed to forestall such events in the future. Chemical releases affecting a population may be difficult to detect. Some epidemiologic clues may include (Patel et al., 2003):

- An unusual increase in the number of people seeking care for a particular illness
- Unexplained deaths among the young or healthy adults
- Emission of unknown odors by patients
- Clusters of cases with a potential common point source of exposure
- Rapid onset of symptoms after an exposure to a potentially contaminated medium
- Unexplained deaths of plants, fish, and animals
- Syndrome consistently present in patients reminiscent of a specific chemical exposure (e.g., cholinergic crisis, anti-cholinergic syndrome, cellular hypoxia)

There are some common denominators in public health responses commensurate to the needs of a community impacted by a chemical disaster. Deployment of adequate resources to attend to the medical needs of the injured is of immediate importance. Notification with warnings, advisories and evacuation routes, and the location of public shelters must be provided. Inter-agency cooperation and integrated emergency response systems are essential. Evacuation of survivors to a safe perimeter, and the provision of safe food, water, and shelter for refugees or victims in the immediate area.

Such events occasion many other challenges: disrupted essential public services; lack of telecommunications and electricity, water and other utilities; damaged roads and poor access to remote communities; lack of adequate manpower and resources for deployment. After the acute emergency, there is even more work to restore the community's services and elements of normality to daily life. The aftermath of toxic exposures at both the individual and community levels may extend for months to years. The costs of post-event clean-up, restitution and reconstruction can be enormous, and both the short and long-term population needs are daunting. Anxiety and depression, post-traumatic stress syndrome (PTSD) and other mental health issues are of great consequence in every disaster, no matter its intensity and magnitude, and often go unaddressed by health authorities. The organization and planning of first response emergency medical services, surge capacities of poison control centers, hospitals and other treatment centers, and the integration of local agencies could put into action a coordinated response; the lack of these would make extreme conditions worse.

The reader is forewarned that we choose to include here only a few examples in this section. We will not discuss radiation events that occur all too frequently. The nuclear facility disasters at Three Mile Island (1979), Chernobyl (1986), and Fukushima Daiichi (2011) are all illustrative of the "ultra-hazardous" category of activities within the nuclear industry. All three events released uncontrolled and dangerous amounts of radiation in the vicinity of a nuclear reactor that posed a great threat to the surrounding communities. Nor have we included other instances of the mishandling of radioactive materials early after the discovery of radium, such as luminous watch dial-making that occurred in the United States in the early 1900s. (readers are referred to the excellent retelling of that story in the book: *Radium Girls* by Kate Moore).

And we have not included such long-standing environmental toxic exposures related to decades-long industrial pollution, typified in America by chromium pollution of the water in Woburn Massachusetts (1979) and by Superfund sites such as Love Canal in New York (1940s–50s), Times Beach PCBs and dioxin contamination in Missouri (1971), and Anniston PCB contamination in Alabama (1980s). Epidemics from long-standing local activities such as fluorosis from coal-burning used for heating in rural homes in China are also too numerous to include. Natural disasters are also not covered in this section, although they challenge toxicologists around the world. For example, a presumed volcanic eruption in the bottom of Lake Nyos in Cameroon on August 21, 1986, killed 1746 people and 3500 livestock. They were asphyxiated by the sudden release of thousands of tons of carbon dioxide which, heavier than air, settled around the lake region and spread into nearby valleys where people were living.

In this section, we illustrate only a few infamous examples of discreet community-wide toxic exposure events which led to new programs or agencies, new knowledge contributing to future safety measures and precautions, or important changes in policies or regulations. We acknowledge that these are only examples; there are many other such pivotal events that have occurred (or are occurring) around the world. A timeline of recent events described in this section is depicted in (Fig. 1).

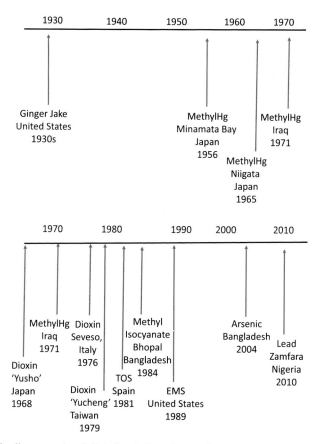

FIG. 1 Timeline: examples of clinical toxicology disasters from around the world.

Reference

Patel M, Schier J, Belson M, Rubin C, Garbe P. Recognition of illness associated with exposure to chemical agents – United States, 2003. CDC, MMWR 2003;52(39):938–40.

Chapter 1.1

Triortho cresyl phosphate "Ginger Jake" disaster—United States, 1930s

Alan D. Woolf

Boston Children's Hospital & Harvard Medical School, Boston, Massachusetts, United States

Prohibition, the "noble experiment," ushered in "speak-easys," gangsters, and bath-tub gin in the "Roarin" 1920s in the United States. However, for many Americans, the Market Crash in 1929 and the subsequent Great Depression led to a prolonged period of joblessness, hard times, and austerity during the 1930s (Fig. 1.1.1).

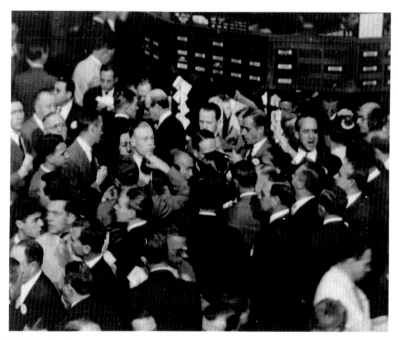

FIG. 1.1.1   Traders on the Floor of the New York Stock Exchange—1930s. *(Creative Commons Source: public domain pingnews.com (https://www.flickr.com/photos/39735679@N00/2884233032))*

History of Modern Clinical Toxicology. https://doi.org/10.1016/B978-0-12-822218-8.00044-2

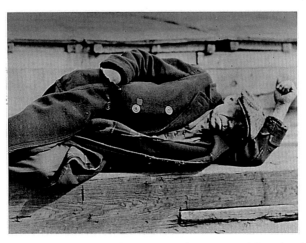

FIG. 1.1.2   Poverty-stricken men in the Great Depression were especially vulnerable to Ginger Jake poisoning. *(https://commons.wikimedia.org/wiki/File:Man_lying_down_on_pier_during_Great_Depression_New_York_City_USA_1935.gif. Attribution: Franklin D. Roosevelt Presidential Library and Museum: photo by Lewis W. Hine.)*

The "Ginger Jake disaster" of the 1930s was a predictable event related to the combination of the loss of self-esteem and clinical depression brought about by job loss and extreme poverty, the prohibition on alcoholic beverages, and the ever-present unsavory types eager to make a buck. Jake poisoning struck adults, mostly poor middle-aged vagrants with little medical care or social standing. These "invisible" Americans suffered an enduring tragic legacy of irreversible paralysis. The public had little thought of compensating the victims and little pity for their plight. They were resigned to a fate of their own doing (Fig. 1.1.2).

Extract of ginger

Jamaican ginger extract, known simply as "Ginger Jake," was a cheap alcoholic "tonic" produced and distributed as early as 1863. "*Extractum Zingiberis Fluidum*" contained ethanol as a solvent and, as an "extract" of the very pungent oleoresin of ginger, was about four times stronger than tincture of ginger. It was entered into the US Dispensary of medicinal products by 1880 (Stillé and Maisch, 1880). Ginger extract, diluted in coffee or soda pop, was commonly used for a variety of medicinal purposes (as a carminative, to aid digestion or to treat headaches, upper respiratory infections, stomach pains, or poor menstrual flow). It was manufactured legitimately to meet USP standards of purity as an extract by such reputable companies as Eli Lilly & Co, Smith Kline & French Laboratories, Upjohn Co., Norwich Pharmaceuticals, Wyeth Inc., and Sharp and Dohme Co. It was an especially popular tonic in Southern "dry" states, such as Tennessee, Kentucky, Mississippi, Oklahoma, and Kansas (Harris, 1930).

Prohibition and the rise of Ginger Jake

Jamaica ginger extract, containing 60%–90% ethanol by volume, was known as "Ginger Jake" or simply "Jake." Prohibition in the U.S. began on January 17 1920 with the passage of the Volstead Act (18th Amendment) and ended on December 5th 1933 with its repeal by the ratification of the 21st Amendment. During Prohibition, the price of other legal alcohol-containing medicines, such as castor oil, skyrocketed. Because of its concentrated potency, the Prohibition Bureau declared USP. Jamaica ginger extract to be "nonpotable" and was a "medicine" and exempted it from laws restricting the sale of alcohol. Ginger Jake sold for 35 cents for a 2 oz. bottle. Its popularity increased during Prohibition as a substitute for liquor, to circumvent federal laws prohibiting legal alcohol sales while avoiding the more costly and illicit bootleg ethanol. Brands of Jamaica ginger extract, such as "Queen City" and "Land," flooded the marketplace. Jake was sold in grocery or drug stores, barber shops, or even at roadside stands around the country. It was commonly mixed with cola or coffee, often with a wink and a nod from local law enforcement authorities (Harris, 1930; Morgan, 1982). It became the beverage of choice among working poor, middle-aged men, especially in the southern United States.

Tainted Ginger Jake

Sensing the possibility of a quick cash windfall, Harry Gross, president of Hub Products Inc. at 65 Fulton Street in Boston substituted 135 gal of the cheaper Lindol adulterant, a plasticizer and ingredient in varnishes, as a cheaper solvent for his batches of Ginger Jake in January 1930. Supplier Martin Swanson and chemist Harry Mandel at the Deluxe Drug Company in Brooklyn, NY, concocted the product (Morgan, 1982). The purpose of adding the solvent was to substitute inexpensive inert solids for the true oleo-resin of ginger present in pure, USP quality Ginger Jake medicinals. The result would be more dilute and palatable to drink when its purpose was diverted to that of a bootleg beverage. Distributors such as the Jordan Brothers Inc. took delivery of the poisonous extract in their Brooklyn, New York warehouse, and it was shipped out on February 15th. Other shipping points included Cincinnati, Oklahoma City, and Kansas City. By February, more than 500 gal had been produced and 640,000 bottles of the extract had been distributed all over the country (Morgan, 1982).

On February 27th, Oklahoma doctor W.H. Goldfain observed a patient at Reconstruction Hospital in Oklahoma City with unusual symptoms of multiple neuritis without evidence of infection or exposure to heavy metals such as arsenic or lead, or any other clear etiology (Parascandola, 1994). Later that same day, he saw four other patients with similar complaints, among whom was a pharmacist who sold Ginger Jake and also took some himself about 10 days previously. Another of his patients gave him a list of maybe 65 other people with similar complaints. Dr. Goldfain then consulted with the Oklahoma City Health

Supervisor Dr. E. Miles, and they went to see about 30 people on the list, all of whom had consumed Ginger Jake purchased at local drug stores (Parascandola, 1994). Since the extract had been in use for years, it was not immediately obvious to the doctors why it was now associated with sudden onset of neurologic symptoms: numbness, weakness, muscle pain, and then, in some, paralysis. The first newspaper reports of a "strange paralysis" affecting people appeared as early as March and soon implicated Ginger Jake as the cause.

Triortho cresyl phosphate—The adulterant

Unfortunately, the bad batches of Ginger Jake had been manufactured using a cheap solvent containing the organophosphate ester: triortho cresyl phosphate (TOCP; also known as lindol, triaryl phosphate, tricresyl phosphate, phosphorcreosote, tritolyl phosphate, Celluflex, Kronitex). TOCP contaminates the tricresyl phosphates—slightly yellowish, viscous, oily chemicals commonly used industrially in plasticizers, hydraulic fluids, lubricants, glues and adhesives, solvents, and flame retardants. TOCP does not degrade at high temperatures or pressures, and is miscible in a variety of solvents and thinners, as well as castor or linseed or cottonseed oils (Fig. 1.1.3).

TOCP is readily absorbed through the skin, lungs, and gastrointestinal tract and accumulates in target organs, including the liver, kidneys, lungs, and nervous system. Unlike other organophosphates, it does not have cholinesterase enzyme inhibiting activity. The intraneuronal metabolite, 2-0-cresyl-4H-1:3:2 benzodioxaphosphoran-2-one (CBDF) may be the principal neurotoxin, causing degenerative changes and secondary demyelization in a distal motor neuropathy (Vasilescu and Florescu, 1980). Distal large axons of peripheral nerves of both upper and lower extremities are affected first—a pathological process known as a Wallerian-type "dying back" axonopathy, reproducible in rabbit and hen animal models (Parascandola, 1994).

Clinical toxicology

Unlike many other organophosphate compounds, TOCP produces few cholinergic effects clinically, although poisoning is often heralded by gastrointestinal

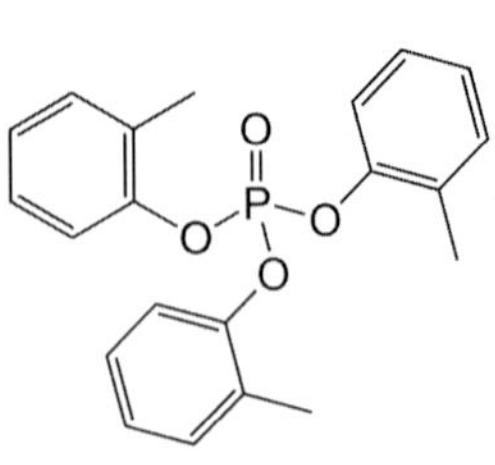

FIG. 1.1.3 Chemical structure of triortho cresyl phosphate. Source: https://upload.wikimedia. org/wikipedia/commons/thumb/5/57/Tri-o-cresyl_phosphate.svg/534px-Tri-o-cresyl_phosphate. svg.png.

symptoms, including nausea, vomiting, abdominal pain, and diarrhea. Many patients early on experienced muscle pain, aching, calf tenderness, myoclonic jerks, weakness, and fatigue. In the Ginger Jake disaster, infectious causes of a reversible polyneuritis were at first mistakenly suspected as the etiology of the illness. Within weeks of the ingestion, symmetrical motor dysfunction can affect both the upper and lower extremities of the poisoning victims, although the legs are more often involved, with flaccidity and difficulty walking. These motor signs were accompanied by paresthesias, with sensations of coldness and tingling. In mild cases, where people had only imbibed small amounts of the extract, resolution of the symptoms and signs of toxicity might take place over the ensuing weeks or months.

In moderately-to-severely affected individuals, neuropathies progressed to include spasticity, foot and wrist drop, hypoactive reflexes, and eventually muscle atrophy, especially in extensors and intrinsic muscles of both hands and feet, resembling amyotrophic lateral sclerosis. The typically altered gait ("scissored" walking or hip walking) with ataxia, foot drop, and limping associated with the motor neuritis, was known as the "Jake walk" or "Jake leg." Bulbar dysfunction, occurring in severe cases, included facial weakness, difficulty handling secretions, and loss of gag reflex. More severely affected patients experienced depressed consciousness or even coma (Goldstein et al., 1988). Antidotes such as atropine or the oximes, while effective in the treatment of organophosphate pesticide poisoning, did not affect the course of TOCP poisoning. Those victims ingesting larger doses were more severely affected; some suffered permanent quadriplegia and its accompanying disability.

Recall of tainted Ginger Jake

Newspapers documented the growing epidemic as early as February and March in 1930. More than 400 patients were admitted to Cincinnati General Hospital over a 6-month period in 1930, all with similar complaints of muscle pain and weakness (Morgan and Tulloss, 1976). Between March and July, before the source of the contamination could be uncovered, more than 20,000 individuals had been affected by Ginger Jake paralysis (Valaer, 1930). Many victims were blue-collar, low wage or jobless, middle-aged rural white men with little medical care or social standing. Some were vagrant wanderers without families, rootless, and alcoholic. It was thought to be largely a white man's illness and there was speculation that pigmented skin might be protective. However, it was more likely that the only patients who were counted as victims in the epidemic were those seen in the segregated hospitals or clinics of the South, serving whites only (Morgan and Tulloss, 1976).

Hundreds of samples of the bootleg version of Jamaica ginger extract were sent to the Treasury Department's Bureau of Industrial Alcohol (BIA) for pharmacologic and toxicological analysis in 1930. The chemists there, led by Senior Pharmacologist Dr. Maurice Smith and including chemists Peter Valear

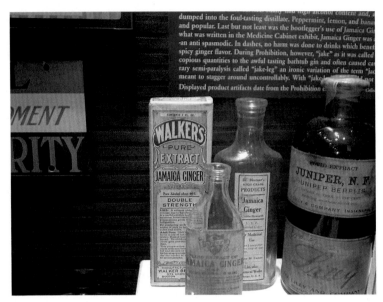

FIG. 1.1.4   Walker's Pure Extract—Jamaica Ginger. Source: https://upload.wikimedia.org/wikipedia/en/thumb/c/c8/Jamaican_ginger.jpg/1200px-Jamaican_ginger.jpg. Attribution: Deltabeignet

and Elias Elvove, found an adulterant in discarded bottles of Ginger Jake associated with the afflicted patients; they found a cresol compound identified as TOCP (Valaer, 1930; Parascandola, 1994). Drs. Smith and Elvove of the BIA published their results regarding an outbreak from Ginger Jake shipped to California outlets in *Public Health Reports* in 1931 (Smith and Elvove, 1931). Experiments by other investigators confirmed that chickens could be paralyzed by the tainted Jake, whereas the animals were unaffected by USP Jake or alcohol alone (Valaer, 1930) (Fig. 1.1.4).

Over 2000 gal of tainted Ginger Jake were confiscated by December 1930, and still a cluster of Jake paralyzed patients was newly discovered in California in 1931. Cases of "polyneuritis" from an unknown adulterant in the ginger extract were documented in medical journals as early as June 1930, with Dr. Benjamin Burley describing 50 cases in the *New England Journal of Medicine* (Burley, 1930) and Dr. Peter Valaer reporting additional cases in the October of the same year. He also implicated cresyl chemical adulterants in the ginger extract, in concentrations as high as 2% by volume, as causing the neurotoxicity (Valaer, 1930).

Stigma of "JakeLeg"

Victims of Ginger Jake poisoning were stereotyped as shiftless alcoholics. Their steppage gait was visible to a disapproving community; and they often could find neither understanding nor employment. The symptoms and stories of victims were told not only in medical journals but also in song (Morgan and Tulloss, 1976; Woolf, 1995). Hillbilly jazz and blues artists sang of the "Jake Leg Blues" with a resignation to the fate of their own doing, brought on by the intemperance of a wasted life. The Allen Brothers released the song JAKE WALK BLUES on May 30, 1930, in Memphis, Tennessee (Victor V-40303 Reissue Folk Variety FV 12501©1977 Jazz Records). Many more artists documented in song the despair of the victims.

JAKE LEG BLUES
Willie Lofton
I said Jake Leg Jake Leg Jake Leg Jake Leg
Tell me what in the world you gonna do
I said Jake Leg Jake Leg Jake Leg
Tell me what in the world you gonna do
I say I gone done drunk so much Jake oh Lawd
That it done give him the limber leg yeah!
I say I know this Jake oh Lawd!
I say done give him the walk
I say these people drink this Jake on the road
They even throw they bottle away
I say these people drink this Jake on the road oh Lawd!
They even throw they bottle away
Cause this Jake leave 'em wid a present
That keep 'em company every day.

(Chicago, IL September 24, 1934 Decca, 1976 Collector: Joseph Bussard Jr.)

Aftermath

An examination of 11 patients aged 64–81 years old even 47 years after the original Jake exposure revealed continuing evidence of severe motor neuron syndrome with spasticity, hyperactive reflexes, foot drop, and claw hand. While all had largely recovered upper limb function, 10 of 11 men still had a noticeable high steppage gait disturbance and needed assistance to walk (Morgan and Penovich, 1978). Some had developed mild dementia; others were still so shamed by the experience that they denied it, offering that they had suffered a stroke rather than admit to having Jake leg.

Many of the Jake dealers and distributors were indicted and prosecuted, although these cases often resulted in little more than small fines as punishment. Those responsible denied culpability; they claimed that their product was "misused" as it was never intended nor labelled as a beverage. Harry Gross succeeded in delaying the judicial process, vowing to "find the real poisoner" in New York. He and his associate, Harry Reisman, were eventually tried and convicted receiving a $1000 fine and a 2-year suspended sentence (Morgan, 1982). The FDA later determined that there was no elusive "bootlegger" in New York, that Gross himself had mixed the poisoned Jake. When his probation was later revoked, Harry Gross did serve some jail time.

The postscript of Ginger Jake was grim. Those who were responsible for the epidemic received little punishment and many who drank the poisoned Jake were left both uncompensated and crippled by irreversible paralysis for the rest of their lives (Table 1.1.1).

TABLE 1.1.1 TimeLine: American Ginger Jake disaster.

1863—Extract of ginger developed
1880—Ginger extract in US Dispensary
1920—18th U.S. Constitutional Amendment passed—Prohibition begins
1920s—"Roarin" Twenties
1929—Stock Market Crash
1929—Price of castor oil skyrockets
1929—Harry Gross: Hub Products Company, Boston, MA
1929—Great Depression
January 1930—Lindol adulterant added (first 135 gal of ginger extract)
February 1930—640,000 bottles of "Ginger Jake" distributed mostly in South, Southwest United States
March 1930—Newspaper reports of tainted Jake in Mississippi, Kansas, Oklahoma, Tennessee
March to August 1930—50,000 people poisoned by Ginger Jake
March, 1930—Jake Liquor Blues song released by Ishman Bracey
May 1930—Jake Leg Blues song released by the Allen Brothers
June 1930—New York Times newspaper article warns of tainted extract
1930—First medical journal reports of Ginger Jake toxicity
November to December 1930—2000 gal of Jake confiscated
January 1931—Cluster of Jake poisoning reported in California
1932—Franklin Delano Roosevelt (FDR) elected
1933—18th Amendment repealed—Prohibition ends
1933—FDR's First "New Deal" to put people back to work
September, 1934—Jake Leg Blues song released by Willie Lofton
1941—America enters World War II, effectively ending the Great Depression

Table created by author.

Other triortho cresyl phosphate adulterant disasters

By 1933, the 18th Amendment to the Constitution and Prohibition were repealed, and that, along with the previous product recall efforts, effectively curtailed any further exposure to adulterated Ginger Jake extract in the United States. However, unfortunately that was not the end of mass poisonings caused by TOCP adulteration of foods and beverages. Other instances included an epidemic of poisoning 25 years later in Morocco in which a dark lubricating oil containing TOCP was being sold by a wholesaler as cheap "olive oil" (Smith and Spalding, 1959). Between August and October 1959, the tainted cooking oil affected as many as 2000 victims (later tallies estimated greater than 10,000 victims), with the lower extremity pain, paresthesias, stocking-glove distribution numbness, and paralysis typical of the toxic effects of TOCP. Again some 45 years later a cluster of TOCP poisoning cases were reported in Vietnam (Dennis, 1977). A group of poor Vietnamese people had purchased black market hydraulic fluid intended for U.S. jet fighters during the Vietnam war and used it as a cooking oil.

An English physician reported 17 cases of polyneuritis, paralysis, and foot drop caused by TOCP poisoning traced to contaminated cottonseed cooking oil in Merseyside, Great Britain, in 1945 and 1946 (Hotston, 1946). The cooking oil was probably contaminated when it was transferred for distribution to second-hand containers which had previously been used for industrial purposes and had contained TOCP-containing varnishes or lacquers.

Three outbreaks of TOCP were reported from the West Bengal area of India: one from contaminated flour in 1962 resulted in over 400 cases of paralysis; another in the Kankinara District involved cooking oil that poisoned 25 people; a third instance in the Dum Dum Municipality in August 1972 involving contaminated mustard oil affected more than 36 people, including the grocer himself (Sarkar, 1974).

In total, more than a dozen instances of TOCP poisoning were recorded around the world between the 1930s and 1970s (Morgan, 1982). Such episodes point out the continuing need for strict governmental policies in all countries regarding the manufacture and sale of safe foodstuffs. Public health ministries and agencies must maintain heightened vigilance to curtail the distribution of adulterated products through sophisticated, well-funded programs of surveillance efforts to ensure the public of the safety and purity of foodstuffs and medicinal products.

References

Burley BT. The 1930 type of polyneuritis. N Engl J Med 1930;202(24):1139–42.

Dennis DT. Jake walk in Viet Nam. Ann Intern Med 1977;86:665–6.

Goldstein DA, McGuigan MA, Ripley BD. Acute tricresylphosphate intoxication in childhood. Hum Toxicol 1988;7:179–82.

Harris S. Jamaica ginger paralysis. South Med J 1930;23(5):375–6.

Hotston RD. Outbreak of polyneuritis due to orthotricresyl phosphate poisoning. Lancet 1946;9:206–7.

Morgan JP. The Jamaica ginger paralysis. JAMA 1982;248(15):1864–7.

Morgan JP, Penovich P. Jamaica ginger paralysis—forty-seven-year follow-up. Arch Neurol 1978;35:530–2.

Morgan JP, Tulloss TC. The Jake Walk Blues—a toxicological tragedy mirrored in American popular music. Ann Intern Med 1976;85:804–8.

Parascandola J. The Jamaica ginger paralysis episode of the 1930s. Pharm Hist 1994;36(3):123–43.

Sarkar JK. Outbreaks of paralytic disease in West Bengal due to tricresyl phosphate poisoning. J Indian Med Assoc 1974;63(11):359–61.

Smith HV, Spalding JMK. Outbreak of paralysis in Morocco due to ortho-cresyl phosphate poisoning. Lancet 1959;2:1019–21.

Smith MI, Elvove E. The epidemic of so-called ginger paralysis in Southern California in 1930–31. Public Health Rep 1931;46:1227–35.

Stillé A, Maisch JM. The national dispensatory. 2nd ed. Philadelphia, PA: Henry O Lea's Son & Co; 1880.

Valaer P. The examination of cresyl-bearing extracts of ginger. Am J Pharm 1930;571–4.

Vasilescu C, Florescu A. Clinical and electrophysiological study of neuropathy after organophosphate compounds poisoning. Arch Toxicol 1980;43:305–15.

Woolf AD. Ginger Jake and the blues: a tragic song of poisoning. Vet Hum Toxicol 1995;37(3):252–4.

Chapter 1.2

Three methylmercury poisoning disasters

Alan D. Woolf

Boston Children's Hospital & Harvard Medical School, Boston, Massachusetts, United States

Chapter 1.2.1

Minamata Bay, Japan

Mercury is a ubiquitous, naturally present metal found in the earth's crust. The metal exists in three forms: as elemental mercury, as inorganic mercury salts, and in organic mercury-containing compounds. Mercury has a long history of use in industry, in the manufacture of commercial products, in agriculture, and in medicine. The metal has been found in small amounts in many types of animals, including birds and fish, and in man, where it has no physiological role. Organomercury compounds specifically have an unfortunate history of notorious mass poisonings.

Minamata Bay, Japan, 1956

The tragic story of the Minamata Bay contamination in Japan by an industrial concern shocked and horrified the world. The Chisso Chemical Plant began operations in Minamata, in the Kumamoto Prefecture, in 1908. (Fig. 1.2.1) It first manufactured fertilizers, but in the 1930s, it expanded and diversified its product line to include a variety of chemicals used commercially. The company began using mercury sulfide as a catalyst in the manufacture of aldehydes, used in paper processing and as intermediary compounds in the production of plastics, perfumes, dyes, pharmaceuticals, synthetic rubber manufacture, resins, formaldehyde, and other products. The plant began to dump a by-product of the reactions, methylmercury, in its waste effluent directly into Minamata Bay,

History of Modern Clinical Toxicology. https://doi.org/10.1016/B978-0-12-822218-8.00037-5

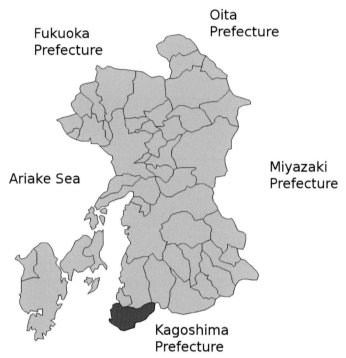

FIG. 1.2.1   Chisso Factory and Minamata Bay in Japan. *(From https://it.wikipedia.org/wiki/ Malattia_di_Minamata#/media/File:Minamata_map_illustrating_Chisso_factory_effluent_ routes2.png.)*

a common practice of the time. Over the next several decades, it would discharge over 150 t of methylmercury into the river (Powell, 1991).

By the 1940s, people living in the area began to notice bizarre behaviors of pet cats who were acting strange and dying in large numbers. By the 1950s townspeople noticed a variety of other animals and pets similarly affected and dying for unknown reasons. Birds dropped from the sky; oysters vanished; fish floated dead in the water (Powell, 1991).

Historical context

The historical context of this event is important. People living in the Minamata Bay were workers, friends, or family members of workers at the Chisso plant, or else they were indigenous fishermen and farmers. Culturally, Japanese people identified closely with the success of private companies; virtues of loyalty and fealty to an employer were prominent in the national character. Also, it was a defeated Japan after World War II; the shaky new government desperately needed food and jobs for its struggling, starving citizens. The Chisso Chemical Company was the prominent employer in the region whose success was encouraged by

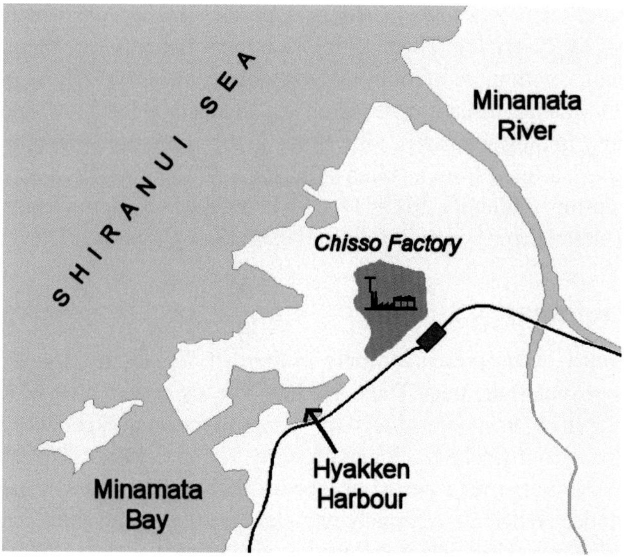

FIG. 1.2.2 Map of Chisso Chemical Plant in Relation to Minamata City at Hyakken Harbor and Shiranui Sea. (Wikimedia commons: public domain. https://commons.wikimedia.org/w/index.php?curid=1443750). Attribution: FDL (Free Documentation License).

the government and celebrated by the people living in the "company town." Approximately one-half of the townspeople depended either directly or indirectly on the plant for their livelihoods (Normile, 2013) and were intensely loyal to its owners. It was inconceivable to the Japanese that the company itself could be responsible for people's health problems by polluting the bay (Fig. 1.2.2).

First suspicions

The people living in the Minamata Bay region ate large amounts of fish and shellfish as a dietary staple—up to three meals daily. In 1953, they began to experience signs of a progressive neurodegenerative disease, such as numbness of hands and feet, dysarthria, altered mental status, and ataxia. They presented themselves to hospitals, but doctors could not determine a known etiology for such complaints. Dr. Hajime Hosokawa, Chief Medical Officer of the Chisso Corporation Factory Hospital, filed a report on May 1, 1956, describing the neurodegenerative disorder affecting four fishermen (O'Malley, 2017). Increasing numbers of cases and deaths were subsequently documented. It was some months before the cause of "Minamata disease" was found to be the methylmercury accumulating in the effluent discharged into the bay. The fish and shellfish harvested from the bay had bio-accumulated the methylmercury contamination from the plant to as much as 60× above comparative background levels and were shown to be the source of the toxic exposure of the populace. Methylmercury levels in the bay's sediments were highest near the wastewater discharge site. The cats in the town, feeding off dinner table scraps, were the ones to die first. They exhibited bizarre behaviors and seizures, known locally as *neko odori byo* or "cat dancing disease" (O'Malley, 2017). By the fall of 1956, 89 human patients had been identified, with 39 deaths, with more to follow (Matsumoto et al., 1965). Those people who developed Minamata disease were feared and shunned by local townspeople; they had difficulty finding spouses or jobs. Some in the community thought they were contagious or suffered from a "tatari" (Japanese for a curse) because of the sins of their ancestors (Gilhooly, 2015). Despite being the blameless victims of a mass poisoning, their shame and guilt followed them throughout their lives.

Clinical findings

Methylmercury, when presented orally in the diet, has almost 100% absorption from the gastrointestinal tract. There is a long latency period, after which toxicity targets multiple organ systems. Early on, some patients may experience abdominal pain, myalgias, and weakness. Methylmercury is converted to divalent inorganic mercury in the brain over a period of months. Pathological changes include brain cell loss in the cerebellum, especially granular layer cells, and extensive nerve degeneration in the cerebral cortex and the visual cortex (Weiss et al., 2002). Patients may develop narrowed peripheral vision, decreased hearing, and neurological symptoms including sensory loss on the lips and tongue, limb paresthesias, memory loss, ataxia, delirium, incoherence, and loss of motor control (Ekino et al., 2007). In severe intoxications, patients may experience hallucinations, stupor, and coma. Electroencephalogram studies can show prominent changes in brain function in children (Harada, 1968), and they too may experience seizures and motor deficits.

Women experienced an increasing number of stillbirths, and their babies with "fetal Minamata disease" had generalized neurological problems and seizures typical of the chronic static encephalopathy known as cerebral palsy. Japanese doctors were the first to report two cases of fetal Minamata disease, infants with cerebral palsy exposed to methylmercury only via vertical transmission through the placenta of their otherwise healthy-appearing mothers during their pregnancies (Matsumoto et al., 1965). They documented malformations of different brain areas and generalized atrophy of both the cerebral cortex and cerebellum, as well as neuronal degeneration and elevated mercury content in brain, liver, and kidneys. Although mothers thought their babies were just being good, doctors began to realize that the "quiet baby syndrome" was an indication of the severe brain damage wrought by fetal mercury poisoning (Table 1.2.1).

Community tensions rise

The population was ill-equipped to cope with this poisoning and the government was slow to intervene and offer resources and remediation. Victims were feared and shunned by the people of Minamata; they refused to associate with them and ridiculed them. People of Minamata were horrified and in disbelief when it became public knowledge that the Chisso factory itself could have been responsible for the long-term environmental poisoning. Officials avoided probing

TABLE 1.2.1 TimeLine—Minamata Japan methylmercury disaster.

1907—Chisso Corporation established at Minamata

1930—Chisso builds plant in Korea

1932—Aldehyde production begins at Chisso plant in Japan

Mercury is contained in plant discharge effluent

1952–60—Post-World War II demand for aldehyde increases; height of Chisso operations

1956—Cats start to disappear

1956—First evidence of neurological disease in local people

1957—Fishing banned

1959—Methylmercury identified as the cause of Minamata disease

1960—Chisso factory identified as source of mercury

1964—Chisso offers "sympathy settlement" to victims

1968—Chisso production of aldehyde ends

1968—Citizen's Council for Minamata Disease formed

1971—Story in Life Magazine

1971—Japanese government establishes "kankyo-cho": the first Environmental Agency

1974—Over 798 cases certified by Japanese government for compensation purposes

1975—Minamata Bay closed to fishing

1994—Minamata mayor offers formal apology to the victims

1996—Final Settlement (Wakai Kyotei) reached for 2200 registered victims

1997—Fishing ban in Minamata Bay lifted after massive dredging removes mercury-laden sediment

2013—Minamata Convention on Mercury treaty—ratified by 50 nations

Table created by author.

into the root causes of the disease outbreak, deferring to the company and fearing the possibility of economic losses. Responding to these early accusations, Chisso had installed a Cyclator-based wastewater treatment system at the plant in 1959. Company officials claimed the process centrifuged and precipitated effluent solids purifying the effluent, but it was later determined that the system was useless in removing methylmercury from the waste stream (Powell, 1991; Normile, 2013). The company continued to deflect blame and a growing environmental disaster was ignored. The plant continued to put out mercury in the effluent. Without admitting its own role or guilt as the cause of poisoning, Chisso Corporation officials offered "sympathy settlements" to some of the affected populace in 1964 and ended its production of acetaldehyde and its use of mercury four years later, in 1968 (Normile, 2013). It refused to disclose its production processes or disclose any information about its waste discharges.

Community activists formed the Citizen's Council on Minamata Disease in 1968 and began to press company and government officials legally for an acknowledgement of responsibility, assigning blame and providing recourse for victims. Only later, during lengthy litigation proceedings, was it learned that there had been internal memos produced by the company's health officer, Dr. Hideyo Matsumoto, years earlier warning that the plant's mercury-laden effluent could be responsible for the human cases of neurotoxicity seen in Minamata. The company had suppressed the in-house scientific evidence, deflecting a focus on its responsibility by offering other theories of causation.

And then the tide turned. Two influential books were published in English in the 1970s—one a scholarly work on the toxicity of methylmercury and the other, by photojournalists W. Eugene and Aileen Smith, documented the tragedy in photographs (Tsubaki and Irukayama, 1977; Smith and Smith, 1975). These publications were widely read and opened the eyes of the world to the consequences of environmental pollution. A feature story in Life Magazine in 1971 included a startling picture of a young girl with cerebral palsy: "Tomoko Uemura at her bath" taken by one of the authors, W. Eugene Smith. The article also focused worldwide sympathy and attention on this manmade environmental disaster.

Japan acknowledges tragedy

Japan only belatedly acknowledged the human consequences of this preventable disaster and the resulting incurable disease foisted on the area's inhabitants. Fishing in Minamata Bay continued until the government issued a ban in 1975, exposing many more people to the possibility of chronic poisoning. Minamata disease devastated peoples' lives. Those afflicted, who suffered various levels of the functional disabilities through no fault of their own, were stigmatized and isolated socially by others in their community. People were afraid that they could "catch" the illness and they shunned and were hostile to their neighbors with Minamata disease. Shopkeepers would not take their money and banished them from their shops (O'Malley, 2017).

The Japanese government designated criteria to be met by patients stigmatized with "Minamata disease" for purposes of compensation, and it continued to make payments to the victims of this tragedy and their long-lasting health sequelae for the next 50 years. In 1971, as a result of the tragedy Japan also enacted 14 laws to stem pollution and created its first official Environmental Agency (Kankyo-cho), recognizing the critical importance to its citizens of preserving a clean environment (O'Malley, 2017). The government "certified" 2260 patients with Minamata disease using the strict criteria it had laid out in 1977 (Normile, 2013). Another 11,000 people with less severe injuries later qualified for limited payments under a revised 1995 law. Additional patients, as many as 65,000, may qualify for compensation under a new program initiated in 2009 (Normile, 2013).

Aftermath of Minamata disease

Controversies remain in the Minamata Bay area of Japan. While a final settlement was offered to 2200 registered victims by the government in 1996, activists continue to maintain that up to 200,000 people were adversely affected by the contamination, many of whom have subtle neurological symptoms not qualifying them to be officially designated as a registered victim eligible for compensation (O'Malley, 2017). The ban on fishing was lifted in 1997, after extensive dredging of the toxic sediments from the harbor's seabed was completed. However, fishermen would still have difficulty making a living; the label Minamata had acquired an unenviable association with pollution. People would not buy fish taken from the Minamata Bay even though it was shown to be safe; they thought it might still be tainted with mercury.

The Minamata Convention on Mercury treaty was ratified by 50 nations in 2013, resolving to address, remediate, and eradicate environmental sources of mercury (McNutt, 2013; Normile, 2013). The two largest industrial sources of mercury emissions in the world now are artisanal gold mining and coal-fired power plants. Today, Minamata is the site of two museums and a memorial to the victims of the tragedy, which changed the way Japan addresses environmental concerns and its obligations to its citizens (O'Malley, 2017).

Shiranui Sea coastal areas

It is still unclear if there is such a thing as a "safe" chronic dose of human methylmercury contamination from background environmental sources. Subsequently, it was discovered that the Chisso Corporation expanded operations to meet the growing demand for acetaldehyde to make plastics. It had changed its factory's drainage site from Minamata Bay to the mouth of the Minamata River leading into the Shiranui Sea and continued discharging methylmercury there until 1968. People living in the surrounding coastal areas were exposed to low doses of the metal chronically through consumption of contaminated fish and over the following 30 years manifested paresthesias, visual field defects, and other evidence of subtle somatosensory damage (Ekino et al., 2007).

References

Ekino S, Susa M, Ninomiya T, Imamura K, Kitamura T. Minamata disease revisited: an update on the acute and chronic manifestations of methyl mercury poisoning. J Neurol Sci 2007;262:131–44.

Gilhooly R. Mercury rising: Niigata struggles to bury its Minamata ghosts. Japan Times; June 2015. https://www.japantimes.co.jp/news/2015/06/13/national/history/mercury-rising-niigata-struggles-bury-minamata-ghosts/#.XXzhZCV7mu4. [Accessed 14 September 2019].

Harada Y. Electroencephalographic studies of Minamata disease in children. Dev Med Child Neurol 1968;10(2):257–8.

Matsumoto H, Koya G, Takeuchi T. Fetal Minamata disease. A neuropathological study of two cases of intrauterine intoxication by a methyl mercury compound. J Neuropathol Exp Neurol 1965;24(4):563–74.

McNutt M. Mercury and health. Science 2013;341(6153):1430.

Normile D. In Minamata, mercury still divides. Science 2013;341(6153):1446–7.

O'Malley GF. The blood of my veins—mercury, Minamata and the soul of Japan. Clin Toxicol 2017;55(8):934–8.

Powell PP. Minamata disease: a story of mercury's malevolence. South Med J 1991;84(11):1352–8.

Smith WE, Smith AM. Minamata—words and photographs. New York: Holt Rinehart & Winston; 1975.

Tsubaki T, Irukayama K, editors. Minamata disease: methylmercury poisoning in Minamata and Niigata, Japan. Tokyo: Kodansha Ltd; 1977.

Weiss B, Clarkson TW, Simon W. Silent latency periods in methylmercury poisoning and in neurodegenerative disease. Environ Health Perspect 2002;110(Suppl 5):851–4.

Chapter 1.2.2

Niigata, Japan, 1965

Industrial contamination of the environment by discharges of methylmercury in effluent wastes was revisited in Japan less than a decade after the Minamata Bay disaster. The details were eerily similar to what had happened at Minamata previously, so much so that the poisoning of Niigata was often referred to as the "Second Minamata disease." Again, it was the odd behavior and strange death of cats, a harbinger of bad things to come, that was first noticed by townspeople living in the Niigata Prefecture on the banks of the Agano (Aganogawa) River in 1964. Once again, it was discovered that an industrial giant—the Shōwa Denkō Electrical Company's chemical plant in Kanose Village—was using mercury sulfate as a catalyst in its production of acetaldehyde. Untreated waste containing methylmercury was settling downstream in the sediment of the river bed near Niigata, some 50 km away from the plant (Fig. 1.2.3).

"Second Minamata Disease" discovered in Niigata

Fish of the Agano River accumulated high concentrations of the metal in their tissues, slowly poisoning the people who caught and ate them. Fish samples collected in the lower Agano River basin in June 1965 had elevated mercury amounts in their tissues up to 41 ppm (Maruyama et al., 2012). Dr. Koichi Hirota, a newly trained 26-year old neurologist at the Brain Research Institute of Niigata University, diagnosed the first patient in Niigata, who had numbness and tingling of the extremities and other signs, as having Minamata disease in January, 1965. Mercury in his hair sample was elevated to 765 ppm (765 × higher than the EPA's reference level). Partnering with his mentor, Professor Tadao Tsubaki from Niigata University, Dr. Hirota diagnosed two additional patients. These clinical toxicologists made the first public announcement of their clinical findings on June 12, 1965 (Maruyama et al., 2012). Dozens of additional patients came forward with similar complaints in the ensuing months (Fig. 1.2.4).

Niigata community support

Unlike the people living in the shadow of the Chisso plant in Minamata, the affected populace here lived some distance from Shōwa Denkō plant along the lower Agano River basin and for the most part did not work for the electric company. Those people who were affected manifested the same clinical symptoms and signs of neurological dysfunction as those seen elsewhere in mercury poisoning outbreaks. While the company officials tried to deflect blame for the contamination, offering an alternative explanation of "agricultural run-off" and denying the science, this time, after the Minamata story had unfolded,

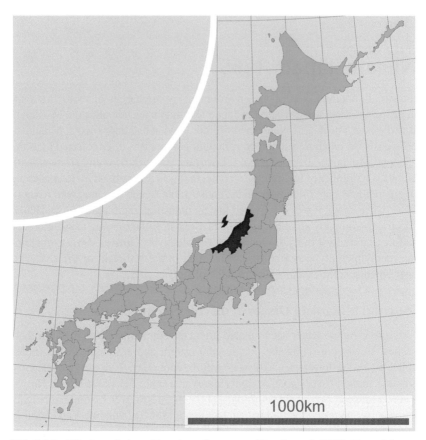

FIG. 1.2.3 Niigata prefecture. *(From https://commons.wikimedia.org/wiki/File:Map_of_Japan_ with_highlight_on_15_Niigata_prefecture.svg.)*

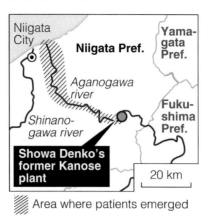

FIG. 1.2.4 Shōwa Denkō's Kanose Plant on the Aganogawa River. *Source: Ekino et al. J Neurol Sci 2007.*

the public was not accepting it. A collaboration was formed with researchers from the Kumamoto University Research Group and Dr. Hajime Hosokawa from Minamata, Professor Tadao Tsubaki (Niigata University), local medical practitioners (neurologist Koichi Hirota at the Brain Research Institute), the local government's health officials, and community activists. They all worked together to uncover and document the Shōwa Denkō company's role in this disaster.

Shōwa Denkō held accountable

By March 1966, wastewater from the chemical factory was suspected as the source, and in September local governmental officials confirmed the presence of mercury in the river at the outlet of the Shōwa Denkō plant upstream from Niigata. It was also known that in the 1950s, Shōwa Denkō's use of mercury at its plant was increased from 2500 to 4500t, and so the pollution had been going on unnoticed for years (Gilhooly, 2015). Public outrage soon turned against the company's officials. While it took 13 years for the officials at Chisso in Minamata to be held accountable legally, a lawsuit was filed against Shōwa Denkō leaders in 1967, less than 3 years after the outbreak. The adjudicated outcome in favor of the victims was reached by 1971, with substantial financial compensation. At least 702 people in Niigata were eventually identified as suffering from "Minamata disease": the effects of mercury contamination (Gilhooly, 2015). And researchers have shown that some mildly affected adults in Niigata had lingering effects, such as hearing loss, sensory disturbances, and disequilibrium, even though their hair mercury levels did not meet the WHO-set standard (50 υg/g) for environmental exposure (Maruyama et al., 2012). Thus, Niigata became known as the "second Minamata" in the annals of environmental methylmercury disasters.

Lessons learned

The disasters at Minamata Bay and Niigata demonstrated to the world for the first time that unchecked environmental pollution by industrial chemicals over time could devastate an ecosystem and lead to catastrophic effects on the health and well-being of entire populations of people living in the affected communities. It introduced for the first time the legal principle that a company had a duty and responsibility to ensure that its operations would not harm the environment or people living in the vicinity of its manufacturing plants, power generators, mines, smelters, or other industrial concerns. A company could and would be held legally liable and accountable for any transgressions.

A commonality in all of the methylmercury chronic poisoning outbreaks was the difficulty in making (and certifying, for compensation purposes) the diagnosis in people who were only exposed to relatively low environmental concentrations of the metal. The severity of mercury poisoning was dependent on dose and duration of exposure. Some victims in both Minamata and Niigata had only subjective symptoms and/or very subtle neurological findings. Those with only mild neurological findings initially and no continuing exposure to mercury could improve over time and be left later on with only subjective findings of paresthesias, headaches, limb pain, and weakness, with little objective findings on neurological exam. While they were still victims of a mass poisoning, they would not meet the government's strict definition of methylmercury poisoning used to determine certification for compensation. Another lawsuit was filed in the Niigata District Court against the government and Shōwa Denkō pleading the cases of 2400 additional, newly discovered victims in 2013 (Gilhooly, 2015).

References

Ekino S, Susa M, Ninomiya T, Imamura K, Kitamura T. Minamata disease revisited: an up-date on the acute and chronic manifestations of methyl mercury poisoning. J Neurol Sci 2007;262:131–44.

Gilhooly R. Mercury rising: Niigata struggles to bury its Minamata ghosts. Japan Times; 2015. https://www.japantimes.co.jp/news/2015/06/13/national/history/mercury-rising-niigata-struggles-bury-minamata-ghosts/#.XXzhZCV7mu4. [Accessed 14 September 2019].

Maruyama K, Yorifuji T, Tsuda T, Sekikawa T, Nakadeira H, Saito H. Methylmercury exposure at Niigata, Japan: results of neurological examinations of 103 adults. J Biomed Biotechnol 2012:7. https://www.hindawi.com/journals/bmri/2012/635075/.

Chapter 1.2.3

IRAQ, 1971

Organomercury fungicides

Fungicides have been used to treat (or dress) seeds of grains for centuries to prevent disease and improve crop yields. Typically, such chemicals have included alkyl mercury compounds (e.g., methylmercury and ethylmercury), alkoxyalkyl mercuric compounds (e.g., methoxyethyl mercury, ethoxyethyl mercury), and aryl mercuric compounds (e.g., phenyl mercury, p-tolyl mercury). Use of these mercurial fungicides grew during the 1940s and 1950s, and reached their zenith worldwide in the 1960s. Methyl and ethyl mercury were used as a pesticide and a fungicide to protect the seeds from deterioration and spoilage before they could be planted. In this way, methylmercury-coated wheat seeds were intended to improve crop yields; the methylmercury dissipated in soil once the wheat or barley plants were growing. Methylmercury-containing compounds, in the form of the fungicide products "Granosan" or "Panogen" or "Ceresan," had been added at about 7.9 µg/g, with a range of 3.7–14.9 µg/g; and the seeds were colored reddish-pink as a visible warning to discourage direct consumption (Greenwood, 1985; Al-Mufti et al., 1976). However, the dye could be washed off the seed, perhaps falsely reassuring some farmers that the methylmercury was also being washed away, when it was not.

1970 Iraqi famine

In 1971, wheat and barley seeds were shipped to Iraq in large quantities from the United States. At the time, the country was in the midst of one of its worst droughts resulting in wheat and other crop failures in 1970. The resulting food shortage was a human catastrophe. Thousands of people were weakened from nutritional deficiencies or died. Four years of poor crops forced the Iraqi government to contract with an American grain exporter, Cargill Inc., in California. The Iraqi government acquired a total of 73,201 metric tons of imported 50 kg bags of US wheat seed and 22,262 tons of barley seed (Skerfving and Copplestone, 1976; Clarkson et al., 1976; Greenwood, 1985). The seed was treated with pink-colored "Granosan" organomercurial pesticides. The sacks were widely distributed in the cereal farming areas of northern, central, and southern rural Iraq.

There were clear warnings imprinted on the bags that the seed contained methylmercury and should not be consumed. However, the warnings were stenciled either in Spanish (since most bags of wheat seed were shipped from Mexico) or English (barley seed came from California) and sent to rural Iraq where the language was Arabic. The western "skull and crossbones" warning

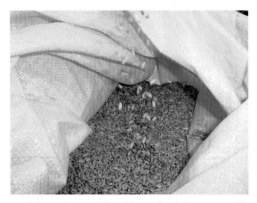

FIG. 1.2.5 Sack containing wheat grain. *(From https://commons.wikimedia.org/w/index. php?search=Wheat&title=Special%3ASearch&profile=advanced&fulltext=1&advancedSearch-current=%7B%7D&ns0=1&ns6=1&ns12=1&ns14=1&ns100=1&ns106=1#/media/File:Wheat_in_sack.jpg.)*

logo stenciled on some bags was not recognized culturally by Iraqis as a symbol of poison. The Iraq Ministry of Agriculture estimated that the treated grain would have been distributed to about 200,000 people between October and December, 1971.

Instead of being planted in the fields as was intended, the seeds were ground into flour for making homemade unleavened bread; the barley was fed to livestock. The fact that animals fed the seed did not experience any symptoms right away also probably gave people false reassurance that it was safe to eat. Bread made from the contaminated flour was consumed by large numbers of farming families in rural Iraq. The adults might eat up to six to eight 220 g loaves of bread daily, while young children may typically eat two to three loaves (Greenwood, 1985). The methylmercury content was about 7.9 µg/g of flour (range 3.7–14.9 µg/g); so typically, patients ingested between 50 and 400 mg as methylmercury in the homemade bread (Bakir et al., 1973; Al-Mufti et al., 1976). As a result, widespread mercury poisoning ensued throughout rural areas of Iraq until the mistake was discovered and warnings first issued 32 days after the distribution (Fig. 1.2.5).

Clinical toxicology

The first poisoning cases were diagnosed in the northern province of Kirkuk in December 1971 (Clarkson et al., 1976). After a latency period of about 2–6 weeks, people began to suffer symptoms and signs of mercury poisoning. Early symptoms, usually weakness and limb paresthesias occurred when an individual had accumulated a body burden of 25–40 mg of mercury (Bakir et al., 1973). The first cases were recognized by Drs. Saadoun Tikriti and Salem Damluji of the Medical City Teaching Hospital in Baghdad (Al-Damluji, 1976;

Greenwood, 1985). By February 1972, there were already an estimated 5500 cases of mercury poisoning (Clarkson et al., 1976). In one district, a case fatality rate of 22% was reported (Al-Mufti et al., 1976). By March 1972, there were more than 6148 hospital admissions and 452 deaths attributed to the Iraq grain disaster (Skerfving and Copplestone, 1976).

Patients presented to clinics or hospitals with vomiting, dehydration and abdominal pain and cramping. Neurotoxicity included peripheral neuropathy with stocking-glove numbness and loss of sensation, unsteady gait (ataxia), frequent falls, blurred vision, narrowed visual fields, deafness, astereognosis, and slurred speech (dysarthria) (Al-Mufti et al., 1976). Those with severe poisoning who survived had irreversible damage to the cerebral cortex and cerebellum; their disability did not improve much over time. Severely poisoned patients lost weight, became blind and deaf, and were bedridden. They had brisk reflexes, developed tremors and myoclonic jerks, and progressed to incapacitating spasticity and quadriplegia. Personality changes (e.g., excitability, irritability, apathy, confusion) and memory loss preceded a deteriorating level of consciousness into coma and death.

There were two other routes of exposure in Iraqi families besides the home-made bread: prenatal transmission and lactation (Bakir et al., 1980). Methylmercury readily crosses the placenta and is highly fetotoxic, although the pregnant woman herself might have minimal symptoms. Stillborn infants had an almost complete lack of neuronal development, while infants who survived were born with severe developmental delays and a static encephalopathy similar to that seen in births after the Minamata Bay disaster in Japan. The lipophilic alkyl metal also concentrates in breast milk at a concentration of 3% of the mercury level in the mother's blood, conveyed to infants during lactation (Bakir et al., 1973).

Dose vs. severity of poisoning

The daily mercury intake could be calculated from how much bread the people ate. Clearance half-lives for the absorbed mercury varied between 64 and 120 days, so that the hazard from accumulating a body burden of mercury from chronic dosing varied between individuals (Clarkson et al., 1976). Epidemiologic studies showed that those who had eaten the most bread suffered the most severe effects (Clarkson et al., 1976; Al-Mufti et al., 1976). The severity of poisoning varied depending on mercury dose: those ingesting 2.4 mg/kg of mercury had mild-to-moderate symptoms, whereas those ingesting 3.6 mg/kg or more experienced a severe, life-threatening poisoning. In one study, those eating contaminated bread had a higher mean blood mercury level 34 ng/mL and higher mean hair mercury 136 µg/g versus 7 ng/mL and 5 µg/g, respectively, in controls who did not eat the bread (Kazantzis et al., 1976a). Maximum hair concentrations correlated with estimates of the amount of contaminated bread eaten; the most severely disabled had hair mercury concentrations as high as 2130 µg/g (Kazantzis et al., 1976a). Hair mercury levels above 5 µg/g were used to determine those exposed to the contaminated grains (Greenwood, 1985).

Clinical outcomes

Those with only mild or moderate poisoning could make a considerable recovery, especially with the aid of physical therapy. They might be left with only subjective symptoms, such as headaches, fatigue, and weakness or paresthesias (Al-Damluji, 1975; Kazantzis et al., 1976b; Skerfving and Copplestone, 1976). Children suffered the same neurotoxicity as adults. In one 2-year follow-up study of 49 children, most with mild or moderate poisoning regained at least some partial functions. Of the 18 children with severe poisoning, 7 (39%) were left with severe, incapacitating disability (Amin-zaki et al., 1978).

Iraqi poisonings compared with Minamata poisonings

In 1972, the Iraqi government issued a warning making it illegal for continued possession or consumption of the treated grain. It was hypothesized that the Iraqi disaster differed from the Minamata disease, in that it was a more concentrated dose of methylmercury over a short period of time of a few months versus the chronic, repeated, smaller dosing among Japanese families during their everyday consumption of foods over months to years. Table 1.2.2 illustrates the comparison of the two epidemics.

TABLE 1.2.2 Comparison of Clinical Findings: Iraq versus Minamata, Japan.

Symptom or sign	Minamata disease ($N = 34$)	Iraqi cases ($N = 66$)
Constricted visual fields	100%	44%
Yellow vision	0	12%
Ataxia	80%–90%	62%
Impaired hearing	85%	36%
Speech disturbance	88%	61%
Dysphagia	94%	5–9%
Tremor	76%	38%
Mental disturbance	71%	8%–9%
Impaired superficial sensation	100%	23%
Brisk reflexes	38%	56%
Abdominal pain	0	52%
Nausea/vomiting	0	33%

Adapted from Al-Damluji, 1976.

Thus there was a longer lapse of time prior to the onset of symptoms and signs of poisoning in Minamata disease. With a much higher cumulative body burden of mercury, many more victims of Minamata disease suffered permanent disabilities than did Iraqis (Amin-zaki et al., 1978).

Lessons learned

Lessons from the Iraqi methylmercury-related toxic epidemic were set forth at a conference held in Baghdad Iraq in 1974 (Skerfving and Copplestone, 1976). Recommendations included the following:

- Use of safer alternative compounds as seedling dressings
- Stricter controls over treated grain seeds
- Establish national poison control centers
- Hold stocks of antidotes
- Encourage local doctors and health organizations to report cases or clusters of poisoning
- Early notification of health organizations and the public of an outbreak
- Early epidemiological field surveys and extensive sampling
- Improved availability of sophisticated, reliable, precise laboratory analyses
- Access to early emergency assistance from WHO and other international agencies and experts

The Iraqi disaster could have been prevented with a more informed approach to the warnings (in the appropriate language) supplied with the imported grain and a more coordinated governmental policy to ensure safe distribution to farmers who would use it as intended. The strategy of coloring the grain as a warning against its consumption did not work to prevent this epidemic. In the end, a switch to safer fungicides than mercurial compounds that was made by agricultural concerns in the 1970s helped to prevent additional epidemics.

Methylmercury in foodstuffs—A global public health issue

Table 1.2.3 presents some of the mass poisoning occurrences involving methylmercury from around the world. In 1969, a New Mexico family in Alamagordo mistakenly fed mercury-preserved grains to their pigs and subsequently several family members suffered serious mercury neurotoxicity. In 1970, the United States banned the use of methylmercury as a fungicide treatment of seeds used in agriculture, noting that improper, unsafe uses could not be prevented. Other countries had previously banned alkylmercury-based fungicides for the same reasons; there were less toxic, less expensive and equally effective alternatives for agricultural use.

TABLE 1.2.3 Epidemics of methylmercury poisoning world-wide.

Location	Year	Victims	Deaths	Foodstuffs
Minamata, Japan	1956	2262	Unknown	Fish, shellfish
Northern Iraq[a]	1956	100	14	Grain seed
Iraq[b]	1960	1000	Unknown	Grain seed
West Pakistan[c]	1963	34	4	Grain seed
Guatemala[d]	1966	45	20	Grain seed
Niigata, Japan[e]	1965	702	Unknown	Fish, shellfish
New Mexico, USA[f]	1969	4	0	Pigs
Iraq[b]	1972	6530	459	Grain seed

[a] Takizawa Y. Mercury-contaminated grain in Iraq. Environ. Toxicol. Hum. Health, volume 1. UNESCO.EOLSS. Accessed 12 September 2019, https://www.eolss.net/ebooklib/cart.aspx.
[b] Bakir F, Damluji SF, Amin-Zaki L, Murtadha M, Khalidi A, Al-Rawi NY, Tikriti S et al. Mercury poisoning in Iraq. Science 1973;181:230–41.
[c] Haq IU. Agosan poisoning in man. Br Med J 1963;(1):1579–82.
[d] Ordonez JV, Carillo JA, Miranda M, Gale JL. Epidemiological study of an illness in the Guatemala highlands believed to be encephalitis. Boletin de la Oficina Sanitaria Panamericana 1966;60:18–24.
[e] Gilhooly R. Mercury rising: Niigata struggles to bury its Minamata ghosts. The Japan Times. June 13, 2015. Accessed 14 September 2019, https://www.japantimes.co.jp/news/2015/06/13/national/history/mercury-rising-niigata-struggles-bury-minamata-ghosts/#.XXzhZCV7mu4
[f] Snyder RD, Seelinger DF. Methylmercury poisoning. J Neurol, Neurosurg, Psych 1976;39:701–04.

References

Al-Damluji SF. Intoxication due to alkylmercury-treated seed—1971–72 outbreak in Iraq: clinical aspects. Bull World Health Organ 1976;53(Suppl):65–81.

Al-Damluji SF & the Clinical Committee on Mercury Poisoning. Intoxication due to alkylmercury-treated seeds-1971–72 outbreak in Iraq: clinical aspects. Bulletin of the World Health Organization December 1975;53(Suppl):65–81.

Al-Mufti AW, Copplestone JF, Kazantzis G, Mahmoud RM, Majid MA. Epidemiology of organomercury poisoning in Iraq. I. Incidence in a defined area and relationship to the eating of contaminated bread. Bull World Health Organ 1976;53(Suppl):23–36.

Amin-zaki L, Majeed MA, Clarkson TW, Greenwood MR. Methylmercury poisoning in Iraqi children: clinical observations over two years. Br Med J 1978;1(6113):613–6.

Bakir F, Damluji SF, Amin-Zaki L, Murtadha M, Khalidi A, Al-Rawi NY, Tikriti S, Dahahir HI, Clarkson TW, Smith JC, Doherty RA. Methylmercury poisoning in Iraq. Science 1973;181(4096):230–41.

Bakir F, Rustam H, Tikriti S, Al-Damluji SF, Shihristani H. Clinical and epidemiological aspects of methylmercury poisoning. Postgrad Med J 1980;56(651):1–10.

Clarkson TW, Amin-Zaki L, Al-Tikriti SK. An outbreak of methylmercury poisoning due to consumption of contaminated grain. Fed Proc 1976;35(12):2395–9.

Greenwood MR. Methylmercury poisoning in Iraq. An epidemiological study of the 1971–1972 outbreak. J Appl Toxicol 1985;5(3):148–59.

Kazantzis G, Al-Mufti AW, Al-Jawad A, et al. Epidemiology of organomercury poisoning in Iraq. II. Relationship of mercury levels in blood and hair to exposure and to clinical findings. Bull World Health Organ 1976a;53(Suppl):37–48.

Kazantzis G, Al-Mufti AW, Copplestone JF, Majid MA, Mahmoud RM. Epidemiology of organo-mercury poisoning in Iraq. III. Clinical features and their changes with time. Bull World Health Organ 1976b;53(Suppl):49–57.

Skerfving SB, Copplestone JF. Poisoning caused by the consumption of organomercury-dressed seed in Iraq. Bull World Health Organ 1976;54(1):101–12.

Chapter 1.3

Community dioxin disaster—Seveso Italy, 1976

Alan D. Woolf

Boston Children's Hospital & Harvard Medical School, Boston, Massachusetts, United States

The explosion

The Industrie Chimiche Meridionali Societá Anonima (ICMESA) chemical factory located in Meda, Italy, near Seveso in the *Lombardia* region of Italy about 74 km north of Milan, was involved in the manufacture of chlorine compounds, such as trichlorophenol, used in the production of cosmetics and pharmaceuticals (Fig. 1.3.1).

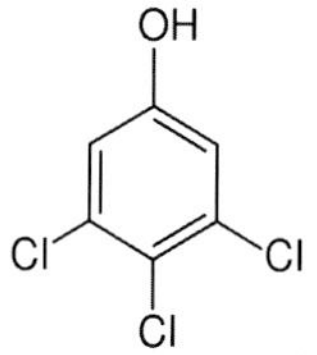

FIG. 1.3.1   Trichlorophenol. *(Source: wikimedia commons)*

The unwanted, intermediate by-products of this manufacturing process included a compound within a common chemical family: dioxins. On July 10, 1976, an unexpected chemical exothermic reaction went out of control in the trichlorophenol reactor in the ICMESA plant; the mixture reached a temperature of 250°C and a pressure to 4 atm. A safety valve ruptured, resulting in an explosion. The plant accidentally released a large plume containing more than 1500 kg of aerosolized sodium hydroxide, ethylene glycol, sodium trichlorophenate, and 2,3,7,8-tetrachlorobenzo-*p*-dioxin (TCDD) over an 18 km^2 area involving the nearby area of several towns known as the "*Brianza di Seveso*," with a total population at the time of about 220,000 residents. An estimated 34 kg of dioxin was released and dispersed over a wide area (Bertazzi et al., 1998) (Fig. 1.3.2).

History of Modern Clinical Toxicology. https://doi.org/10.1016/B978-0-12-822218-8.00004-1

35

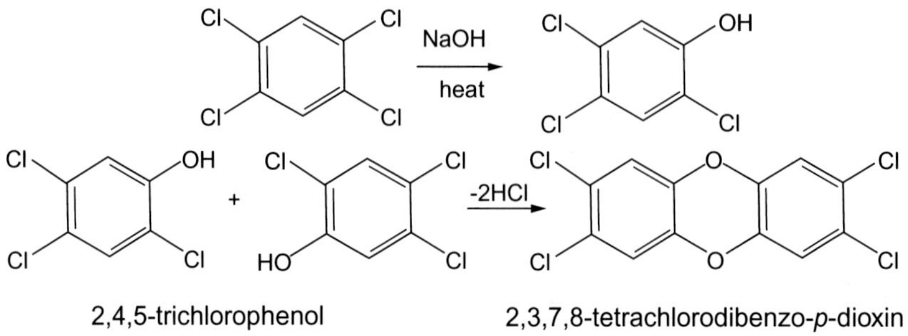

2,4,5-trichlorophenol   2,3,7,8-tetrachlorodibenzo-*p*-dioxin

FIG. 1.3.2 2,3,7,8-Tetrachlorodibenzo-*p*-dioxin (TCDD) as a by-product of trichlorophenol production. *(Source: wikimedia commons)*

The plume spread quickly via prevailing conditions, facilitated by ambient humid, warm weather conditions and a 5 m/s wind blowing south-eastward. The cloud contained relatively pure TCDD. It covered a populated area surrounding the town of Seveso, exposing more than 37,000 residents directly, by inhalation and dermal absorption in the acute event. Although at the time TCDD could not be measured in humans, it could be measured in soil. Investigators, guided by the presence of dead animals and killed vegetation, took systematic samples of the soil in the area under the plume. This initial survey allowed investigators to separate areas into zones of the level of contamination risk to the inhabitants, based on the concentration of dioxin in the soil (Fig. 1.3.3).

In Zone A (0.3 mile^2)—the very high exposure, an estimated 1.3–2 kg of TCDD was dispersed unevenly (Pocchiari et al., 1979; Mocarelli et al., 1988). Some animals, such as rabbits and poultry, in this area died soon after the accident, especially those eating contaminated plants. There were 736 residents (212 families) who were evacuated by August 2, 1976, and who were not allowed back in the area. This most contaminated zone was divided into subzones A1–A7, with the highest TCDD concentrations in soil in closest proximity to the factory (Pocchiari et al., 1979). Subsequently, some homes and commercial buildings were destroyed as part of the clean-up and an entire 40-cm deep layer of top soil was removed and buried elsewhere, in two designated toxic waste dumps (Signorini et al., 2000).

Zone B (1.0 mile^2) residents—about 4800 people—were also in a contaminated area but were not evacuated by the Lombardia Regional Government. Much less TCDD, about 20 g, was estimated to have been dispersed over a larger area of ground than Zone A (Pocchiari et al., 1979). Access to some contaminated grounds was restricted and contaminated food was destroyed (Mocarelli, 1986). Residents were warned against eating locally produced foods.

Zone R (5.5 mile^2) residents—about 22,000 people—lived in the least contaminated area and were allowed to remain but were still warned not to eat locally produced foods or produce. An estimated 20 g of TCDD was dispersed over this much larger area of land than the other two zones (Pocchiari et al., 1979).

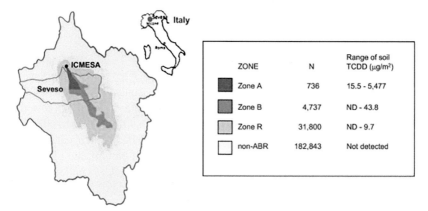

ZONE	N	Range of soil TCDD (µg/m²)
Zone A	736	15.5 - 5,477
Zone B	4,737	ND - 43.8
Zone R	31,800	ND - 9.7
non-ABR	182,843	Not detected

FIG. 1.3.3 Zones of contamination relative to plant at Seveso, Italy. *(From Eskenazi et al., 2018, Environ Int)*

Specimens of soil from Zone A contained TCDD at concentrations of 15.5–5447 µg/m² of soil (mean 530 µg/m²); Zone B contained from a low of nondetectable amounts to 43.8 µg/m² (mean 3 µg/m²); Zone R some soil samples contained some TCDD (up to 9 µg/m²) but mostly nondetectable amounts (Signorini et al., 2000). Dioxin levels measured in plants in each of the zones correlated well with soil levels. However, in retrospect, it was thought that many of the soil measurements may have underestimated the amount of contamination by as much as 25- to 60-fold (Bertazzi et al., 1998).

A reference zone of about 183,000 people living in 28.8 mile² near Seveso was uncontaminated by the explosion plume and was designated as a control population by investigators. The health of people living there was monitored longitudinally for comparison purposes in the numerous post-explosion, population-based health studies that ensued.

Serum TCDD levels and half-life

In the weeks after the explosion, more than 30,000 serum or plasma samples were collected, frozen, and stored carefully labeled with the victim's name and whether they lived in Zone A, B, R, or an unaffected area. The ability to measure TCDD in serum was not technically possible until laboratory techniques using gas chromatography-high performance mass spectrometry became available in 1986. Thus some of the most informative environmental epidemiologic toxicology studies could not be completed until over a decade after the explosion. Retrospective cohort studies since the 1980s have correlated well the serum TCDD concentrations of victims with the soil TCDD levels in the geographic zones in which they lived. Analysis of those original samples revealed some extraordinarily high serum TCDD concentrations—as high as 27,821 ppt in residents with severe chloracne (Mocarelli et al., 1988). One analysis of blood samples taken in 1976 reported median TCDD levels in Zone A at 447 ppt (*N*=296), in Zone B at 94 ppt (*N*=80), and in Zone R at 48 ppt (*N*=48) (Needham et al., 1997-1998).

In 1992–93, people in Zone A still had median serum TCDD levels of 72 ppt (back-extrapolated to 379 ppt in 1976) (Steenland et al., 2004). In the Seveso Women's Health Study (SWHS), a historical cohort study, the median TCDD serum concentration was 55 ppt, with an enormous range: from 2.5 ppt to some of the highest serum concentrations ever recorded: 56,000 ppt (Eskenazi et al., 2018). Studies have determined the TCDD half-life to be about 7 years in adolescents and adults and have continued to provide data on both the victims as well as effects on their offspring (Eskenazi et al., 2018). Children under 10 years of age were found to have higher TCDD serum concentrations but shorter half-lives (3–5 years) than adults.

Background—Dioxins

The word, "dioxin" commonly refers to 2,3,7,8-tetrachlorobenzo-*p*-dioxin or TCDD. This is one of the most toxic congeners in this large family of chemicals. However, "dioxins" and dioxin-like substances include many different compounds with related chemical structures. Fig. 1.3.4 shows some of these chemical entities and the numbered areas of substituted R groups on each of the aromatic carbon rings. Dioxin and dioxin-like chemicals have been recognized as widespread, almost ubiquitous environmental contaminants. These pollutants accumulate and are persistent, degrading naturally in the environment only over very long periods of time. Of the family of dioxins, seven are most associated with toxic effects in humans; chief among these is TCDD.

Dioxins are manmade chemicals produced as a by-product of waste incineration and in the manufacture of paper and pulp bleaching and the synthesis of some chlorine-containing organic chemicals, such as herbicides, pesticides, and fungicides. They are environmentally persistent, lipophilic, bio-accumulative pollutants. TCDD was the chemical found in trace amounts as a by-product in "Agent Orange" chemicals: 2,4 dichlorophenoxtacetic acid (2,4 D) and 2,4,5 trichlorophenoxyacetic acid (2,4,5T) used as defoliant herbicides delivered by airplanes over large swaths of land during the Vietnam war (Schecter et al., 2006).

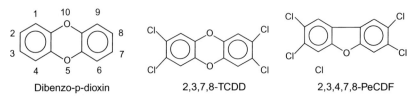

FIG. 1.3.4 Chemical structures of dibenzo-*p*-dioxins, 2,3,7.8 tetrachloro-dibenzo-*p*-dioxin (TCDD) and an example of a dioxin-related furan chemical: 2,3,4,7,8 pentachlorodibenzofurane. *(Source: wikimedia commons)*

These dioxin-containing wartime defoliants contaminated the countryside and subsequently sickened thousands of Vietnamese, as well as American troops.

The most common exposure to dioxins and dioxin-like chemicals today is through eating a diet that includes fatty foods, such as dairy products, meat, fish, and eggs. In 1998, WHO set a "tolerable daily intake" of dioxins and dioxin-like compounds at 1–4 pg TEQ per kilogram body weight per day. Thus most people have dioxins detectable in blood and adipose tissues, although levels have been declining over the past few decades as sources of these compounds are eliminated from the environment. The average lipid-adjusted body burden in people living in North America and Europe in 2000 was about 2 ppt (Aylward and Hays, 2002).

At the time of the Seveso explosion in 1976, not much was known about effects of dioxins in humans. Much of what we know now has since been learned from occupational exposures of workers in electrical and other industries, although accidental exposures of the public, such as those seen at Seveso Italy and in the Yusho and Yu-Cheng cooking rice oil contamination incidents in Japan and Taiwan, have provided additional data on toxicity. The reader will find details on the Yusho and Yu-Cheng disasters in Chapter 1.10 of this book. The poisoning of a Ukrainian politician, Viktor Yushchenko, in which pure TCDD was used, is described in Chapter 2.6.

Since Seveso, the toxicology of dioxin and related compounds has been well-studied, although some details of their subcellular effects remain unclear. One of the principal sites of dioxin action in cells is the aHr (aromatic hydrocarbon receptor), which is present in many cell types and is conserved across a variety of animal species (Schecter et al., 2006). The aHr complex, composed of two proteins—a dimer of aHr and aHr nuclear translocator protein, is involved in diverse biochemical functions. The aHr complex also binds to transcription factors acting to regulate gene expression. The toxicity of dioxin is linked to its ability to bind to aHr, perturbing endogenous subcellular signaling pathways. One major function of aHr is to regulate the induction of specific forms of the cytochrome P-450 complex. The Seveso incident as well as animal and occupational studies have demonstrated that the acute effects of dioxin are to upregulate aHr, whereas later on the chronic exposure of cells to dioxin leads to permanent down-regulation of aHr (Rysavy et al., 2013). Dioxin also has non-aHr associated cellular effects, with formation of active ligands that induce toxin-specific novel pathways and inhibit or activate some enzyme systems. Dioxin may affect downstream cell functions through: (1) non-genomic signaling via calcium and other targets mediating cellular effects outside of transcription, (2) aHr-mediated genomic signaling of calcium-dependent genes, and (3) genomic signaling associated with other genes that are targets of aHr plus other transcription factors (Skene et al., 1989; Rysavy et al., 2013). Through its direct and indirect effects on DNA transcription and gene activity, dioxin quite possibly acts as a mutagen and promoter of carcinogenesis (Skene et al., 1989).

Immediate symptoms and signs of toxicity

Small animals such as rabbits and chickens in Zone A died and plants turned yellow and withered after the Seveso incident. Although the mayor of Seveso was notified of the explosion the next day, the release of dioxin as the major contaminant in the cloud was not confirmed until 10 days later (Bertazzi et al., 1998). This resulted in an unfortunate delay in the mobilization of an appropriate governmental response to the disaster. People living in Zone A were evacuated only on days 16–23. At the time of the explosion, victims in the path of the plume were exposed directly to TCDD by inhalation and by absorption through eyes, skin, and mucous membranes. Not much was known about the toxicity of dioxin in humans prior to the time of this incident, except what was learned from animal studies and a few small studies of occupational exposures. Some of the immediate symptoms of the Seveso residents included headaches, nausea, and eye irritation; within 6 days, 14 children were hospitalized and treated for chemical burns (Eskenazi et al., 2018). Subacute effects included possible reduced nerve conduction velocity but no other significant differences in neurological function. No effects on the immune system or higher rates of congenital malformations or spontaneous abortions could be appreciated (Pocchiari et al., 1979).

Skin lesions and chloracne

Insidious symptoms and signs of TCDD toxicity were manifest subsequently in the population, including chloracne soon after the exposure. Of 1600 people examined 20–40 days after the incident, 447 had early, irritative cutaneous lesions (edema, erythema, papulonodular lesions, and bullae) attributable to direct exposure to the cloud (Caputo et al., 1988). All these early lesions disappeared within a month, leaving only mild hyperpigmentation.

By April 1977, 187 cases of chloracne had been documented; 164 (88%) of those were children (Bertazzi et al., 1998). Chloracne is not true "acne," but rather an inflammatory response to fat-soluble chloracnegen chemicals, with hyperplasia and hyperkeratosis of the interfollicular epidermis and sebaceous follicles, comedones, cysts, and squamous metaplasia of the sebaceous glands. Chloracne is a cardinal feature of exposure to dioxin, although it is not universal among victims (Steenland, 2004). One can be exposed to a significant dose of TCDD without manifesting chloracne of the skin. The keratogenic plugs and pustules in skin pores begin within days or as late as 3–4 weeks after exposure and can affect any part of the body, including the face, shoulders, back, chest, and abdomen. The exposed children of Seveso were especially prone to manifesting, early on, the skin lesions of chloracne. One study monitored 193 chloracne patients from Seveso over the subsequent 2-year period after the accident, and specifically studied the course of 44 children and adolescents (Caputo et al., 1988). Most skin lesions had regressed and attenuated over the 2 years of study, leaving atrophic scarring (Fig. 1.3.5).

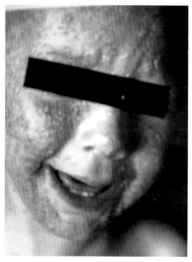

FIG. 1.3.5   Chloracne and hyperpigmentation in a child in Seveso, Italy. *(Source: (Schecter et al., 2006, Environ Res) Courtesy Professor Paolo Mocarelli)*

Carcinogenesis

Dioxins have been known to be carcinogenic from animal studies for some time. TCDD is thought to be a cancer promoter and has been designated as a probable carcinogen by both the EPA and IARC since 1997. Among men 20 years after the Seveso incident, risk rates of all-cancer, rectal cancer and lung cancer were already higher than expected (Steenland, 2004). One cancer mortality study of 278,108 subjects (Seveso victims, in-migrants, and children born after the event) carried out 25 years after the event (Consonni et al., 2008) as well as a 15-year follow-up study of Seveso residents who were originally exposed (Pesatori et al., 2009) both found increased rates of hematopoietic and lymphatic neoplasms (e.g., non-Hodgkin's lymphoma) and breast cancer in women, as well as other illnesses, such as chronic obstructive lung disease, diabetes, and circulatory diseases (Eskenazi et al., 2018).

The Seveso Women's Health Study, a retrospective cohort study, recruited over 981 women aged 0–40 years old residing around Seveso at the time of the explosion; it is the largest study of a female population with known exposure to TCDD. A report published in 2011 found the hazard ratio for all cancers was significantly associated with a 10-fold increase in serum TCDD concentration; that for breast cancer was also elevated, though not to a statistically significant level (Warner et al., 2011). Authors pointed out their numbers were still small (66 cancers), and many women enrolled (about half) were still not of the age of greatest breast cancer risk yet (i.e., post-menopausal).

Aftermath

Residents as well as in-migrants to the Seveso region and children born to women after the event, were also exposed to TCDD indirectly long after the event by the ingestion of contaminated foodstuffs. Dioxin permeated the soil and bio-accumulated in cow's milk, fish, and other foods important in the diet of Seveso inhabitants. Research scientists and clinical toxicologists collaborated in the aftermath of the incident to enroll cohorts of victims to monitor their health longitudinally (Pocchiari et al., 1979). Early studies of blood taken from children found only slight alterations of liver transaminases and no appreciable alterations in lipid profiles (Mocarelli, 1986).

Extremely high levels of TCDD continued to be found in blood and milk of the Seveso residents for years after the incident. Thus it is not surprising that some adverse health outcomes in humans only became apparent after a long latency period from the original exposure. Health concerns included induction of liver enzymes, diabetes and endocrine disruption, altered semen activity and other reproductive effects, and increased female:male birth ratios (Bertazzi et al., 1998; Pesatori et al., 2003). Speculation about increased rates of cardiovascular and respiratory disease suggested that, rather than direct chemically-induced toxicity, such illnesses might also be related to the psychological stressors associated with the long-lasting disruptions in daily life associated with such a traumatic event (Pesatori et al., 2003).

After the Zone A area of extreme contamination near Seveso had been completely evacuated and the buildings razed and topsoil removed in 1976, a large expanse of scarred, open land remained. This area was later reconstructed environmentally into an urban park, named the *Bosco delle Querce*. Woods and meadows subsequently flourished there; more than 26 species of birds were identified as inhabitants. The ecology and wildlife of the park were studied systematically more than 20 years later, in 1998–99 (Garagna et al., 2001). TCDD measured in the soil at that time was low at 16 pg/gm dry soil. Mammals such as rabbits and mice, birds, insects, and arthropods showed biological diversity similar to those living in unaffected parks. No mutagenic effects of TCDD or effects on reproductive morphology of the animals living there could be detected.

Lessons learned

The Seveso disaster provided important lessons for clinical toxicologists. There were delays in the immediate aftermath of the explosion in the recognition of the nature and scope of the disaster. The government's response was not begun for some days, with people in the affected area continuing to be exposed and continuing to eat contaminated foods. This event illustrated the necessity to begin enrolling victims in a surveillance program within hours of a disaster whenever possible, and to evacuate them immediately so as to limit the health consequences. The careful recording of the victims' demographic information, the circumstances and details of exposure, symptoms and signs of toxicity, and the collection and storage of biologic samples for later analysis are all critically important.

The lack of a quantitative laboratory technology for measuring TCDD in blood in 1976 proved an important barrier in defining the exposure dose in individuals and limited an understanding of the true scope of the disaster and its impact on the affected population. Frozen blood samples were only able to be analyzed years later, in the 1980s.

The creation of health, cancer, birth defects, and other registries of the victims facilitated longitudinal epidemiological studies of medical issues related to the exposure arising years after the event. The foresight of the public health officials and scientists involved in Seveso in creating and maintaining these prospective registries has shed light on the aftermath of the largest human exposure to TCDD ever recorded.

Finally, the subsequent restoration of woods and fields in creating a park in Zone A in Seveso confirmed that small–medium metropolitan areas, even when heavily polluted, could recover ecologically with good environmental planning and policies (Garagna et al., 2001).

References

Aylward LL, Hays SM. Temporal trends in human TCDD body burden: decreases over three decades and implications for exposure levels. J Expo Anal Environ Epidemiol 2002;12:319–28.

Bertazzi PA, Bernucci I, Brambilla G, Consonni D, Pesatori AC. The Seveso studies on early and long-term effects of dioxin exposure: a review. Environ Health Perspect 1998;106(Suppl 2):625–33.

Caputo R, Monti M, Ermacora E, Carminati G, Gelmetti C, Gianotti R, Gianni E, Puccinelli V. Cutaneous manifestations of tetrachlorodibenzo-*p*-dioxin in children and adolescents. J Am Acad Dermatol 1988;19(5 part 1):812–9.

Consonni D, Pesatori AC, Zocchetti C, Sindaco R, D'Oro LC, Rubagotti M, Bertazzi PA. Mortality in a population exposed to dioxin after the Seveso, Italy, accident in 1976: 25 years of follow-up. Am J Epidemiol 2008;167(7):847–58.

Eskenazi B, Warner M, Brambilla P, Signorini S, Ames J, Mocarelli P. The Seveso accident: a look at 40 years of health research and beyond. Environ Int 2018;121(Pt 1):71–84.

Garagna S, Zuccotti M, Vecchi ML, Rubini PG, Capanna E, Redi CA. Human-dominated ecosystems and restoration ecology: Seveso today. Chemosphere 2001;43(4–7):577–85.

Mocarelli P. Clinical laboratory manifestations of exposure to dioxin in children. JAMA 1986;256(19):2687–95.

Mocarelli P, Pocchiari F, Nelson N. Preliminary report: 2,3,7,8-tetrachlorodibenzo-*p*-dioxin exposure in humans – Seveso, Italy. Morb Mortal Wkly Rep 1988;37(18):733–6.

Needham LL, Gerthoux PM, Patterson Jr DG, Brambilla P, Turner WE, Beretta C, Pirkle JL, Colombo L, Sampson EJ, Tramacere PL, Signorini S, Meazza L, Carreri V, Jackson RJ, Mocarelli P. Serum dioxin levels in Seveso, Italy, population in 1976. Teratog Carcinog Mutagen 1997-1998;17(4–5):225–40.

Pesatori AC, Consonni D, Bachetti S, Zocchetti C, Bonzini M, Baccarelli A, Bertazzi PA. Short- and long-term morbidity and mortality in the population exposed to dioxin after the "Seveso accident". Ind Health 2003;41(3):127–38.

Pesatori AC, Consonni D, Rubagotti M, Grillo P, Bertazzi PA. Cancer incidence in the population exposed to dioxin after the "Seveso accident": twenty years of follow-up. Environ Health 2009;8:39.

Pocchiari F, Silano V, Zampieri A. Human health effects from accidental release of tetrachlorodibenzo-p-dioxin (TCDD) at Seveso, Italy. Ann N Y Acad Sci 1979;320:311–20.

Rysavy NM, Maaetoft-Udsen K, Turner H. Dioxins: diagnostic and prognostic challenges arising from complex mechanisms. J Appl Toxicol 2013;33(1):1–17.

Schecter A, Birnbaum L, Ryan JJ, Constable JD. Dioxins: an overview. Environ Res 2006;101:419–28.

Signorini S, Gerthoux PM, Dassi C, Cazzaniga M, Brambilla P, Vincoli N, Mocarelli P. Environmental exposure to dioxin: the Seveso experience. Andrologia 2000;32(4–5):263–70.

Skene SA, Dewhurst IC, Greenberg M. Polychlorinated dibenzo-p-dioxins and polychlorinated dibenzofurans: the risks to human health. A review. Hum Toxicol 1989;8:173–203.

Steenland K, Bertazzi P, Baccarelli A, Kogevinas M. Dioxin revisited: developments since the 1997 IARC classification of dioxin as a human carcinogen. Environ Health Perspect 2004;112(13):1265–8.

Warner M, Mocarelli P, Samuels S, Needham L, Brambilla P, Eskenazi B. Dioxin exposure and cancer risk in the Seveso Women's health study. Environ Health Perspect 2011;119(12):1700–5.

Chapter 1.4

Arsenic in tube well water— Bangladesh, 1970s–1990s

Alan D. Woolf

Boston Children's Hospital & Harvard Medical School, Boston, Massachusetts, United States

Bangladesh lies in the confluence of the Ganges, Brahmaputra, and Meghna plains with some of the most fertile soils in the world. The low-lying country, crisscrossed by more than 230 rivers and tributaries, is subjected to torrential monsoon rains, sometimes causing catastrophic flooding. It is one of the most densely populated and poorest countries in the world. A 2002 report estimated 70 million (55%) of its people were living below the poverty line, about 20 million of them living in extreme poverty. In its agrarian society, over 53% are landless (Alam et al., 2002) (Fig. 1.4.1).

Clean, safe water has long been an unattainable goal for many people living in Bangladesh, especially those in its rural areas. Dhaka, the capital of Bangladesh, and other major cities in the country had access to clean water from deeper aquifers or treated surface water. But people living in dire poverty in rural Bangladesh, a majority of its large population, did not. Their primary source of water for decades was surface waters which were easily contaminated by agricultural wastes (e.g., fertilizers, pesticides, and insecticides), untreated sewage, and human and animal wastes. Both the quality and the quantity of surface water were often unstable in periods of drought or flooding. Thousands of people would die each year due to infections such as dysentery, typhoid, and cholera. Life-threatening gastrointestinal illnesses of both the young and the old could be traced to their drinking fecal-contaminated, untreated, stagnant surface pools and pond water.

Clean drinking water initiatives

Thus the government of Bangladesh welcomed an innovative effort by UNICEF and international non-governmental organizations (NGOs) beginning in the 1970s to provide access to clean, safe drinking water. This initiative mobilized extensive resources to provide access to more stable, uncontaminated groundwater sources through the drilling of inexpensive small diameter (less than

History of Modern Clinical Toxicology. https://doi.org/10.1016/B978-0-12-822218-8.00049-1

45

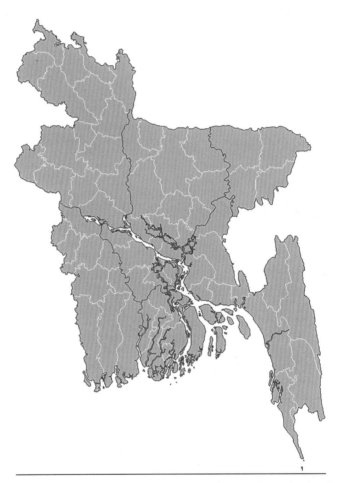

FIG. 1.4.1 Map of Bangladesh. https://commons.wikimedia.org/w/index.php?title=Special:Sea rch&limit=20&offset=20&profile=default&search=map+of+bangladesh&advancedSearch-current ={}&ns0=1&ns6=1&ns12=1&ns14=1&ns100=1&ns106=1#/media/File:Bangladesh_districts.png

5 cm) hand-pumped tube wells into shallow (less than 150 m deep) ground-water aquifers. Using these tube wells, people were able to draw large amounts of clean water for personal use in their homes without the threat of microbial contamination. Government agencies and international NGOs pooled resources to drill more than 1.8 million such shallow, hand-pumped wells, mostly in the rural areas (Fazal et al., 2001). UNICEF declared in its 1997 country report that it had surpassed its goal of providing 80% of the population with "safe" drinking water from groundwater sources by year 2000 (Smith et al., 2000). Also during the 1970s–1980s, the government installed a number of large bore (16–20 cm) wells for agricultural irrigation purposes, placing additional environmental pressures impacting the groundwater hydrology and causing extreme

fluctuations in groundwater levels. Standard water testing practices for any of the new wells did not include testing for arsenic. More than 90% of the extracted groundwater from wells in Bangladesh was used for irrigation purposes (Fazal et al., 2001). While the total number of wells in Bangladesh is unknown, it has recently been estimated at about 8–12 million (Chakraborti et al., 2015).

However, no one at the time that tube wells were proposed as a solution to the lack of clean drinking water appreciated the ancient geological history of the land mass now known as Bangladesh. Large rock masses containing high concentrations of arsenic and other minerals had migrated from the Himalayan mountains south to the coastal plains of Bangladesh and India millions of years ago forming the Himalayan Tableland Plain. Alluvial lacustrine sediments laid down during the Holocene period included common arsenic-containing minerals such as arsenopyrite (FeAsS), realgar (As_4S_4), and orpiment arsenic trisulfide (As_2S_3). Deltaic and alluvial soils cover about 85% of Bangladesh; an estimated 2.4 billion tons of sediments are deposited in the river delta annually (Alam et al., 2002). Arsenopyrite is the ore that is thought to be mostly contributing the arsenic contaminating the water of Bangladesh. The arsenic-contaminated water and soils are concentrated in western Bangladesh and the adjacent areas of West Bengal, India.

Early detections of arsenic in tube wells

The presence of high levels of arsenic in drinking water was first discovered in six districts in neighboring West Bengal, India, in July 1983 by Dr. K.C. Saha of the School of Tropical Medicine in Calcutta (Alam et al., 2002). He found arsenic levels in water serving a population of 30 million were higher than the WHO limits for potable water (50 µg/L at the time). The natural contamination of Bangladeshi groundwater with high levels of arsenic, especially in poverty-stricken rural areas, was not discovered until 1984, when it was first measured and documented to be elevated to alarming levels (Chowdhury et al., 2000). However, even after that discovery, there was no appreciation that this constituted a public health emergency. Only after further water sampling studies by the School of Environmental Studies (SOES) at Jadavpur University based in Kolkata, India, in 1992 serendipitously discovered that people emigrating there from Bangladesh had arsenical skin lesions did the scope of the problem begin to be understood. Researchers informed WHO, UNICEF, and Bangladeshi government officials of their findings. After an International Conference on Arsenic was held in Calcutta in 1995, medical staff from Bangladeshi hospitals reported that they had been seeing many patients with similar skin lesions for some years without the knowledge that these were manifestations of arsenic toxicity (Chakraborti et al., 2010). Detailed surveys by SOES in Bangladeshi districts bordering West Bengal, with sampling of water from 750 tube-wells, began in 1996. Only by then had the enormous scope of widespread contamination begun to be appreciated by governmental agencies and international organizations participating across Bangladesh.

Unprecedented scope of arsenic contamination

In effect, one public health disaster had been replaced with another. The result evolved over the following quarter of a century into the largest mass poisoning of a populace in history. Both Bangladesh and districts in neighboring West Bengal, India, were impacted. As many as 269 of the 464 administrative divisions of Bangladesh, known as *upazilas*, contained elevated levels of arsenic in the water (Khalequzzaman et al., 2005). Generally, the deeper the tube well, the lower the concentration of arsenic in the water, related to geological and hydrological considerations. Wells that were deeper than 350 m were thought to be safe from arsenic contamination but were too expensive to drill. Most of the dug wells in Bangladesh were very shallow; many of the inexpensive ones, affordable even for poor families, were only 20–50 m deep. A 14-year study of 52,202 water samples taken from hand tube-wells reported 27.2% and 42.1% had arsenic levels above the 50 μg/L (Bangladeshi standard) and above 10 μg/L (WHO standard), respectively (Chakraborti et al., 2010). An estimated 30% of 10 million private wells in rural areas of the country were thought to be highly contaminated (Khalequzzaman et al., 2005). Some of the wells had arsenic levels as high as 4730 μg/L (Chakraborti et al., 2015). Of the 125 million residents of Bangladesh in the year 2000, a range of 35–77 million (50% by one estimate) were placed at high risk of drinking contaminated water and developing the illnesses associated with chronic arsenicosis (Smith et al., 2000). Even those results, some of which rely on qualitative field testing kits which may be inaccurate and give falsely low readings, may underestimate the scope of the contamination (Fig. 1.4.2).

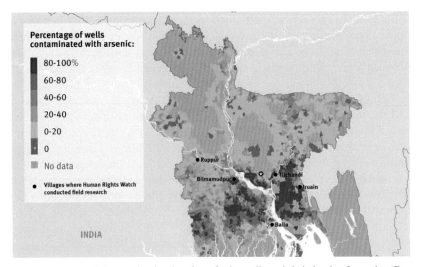

FIG. 1.4.2 Geocoded map showing location of tube wells and their levels of arsenic. *(From Hossain M, Rahman SN, Bhattacharya P, Jacks G, Saha R, Rahman M. Sustainability of arsenic mitigation interventions—an evaluation of different alternative safe drinking water options provided in Matlab, an arsenic hot spot in Bangladesh. Front Environ Sci 2015;3:30. https://doi.org/10.3389/fenvs.2015.00030.)*

Toxicology of arsenic

Arsenic is a brittle grayish metal that exists in nature as mineral compounds. When dissolved in water, it is colorless, tasteless, and odorless. It has no physiological role in the human, but is a cellular poison, interfering with sulfhydryl-containing enzymes, mitochondrial function, and the production of phosphate-containing, high energy compounds. Arsenic also interferes with DNA replication and repair and normal cell division. There is some evidence that it is an endocrine disruptor, interfering with the glucocorticoid receptor function. The trivalent arsenite ions are about 60 times more toxic than pentavalent arsenate ions; both were commonly found in the contaminated water.

Rapidly dividing cells are most affected, such that target organs for toxicity include the mucous membranes, skin, liver, lungs, and the gastrointestinal tract. Arsenic that is not excreted in urine is bound to and accumulates in target body tissues, including the skin, with a progression to increased, aggregated body burdens in deep reservoirs over time. The most common biomarkers used to confirm arsenic exposure include hair arsenic concentrations (normal 80–250 µg/kg with toxic levels > 1000 µg/kg) and fingernails (normal 430–1080 µg/kg) which denote body burden, and urinary arsenic concentrations (normal < 50 µg/L; toxic ≥ 200 µg/L assuming 1.5 L urine/day), denoting recent exposures (Ahamed et al., 2006).

Clinical toxicity

Acute symptoms of arsenic poisoning include anorexia, abdominal pain, and diarrhea, along with tingling sensations or numbness of the extremities. However, the poisoning seen in arsenic exposures at relatively low environmental levels may be insidious, with a delayed onset occurring after a latency period from a few months to as long as 8–14 years, depending on many individual factors such as consumption (dose and chronicity), genotype, lifestyle habits, and nutritional status. Victims of such chronic low-level arsenic poisoning may notice early on reductions in their energy level, stamina, and appetite. The exposure threshold for arsenic contamination of drinking water daily associated with the eventual manifestation of overt skin lesions is thought to be about 300 µg/L (Chakraborti et al., 2010).

Skin lesions

Victims of low-level arsenic poisoning develop spreading pigmented spots on their skin, especially on the palms and soles. There can be a progression of skin disease: from general hyperpigmentation to melanosis (pigmented spots, usually on chest, back, and/or limbs) to leukomelanosis (white and dark spots side-by-side) and more generalized melanosis to keratosis (skin thickenings, especially on the hands and feet) to hyperkeratosis (nodular or spotted keratosis) to squamous cell carcinoma in situ (Bowen's Disease) or gangrene (so-called "Blackfoot Disease") (Ahamed et al., 2006; Chowdhury et al., 2000). Advanced

Skin cancer (below) on the palm of a patient who ingested arsenic over a prolonged period of time from a contaminated well (photo courtesy the Arsenic Foundation).

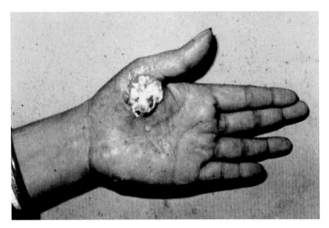

FIG. 1.4.3 Skin cancer in patient drinking contaminated water over a prolonged period. *(Source: U.S. Federal Agency: ATSDR https://www.google.com/search?q=arsenic+skin+cancer&tbm=isc h&sxsrf=ALeKk03VAT6qb0qcd4sq7gocgHmgeH04_A%3A1616659879535&source=hp&biw=13 72&bih=707&ei=p0VcYPHNHuWJggf7goXIBg&oq=arsenic+skin+cancer&gs_lcp=CgNpbWc-QAzICCAA6BQgAELEDOggIABCxAxCDAToECAAQAzoGCAAQCBAeOgQIABAeOgQIABAYUK QJWNYlYL4uaABwAHgAgAHBAYgBwgqSAQQxOC4xmAEAoAEBqgELZ3dzLXdpei1pbWfWc&sclie nt=img&ved=0ahUKEwixvdyu_8rvAhXlhOAKHXtBAWkQ4dUDCAY&uact=5#imgrc=L4SWvc6V zym5hM)*

cracking, rough skin, desquamation on the palms and soles, and nodular keratosis of the extremities can be extremely debilitating, with complications, such as enlarged liver, renal involvement, and secondary infection, requiring medical attention. While children can also develop the skin lesions, there is typically a dose-dependent, latency period of up to 10 years of exposure to arsenic before such skin changes become clinically apparent (Fig. 1.4.3).

Clinical toxicity — Other

Although skin lesions are the most visible signs of poisoning, the victims of chronic low-level arsenic exposure suffer long-term high rates of morbidity and mortality from pulmonary, neurological, reproductive, and cardiovascular diseases associated with arsenicosis (Table 1.4.1). The skin lesions can also become secondarily infected, and pulmonary complications can be worsened by exposure to such infections as tuberculosis. One 2005 survey of a small rural village in Bangladesh where the drinking water was contaminated with arsenic found

TABLE 1.4.1 Toxic effects of arsenic.

Target Organ	Health effects
Skin	Hyper-pigmented lesions, especially on palms of hands and soles of feet Skin cancer Gangrene
Newborn	Increased infant mortality Reduced birth weight
Nervous system	Neurological abnormalities Impaired cognitive function (children and adults) Impaired motor function Peripheral sensory neuropathies Hearing loss Psychiatric (anxiety, apathy, depression)
Reproductive	Spontaneous abortion Stillbirth Low birth weight Increased infant mortality
Respiratory system	Restrictive pulmonary disease Bronchiectasis Increased mortality from pulmonary TB
Cardiovascular system	Coronary artery disease Myocardial infarction Hypertension Ischemic peripheral vascular disease ('Blackfoot' disease)
Cancers	Liver Kidney Bladder and urinary tract Prostate Lung Skin
Immune function	Altered immune function Inflammation Increases infantile infectious disease morbidity
Liver	Noncirrhotic portal fibrosis
Endocrine	Diabetes Impaired glucose tolerance test (GTT) in pregnancy

Modified from Naujokas MF, Anderson B, Ahsan H, Aposhian HV, Graziano JH, Thompson C, et al. The broad scope of health effects from chronic arsenic exposure: update on a worldwide health problem. Environ Heal Perspect 2013;121(3):295–302.

that 25% of 1580 adults examined had skin lesions and 10% exhibited peripheral neuropathies; there were also anecdotal accounts of high rates in the village of spontaneous abortions, stillbirths, and neonatal deaths (Ahamed et al., 2006).

There is good scientific evidence that the occurrences and severity of adverse health effects are also related to a variety of other factors: concentration of arsenic in the water, daily water intake, duration of exposure, and an individual's genetic make-up and nutritional status. Arsenic-associated illnesses are more likely in people who are undernourished, especially those lacking adequate sources of vitamin A, methionine, zinc, and selenium. Arsenic metabolism and detoxification is facilitated by methylation to form metabolites excreted in urine; those with poor nutrition may have impaired capacity for methylation of the metal's toxic ions and intermediary compounds.

Arsenic and cancers

High body burdens of arsenic are associated with the development of lung, liver, kidney, skin, prostate, and urinary bladder cancers. An estimated 1 in 10 people drinking 1 L of water daily with 500 ug/L arsenic will ultimately die from an arsenic-associated cancer (Smith et al., 2000). The US National Research Council estimated that chronic consumption of water containing 50 ug/L arsenic would result in a combined cancer risk of 1 in 100 people (National Research Council, 1999). One follow-up cohort study of 811 Bangladeshi people with arsenical skin lesions 9–12 years later reported 16.6% had died of cancers within that time frame (Chakraborti et al., 2010).

Arsenic concentration limits — Drinking water

While the Bangladeshi government's threshold limit for arsenic in drinking water has remained at 50 µg/L, WHO lowered its standard to 10 µg/L in 1993. The SOES team from Jadavpur University reported in 2000 that about 25 million people were exposed to water exceeding the 50 µg/L arsenic limit and about 52 million were drinking water with contamination exceeding 10 µg/L (Fazal et al., 2001). Moreover, the WHO and Bangladeshi standards assumed daily consumption rates of about 1–2 L/day. However, scientific studies have reported usual daily water consumptions of Bangladeshi people living in arsenic-contaminated districts to be closer to 3–4 L/day; those engaged in strenuous agricultural work were drinking as much as 4–6 L of water daily (Chakraborti et al., 2010). Thus even the lower WHO standard may not be adequately protective of the entire populace.

Government agencies respond to contaminated drinking water

The first cases of arsenicosis specifically linked to tube well contamination were reported starting in 1993; and more than 2900 cases had been documented over the next 6 years, although thousands of *undocumented* cases were also occurring in rural areas (Josephson, 2002). By the mid-1990s, more than 5 million tube wells had been field-tested by the Bangladeshi government, with the support of the World Bank, donors, and Non-Governmental Organizations (NGOs) in a massive effort known as the Bangladesh Arsenic Mitigation Water Supply Project (BAMWSP). Maximum arsenic concentrations as high as 2000–3000 µg/L were documented in tube-well water in some districts (Chakraborti et al., 2010).

Arsenic contamination was mitigated by prohibiting use of those wells with levels exceeding the safe limit of 50 mcg/L set by the government. UNICEF and other organizations painted those carrying "safe" water (arsenic < 50 ug/L) green and those carrying arsenic-laden water (arsenic ≥ 50 ug/L) as red and in a public education campaign urged villagers to take drinking water only from green wells. By 2005, more than 1.5 million tube wells had been painted red. BAMWSP would also eventually document some 38,000 cases of suspected arsenicosis within the 270 upazilas where field tests were conducted (Pearshouse et al., 2016).

The Department of Public Health Engineering (DPHE), within the Ministry of Local Government, Rural Development, and Cooperatives, was charged with implementing safe supplies of drinking water and proper sanitation in rural areas. The second phase of mitigation, the "National Policy for Arsenic Mitigation" adopted in 2004 was to install deeper wells to provide water points accessible to all rural communities. "Very high priority" rural areas were those where over 80% of water points are contaminated and less than 20% of the population had access to safe water devices.

Evolving arsenic-contaminated water crisis — 2000s

In the early 2000s, using funds largely donated by UNICEF and the World Bank, DPHE installed several hundred thousand new tube wells, drilled deeper to tap safer groundwater aquifers. However, these "deep" wells, even while they are safer, less prone to microbial contamination and easier to maintain for many years, are also costlier to install. Shallow tube wells were also installed. Of the 125,000 wells installed by DPHE from 2006 to 2012, 5% were found to be still contaminated by arsenic above the national Bangladeshi standard of 50 ug/L (Pearshouse et al., 2016). And many rural areas in highest need of convenient safe drinking water were neglected by these governmental programs.

Unfortunately, once the BAMWSP effort ended in 2007, there was no subsequent national program aimed at screening wells and mitigating the risks at a community level. Since that time, government resources needed and concerns over the public health issue have both waned. There is no longer a sense of urgency and progress has slowed (Pearshouse et al, 2016). For political and other reasons, the Bangladeshi government has concentrated its efforts to dig new, clean shallow wells in areas that may not have the highest need, ignoring areas with the highest arsenic contamination. In some locales, there are also geological and hydrological challenges to reach clean aquifers. The result is that DPHE efforts are still not matched to local rural needs (Fig. 1.4.4).

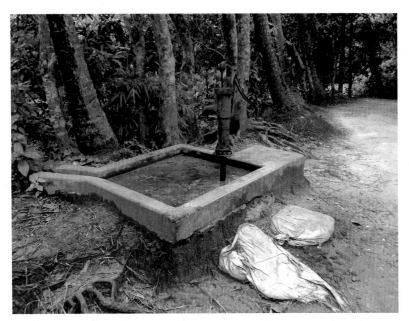

FIG. 1.4.4   Tube well for fresh water. *(Source: wikimedia commons https://commons.wiki-media.org/w/index.php?search=tube+well&title=Special:MediaSearch&go=Go&type=image Attribution: Asive Chowdhury)*

Many rural villagers have dug their own cheap shallow tube wells privately and are relying on untested water for all their household uses. Some of the government sponsored tube wells recently dug in many locales turn out to be contaminated with arsenic. The public education warnings about arsenic contamination ended years ago. Many people simply do not care and ignore the red-painted warnings on the tube wells convenient to their homes to obtain their drinking water. A 2008 survey in rural Bangladesh found that lower income villagers were more likely to suffer arsenicosis, although about 70% of women were willing to walk between 1 and 5 minutes: to obtain safe drinking water (Nahar et al., 2008).

Continuing threats to clean drinking water

In addition, the dynamic nature of hydrology was not appreciated; heavy extraction of groundwater for irrigation and other purposes caused movement and altered composition of the water table. Such heavy water usage could change its acidity, leading to greater leaching of arsenic from the pyrite-containing sediments. Some "green" tube-wells were later found to have unacceptable levels of arsenic contamination due to temporal changes in the ground-water flow; these wells were no longer a safe source of drinking water. There exist enormous long-term challenges to be faced in assuring the people of sustainable clean water. There was and continues to be an urgent unmet need to properly administer the wells, monitor the water quality, manage extraction practices in the watershed, and seek better long-term solutions to the demands for clean water. Moreover, other metals occur naturally in Bangladesh groundwater in concentrations exceeding WHO guidelines, including manganese, molybdenum, antimony, boron, chromium, barium, lead, and others (Frisbie et al., 2002). The scope of the contribution of these other metals to adverse health effects seen in the populace remains largely unmeasured and unknown. Unfortunately, the water and soils in Bangladesh were found to be deficient in minerals such as selenium and zinc, which can have a protective effect, facilitating the metabolism of arsenic to less toxic metabolites and attenuating some of its potential adverse effects (Frisbie et al., 2002).

Contamination of agricultural crops

A related issue in addition to the Bangladesh water contamination is that of contamination of foods and crops grown in arsenic-rich soil and nourished with arsenic-contaminated irrigation. Arsenic is actively translocated in many vegetables and can bioaccumulate in some animals such as cattle and some species of fish. Rice, a staple food in the diet of most Bangladeshi families, easily accumulates arsenic during its growth in arsenic contaminated soils in paddies. Some Bangladeshi agricultural soils contained as much as 1000 mg/kg of arsenic (Alam et al., 2002). Rice makes up two-thirds of the cereals grown in Bangladesh, with a per capita consumption of 150 kg/year (Alam et al., 2002; Duxbury et al., 2003). Arsenic concentrations in polished rice were measured to be very high (0.16–0.58 µg/g); and arsenic was also present in other vegetables, including lentils, beans, peas, and grass pea. Thus foods grown in highly contaminated rural areas provided yet another pathway for exposure.

Social and health consequences

The investigation of health consequences of chronic exposure to arsenic in the drinking water of affected areas of Bangladesh (and neighboring West Bengal in India) were complicated by cultural and social factors. Many of the people living in rural areas were too weak to travel or lived too far away to come to the medical camps investigating the epidemic. In many villages, people were unaware of the risk or attached a stigma to those with obvious skin lesions, fearing that the disease was contagious, leading to social isolation of the victims (Ahamed et al., 2006). Some believed that the dark skin spots were not due to arsenic but due to past sins from a prior birth. There were also cultural constraints to the epidemiological investigations: many women would not allow themselves to be examined and some were reluctant to give a reproductive history of spontaneous abortions or stillborn children. Health workers held meetings or clinics during the daytime, when many villagers were working in the fields and unavailable to be examined (Ahamed et al., 2006).

The social and health consequences of chronic arsenic exposure in Bangladesh have been enormous; it continues to be a disease associated with rural poverty. Many people in affected areas of the country noticed the pigmented keratosis on the skin, one very visible indicator of arsenic poisoning, which in some villages carried considerable social stigma. The villagers, illiterate and without good information, often mistook the skin lesions for leprosy, which was feared as highly contagious. People with skin lesions of arsenicosis were shunned; employers immediately dismissed them from their job. Children were kept from attending school. Women were divorced or sent by their husbands back to their parents. Single women with skin lesions could not find partners; divorced women were ostracized, no longer had a social role, and became destitute (Alam et al., 2002). Victims were not allowed to appear in public and people avoided direct contact with them.

The Bangladeshi DHPE still estimates the scope of the public health problem and gauges its response using a definition of an "arsenic victim" as one with visible skin lesions. But many victims suffer life-threatening toxicity from chronic arsenic exposure and do not develop the tell-tale skin lesions. Many have died from arsenic-associated cancers or pulmonary, cardiovascular or other diseases attributable to chronic arsenic poisoning without being counted by the DPHE as arsenic victims. It has been estimated that 43,000 Bangladeshi people die each year from arsenic-related illness (Pearshouse et al., 2016). An additional 1–5 million children of the 90 million born between 2000 and 2030 will die from arsenic-related causes, given the slow progress in correcting the tube well-related contamination in poverty-stricken, rural parts of the country (Pearshouse et al., 2016).

Moreover, in 1993, WHO had lowered its standard of arsenic concentration from 50 to $10\,\mu g/L$ as the level at which drinking water is safe (WHO, 1993). However, the Bangladeshi government ignored this action, maintaining the national reference ceiling for arsenic in drinking water at 50 ʊg/L, even though some research documents a dangerously higher risk of arsenic-related morbidity and mortality resulting from chronic exposures to levels of 10–$50\,\mu g/L$ (Ahsan et al., 2006). And so, there is little effort by the government to measure or address the true health consequences from arsenic-contaminated water in the country. It can claim success of what some considered to be underfunded, under-resourced, and inadequate remediation efforts (Pearshouse et al., 2016).

Other solutions

The Bangladeshi government has been criticized for many administrative and policy mistakes which have delayed or ignored remedial actions that might be effective solutions. Strategies offered have included a return to traditional surface water sources such as wetlands, rivers, or lakes in some areas, with proper watershed managerial controls in place to assure the safety of the drinking water. Bangladesh has some of the wettest weather seasons on the planet; effective rain-water capture and conservation as a source of household water has also been proposed. Arsenic removal plants (ARPs) using filters to make water safe have been proposed, but are expensive and require adequate maintenance and routine filter replacements (Chakraborti et al., 2015). Access to deeper ground-water aquifers (where the geology confirms a clay cap barrier from seepage of arsenic-contaminated shallow groundwater) would be an effective albeit expensive strategy. More effective management of extraction of ground-water from the safe tube-wells already in place is imperative to control the hydrology of water tables so that wells are not newly contaminated by further leaching from arsenopyrite.

Lessons learned

The unfolding and continuing tragic legacy of arsenic water pollution in Bangladesh has served as a lesson in the complexity of solving community-wide issues in economically weak countries relying on external aid. In Bangladesh, the quest for more data and research precluded an adequate response to the poisoning; it was not treated as an immediate and compelling national emergency. As Bangladesh has shown, a data-driven search for a "perfect solution" should not be allowed to delay immediate efforts at mitigation and remediation when lives are at stake. The response in Bangladesh also illustrates the need to mobilize existing systems and government agencies as the most effective public health strategy in responding to a community-wide toxic emergency (Smith et al., 2000).

The insidious nature and sometimes long latency period to the onset of clinically apparent health effects associated with environmental pollutants such as arsenic again illustrate the challenges in determining the scope of impact of toxic disasters. Use of overly narrow and imprecise clinical symptoms and signs of poisoning can lead to erroneously under-counting exactly who is a "victim" for epidemiological and governmental relief purposes.

Finally, the need to be persistent in public health messaging at the local level was evident in the rural communities. One-time warnings to people in need of convenient access to water were sometimes ignored. Old habits, cultural traditions, and behaviors are hard to change. Many people, either because of convenience or necessity, soon after went back to drinking contaminated water, ignoring the clear and present hazard, even if the well spigots were painted red. Efforts must be persistent at engagement of the community in addressing the reality of the contamination and its health implications, with participation of community leaders in finding local and/or regional solutions.

Global arsenic contamination

Arsenic is ubiquitous, present in about 1% of the earth's crust. While Bangladesh is the most dramatic example, it is not the only country affected by contamination of drinking water by natural sources of arsenic in groundwater. Instances of arsenic in drinking water as a public health concern, albeit on a smaller scale, have been documented in diverse locales, including Taiwan, India, Argentina, Chile, China, Japan, Philippines, Mongolia, Thailand, Mexico, and parts of the United States (Fazal et al., 2001).

References

Ahamed S, Sengupta MK, Mukherjee SC, Pati S, Mukherjeel A, Rahman MM, Hossain MA, Das B, Nayakl B, Pal A, Zafar A, Kabir S, Banu SA, Morshed S, Islam T, Rahman MM, Quamruzzaman Q, Chakraborti D. An eight-year study report on arsenic contamination in groundwater and health effects in Eruani village, Bangladesh and an approach for its mitigation. J Health Popul Nutr 2006;24(2):129–41.

Ahsan H, et al. Arsenic exposure from drinking water and risk of premalignant skin lesions in Bangladesh: baseline results from the health effects of arsenic longitudinal study. Am J Epidemiol 2006;163(12):1138–48.

Alam MG, Allinson G, Stagnitti F, Tanaka A, Westbrooke M. Arsenic contamination in Bangladesh groundwater: a major environmental and social disaster. Int J Environ Health Res 2002;12(3):235–53.

Chakraborti D, Rahman MM, Das B, Murrill M, Dey S, Chandra Mukherjee S, Dhar RK, Biswas BK, Chowdhury UK, Roy S, Sorif S, Selim M, Rahman M, Quamruzzaman Q. Status of groundwater arsenic contamination in Bangladesh: a 14-year study report. Water Res 2010;44(19):5789–802.

Chakraborti D, Rahman MM, Mukherjee A, Alauddin M, Hassan M, Dutta RN, Pati S, Mukherjee SC, Roy S, Quamruzzman Q, Rahman M, Morshed S, Islam T, Sorif S, Selim M, Islam MR, Hossain MM. Groundwater arsenic contamination in Bangladesh-21 years of research. J Trace Elem Med Biol 2015;31:237–48.

Chowdhury UK, Biswas BK, Chowdhury TR, Samantha G, Mandal B, Basu GC, et al. Groundwater arsenic contamination in Bangladesh and West Bengal, India. Environ Health Perspect 2000;108:393–7.

Duxbury JM, Mayer AB, Lauren JG, Hassan N. Food chain aspects of arsenic contamination in Bangladesh: effects on quality and productivity of rice. J Environ Sci Health 2003;38(1):61–9.

Fazal MA, Kawachi T, Ichion E. Extent and severity of groundwater arsenic contamination in Bangladesh. Water Int 2001;26(3):370–9.

Frisbie SH, Ortega R, Maynard DM, Sarkar B. The concentration of arsenic and other toxic elements in Bangladesh's drinking water. Environ Health Perspect 2002;110(11):1147–53.

Josephson J. The slow poisoning of Bangladesh. Environ Health Perspect 2002;110(11):A690–1.

Khalequzzaman M, Faruque FS, Mitra AK. Assessment of arsenic contamination of groundwater and health problems in Bangladesh. Int J Environ Res Public Health 2005;2(2):204–13.

Nahar N, Hossain F, Hossain MD. Health and socioeconomic effects of groundwater arsenic contamination in rural Bangladesh: new evidence from field surveys. J Environ Health 2008;70(9):42–7.

National Research Council. Arsenic in drinking water. Washington, DC: National Academy Press; 1999.

Pearshouse R, Root B, et al. Nepotism and neglect: the failing response to arsenic in the drinking water of Bangladesh's rural poor. Human Rights Watch; 2016, ISBN:978-1-6231-33399. https://www.hrw.org/report/2016/04/06/nepotism-and-neglect/failing-response-arsenic-drinking-water-bangladeshs-rural#page. [Accessed 1 October 2019].

Smith AH, Lingas EO, Rahman M. Contamination of drinking-water by arsenic in Bangladesh: a public health emergency. Bull World Health Organ 2000;78(9):1093–103.

WHO. Guidelines for drinking water quality. 2nd ed. Geneva, Switzerland: WHO; 1993.

Chapter 1.5

Toxic oil syndrome — Spain, 1981

Alan D. Woolf

Boston Children's Hospital & Harvard Medical School, Boston, Massachusetts, United States

Toxic oil syndrome: The index case

Sometimes a single case of poisoning—what we often call an index or sentinel case—becomes a teaching moment for astute clinicians and researchers and turns out to have much broader public health implications. The toxic oil syndrome (TOS), a severe progressive multisystem disease, is said to have been originally described in Torrejon de Ardoz, Spain, on May 1, 1981, when an 8-year-old boy, Jaime Vaquero, suffered a bizarre pneumonia and presented to a Madrid hospital in acute respiratory failure. His condition unexpectedly deteriorated, leading to an untimely, precipitous death (Kilbourne et al., 1991). This first victim heralded the rapid spread of the condition through the community, with many other patients presenting to the hospital with similar complaints in the following days and weeks. The epidemic of TOS seemed to peak in May and June in 1981. At first, an infectious agent was thought to be responsible for the outbreak, and micro-organisms such as Legionella and mycoplasma were investigated but proved to be uninvolved. Investigation of organophosphate pesticide-contaminated vegetables, another hypothesis vigorously pursued, also proved to be an untenable explanation.

Most cases occurred in 14 provinces in Central and Northwestern Spain, according to a central registry developed by the government. An initial dietary study with rather general questions did not reveal oil as a possible cause. However, an astute Spanish clinician, Dr. Juan Manuel Tabuenca-Oliver noticed that TOS suffered by family members excluded infants under 6 months of age who were being exclusively breast-fed. However, one of his little patients who was younger than 6 months developed TOS and he investigated further why this had happened. It turns out that the baby's grandmother was adding oil to his formula as a dietary supplement. The oil came from a plastic container sold to her by a street vendor (Kilbourne et al., 1991). The doctor's own epidemiological studies suggested an association between a family's use of this rapeseed oil for cooking and the occurrence of TOS. Subsequently, case-control studies confirmed that a suspect

History of Modern Clinical Toxicology. https://doi.org/10.1016/B978-0-12-822218-8.00010-7

cooking oil was used much more often by families with TOS-afflicted family members than by control families (Doll, 2004).

Epidemiology

Remarkably, TOS was confined to Spain; there were no reports of cases occurring outside of the country. Victims numbered more than 12,000 by August 31st and 121 had died. TOS was suspected in a total of over 20,000 cases in Spain, accounting for more than 12,000 hospital admissions and >300 deaths (Kilbourne et al, 1991) during the initial 1980s surveillance period by public health officials. Middle-aged people, typically women 20–50 years old, were disproportionately more affected; about 20% of the victims were children aged 8–15 years old. TOS was associated with lower educational and socioeconomic status in the Madrid area and surrounding province (Figs. 1.5.1 and 1.5.2). Later studies estimated that there was approximately a 1% rate of death, mostly in the acute phase and from respiratory failure. A total of 1663 persons of the 19,904 people in the Official TOS Census or 8.3%, had died by December 31, 1994, due to cardiovascular and pulmonary diseases and malignancies (Posada de la Paz M et al., 2001).

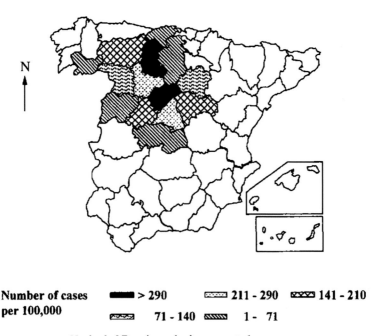

| Number of cases | ■ > 290 | ▨ 211 - 290 | ▨ 141 - 210 |
| per 100,000 | ▨ 71 - 140 | ▨ 1 - 71 | |

Unshaded Provinces had no reported cases

FIG. 1.5.1 Geographic distribution of TOS in northern parts of Spain. From: Posada de la Paz, Epidemiologic Reviews 2001.

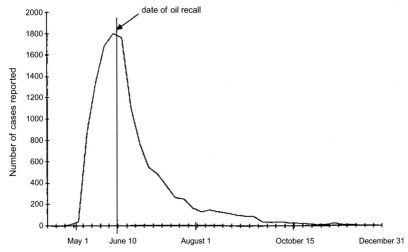

FIG. 1.5.2 Distribution of cases of toxic oil syndrome over time in 1981. *(From Posada de la Paz. Epidemiologic Reviews, 2001)*

Etiology of toxic oil syndrome—Rapeseed oil

Rapeseed oil is a pale yellow-colored, inexpensive oil with characteristics (taste-less, a low smoking temperature) that made it widely used in Spain for cook-ing, despite the Spanish government's efforts to protect its olive oil industry by making it illegal to import rapeseed oil for human consumption. One study (Cañas and Milbourne, 1987) in the barrio of Orcasur found that 5 household cases [35 people of whom 14 (40%) developed TOS], all had purchased oil from traveling salesmen whereas only 34% of noncase families did so. Buying oil from door-to-door vendors or traveling salesmen from outside the district was positively associated with the development of illness. In all, more than eight subsequent case-control studies affirmed the association between TOS and use of the adulterated cooking oil (Posada de la Paz et al., 2001).

RAELCA oil distributor

Other investigators published reports putting forth the same theory of causation as adulterated oil. Itinerant salesmen would sell the tainted cooking oil in unla-beled 5-L plastic containers claiming it was olive oil. The oil was manufactured originally for use in industrial processes but diverted for sale to the public as a cheap cooking oil. Residents could also purchase it in open marketplaces. Based on these early suspicions and in an effort to halt the spread of the epidemic, the Spanish Ministry of Health and Consumer Affairs alerted the public on June 10, 1981, about the relation between TOS and the consumption of unlabeled adulterated oil. The government orchestrated and financed a recall program of the illegal oil, replacing it with pure olive oil. That program collected almost 100,000 plastic containers of adulterated rapeseed oil. The incidence of TOS thereafter rapidly declined after the identification of a cooking oil product associated with the outbreak (Figure 1.5.2). Subsequent trace-back of the origins of the oil identified a Spanish oil distributor, RAELCA, as the source of the fraudulent cooking oil. RAELCA imported rapeseed oil intended for industrial uses from France and then used its own commercial networks to refine the oil, using aniline to denature the oil and then mixing it with other oils after refining. It was then relabeled as rapeseed oil suitable for human consumption as an inexpensive cooking oil. RAELCA was the only company that routinely distributed its product for sale to customers by itinerant salesmen off the street.

An elusive culprit

A report published in *Lancet* reported that the denatured oil was contaminated with 2% aniline used in the denaturing process during its manufacture (Tabuenca, 1982). Later studies outlined the immuno-toxicological mechanisms (Yoshida et al., 1994). When the oil was used in frying, it could generate oxidized anilide derivatives (Ruiz-Mendez et al., 2001) thought to be more toxic in murine experiments. The process produced anilide fatty acids, such as oleic anilide, that were thought to provoke an immune response. Additionally, fatty acid esters of 3-(*N*-phenylamino) propane-1,2-diol (PAP esters) generated via the reaction of triglycerides and aniline in the deodorization step in the refining of the industrial oil were also implicated as provoking similar immune responses (Morató et al., 2005). These PAP esters and fatty acid anilides have both been considered as strong biomarkers for TOS. PAP and its mono-oleoyl and di-oleoyl esters (OPAP and OOPAP) have been identified in the tainted cooking oil.

Bioavailable anilides could travel through lymphatics to the lungs where oxidative stress of alveolar endovascular cells ensued, causing some of the early pulmonary signs of TOS. Pathologic studies revealed degenerative changes in myelinated axons, extensive injury to peripheral nerves, chromatolysis of anterior horn cells, an inflammatory myopathy, and endomysial fibrosis in atrophied muscle cells (Ricoy et al., 1983). Free radicals and cytotoxic peroxidases could injure cells and underlie the pathogenesis of disease. Statistically significant higher amounts of oleyl anilide, linoleyl anilide, and palmityl anilide were detected in the RAELCA products purchased by families whose members developed TOS, and very few non-RAELCA bottles contained any contaminants (Posada de la Paz et al, 2001).

Lack of a true animal model

What seems clear is that TOS is an inflammatory response of the immune system to oxidative stress and cell injury induced by a toxic chemical. Early oxidative damage to the microvasculature endothelial cells by anilides acting as immunogens has been postulated (Philen and Posada, 1993; Yoshida et al., 1994). This nonnecrotizing endothelial cellular injury may provoke a broader cascade of inflammatory reactions involving activated T cells and the elaboration of cytokines. However, it remains unclear which of these chemical compounds in the oil was actually the principal factor in producing disease. Even after hundreds of research reports investigating the etiology of TOS, many questions surrounding the disease remained years later. Scientists were never able to reproduce the disease successfully in experimental animals although Rodrigo et al. (1983) showed that in rabbits, fatty acid anilides administered intraperitoneally or by gavage produced lung eosinophilic infiltrates and interstitial pneumonia, as well as degenerative changes in the brain consistent with neurotoxicity. They postulated an indirect effect, with the tissue inflammation and injury being mediated by antibodies produced against the anilides. The Ministry of Health and Social Affairs of Spain, the European Office of WHO, and the WHO, Joint WHO/CISAT Scientific Committee for the Toxic Oil Syndrome published an update of research findings concerning the pathogenesis of the disease in 2004 (WHO, 2004).

Clinical toxicology

The disease could be described in three phases (Noriega et al., 1982; Kilbourne et al., 1983; Yoshida et al., 1994):

- Acute—fever, respiratory illess, asthenia, pruritus, elevation in peripheral blood eosinophils.
- Intermediate—neuromuscular weakness, occasional paralysis, patchy sensory deficits.
- Chronic—functional neuromuscular and cognitive disabilities, scleroderma-like permanent scarring and skin changes, joint contractures.

Prodromal acute phase

In retrospect, studies found there to be a latency period of about 4–7 days between the date of oil consumption and the onset of symptoms, depending on the dose and concentration.

The initial clinical manifestations were usually respiratory in nature, and included low-grade fever, cough, hypoxemia (sometimes progressive, requiring ventilator support), precordial tightness, and pleuritic chest pain. Chest X-rays often showed pulmonary interstitial/alveolar infiltrates and/or pleural effusions or signs of a noncardiogenic pulmonary edema. A maculopapular skin rash, scalp itchiness and/or malar erythema were also prominent features in the presentation of some, but not all patients. Laboratory abnormalities included a characteristic rise in the eosinophil count in the peripheral blood, in the range of

500–2000 per mm^3 or higher, early in the acute phase. Many patients also complained of facial edema, muscle aches and pains, numbness in the extremities, and an ascending paresis. About 78% of patients developed eosinophilia, 80% complained of myalgias, 70% had pulmonary findings, and 39% developed a rash (Gómez de la Cámara et al., 2004) (Table 1.5.1).

Intermediate phase

About 1–3 months after the acute phase, an intermediate phase of intense muscle pain and tenderness to palpation was manifest, with even higher levels of eosinophilia. This development portended a chronic phase of anorexia and weight loss, muscle atrophy, chronic pain syndrome, sicca syndrome, contractures, scleroderma-like skin manifestations, and progressive pulmonary hypertension. Life-threatening thrombo-embolism was observed in a few severely affected patients, and resulted in some deaths. More than 300 patients diagnosed with TOS died in the first 2 years (Gómez de la Cámara et al., 2004).

Laboratory evaluations were notable for the presence in many patients of a prominent eosinophilia, as well as an elevation in the levels of immunoglobulin E in their peripheral blood, suggesting an immune and/or allergic component to the pathogenesis of the disease. Administration of glucocorticoids seemed to benefit patients with respect to their pulmonary symptoms, also supporting the hypothesized etiology as an auto-immune or allergic reaction. The lack of efficacy of antibiotics in changing the clinical course seemed to rule out common pulmonary pathogens as etiologic agents. Moderate elevations in serum transaminases and bilirubin signaled liver involvement in some patients (Kilbourne et al., 1991).

Chronic phase

In as many as 59% of patients, the disease progressed to a late, chronic phase with residual neuromuscular disabilities and functional limitations. Complaints included scleroderma-like skin changes and scarring, joint contractures of the jaw and extremities, muscle cramps, carpal-tunnel syndrome, myalgias, and weakness. Chronic neurological changes included motor and sensory axonal neuropathies (mononeuritis multiplex), paresthesias, memory loss, and depression. A study conducted 18 years after the epidemic on 79 adults suffering TOS compared with age- and sex-matched controls found a significant number of central and peripheral nervous system adverse effects and deficits still evident in the victims of TOS (Posada de la Paz et al., 2003). No treatments, such as steroids, analgesics, antiinflammatory medicines, or vitamin E, had any lasting beneficial effect on the course of the disease. Individual patient management focused on symptomatic treatment and physical rehabilitation (Gómez de la Cámara et al., 2004).

TABLE 1.5.1 Clinical manifestations of toxic oil syndrome.

Acute phase (1–2 months)	Intermediate phase (2–4 months)	Chronic phase (≥4 months)
Eosinophilia	Myalgia	Peripheral neuropathy
Tissue edema	Weight loss	Hepatopathy/hepatitis
Myalgia	Sicca syndrome	Scleroderma
Arthralgia	Raynaud's syndrome	Pulmonary hypertension
Pruritis	Alopecia	Sicca syndrome
Malaise	Pulmonary hypertension	Osteoporosis/osteonecrosis
Mortality (respiratory failure)	Mortality (thromboembolism and ischemic colitis)	Mortality (respiratory failure, secondary infections, and hemorrhagic complications)

(Table adapted from Table 1, Academic Press, Inc. Yoshida SH, German JB, Fletcher MP, Gershwin ME. The Toxic Oil Syndrome: a perspective on immunotoxicological mechanisms. Reg Toxicol Pharmacol 1994;19(1):60–79. PMID: 8159816.)

Implications

This Spanish epidemic illustrated political and social implications of such a disaster. Oil company officials and governmental agents who allowed the oil importation despite knowledge of its illegality and the existence of regulations intended to prevent such imports were brought to justice. More than 40 businessmen were brought to trial for public health offenses and fraud. The outbreak revealed serious gaps in the control of the food oil market and the monitoring of food safety in Spain. It also highlighted the government's responsibilities in such epidemics. Victims of TOS were eventually compensated, but not without advocacy and controversies. Only those who were officially registered as TOS victims were eligible, which excluded many who did not meet the criteria or were too stigmatized to even apply. Social justice inequities existed; those with jobs were compensated at first, whereas those unemployed were not (Terracini and Martin-Arribas, 2004).

TOS caused societal upheaval with enormous economic and social and psychological costs. Some families lost several family members, sometimes including the family's principal breadwinner, to TOS. In others, severe disabilities brought on by TOS led to job loss as well as considerable medical expenses. These were new economic hardships for desperate families who had been living precariously on the economic edge of destitution beforehand (Posada de la Paz et al., 2001). Many victims suffered lifelong functional disabilities and reduced life-spans due to the disease. There was social stigma attached to the illness, so many were ashamed and would keep the diagnosis secret from friends and even family. This stigma led to difficulties for researchers in obtaining consent from TOS victims to participate in studies of the epidemiology or natural history of the disease (Terracini and Martin-Arribas, 2004). The accuracy of the results in some epidemiological studies was uncertain due to selection bias; the actual number of TOS-afflicted people was most certainly undercounted.

Subsequently the Spanish government changed its monitoring of compliance with food safety regulations and increased the resources available to those administrators charged with safeguarding the food supply for its people.

Unfortunately, this has not been the only epidemic of illness secondary to contaminated cooking oil in the world. A serious outbreak associated with the diversion of expired, TOCP-containing jet aircraft lubricating oil mixed in with vegetable oil was fraudulently sold in Morocco as olive oil suitable for cooking in September 1959. This outbreak resulted in the paralysis of more than 10,000 people (Smith and Spalding, 1959). In Japan, the onset of an illness complex known as "Yusho," and in Taiwan, an illness known as "Yucheng" were both associated with the use of rice oil inadvertently contaminated with PCBs, has been documented (see Chapter 1.10 for details on the Yusho and Yucheng disasters).

References

Cañas R, Milbourne E. Oil ingestion and the toxic-oil syndrome: results of a survey of residents of the Orcasur neighbourhood in Madrid, Spain. Int J Epidemiol 1987;16(1):3–6.

Doll R. The etiology of the Spanish toxic syndrome: interpretation of the epidemiologic evidence. In: Terracini B, editor. Toxic oil syndrome: ten years of progress. WHO (World Health Organization); 2004. p. 99–124, ISBN:92 890 1063 0.

Gómez de la Cámara A, Posada de la Paz M, del Mar Plaza Cano M, Estirado de Cabo E, Garcia de Aguinaga ML, Matin-Arribas C, Pozo Rodriguez F. Clinical aspects. In: Terracini B, editor. Toxic oil syndrome: ten years of progress. WHO (World Health Organization); 2004. p. 99–124, ISBN:92 890 1063 0 [Chapter 3].

Kilbourne EM, Posada de la Paz M, Borda IA, Ruiz-Navarro MD, Philen RM, Falk H. Toxic oil syndrome: a current clinical and epidemiologic summary, including comparisons with the eosinophilia-myalgia syndrome. J Am Coll Cardiol 1991;18(3):711–7. ISSN 0735-1097 1869734.

Kilbourne EM, Rigau Pérez JG, Heath CW, Zack MM, Falk H, Mafrtin-Marcos M, de Carlos A. Clinical epidemiology of toxic oil syndrome: manifestations of a new illness. N Engl J Med 1983;309:1408–14.

Morató A, Escabrós J, Manich A, Reig N, Castaño Y, Abián J, Messeguer A. On the generation and outcome of 3-(N-phenylamino) propane-1,2-diol derivatives in deodorized model oils related to toxic oil syndrome. Chem Res Toxicol 2005;18(4):665–74.

Noriega AR, Gomez-Reino J, Lopez-Encuentra A, et al. 'Toxic Epidemic Syndrome Study Group'. Toxic epidemic syndrome Spain 1981. Lancet 1982;2:697–702.

Philen RM, Posada M. Toxic oil syndrome and eosinophilia-myalgia syndrome: May 8–10 1991, World Health Organization meeting report. Semin Arthritis Rheum 1993;23(2):104–24.

Posada de la Paz M, Philen RM, Borda IA. Toxic oil syndrome: the perspective after 20 years. Epidemiol Rev 2001;23(2):231–47.

Posada de la Paz M, Philen RM, Gerr F, Letz R, Ferrari Arroyo MJ, Vela L, Pareja J. Neurologic outcomes of toxic oil syndrome patients 18 years after the epidemic. Environ Health Perspect 2003;111(10):1326–34.

Ricoy JR, Cabello A, Rodriguez J, Téllez I. Neuropathological studies on the toxic syndrome related to adulterated rapeseed oil in Spain. Brain 1983;106(Pt 4):817–35.

Rodrigo J, Robles M, Mayo I, Pestaña A, Marquet A, Larraga V, Muñoz E. Neurotoxicity of fatty acid anilides in rabbits. Lancet 1983;19:414–6.

Ruiz-Méndez MV, Posada de la Paz M, Abian J, Calaf RE, Blount B, Castro-Molero N, Philen R, Gelpí E. Storage time and deodorization temperature influence the formation of aniline-derived compounds in denatured rapeseed oils. Food Chem Toxicol 2001;39(1):91–6. 11259855.

Smith HV, Spalding JMK. Outbreak of paralysis in Morocco due to ortho-cresyl phosphate poisoning. Lancet 1959;2(7110):1019–21.

Tabuenca JM. Toxic-allergic syndrome caused by ingestion of rapeseed oil denatured with aniline. Lancet 1982;2:697–702.

Terracini B, Martin-Arribas C. Ethical and social issues. In: Terracini B, editor. Toxic oil syndrome: ten years of progress. WHO (World Health Organization); 2004, ISBN:92 890 1063 0. http://www.euro.who.int/__data/assets/pdf_file/0005/98447/E84423.pdf. [Chapter 7].

World Health Organization. In: Terracini B, editor. Toxic oil syndrome: ten years of progress. Copenhagen, Denmark: WHO Regional Office for Europe; 2004. ISBN: 9289010630.

Yoshida SH, German JB, Fletcher MP, Gershwin ME. The toxic oil syndrome: a perspective on immunotoxicological mechanisms. Regul Toxicol Pharmacol 1994;19(1):60–79.

Chapter 1.6

Eosinophilia-myalgia syndrome—United States, 1989

Alan D. Woolf

Boston Children's Hospital & Harvard Medical School, Boston, Massachusetts, United States

L-Tryptophan (LT) is an essential amino acid (Fig. 1.6.1) that is absorbed from food and cannot be synthesized by the human body. Tryptophan deficiency is associated with an inability to synthesize niacin (vitamin B_3) which leads to the disease: pellagra. However, it is present in plentiful amounts in chocolate, red meat, cottage cheese, yoghurt, whole grains, eggs, potatoes, bananas, and other foods. While normal dietary sources contribute about 1 g LT per day, it was introduced as a separate product to the American market in about 1974 as an over-the-counter, dietary supplement. LT is metabolized by hydroxylase to 5-hydroxytryptophan and then by pyridoxine-dependent decarboxylase to serotonin. Serotonin is a multifaceted neurotransmitter thought to affect emotions, cognition, memory, reward, and well-being. Health benefit claims for supplemental LT, in doses of 1–15 g/day, included the treatment of anxiety and depression, insomnia, premenstrual syndrome, and obsessive-compulsive disorder. In peripheral tissues, tryptophan is metabolized mainly via the kynurenine pathway to nicotinamide dinucleotide.

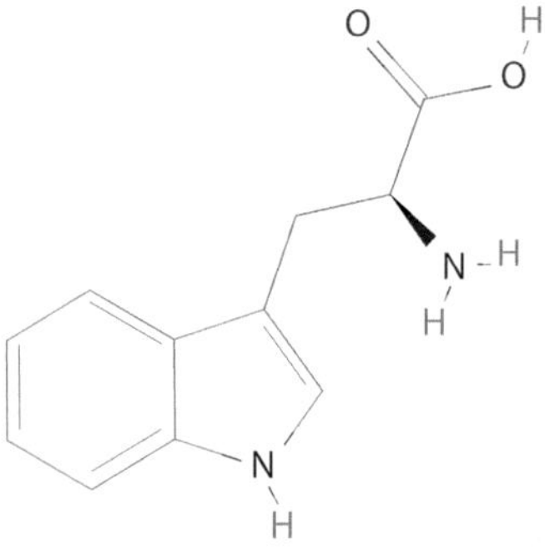

FIG. 1.6.1 Chemical structure of L-tryptophan. *(From PubChem—NLM.)*

History of Modern Clinical Toxicology. https://doi.org/10.1016/B978-0-12-822218-8.00008-9

New disease: EMS

A new disease entity was first described in three patients by Dr. Philip A. Hertzman and his colleagues in New Mexico in October of 1989 (Hertzman et al., 1990). These clinicians noted all three patients complained of myalgias, mouth ulcers, rashes, and abdominal pain. Laboratory tests revealed elevated serum aldolase levels and a striking eosinophilia in peripheral blood. The physicians quickly linked these symptoms to the ingestion of the dietary supplement LT which all three patients took regularly. They reported their findings to the New Mexico Department of Public Health and the CDC. News media outlets publicized this new disease and its victims in feature stories; and more cases quickly emerged in New Mexico within weeks. By November 13, 1990, 30 cases had been identified. The CDC had officially named the new disease entity: "eosinophilia-myalgia syndrome (EMS)" (CDC, 1989). Common symptoms in the patients described initially included pulmonary findings, muscle pain, fever, and lymphadenopathy, with biopsy findings of scleroderma, small-vessel vasculitis, fasciitis, and myopathy, along with remarkable peripheral eosinophilia (Clauw et al., 1990) (Table 1.6.1).

TABLE 1.6.1 Symptoms and physical signs of eosinophilia-myalgia syndrome.

Musculoskeletal
Weakness
Myalgias and arthralgias
Joint pain and swelling
Muscle pain
Muscle cramping
Nonpitting peripheral limb edema
Skin and mucous membranes
Pruritus
Rash, urticarial, or maculopapular
Mouth ulcers
Alopecia
Cardiac
Coronary artery spasm (rare)
Myocarditis (rare)

TABLE 1.6.1 Symptoms and physical signs of eosinophilia-myalgia syndrome—cont'd

Pulmonary

Dyspnea on exertion

Cough

Pleural effusion

Interstitial pneumonia (uncommon)

Gastrointestinal

Anorexia

Abdominal pain

Hepatomegaly

Diarrhea

Neurologic

Fatigue

Headache

Loss of focus, poor concentration

Incoordination

Dysphoria

Anxiety, depression

Peripheral neuropathies

Encephalopathy (rare)

Other

Menstrual changes

Vision changes

Sicca syndrome

Polyserositis

Late Findings

Scleroderma-like scarring—*morphea* lesions

Contractures

Memory loss

Cognitive decline

Table created by author.

Epidemiology

A voluntary national, state-based surveillance system was established within a week of the reported New Mexico outbreak. Case inclusion criteria for epidemiologic research purposes were initially set to include eosinophil counts > 2000 cells/mm^3 (later changed to > 1000 cells/mm^3) and generalized myalgia plus exclusion of trichinosis or any other infection or neoplasm. The rarity of trichinosis in the United States and the fact that this event was obviously not an outbreak of the parasite soon led to its exclusion from the case definition. The usual daily dose of LT in EMS patients ranged from 10 mg to 15,000 mg (median 1500 mg; 90th %tile 4000 mg), although 11 patients reported daily doses <250 mg (Swygert et al., 1990).

EMS seemed to affect predominantly women (up to 84% of reported cases), although that was thought to be more likely related to supplement buying patterns rather than gender differences in metabolism or physiology. Over 97% of patients were non-Hispanic whites and they tended to be middle-aged. The median age of EMS patients was around 48 years; less than 2% of cases involved persons ≤24 years and 14% were older than 65 years (Kilbourne, 1992). LT users over the age of 58 years were nearly twice as likely to get EMS as those younger than 35 years (Silver, 1993).

The daily dose of LT taken correlated with the likelihood of developing the illness. The attack rate for EMS for all LT users was 9.3%, but in one case-control study, people taking more than 4 g daily had a 50% risk of developing EMS (Kamb et al., 1992). On November 11, 1989, the FDA warned consumers to discontinue taking LT in amounts greater than 100 mg per day, but on November 17th the FDA expanded the warning and recalled all LT products regardless of concentration, with a few exceptions such as baby formulas, intravenous nutrient solutions, and protein supplements in which small amounts of LT were used. By January 9, 1990, 1046 cases had been reported to the CDC from 49 states, Washington DC, and Puerto Rico, with 139 (32%) patients requiring hospitalization (CDC, 1990).

By July 9th, 1990 there were 1531 cases and 27 deaths reported (Swygert et al., 1990). By August 1st, 1992, 38 deaths attributable to EMS from neurologic, cardiac, and pulmonary complications were reported; more than 3000 people may have been experiencing EMS symptoms without meeting the full CDC surveillance criteria for the disease (Silver, 1993).

Cases of EMS were not confined to the United States; additional cases were reported in Canada, Germany, Belgium, France, Israel, Japan, and the United Kingdom.

Clinical toxicology—EMS

Symptoms of EMS sometimes began within 1–2 weeks of starting LT supplements, although one national surveillance investigation reported a mean latency period before onset of symptoms of 275 days (range: 0–3668 days; median

127 days) (Swygert et al., 1990). However, such figures should be approached cautiously, since people were surveyed as to when they began supplemental LT, not necessarily when they began taking *tainted* LT.

Many patients with EMS had symptoms and signs of illness similar to those of toxic oil syndrome (TOS) patients (see Chapter 1.5), and similar to findings seen in a third, rare rheumatologic condition called diffuse fasciitis with eosinophilia (DFE). Both TOS and EMS often manifested early prodromal symptoms: influenza-like in the case of EMS and atypical pneumonia in TOS; many patients noticed a short-lived, maculopapular or urticarial pruritic rash. The most prominent clinical manifestations of EMS were severe, incapacitating myalgias, arthralgias, and swollen joints. Patients experienced muscle cramping, and weakness affecting the lower limbs more often than the arms, often with accompanying nonpitting limb edema.

Physical exam findings

Signs of illness included tachycardia, elevated temperature, rash and/or alopecia, palpable muscle tenderness, hepatomegaly, abdominal tenderness, peripheral limb edema, and decreased strength or sensation. Skin rashes were often noted, including a morphea-like, tight thickening of the skin with induration similar to the scleroderma-like lesions see in TOS. Peri-orbital and/or peripheral edema, alopecia, pruritus, and later on, contractures were other findings. Some patients had prominent gastrointestinal symptoms, with malabsorption and weight loss associated with eosinophilic infiltration in the stomach, small bowel, and colon (Silver, 1993). Serious cardiac signs of EMS usually resulted from the pulmonary hypertension seen in some cases and also included coronary artery spasm (Hertzman et al., 1992) and restrictive cardiomyopathy (Berger, 1994).

Unlike TOS in which pulmonary complications were prominent, respiratory symptoms in EMS were generally mild or even nonexistent. In some cases, cough, mild dyspnea, hypoxemia and pulmonary infiltrates and/or pleural effusions on X-ray were evident. Lung biopsies in some patients showed interstitial pneumonitis with eosinophilia and perivascular inflammation.

Neurologic and psychiatric findings

Eosinophil-derived neurotoxin and products of LT metabolism (quinolinic acid) can be neurotoxic, and a few patients with EMS had life-threatening central nervous system manifestations, such as stroke or acute encephalopathy (Silver, 1993). Peripheral neuropathies were reported in up to 60% of EMS patients and an ascending polyneuropathy-associated respiratory paralysis resulted in some deaths.

An early report from New York (CDC, 1991) highlighted the prominent neurocognitive features of EMS. Authors noted changes in the mental status in these patients, including onset of anxiety and depression, fatigue, poor attention span, difficulty concentrating, poor word finding ability, and possible cognitive effects with lowered IQ. Selective neurocognitive and executive function impairments were confirmed in another case series of EMS patients (Armstrong et al., 1997). It was unclear whether such findings were related to the stress associated with the recent onset of a chronic disease or were due to a primary effect of the contaminant itself, an inflammatory reaction in the central nervous system. Later magnetic resonance (MR) imaging and proton MR spectroscopy case-control studies reported findings of subcortical focal lesions, lesions in deep white matter, cortical atrophy, widened ventricles, and periventricular white matter abnormalities, with spectroscopic evidence of inflammatory cerebrovascular disease (Haseler et al., 1998).

Laboratory findings

EMS was remarkable for strikingly elevated numbers of eosinophils in the peripheral blood—various criteria required a peripheral eosinophil count $> 1000/mm^3$ (patients sometimes had eosinophilia up to $13,000/mm^3$). Other laboratory findings often included a low serum albumen and sometimes increased markers of inflammation: erythrocyte sedimentation rates (ESR) and/or c-reactive protein (CRP). In one report, 85% of patients had a leukocytosis, 46% had elevated aldolase levels, 43% had elevated liver function tests, 33% had an elevated ESR, 17% had an elevated serum IgE level, and 10% had an elevated creatine kinase (Swygert et al., 1990).

Progression of disease

Sometimes symptoms of EMS did not abate (or even worsened) after the patient discontinued taking LT supplements. Resolution of the toxic effects was slow. The most persistent sequelae—myalgias, fatigue, neuropsychiatric, memory and cognitive effects, and sclerodermiform skin changes—lasted for months or even years in some patients. Some patients developed an unremitting hemiplegia affecting their mobility. Morphea-like skin changes, muscle contractures, chronic fatigue, and psychological and emotional impairments contributed to long-lasting disability in some patients. Death associated with EMS most often was seen when a patient developed a Guillain-Barre-type, ascending paralysis with respiratory failure.

The only effective treatment for EMS was discontinuation of the ingestion of supplemental LT. Early administration of steroids seemed to improve some, but not all, symptoms such as muscle pain and weakness. Steroids did not seem to alter the overall course or duration of their illness (Philen et al., 1991; Hertzman et al., 1990; Silver et al., 1990; Kilbourne, 1992).

Pathology

Pathologically, perivascular, perineural inflammatory responses in the subcutaneous fat, fascia and dermis were seen without immune complexes. Muscles were infiltrated with abundant eosinophils, plasma cells, and lymphocytes, with excessive deposits of collagen. Common pathologic features included hyaline sclerodermoid collagen in the dermis, septa and fascia, with edema, focal mucinosis and macrophage inflammation (Winkelmann et al., 1991; Medsger, 1990). The presence of lymphocytic infiltration of lesions in both TOS and EMS was notable (Medsger, 1990). Papular mucinosis was a histopathologic finding common to all three conditions: TOS, EMS, and diffuse eosinophilic fasciitis.

Differential diagnosis

Differential diagnoses to be ruled out included parasitic infection (e.g., trichinosis), polyarteritis nodosa, neoplasia, diffuse eosinophilic fasciitis, drug allergy, hypersensitivity pneumonitis, vasculitis, immunodeficiency state, idiopathic hyper-eosinophilic syndrome, and scleroderma. But exposure to LT was the key element in the patient history.

Etiology

Early in the epidemic, the occurrence of EMS was linked to frequent ingestion of dietary supplements, specifically LT. While there were as many as 800–1000 brands of LT containing products on the US market at the time, the occurrence of this syndrome was soon associated with the ingestion of a single dietary supplement, LT, from a particular manufacturer, Showa-Denko KK, Tokyo, Japan (Swygert et al., 1990; Slutsker et al., 1990; Kamb et al., 1992). In Japan, anthranilic acid was used in its manufacture via a high-yield bacterial (*Bacillus liquefaciens* and *B. amyloliquefaciens*) fermentation process, and it was suspected that indoles and indole-like contaminants were generated in that process (Belongia et al., 1990). It was notable that the company had made changes in its manufacturing process: reduced quantities of powdered charcoal were being used in the purification process and a new strain (Strain V) of *B. amyloliquefaciens* was introduced. Lots of the company's retail product distributed from January through June 1989 at the peak of the supplement's popularity as a health aide were identified as the source of the impure LT (Slutsker et al., 1990).

There was evidence early on that the supplement was contaminated with a responsible chemical agent; the manufacturer's specific brand of LT product was found to contain more than 60 micro-contaminants. Identification of which chemical or chemicals might be the etiology of EMS proved challenging. CDC analyses of suspected LT from Showa-Denko KK identified "peak 97" in high-performance liquid chromatography (HPLC) profiles as the di-tryptophan aminal of acetaldehyde (DTAA) as one possible candidate, although animal studies could not confirm its role (CDC, 1990). Another impurity, 1,1′-ethylidenebis LT (EBT) was also considered, although its investigation in animal models could reproduce fascial changes but not the robust eosinophilia typical of EMS.

Another contaminant, 3-(phenylamino)alanine (PAA), similar in structure to the essential amino acid, phenylalanine was measured at 89 ppm (0.0089%) (Mayeno et al., 1992) (Figs. 1.6.2 and 1.6.3). PAA was somewhat similar chemically to the 3-phenylamino-1,2-propanediol (PAPD) associated with TOS. It is possible that one or more of these compounds, or their metabolites, might be responsible (Posada de la Paz et al., 2001; Mayeno et al., 1992, 1995).

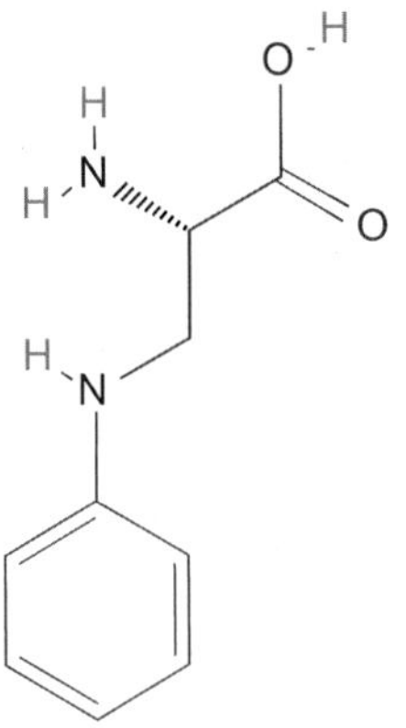

FIG. 1.6.2 3-(Phenylamino)alanine (PAA). *Source: PubChem, NLM.*

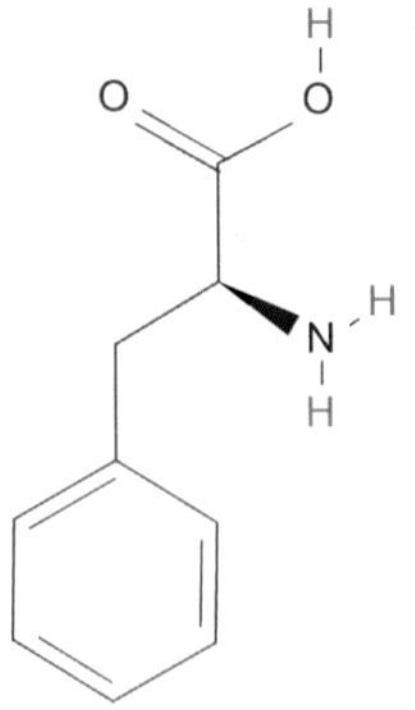

FIG. 1.6.3 Phenylalanine. *Source: PubChem, NLM.*

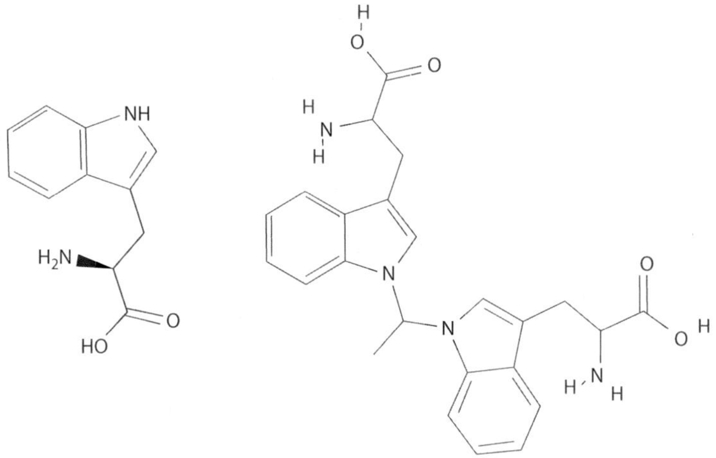

FIG. 1.6.4 (A) Comparison of L-tryptophan and EBT. (B) 1,1'-Ethylidenebis (L-tryptophan). *Source: PubChem, NLM.*

However, other LT contaminants in the Showa-Denko KK product included 1,1'-ethylidenebis (LT) or (EBT). EBT was isolated in only trace amounts but was also postulated to be responsible (Fig. 1.6.4).

It was also theorized that perhaps PAA, PAPD, and EBT shared a common metabolic pathway (e.g., kynurenine pathway or quinolinic acid) and shared a mechanism in the pathogenesis of the syndromes. Some EMS patients (but not all) had increased levels of both L-kynurenine and quinolinic acid in their blood, consistent with activation of the indoleamine-2,3-dioxygenase enzyme system (Silver et al., 1990). Advanced structural analyses later showed that as many as six contaminants in the Showa-Denko KK LT were implicated in cases of EMS, including both indole and indoline compounds. It was speculated that the reactivity of the one or several of the indoline ring structures might play a role in etiology, but this could not be confirmed in animal models (Williamson et al., 1998b). More recently, eight new members of the AAA fatty acid homolog class of contaminants found in the Showa-Denko KK LT product were identified and shown to be structurally similar to the O-PAP and OO-PAP chemicals associated with toxic oil syndrome (Klarskov et al., 2018).

EMS compared with TOS

There have been dozens of research papers and reviews comparing the epidemics of EMS and the TOS in Spain in 1981 (see Chapter 1.5). There are remarkable similarities between the two, in terms of the distribution of contaminated products, the clinical manifestations of illness, and histopathological comparisons. Once the implicated LT was withdrawn from the market in the

United States and the rapeseed oil recalled in Spain, reports of new cases of EMS and TOS rapidly diminished in the two countries. The symptoms and physical signs of illness in EMS and TOS were similar, although not identical (see Table 1.6.2). Both illnesses are suspected to have a pathogenesis involving immune activation precipitated by a toxic contaminant or a toxic metabolite; and both seem to be auto-immune responses (Philen and Posada, 1993). In both syndromes, pathology seen at biopsy or autopsy included widespread perivascular lymphocytic and eosinophilic infiltration of affected tissues. The commercial products implicated in both illnesses contained impurities that were similar in chemical structures. Both the PAP found in LT and the PAPD found in some samples of rapeseed oil might be either interconverted metabolites in the body or simply members of a class of etiologically responsible toxic chemicals (Mayeno et al., 1995; Philen and Hill, 1993).

TABLE 1.6.2 Comparing some clinical features of TOS and EMS.

Feature	Toxic oil syndrome (rapeseed oil)	Eosinophilia-myalgia syndrome (L-tryptophan)
Prodrome	Atypical pneumonia	Influenza-like
Fever	XXX	XXX
Eosiniphil $> 1000/mm^3$	XXX	XXXX
Myalgia/Athralgia	XX	XXXX
Weight loss	XX	XXX
Scleroderma	XX	XXX
Edema	XX	XXX
Headache	XXX	XXX
Cough	XXX	XXX
Cramps	XXX	XXX
Sicca syndrome	XX	XX
Clinical depression	X	X
Neuropathies	X	X
Death rate	2.3%	2.7%
Animal model	No	No

Adapted from Philen & Posada: Sem Arth Rheum (Elsevier Publisher), 1993.

Lessons learned from EMS and TOS

The public health comparisons of the two outbreaks are worth noting as lessons learned. Both epidemics involved consuming so-called "natural" substances. In both instances, the lack of regulatory standards and/or enforcement resulted in contaminated products reaching the marketplace when they should have been interdicted. However, this lesson may not have been learned: melatonin is a dietary supplement and "natural" hormone taken frequently by consumers as a sleep-aide and to alleviate symptoms of "jet lag." Later in the 1990s, cases of melatonin-associated eosinophilia were linked to melatonin-formaldehyde condensation contaminants that were structural analogues of the LT contaminants (Williamson et al., 1998a). And a few years after the LT epidemic, the Dietary Supplement Health & Education Act of 1994 was passed by the US Congress. This law removed herbs, biologicals, and dietary supplements from the oversight and regulations of the FDA, regulations intended to keep individuals safe if they chose to use such products. The ban on the sale of LT products was lifted by the FDA in 2005; one case of postepidemic EMS involving supplemental LT was again reported in 2011 (Allen et al., 2011).

In both the EMS and TOS epidemics, the first cases were not discovered by public health officials through population-based illness surveillance. They were discovered by astute clinicians working in their offices and recognizing the importance of these sentinel cases as a threat to the wider populace. Once the threat to the public's health was made apparent through the efforts of these doctors, then governmental agencies took the lead to organize the broader investigation and mitigate the risk to people's health.

The investigation of the epidemiology of TOS was aided by the creation of a national registry using consensus-based criteria to define a victim, although the original use of geographic and clinical descriptors resulted in some confusion and possible case omission or misclassification. The exploration of epidemiologic characteristics of EMS was hampered by the lack of an agreed-on clinical definition and the absence of a national registry of cases in the United States, although there were efforts by the CDC to aggregate state-level data (Kilbourne, 1992).

In both these epidemics and in others involving a toxic exposure, the spectrum of resulting clinical illness might range from very mild-to-severe in the affected population, depending on dose, genetic predisposition, and other factors promoting either vulnerability or resilience. Thus restrictive criteria in the case definition may have under-counted affected individuals who had more subtle forms of EMS or TOS and thereby could have grossly underestimated the public health impacts of the event.

References

Allen JA, Peterson A, Sufit R, Hinchcliff ME, Mahoney JM, Wood TA, Miller FW, et al. Postepidemic eosinophilia-myalgia syndrome associated with L-tryptophan. Arthritis Rheum 2011;63(11). https://doi.org/10.1002/art.30514.

Armstrong C, Lewis T, D'Esposito M, Freundlich B. Eosinophilia-myalgia syndrome: selective neurocognitive impairment, longitudinal effects, and neuroimaging findings. J Neurol Neurosurg Psychiatry 1997;63:633–41.

Belongia EA, Hedrero CW, Gleich GJ, et al. An investigation of the cause of the eosinophilia-myalgia syndrome associated with tryptophan use. N Engl J Med 1990;323(6):357–65.

Berger PB, Duffy J, Reeder GS, Karon BL, Edwards WD. Restrictive cardiomyopathy associated with the eosinophilia-myalgia syndrome. Mayo Clin Proc 1994;69(2):162–5.

CDC. Eosinophilia-myalgia syndrome—New Mexico. MMWR 1989;38:765–7.

CDC. Analysis of L-tryptophan for the etiology of eosinophilia-myalgia syndrome. MMWR 1990;39:589–91.

CDC. Eosinophilia-myalgia syndrome: follow-up survey of patients—New York, 1990–1991. MMWR 1991;40(24):401–3.

Clauw DJ, Nashel DJ, Umhau A, Katz P. Tryptophan-associated eosinophilic connective tissue disease. JAMA 1990;263(11):1502–6.

Haseler LJ, Sibbitt WL, Sibbitt RR, Hart BL. Neurologic, MR imaging, and MR spectroscopic findings in eosinophilia myalgia syndrome. Am J Neuroradiol 1998;19:1687–94.

Hertzman PA, Blevins WL, Mayer J, et al. Association of the eosinophilia-myalgia syndrome with the ingestion of tryptophan. N Engl J Med 1990;322(13):869–73.

Hertzman PA, Maddoux GL, Sternberg EM, Heyes MP, Mefford IN, Kephart GM, Gleich GJ. Repeated coronary artery spasm in a young woman with the eosinophilia-myalgia syndrome. JAMA 1992;267(21):2932–4.

Kamb ML, Murphy JJ, Jones JL, et al. Eosinophilia-myalgia syndrome in L-tryptophan-exposed patients. JAMA 1992;207(1):77–82.

Kilbourne EM. Eosinophilia-myalgia syndrome: coming to grips with a new illness. Epidemiol Rev 1992;14:16–36.

Klarskov K, Gagnon H, Racine M, Boudreault PL, Normandin C, Marsault E, et al. Peak AAA fatty acid homolog contaminants present in the dietary supplement L-tryptophan associated with the onset of eosinophilia-myalgia syndrome. Toxicol Lett 2018;294:193–204.

Mayeno AN, Belongia EA, Lin F, Lundy SK, Gleich GJ. 3-(Phenylamino) alanine, a novel aniline-derived amino acids associated with the eosinophilia-myalgia syndrome e: a link to the toxic oil syndrome? Mayo Clin Proc 1992;67:1134–9.

Mayeno AN, Benson LM, Baylor S, et al. Biotransformation of 3-(phenylamino)-1,2-propanediol to 3-(phenylamino)alanine: a chemical link between toxic oil syndrome and eosinophilia-myalgia syndrome. Chem Res Toxicol 1995;8:911–6.

Medsger TA. Tryptophan-induced eosinophilia-myalgia syndrome. N Engl J Med 1990;322(13):926–7.

Philen RM, Hill RH. 3-(Phenylamino)alanine – a link between eosinophilia-myalgia syndrome and toxic oil syndrome? (editorial). Mayo Clin Proc 1993;68:197–200.

Philen RM, Posada M. Toxic oil syndrome and eosinophilia-myalgia syndrome: May 8–10 1991, World Health Organization meeting report. Semin Arthritis Rheum 1993;23(2):104–24.

Philen RM, Edison M, Kilbourne EM, Sewell M, Voorhess R. Eosinophilia-myalgia syndrome: a clinical case series of 21 patients. Arch Intern Med 1991;151:333–7.

Posada de la Paz M, Philen RM, Borda IA. Toxic oil syndrome: the perspective after 20 years. Epidemiol Rev 2001;23(2):231–47.

Silver RM. Eosinophilia-myalgia syndrome, toxic oil syndrome, and diffuse fasciitis with eosinophilia. Curr Opin Rheumatol 1993;5:802–8.

Silver RM, Heyes MP, Maize JC, et al. Scleroderma, fasciitis, and eosinophilia associated with the ingestion of tryptophan. NEJM 1990;322:874–81.

Slutsker L, Hoesly FC, Miller L, et al. Eosinophilia-myalgia syndrome associated with exposure to tryptophan from a single manufacturer. JAMA 1990;264(2):213–7.

Swygert LA, Maes EF, Sewell LE, et al. Eosinophilia-myalgia syndrome. Results of national surveillance. JAMA 1990;264:1698–703.

Williamson BL, Johnson KL, Tomlinson AJ, et al. On-line HPLC-tandem mass spectrometry structural characterization of case-associated contaminants of L-tryptophan implicated with the onset of eosinophilia-myalgia syndrome. Toxicol Lett 1998a;99:139–50.

Williamson BL, Tomlinson AJ, Mishra PK, Gleich GJ, Naylor S. Structural characterization of contaminants found in in commercial preparations of melatonin: similarities to case-related compounds from L-tryptophan associated with eosinophilia-myalgia syndrome. Chem Res Toxicol 1998b;11:234–40.

Winkelmann RK, Connolly SM, Quimby SR, Griffing WL, Lie JT. Histopathologic features of the L-tryptophan related eosinophilia-myalgia (fasciitis) syndrome. Mayo Clin Proc 1991;66:457–63.

Chapter 1.7

Methyl isocyanate—Bhopal, India, 1984

Rose Goldman[a,b,c] and Gabriel C. Gaviola[d]

[a]Associate Professor of Medicine, Harvard Medical School, Boston, MA, United States, [b]Associate Professor in the Department of Environmental Health, Harvard T.H. Chan School of Public Health, Boston, MA, United States, [c]Department of Medicine, Cambridge Health Alliance, Cambridge, MA, United States, [d]Resident Physician, Harvard T.H. Chan School of Public Health, Boston, MA, United States

Background

In 1969, the American company, Union Carbide Corporation (UCC), agreed to establish a plant in Bhopal, the capital of the Indian state of Madhya Pradesh, to manufacture carbaryl, a pesticide commonly used in Asia. The Indian government initiated the request to attract foreign investment in local industry. The agreement included local shareholders retaining a substantial percentage of the investment through a subsidiary, Union Carbide India Limited (UCIL) (Fig. 1.7.1).

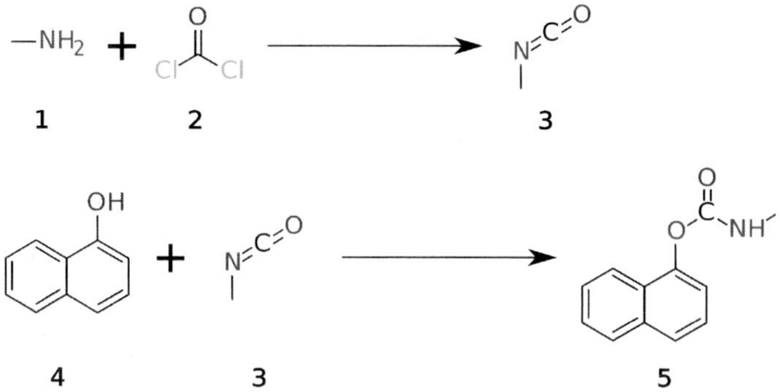

1=methylamine 2=phosgene 3=methyl isocyanate 4=1-naphthol
5=carbaryl

FIG. 1.7.1 Synthesis of carbaryl, which uses methyl isocyanate. (*https://commons.wikimedia.org/w/index.php?sort=relevance&search=bhopal+disaster&title=Special:Search&profile=advanced&fulltext=1&advancedSearch-current=%7B%7D&ns0=1&ns6=1&ns12=1&ns14=1&ns100=1&ns106=1#/media/File:Preparation_of_carbaryl_as_in_Bhopal.svg*).

History of Modern Clinical Toxicology. https://doi.org/10.1016/B978-0-12-822218-8.00036-3

Initially, the plant formulated carbaryl from imported precursor chemicals, including methyl isocyanate (MIC), synthesized by UCC. Increased competition led the plant to expand its capacity in 1979 to include the hazardous process of manufacturing raw materials and intermediate products in addition to the final product (Broughton, 2005; Eckerman, 2011).

Owing to decreased demand for pesticides in the 1980s, UCIL decided to sell the plant. Facing delays in finding a buyer, UCIL began to dismantle key production elements of the facility. During this transition period, the plant continued to operate with substandard safety equipment and procedures (Broughton, 2005). In the years leading up to the disaster, the trade union wrote a letter to management and authorities and distributed posters about potential hazards. Further warnings for a potential large incident included a fire and several leaks in which workers were injured and died. A safety audit performed by UCC in May 1982 cited many safety concerns, but concluded that there was no imminent danger or immediate correction required (Eckerman, 2011).

Though the plant in Bhopal was built centrally and close to transportation, the location was zoned for light industrial and commercial use, not for a hazardous manufacturing plant (Broughton, 2005). The city of Bhopal had a population of about 800,000 people, with an estimated 100,000 living within a 1 km radius of the plant. Much of the population lived in squatter settlements around the plant. The city had 200,000 children below 15 years of age and 3000 pregnant women (Dhara and Dhara, 2002; Mehta, 1990; Eckerman, 2011). The incident to come would be catastrophic to the nearby population (Fig. 1.7.2).

Plant explosion

On the night of December 2, 1984, around 11:00 PM, a faulty valve allowed water to enter a tank containing 40 t of MIC, creating an exothermic reaction. As pressure and heat continued to build, several safety systems failed to contain the reaction. A refrigeration unit containing coolant had been emptied for use in another part of the plant and a gas flare safety system had not been working for several months. Eventually, at 1:00 AM while residents surrounding the plant were asleep, a safety valve failed, sending a plume of MIC gas and by-products into the atmosphere (Broughton, 2005; Mehta, 1990).

Epidemiology

Immediate effects

In the early morning hours, an estimated 40 t of MIC gas and additional chemicals were dispersed over approximately 40 km^2, spreading over the squatter settlements to the south. Low wind speeds and an atmospheric condition of temperature inversion prevented dilution of the gas. More than half a million people were exposed to MIC. An estimated 3800 people died immediately and up to 10,000 people died within 3 days. Reports described streets littered with corpses of humans, buffalo, cows, dogs, and other animals (Broughton, 2005). Of the deaths in

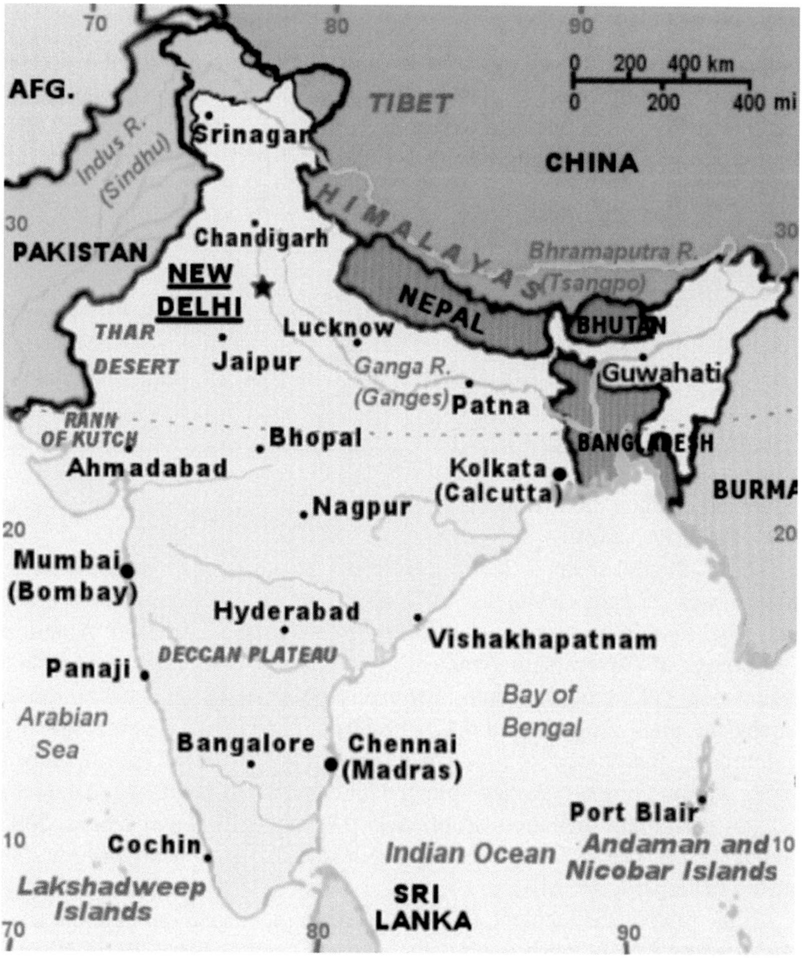

FIG. 1.7.2 Map of India showing location of Bhopal, India. *(Source: Creative Commons Attribution-Share Alike 3.0, https://commons.wikimedia.org/w/index.php?search=Map+of+India& title=Special:MediaSearch&go=Go&type=image).*

the first few weeks, at least 3000 were below 15 years of age. Small children were the most severely affected as their exposure was at a higher concentration per kilogram (Eckerman, 2011). In addition, smaller children have breathing zones closer to the ground, and an increased respiratory rate. Most of the dead and severely injured resided within the 6.65 km^2 area south of the plant (Mehta, 1990).

In the aftermath of the event, 170,000 patients visited hospitals, with 12,000 in very critical condition. Patients presented nearly blind, gasping for breath, foaming at the mouth, and vomiting. In the absence of information about the offending agent, most patients were treated symptomatically. There was a wide variety of symptoms, which was likely due to the presence of different compounds and exposure to increased concentrations closer to the factory (Eckerman, 2011).

Delayed effects

Estimates of morbidity and mortality have ranged widely, and there is no consensus on the number of people who died from the gas leak (Sharma, 2005). The Indian Council of Medical Research (ICMR) estimated there were 22,917 deaths, 508,432 permanently disabled, and 33,781 severely injured (Howard, 2014).

Toxicology—Methyl isocyanate

MIC (chemical formula: C_2H_3NO, with the highly reactive $-N=C=O$ group) is a clear, colorless, flammable liquid that has a pungent odor. An exothermic reaction occurs on contact with water, generating carbon dioxide, methylamine gases, and N,N'-dimethylurea. Methylamines are relatively nontoxic as a single dose unless in extremely high concentrations. At high temperatures, MIC decomposes to hazardous products including hydrogen cyanide (HCN), nitrogen oxides, and carbon monoxide (ATSDR, 2014; Varma and Varma, 1993; Mehta, 1990; U.S. EPA, 2000).

The estimated mean MIC concentration in the cloud that escaped the factory was 27 ppm, which is 1400 times the U.S. Occupational Safety and Health Administration (OSHA) workplace standard and American Conference of Governmental Industrial Hygienists (ACGIH) 8-h threshold limit value (TLV) of 0.02 ppm. Estimates of ground-level concentrations around the plant ranged from 0.12 to 85.6 ppm (median 1.8 ppm). Mucosal and throat irritation occurs at 2–4 ppm (intolerable levels > 21 ppm). Odor is a poor warning property, as the human odor detection for MIC is > 2 ppm and mucous membrane irritation occurs at > 0.4 ppm (Dhara and Dhara, 2002; Mehta, 1990). The U.S. EPA has not established a Reference Concentration or Reference Dose for MIC.

At the time of the incident, there was a single published report about acute MIC toxicity in rats, mice, rabbits, guinea pigs, and humans (Kimmerle and Eben, 1964). MIC was toxic to all animals tested and was irritating to lungs, skin, and eyes at low concentrations. Humans exposed to low concentrations suffered severe eye and throat irritation.

While MIC may be one of the most toxic of all isocyanates, given its extremely high vapor pressure and reactivity, all isocyanates can cause pulmonary toxicity (Varma and Varma, 1993). Major organs affected during the incident were the eyes and respiratory tract, while those body systems less affected were skin and gastrointestinal tracts (MIC dissolved in saliva) (Dhara and Dhara, 2002). MIC is thought to cause injury to exposed tissues by direct reaction with tissue macromolecules, by reaction with functional groups to inhibit certain enzyme activities, or by heat damage through a secondary hydrolysis reaction (Bucher, 1987).

Clinical toxicity in humans

Acute/subacute toxicity

The primary organs affected were the eyes and respiratory tract. Less affected were the gastrointestinal, reproductive, neuropsychiatric, and immunologic systems.

Pulmonary

Though isocyanates can be allergenic in the lung, MIC appears to cause toxicity to the respiratory tract by irritation (Dhara and Dhara, 2002). Irritation of the upper and lower respiratory tract by MIC resulted in cough with frothy sputum (pulmonary edema), a sensation of suffocation, chest pain, breathlessness, and rhinorrhea. Existing diseases were exacerbated, including tuberculosis and chronic bronchitis. Pulmonary function tests showed a reduction in vital capacity (Mishra et al., 2009). Chest radiographs showed extensive interstitial changes (Varma and Varma, 1993). Autopsy studies revealed severe necrotizing lesions in the upper respiratory tract, bronchioles, alveoli, and lung capillaries, as well as cerebral edema and anoxic brain injury. Cause of death was most often acute lung injury or pulmonary edema and acute respiratory distress syndrome, resulting in asphyxia and cardiac arrest (Mishra et al., 2009; Varma and Varma, 1993).

Many chest radiographs performed 3 months after the accident showed abnormal findings, such as haziness, hilar prominence, fine mottling, and reticulation. Some suggested old disease, including tuberculosis, chronic bronchitis, and pneumonitis, was exacerbated by the MIC exposure (Dhara and Dhara, 2002). Lung biopsies of survivors performed 6 months after the incident showed fibrosing bronchiolitis obliterans and chronic restrictive and obstructive disease. Bronchoalveolar lavage of severely exposed patients performed 1–2.5 years after the incident showed alveolitis (inflammation of the lower respiratory tract) (Dhara and Dhara, 2002). Studies performed both several months and 10 years after the accident showed a reduction in respiratory symptoms with increasing distance from the plant (Dhara and Dhara, 2002; Mishra et al., 2009).

Ophthalmic

MIC is intensely irritating to the cornea. Ocular symptoms during the first two months after the accident included intense burning, lacrimation, pain, photophobia, and blurred vision. Exam revealed superficial corneal ulceration, pigmentary deposition on the cornea, conjunctival congestion, and punctate keratopathy (Mishra et al., 2009). Studies conducted 2–3 years postexposure revealed no blindness or evidence of severe damage to internal or external ocular structures. They did show the development of a chronic inflammatory process, with symptoms of persistent lacrimation, burning, itching, and redness, as well as excess cataracts and an increased risk of eye infections. This constellation, termed "Bhopal Eye Syndrome," may have been exacerbated by the living conditions in Bhopal's slum area, characterized by poor ventilation and exposure to dust and smoke (Dhara and Dhara, 2002).

Other

Gastrointestinal findings of superficial esophagitis and gastritis were accompanied by observed symptoms of nausea, vomiting, diarrhea, anorexia, and abdominal pain. **Dermatologic**: MIC is a skin irritant and can cause chemical burns at high levels of exposure. **Neurologic** findings included loss of consciousness, convulsions, impaired auditory and visual memory, muscle weakness, tremors, vertigo, ataxia and persistent numbness and tingling in the extremities. Autopsies revealed that the brains of victims were edematous and red in color, with foci of hemorrhage in white matter and less often intraventricular and intracerebral hemorrhage. **Psychiatric** findings included anxiety, depression, posttraumatic stress disorder (PTSD), and attention deficit. **Immunologic** studies showed reduced T-cell populations along with a decrease in lymphocyte phagocyte activity, suggesting a depression of cell-mediated immunity. It is unclear whether immune system injury was due to MIC or secondary to lung disease. Other **nonspecific symptoms** included fever and muscle fatigue (Mishra et al., 2009; Bucher, 1987; Mehta, 1990; Varma and Varma, 1993; ATSDR, 2014).

Late sequelae

The ICMR, which has conducted much of the research on the health effects of MIC, attributes more than 50% of deaths among exposed victims to respiratory ailments (Eckerman, 2011). Long-term effects and symptoms described by Cullinan et al. (1996) and Eckerman (2011) within 10 years included the following:

- Respiratory: Obstructive or restrictive disease, pulmonary fibrosis, chronic bronchitis, dyspnea, worsening of tuberculosis
- Ophthalmic: Corneal scars and opacities, early cataracts, vision problems, chronic conjunctivitis
- Neurologic: Memory difficulties, numbness, impairment of fine motor skills
- Psychiatric: Posttraumatic stress disorder (PTSD) symptoms

Reproductive and developmental toxicity

High rates of spontaneous abortion, stillbirth, neonatal mortality, and menstrual irregularities were seen after the event. However, the rate of congenital malformations was not found to be higher than baseline (Varma and Varma, 1993). One study conducted 9 months after the accident found that 43% of 865 pregnancies in exposed women resulted in fetal loss compared to the baseline incidence of 6%–10%. Those exposed in the first trimester of pregnancy had a higher spontaneous abortion rate. Of 486 live births, 14% of the infants died within 30 days of birth, a significant increase from the 3% for deliveries during the 2-year period prior to the accident (Varma, 1987). Another study found increased calcification in placentas of premature infants and hydropic degeneration of placental tissue after medical termination of pregnancy, suggesting poor perfusion and anoxia (Kanhere et al., 1987). The mean weight of placentae from full-term exposed women was significantly lower than nonexposed women. Persistent increased rates of spontaneous abortion were reported in Bhopal victims several years after the accident, with higher rates in women with greater exposure (Iyer and Dunn, 2010).

Carcinogenicity

Studies on the genotoxicity and carcinogenicity of MIC have yielded inconclusive results. Chromosomal studies performed 2.5 months after the incident showed a significantly higher number of breaks and gaps in lymphocytes of exposed victims compared with controls. Cytogenetic studies performed 3 years after the incident showed higher levels of chromosomal aberration in the exposed, with higher levels in females than males. A case-control study comparing a cancer registry with a tobacco study in Bhopal showed a marginally increased risk of oropharyngeal cancer after adjusting for age and tobacco use, however, the study was inconclusive as there was short latency between exposure and incidence and no dose-response relationships found with geographic distribution (Dhara and Dhara, 2002). MIC is not classified as to its carcinogenicity either by the International Agency for Research on Cancer (IARC, 2021); or by the United States Environmental Protection Agency (EPA) (U.S. EPA, 2000).

Pediatric effects

Most pediatric clinical studies have been observational with methodological flaws (Mehta, 1990). Children presented acutely with similar respiratory, ophthalmologic, and gastrointestinal symptoms as adults (Irani and Mahashur, 1986). Some had convulsions, hemiparesis, generalized hypotonia and weakness, loss of consciousness, and coma (Mehta, 1990). There is inconclusive evidence that offspring of exposed parents had growth retardation (males only) and menstrual abnormalities (females) (Dhara and Dhara, 2002; Eckerman, 2011).

Animal studies

Acute toxicity

Animal MIC inhalation exposure studies have shown similar respiratory and ophthalmic symptoms to those in humans (Bucher, 1987). Rats exposed to varying levels of MIC via inhalation showed effects in the respiratory system, neurologic system, and eye, with a progressive dose-response relationship for respiratory and nervous system effects. Respiratory effects included respiratory depression, while nervous system effects included sedation and unconsciousness. Effects on the eye were limited to the corneal epithelium, and most severe at intermediate exposure levels (Salmon et al., 1985). Studies of ophthalmic effects in rats showed irritation and lens opacities, but no irreversible damage (Mehta, 1990).

Alteration of ventilation/perfusion in MIC-exposed animals is thought to be due to obstruction of small airways by sloughing of epithelium down to bronchioles along with mucus and fibrin plugging and atelectasis. Ventilation of MIC-exposed guinea pigs did not completely improve hypoxia and low pH resulting from hypercarbia. Pulmonary edema was not found to be significant enough to alter gas exchange (Bucher, 1987). Experimental studies on rabbits and rats showed destruction of alveolar architecture, pulmonary edema, and damage to the epithelial lining of bronchioles, supporting a corrosive effect of MIC. Rats exposed to MIC were found to have impaired alveolar and peritoneal macrophage function and impaired delayed hypersensitivity responses.

Rats exposed to MIC via inhalation showed progressively increasing ataxia, uncoordinated movements, and immobility. Cell cultures isolated from 2-day-old rats exposed to MIC showed death of both fibroblasts and myoblasts, suggesting that MIC directly affects muscle tissue and prevents differentiation (Mehta, 1990).

MIC appears to inhibit erythrocyte ATPase and impair cellular respiration by inhibiting electron transport and acting as an uncoupler in the mitochondria, leading to histotoxic hypoxia. MIC also reduces glutathione levels (Varma and Varma, 1993). Rat and guinea pig studies have shown that MIC does not appear to modify hemoglobin oxygen dissociation, and thus this is not a likely mechanism of tissue hypoxia in Bhopal victims. Rat and guinea pig studies have not shown inhibition of blood or brain cholinesterase, and thus this is not likely a contributing factor to victims' death (Bucher, 1987).

Given its high reactivity, it was thought that inhalation exposure would not result in significant increases in blood levels. However, studies suggest that MIC exposure results in systemic circulation, as inhalation of [^{14}C]MIC by guinea pigs and rats resulted in radioactivity in most organs, including brain, uterus, placenta, and fetus (Varma and Varma, 1993).

Late sequelae

Mortality in rats and mice was seen in several phases: an immediate phase, a subsequent 2-week phase beginning 8–10 days after acute exposure, with occasional deaths as late as 78 days after exposure (Bucher, 1987). Functional studies in rats showed development of severe obstructive airway lesions and gas trapping, as well as increases in right ventricular weight and electrocardiogram changes suggestive of pulmonary hypertension. Restrictive lung lesions were seen at 6 months after exposure (Bucher, 1987). Histopathologic animal studies showed that acute or repeated MIC inhalation did not cause persistent changes in any tissues other than the respiratory tract. Further, following cessation of MIC exposure, eye injury did not persist (Bucher, 1987).

Reproductive and developmental toxicity

Studies of pregnant mice have shown that the fetal toxicity of MIC is partly independent of maternal pulmonary damage and that it can be directly fetotoxic (Mehta, 1990). In male mice, MIC causes temporary reductions in spermatozoa in seminiferous tubules. Animal studies have shown that MIC exposure results in shortening of bones (Irani and Mahashur, 1986).

Carcinogenicity

Despite a negative Ames test, animal and in vitro studies have shown genotoxic potential, with induction of sister-chromatid exchanges, chromosomal breaks, and delay of cell-cycle time. Mice and rat exposure to the highest doses of MIC via inhalation led to marginal increases in pheochromocytomas in both sexes, and pancreatic adenomas in male rats. However, the adrenal medulla and pancreas were not seen as target organs of inhaled MIC (Dhara and Dhara, 2002).

Additional compounds

Though MIC is a potent toxicant, based on the diversity of symptoms observed after the incident, the ICMR concluded that MIC was not the sole agent responsible and that the aerosol of gases contained more than 20 aqueous and thermal decomposition products along with reactant chemicals and polymers of MIC (Sharma, 2005). On investigation of the tanks and residues, Indian scientists inferred that the temperature in the tank rose high enough that MIC would have decomposed into hazardous products including hydrogen cyanide (HCN) (Eckerman, 2011). The controversial diagnosis of acute cyanide poisoning was supported by the cherry-red color of blood and viscera observed in the victims and their response to sodium thiosulfate (an effective therapy for cyanide poisoning) (Mehta, 1990; Broughton, 2005).

Aftermath

UCC attempted to shift culpability for the Bhopal incident to UCIL. The Indian government, acting as sole legal representative for victims to ensure speedy and equitable resolution of claims, eventually reached a $470 million settlement with UCC, a mere fraction of the $3 billion initially claimed as attributable to the event. Bureaucratic corruption absorbed 30% of the settlement money, and half of the sum had not been disbursed as of 2003. The settlement also barred further claims in the United States. A 1999 class-action lawsuit filed by victims against UCC in a US court was dismissed. Ultimately the average amount paid to families of the deceased was $2200 (Broughton, 2005; Howard, 2014; Anonymous, 2000).

UCC discontinued operations at the Bhopal plant after the incident and sold its shares in UCIL to fund the Bhopal Memorial Hospital and Research Center which provided care for the victims. UCIL, renamed Eveready Industries India Limited, leased the site until 1998, when the Madhya Pradesh state government took over the facility (Union Carbide Corporation, 2020). As the site has not been cleaned, MIC, organic pollutants, and heavy metals continue to contaminate the subsoil and groundwater (Howard, 2014; Sharma, 2005).

Lessons learned

The Bhopal Disaster is frequently referred to as the largest industrial catastrophe (Eckerman, 2011). A number of factors contributed to the event; among these, a failure of standard operating practices and engineering controls, repeated disinvestment in the facility by the parent company, lack of skilled local operators, dearth of communication and surveillance by corporate headquarters, lack of an emergency response plan, discontinuation of the safety procedures, proximity to a residential population, and inadequate regulatory policies. Several themes emerged from the disaster, including the placement of industrial facilities near residential areas, the export of hazardous industries to the third world, safety engineering in developing countries, the use of "high tech" hazards like pesticides among "low tech" workers and living conditions, the safety and necessity of pesticides, and poverty and occupational health (Bhopal Working Group, 1987; Eckerman, 2011). The lack of information on the chemicals responsible for the observed health effects was noted to be an impediment in the therapeutic management of victims.

The incident had a pervasive influence beyond the Indian subcontinent. It served as a warning that anywhere hazardous substances are manufactured, stored, or transported, the risk of a similar event is possible (Marwick, 1985). Industrialization in developing countries without improvement in safety regulation could be disastrous from a human, environmental, and economic standpoint (Broughton, 2005). It supported the opinion that businesses had human rights responsibilities, and subsequently, the International Labor Organization (ILO) and other organizations developed conventions (Eckerman, 2011; Howard, 2014).

The event increased environmental awareness and activism in India, leading to the passage of the Environment Protection Act in 1986. This created the Ministry of Environment and Forests which was given responsibility for administering and enforcing environmental laws and policies. Indian states subsequently demanded environmental impact assessments from foreign companies wishing to export industrial operations. For example, DuPont abandoned plans to export a nylon plant from Virginia to Goa and later Chennai (Broughton, 2005). The Indian Ministry of Home affairs set up the National Disaster Management Authority in 2005 to invest in disaster response technology (Howard, 2014). However, the Indian public remains at risk of exposure to harmful chemicals as laws rely on voluntary compliance, officials are susceptible to bribes, and the government remains interested in promoting the chemical industry and has repressed environmental activists (Eckerman, 2011). Pesticides continue to be used widely in India and cause at least 22,000 deaths a year (Broughton, 2005).

In the United States, the Bhopal incident prompted passage of the Emergency Planning and Community Right-to-Know Act (EPCRA, informally known as the "Bhopal Act") in 1986, which was intended to increase the public's access to information on chemicals at industrial facilities, and their release into the environment, and the development of community-wide disaster planning. Per the Act, the governor of each state designates a State Emergency Response Commission (SERC) which in turn designates Local Emergency Planning Committees (LEPCs). EPCRA requires LEPCs to develop emergency response plans and provide information on chemicals and their associated physical and health hazards in the community to citizens. Industrial facilities are required to notify LEPCs and SERCs if there is a release of hazardous substances above a minimum threshold into the community. The EPCRA also established the Toxics Release Inventory, which tracks the management of certain toxic chemicals that pose a threat to human health and the environment (Howard, 2014; U.S. EPA, 2017).

The disaster drew serious attention in industry to the financial liability of adverse health outcomes and prompted a reevaluation of practices and processes by private industry to instill confidence by the public about products and their manufacture. Plant managers were increasingly held responsible by upper management for communicating the plant's activities to the local community. The Chemical Manufacturers Association created a clearinghouse to make communities with chemical plants aware of health and safety protection procedures and expand involvement in community emergency services (Marwick, 1985).

Preventing a future "Bhopal" necessitates that governments and corporations alike understand, anticipate, and prevent the harmful effects of industrial activity on the surrounding community and environment.

References

Anonymous. Has the world forgotten Bhopal? Lancet 2000;356(9245):1863.

ATSDR. Toxic substances portal—methyl Isocyanate. Last modified 21 October 2014 https://www.atsdr.cdc.gov/MMG/MMG.asp?id=628&tid=116; 2014. [Accessed 20 March 2020].

Bhopal Working Group. The public health implications of the Bhopal disaster. Report to the program development board, American Public Health Association. Am J Public Health 1987;77(2):230–6.

Broughton E. The Bhopal disaster and its aftermath: a review. Environ Health 2005;4–6.

Bucher J. Methyl isocyanate: a review of health effects research since Bhopal. Fundam Appl Toxicol 1987;9(3):367–79.

Cullinan P, Acquilla SD, Dhara VR. Long term morbidity in survivors of the 1984 Bhopal gas leak. Natl Med J India 1996;9(1):5–10.

Dhara VR, Dhara R. The union carbide disaster in Bhopal: a review of health effects. Arch Environ Health 2002;57(5):391–404.

Eckerman I. Bhopal gas catastrophe 1984: causes and consequences. In: Nriagu J, editor. Encyclopedia of environmental health. Oxford: Elsevier Publishers; 2011. p. 272–87.

Howard S. Bhopal's legacy: three decades on and residents are still being poisoned. Br Med J 2014;349:g7602.

IARC Monographs on the Identification of Carcinogenic Hazards to Humans, 2021. https://monographs.iarc.who.int/list-of-classifications. [Accessed 22 March 2021].

Irani SF, Mahashur AA. A survey of Bhopal children affected by methyl isocyanate gas. J Postgrad Med 1986;32(4):195–8.

Iyer P, Dunn A. Evidence on the developmental and reproductive toxicity of methyl Isocyanate. California Environmental Protection Agency: Office of Environmental Health Hazard Assessment; 2010. https://oehha.ca.gov/media/downloads/crnr/073010mic.pdf.

Kanhere S, Darbari BS, Shrivastava AK. Morphological study of placentae of expectant mothers exposed to gas leak at Bhopal. Indian J Med Res 1987;86(Suppl):77–82.

Kimmerle G, Eben A. On the toxicity of methylisocyanate and its quantitative determination in the air. Arch Toxicol 1964;20:235–41.

Marwick C. Bhopal tragedy's repercussions may reach American physicians. JAMA 1985; 253(14):2001.

Mehta PS. Bhopal tragedy's health effects. JAMA 1990;264(21):2781.

Mishra PK, Samarth RM, Pathak N, Jain SK, Banerjee S, Maudar KK. Bhopal gas tragedy: review of clinical and experimental findings after 25 years. Int J Occup Med Environ Health 2009;22(3):193–202.

Salmon AG, Muir MK, Andersson N. Acute toxicity of methyl isocyanate: a preliminary study of the dose response for eye and other effects. Br J Ind Med 1985;42(12):795–8.

Sharma DC. Bhopal: 20 years on. Lancet 2005;365(9454):111–2.

U.S. EPA. The emergency planning and community right-to-know act. Last modified 11/2017 https://www.epa.gov/sites/production/files/2017-08/documents/epcra_fact_sheet_overview_8-2-17.pdf; 2017. [Accessed 20 March 2020].

U.S. EPA. Methyl isocyanate. Last modified 01/2000 https://www.epa.gov/sites/production/files/2016-09/documents/methyl-isocyanate.pdf; 2000. [Accessed 22 March 2021].

Union Carbide Corporation. Bhopal gas tragedy information, https://www.bhopal.com; 2020. [Accessed 20 March 2020].

Varma DR. Epidemiological and experimental studies on the effects of methyl isocyanate on the course of pregnancy. Environ Health Perspect 1987;72:153–7.

Varma R, Varma DR. The Bhopal accident and methyl isocyanate toxicity. J Toxicol Environ Health 1993;40(4):513–29.

Chapter 1.8

Zamfara gold mining lead poisoning disaster—Nigeria, Africa, 2010

Mary Jean Brown[a] and Alan D. Woolf[b]

[a]Department of Social and Behavioral Sciences, Harvard T. H. Chan School of Public Health, Boston, MA, United States, [b]Boston Children's Hospital & Harvard Medical School, Boston, Massachusetts, United States

The prospect of earning money from artisanal, small operations gold mining has proven an irresistible way out of poverty for families around the world, from Malaysia to Africa. This is true despite the known dangers posed by the crude methods used in such unregulated, home-based activities, which expose workers and their families to potentially dangerous levels of metals—principally lead, mercury, manganese, and cadmium. This hazard was well illustrated in the poisoning disaster event that involved a poverty-stricken area in Nigeria—the rural Zamfara State in 2010. Small-scale gold ore mining operations there contaminated entire communities with lead, which proved especially deadly for the children.

At the time of the lead poisoning event, Nigeria was a populous country with over 140 million people (2006 census). The country, whose main exports are agricultural products, is divided into 36 states and a Federal Capital Territory, grouped into 6 geopolitical zones and 774 recognized local government areas (NDHS, 2008). Zamfara State is located in the northwest part of Nigeria (Fig. 1.8.1).

2008 Recession and gold mining

During the worldwide economic recession of 2008–12, the price of gold jumped as a safe haven for investments. Whereas in the year 2000, gold sold for about $400, by 2010, gold was trading at $1521 USD per ounce (Macrotrends, 2020). In addition, as a result of climate change, the Sahara Desert was encroaching on formerly arable land and disrupting traditional pastoral farming practices. People in poverty-burdened communities saw this spike in gold prices as an opportunity to generate new income. As much as 50% of the sale of extracted gold from such

History of Modern Clinical Toxicology. https://doi.org/10.1016/B978-0-12-822218-8.00012-0

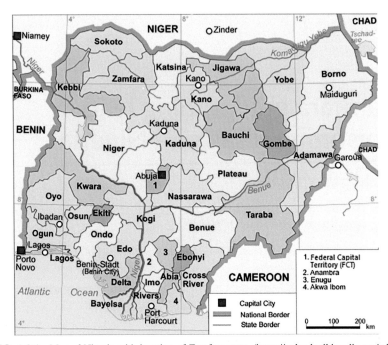

FIG. 1.8.1 Map of Nigeria with location of Zamfara state (https://upload.wikimedia.org/wikipedia/commons/d/d2/Nigeria_political.png). *(Source: Domenico-de-ga, translated and adapted by xandar (https://commons.wikimedia.org/w/index.php?curid=6354185.)*

small artisanal mining activities could be returned to the community. These economic pressures resulted in families turning to artisanal gold mining.

Zamfara State has a population of about 3.7 million, of which 20% are 5 years of age or younger. The population is predominantly Muslim, and the traditional religious leadership system, chaired by local Emirs, has strong political and social influence. Farming is the major livelihood in Zamfara, with greater than 80% of the people participating in agricultural activities. The 2008 Nigeria Demographic and Health Survey found that 18.8% of households had access to electricity, 27.6% to clean water, and 27.5% to improved sanitation facilities (NDHS, 2008).

Quartz (crystalline silica)-rich veins in Zamfara bedrock were mined by hand from near surface workings (Garza et al., 2006). At the mines, ores were sorted into "gold" and "lead" ores based on visual absence or presence of shiny gray lead sulfides. "Gold" ores were transported in cloth bags to villages, where families purchased them for processing. However, these gold ores were heavily contaminated by lead (Plumlee et al., 2013).

Six ore processing activities were used to extract the gold. All produce large amounts of toxic lead dust. They included the following:

1. Breaking ore into gravel-sized pieces using hammers, work often conducted by preteen children.
2. Grinding those pieces into a powder with gasoline-powered flour mills.

3. Washing (sluicing) the powder with water to separate particles of gold.
4. Drying the powder after washing. Often this was done within the family home and children played with the powder with the consistency of wet sand.
5. Hand mixing mercury into the slurry to amalgamate the gold.
6. Vaporizing mercury to remove it from the gold, usually conducted by adults as privately as possible.

Many of the extraction activities were conducted by mothers. Because the families lived under strict *Sharia*, women were not permitted to leave the family compound and the ore processing was an acceptable way for them to contribute to the family income. Thus young children and babies came into close contact with the toxic lead dust generated by the grinding activities. Mothers who ground, washed, or dried the ore were nearly three times more likely to have had a child less than 5 years of age die in a year (Bashir et al., 2014).

Unexplained childhood deaths

Reports of unexplained deaths of children in rural settlements began appearing late in 2009 and early in 2010 in two villages: Dareta and Yarghalma. Typical symptoms included vomiting, colicky abdominal pain, headaches, altered consciousness, and seizures, all unresponsive to both antibiotics and antimalarial drugs. Malaria was suspected at first, because it is endemic to Nigeria. This uncertainty in the diagnosis of the illness lasted for about a year, before doctors from *Médecin Sans Frontières* cooperated with local public health officials to investigate the situation further. Blood lead levels (BLL) from eight symptomatic children in affected villages were initially sent to Europe for analysis. The results were shocking; the children were found to have potentially lethal venous BLL between 168 and 370 µg/dL (Dooyema et al., 2011). By comparison the US Centers for Disease Control and Prevention (CDC) estimates that 97.5% of preschool-age children in the U.S. currently have levels <5 µg/dL. According to CDC guidance, BLL ≥ 70 µg/dL are considered to be Class V life-threatening childhood lead poisoning (CDC, 2019). By May 2010, nearly 300 children in 4 villages had neurological symptoms, with a 48% mortality rate (Greig et al., 2014).

Elevated blood lead levels in children

Concentrations of lead in the blood of children who suffered encephalopathy or who had died were among the highest ever seen. In May to June 2010 the CDC in collaboration with the Nigerian and Zamfara Ministries of Health, conducted a study of children in 119 family compounds where ore processing for gold had occurred. Of 463 children under 5 years, 118 (25%) in the settlement had died the previous year; 82% of these had convulsions prior to their deaths (Dooyema et al., 2011). The same study measured BLL in the remaining children under the age of 5 years and found 97% had an elevated BLL ≥ 45 µg/dL, meeting the CDC and WHO criterion for consideration of chelation therapy. Another cross-sectional survey in the Bagega community in Zamfara State carried out in August to September 2010 found that most of the 185 children ≤5 years of age had BLLs ≥10 μg/dL (Ajumobi et al., 2014). The median BLL was 71 μg/dL (range: 8–332 μg/dL), and 91.4% of children had BLL >45 μg/dL. Another 2010 study of 70 villages in Zamfara found 54 (77%) of them were active in processing ore; those villages processing ore were 3.5 times more likely to have children with lead poisoning than those not involved in mining (Lo et al., 2012).

Soil/dust lead levels

The U.S. EPA has set a standard for allowable lead in residential soil and dust at 400 ppm, although there is evidence that a "safe" level may be considerably lower than that. Of the 37 soil samples collected by investigators in the Bagega district of Zamfara in 2010, 37.8% had lead concentrations 1000–10,000 ppm and 21.6% had soil lead concentrations > 10,000 ppm (Ajumobi et al., 2014). In another study of 116 village compounds, 85% of soil samples had lead concentrations exceeding 400 ppm (average 7959 ppm; range: 421 to > 100,000 ppm) (Dooyema et al., 2011). Water from community wells in two villages analyzed in 2010 also had elevated lead levels with 520 ppb and 1300 ppb, respectively, both 40–100 times higher than U.S. EPA limits for drinking water (15 ppb) (Dooyema et al., 2011). Dust gathered inside 22 households (59.5%) exceeded 400 ppm (Dooyema et al., 2011).

Later testing with advanced technologies of soil samples from ore processing villages in Zamfara found that all village soil samples and most indoor dust sweep samples were ≥400 ppm and ranged from 1200 to as high as 185,000 ppm (Plumlee et al., 2013). In the study reported by Lo, only those villages processing ore had elevated soil/dust lead levels ≥400 ppm and young children with BLLs ≥45 μg/dL (Lo et al., 2012) (Fig. 1.8.2).

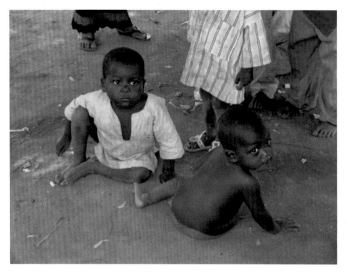

FIG. 1.8.2 Zamfara toddlers playing in soil with 70 times the U.S. EPA lead standard. *(Photo Source: Courtesy Mr. Nasir Umar Tsafe, with permission.)*

Toxicology of lead

Lead is perhaps the most studied metal with regard to its health effects in humans, dating back to the writings of Orfila in the early 1800's (Orfila, 1817). A variety of mechanisms underlie the pathogenesis of human toxicity associated with exposure to high concentrations of lead. But even though it has been the subject of decades of basic research, there are still many unanswered questions regarding the cellular, subcellular, and genetic systems damage associated with lead.

A divalent cation, lead mimics other cations and binds sterically to protein receptors with even greater affinity than calcium or zinc, changing the spatial configuration of protein groups and disrupting cellular physiology and, thereby, their function (Garza et al., 2006).

Lead irreversibly binds to sulfhydryl groups commonly found in many enzyme systems, disrupting their function. Examples include enzymes important for hemoglobin synthesis in the red blood cell: delta-aminolevulinic acid dehydratase which catalyzes formation of the porphyrin ring and ferrochelatase, which catalyzes the penultimate incorporation of iron into the protoporphyrin ring, resulting in functional hemoglobin. If iron cannot enter the ring because of enzyme inhibition, then zinc substitutes and is inserted into the ring, producing nonfunctional zinc-chelated protoporphyrin. Interference with these enzymes contributes to the development of the microcytic, hypochromic anemia typically seen in moderate to severe childhood lead poisoning.

Lead competes with calcium for receptor binding at the subcellular level, which contributes to cellular dysfunction. It binds to and inhibits calcium-activated proteins and calmodulin, and inhibits protein kinase C. It blocks calcium-dependent membrane channels and voltage-gated channels, slowing calcium entry and disrupting intra/extra-cellular calcium homeostasis (Garza et al., 2006). Disruption of the voltage-gated channels changes the permeability of the cell membrane and allows heavy metals, such as lead, to cross into the cytosol. Lead can indirectly alter genetic RNA/DNA transcription fidelity and thereby negatively modulate a number of downstream neuronal pathways (Stansfield et al., 2012). It also can disrupt mitochondrial metabolism as well as the subcellular second messenger system.

In the developing brain, lead can interfere with bidirectional, presynaptic and postsynaptic signaling processes and disrupt neuronal synaptogenesis during development, contributing to changed dendritic morphology, disrupted migration, and reduced spine density (Stansfield et al., 2012). Myelin production and deposition, intracellular synaptic vesicle formation, mobilization, and release, neuronal pruning, astroglia and oligodendroglia cell differentiation, and neural organization are also altered by lead. Lead also interferes with calcium-mediated neurotransmitter release and re-uptake in the neuronal synaptic cleft.

Other body systems besides the neurological system are also affected. Lead interferes with cellular function in the renal glomerulus and tubules and can contribute to chronic renal dysfunction and hypertension. It also is toxic to bone cells (osteoblasts and osteoclasts), leading to interruptions in normal skeletal growth and remodeling. Lead affects cellular function in the endocrine system (e.g., parathyroid gland function and interference with vitamin D-mediated osteocalcin synthesis). Lead is toxic to auditory nerve cells; chronic exposures can be associated with subtle hearing impairment.

CDC and partners offer assistance and environmental remediation

In response to the Zamfara disaster, the U.S. CDC partnered with the government of Nigeria and international nongovernmental organizations to mount an unprecedented campaign of education, environmental remediation, and medical treatment of affected children with chelation. The response required an interdisciplinary, interagency effort. The Zamfara State Ministry of Health, the State Ministry of Mines and Solid Minerals, and the Zamfara State Ministry of the Environment were all mobilized to provide adequate support to address the situation. The federal Ministries of Health and the Environment also provided support for this mission and banned gold mining in June 2010 (Fig. 1.8.3). The ban was lifted in June 2012 and subsequently reinstated in the Fall of 2019.

Terra Graphics and the Blacksmith Institute worked with the Zamfara Emirate to clean contaminated compounds by removing 5 cm of topsoil, allowing soil levels to fall back to a background lead concentration of 15–17 ppm. Contaminated soil was deposited in large waste pits that were given the status of cemeteries by local religious leaders to prevent their being disturbed. The site surveys and remediation were conducted locally.

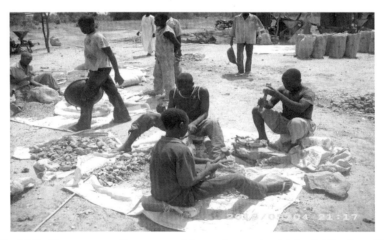

FIG. 1.8.3 Teenagers pounding ore-containing rocks on the jobsite in Zamfara—2010. *(Photo Source: Courtesy Mr. Nasir Umar Tsafe, with permission.)*

Clinical features of childhood Lead poisoning

Children are especially susceptible to hemorrhagic encephalopathy caused by high lead levels. Severe lead encephalopathy is associated with life-threatening seizures and cerebral edema in both children and adults. The brains of young children do not readily exclude the metal and it can damage, through both direct and indirect toxic effects, endothelial cells, microglial function, neurons, and the cerebral microvasculature. Adverse effects associated with BLLs as low as 5 µg/dL are consistent across a wide range of health outcomes, across major physiological systems from reproductive to renal, among multiple groups, and from studies using substantially different methods and techniques.

The U.S. National Toxicology Program (NTP) found sufficient evidence to confirm that, in children, BLLs < 5 µg/dL can cause an increased diagnosis of attention-related behavioral problems, a greater incidence of problem behaviors, and decreased cognitive performance as indicated by (1) lower academic achievement, (2) decreased IQ, and (3) reductions in specific cognitive measures (NTP, 2012). They also found limited evidence that blood lead < 5 µg/dL is associated with delayed puberty and decreased kidney function in children ≥ 12 years of age and sufficient evidence that BLLs < 10 µg/dL in children are associated with delayed puberty and reduced postnatal growth (NTP, 2012).

Changes in other physiological functions in children have been demonstrated at relatively low BLLs, such as signs of reduced hemoglobin formation, slower nerve conduction velocity, and anecdotal description by parents of poor appetite, irritable behaviors, loss of focus and attention, poor sleeping, and constipation. Higher BLLs are associated with intermittent abdominal pain (lead colic), peripheral neuropathies (e.g., wrist-drop and foot-drop, seen more often in adults than children), and frank microcytic anemia with or without basophilic stippling.

BLLs ≥ 45 µg/dL are rare in affluent countries, but children continue to experience very high BLLs in low and middle income countries. Children can experience advanced neurologic toxicity such as encephalopathy, increased intracranial pressure, and seizures at BLL above 70 µg/dL. Venous BLLs well above the lethal dose have been identified in several countries in the past decade and were found as a result of testing numerous Zamfara children. Children who do not die from severe plumbism are often left with significant disabilities including blindness, hearing loss, seizure disorders, severe intellectual disability, motor dysfunction, and erratic behavior. A study of 972 Zamfara children < 5 years of age who had BLL > 45 µg/dL reported a geometric mean BLL of 79.4 µg/dL; 35% had a BLL > 80 µg/dL (Greig et al., 2014). Of the 972 children studied, 9% had some clinically identified neurological features consistent with lead poisoning; but only those with BLL > 105 µg/dL had life-threatening signs, such as seizures or altered consciousness.

Chelation of Zamfara children with succimer

Chelation therapy has proven to be life-saving in the worst cases of lead poisoning. Animal studies on dimercaptosuccinic acid (DMSA; also known as succimer) confirm that it can lower blood and brain lead levels (Smith and Strupp, 2013). However, the neurologic deficits and other harms caused by the lead exposure are not necessarily reversed by the therapy. Succimer is an oral drug that shows binding activity for metals including lead. The bound moiety is subsequently excreted in urine, resulting in a lead diuresis.

In the Zamfara tragedy, many children died before succimer therapy could be initiated. Limited supplies and the concern that adults given succimer would use it while they continued to process ore in illegal mining activities resulted in most of the drug being used therapeutically to treat only the sickest children. One study (Thurtle et al., 2014) documented the outcomes of 3180 courses (up to 15 cycles per patient of either 28 days or 19 days in treatment duration) of treatment with succimer in a cohort of 1156 children aged 5 years and younger. *Médecin Sans Frontières* worked to identify and treat children with BLL ≥ 45 mcg/dL. Many of the children manifested encephalopathy; 36% of the children had BLL ≥ 80 mcg/dL and 6% had BLL ≥ 120 mcg/dL. Succimer reduced lead-related childhood mortality from 65% reported in the literature to 1.5% (20 children). The drug was effective in a net reduction in BLL from the pretreatment level in 71% of children who received it, with no reports of severe adverse events (Thurtle et al., 2014). Authors noted that re-exposure to a home environment that had not yet been remediated, and nonadherence with this oral medication, probably accounted for a lower than expected impact of out-patient treatment.

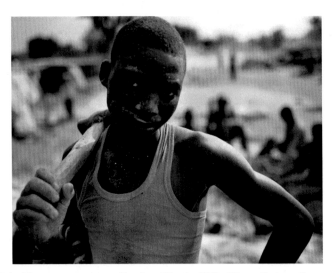

FIG. 1.8.4 Young ore processor, Zamfara, Nigeria 2012. *(Photo Source: Courtesy Marcus Beasdale - Human Rights Watch, with permission)*

Aftermath

Eventually, more than 400 children had died and over 2000 were left permanently disabled from inhalation and ingestion of lead particulates in the Zamfara State mining disaster (Kaufman et al., 2016). After 2011, the international partners and the state and federal government collaboration continued to mitigate the lead crisis in Zamfara and to respond to similar outbreaks in neighboring states. These activities were moderately successful. A representative, population-based study of ore processing and nonprocessing villages conducted throughout Zamfara in 2012 found that only 17.2% families were still engaged in ore processing activities (Kaufman et al., 2016). Although most families had moved their ore processing activities outside the village, children living in villages where anyone participated in ore processing still had significantly higher BLL than those living in villages without ore processing (Fig. 1.8.4). Over 38% of these children still had BLL $\geq 10\,\mu g/dL$. This finding probably represented continued exposure to the hazards of "take home" lead dust on the body and/ or clothing of parents working with ore at the site of the mine. The investigators also found that other sources of lead were widespread in Zamfara including galena-based eyeliner, drinking water, and bricks made from ore wastes (Kaufman et al., 2016). Food contamination was also later identified as another source of lead exposure among both children and adults living in Zamfara State, with concentrations of lead as high as 145 ppm in contaminated foods (Plumlee et al., 2013; Tirima et al., 2018).

In 2015, 28 childhood lead poisoning deaths related to gold ore processing in the same ore vein but in Niger State were reported. The rapid response of Nigerian officials trained during the Zamfara outbreak resulted in no further deaths and a deep reduction in BLLs (Kaufman et al., 2016). As these reports indicate, even after the Zamfara experience children remained at risk for lead poisoning throughout Nigeria from multiple sources. Continued vigilance including routine BLL testing, initiation of safer processing practices, education about the dangers of lead exposure throughout the region and sustained support from federal and state officials are critical to preventing future tragedies. The current tensions and intertribal violence have hampered efforts to sustain these activities and reduced the ability to reach remote villages.

Lessons learned

Small-scale mining provides much needed income to families. The high price of gold poses a continuing threat that ore processing will recommence, and villages will be recontaminated. Given the economic importance and rootedness of small-scale mining in countless rural economies across low and moderate income countries, developing sustainable, transferrable, safer mining practices is of critical importance.

The Zamfara outbreak also reinforces the need for international organizations to respond to complicated environmental disasters based on the following five organizing principles (Tirima et al., 2016):

1. widespread dissemination of education regarding the hazards of lead exposure to the exposed community;
2. reliance on community political and cultural leaders to work with the project staff and community members in the design and conduct of the remediation;
3. a deep respect for cultural norms and practices;
4. wherever possible the use of local residents to conduct the work; and
5. training and active transfer of all aspects of the work to local officials.

The Zamfara lead poisoning experience itself revealed new public health uses of biomonitoring techniques and how medical chelation therapy could be applied to the management of severely lead poisoned victims living in rural conditions of extreme poverty.

The disaster also brought into focus the need for definitive environmental remediation, coupled with more enlightened governmental policies and enforcement, as the only ways to achieve tangible, sustained and long-lasting improvements to the health and safety of the affected population. "Collaboration between governments and the international community can prevent lead poisoning in children. When strategies such as use of processing techniques that control dust and residual ore wastes, continued blood lead surveillance, chelation therapy when warranted, and environmental cleanup of hazardous sites are successfully implemented, a sustained reduction of BLL in children can be achieved" (Bashir et al., 2014).

References

Ajumobi OO, Tsofo A, Yango M, Aworh MK, Anagbogu IN, Mohammed A, et al. High concentration of blood lead levels among young children in Bagega community, Zamfara—Nigeria and the potential risk factor. Pan Afr Med J 2014;18(Suppl 1):14.

Bashir M, Umar-Tsafe N, Getso K, Kaita IM, Nasidi A, Nasir SG, et al. Assessment of blood lead levels among children aged ≤5 years—Zamfara state, Nigeria, June-July 2012. Centers for disease control. MMWR—Morb Mortal Wkly Rep 2014;63(15):325–7.

Centers for Disease Control & Prevention (CDC). Childhood lead poisoning prevention: standard surveillance definitions and classifications, https://www.cdc.gov/nceh/lead/data/case-definitions-classifications.htm; 2019. [Accessed 27 March 2020].

Dooyema CA, Neri A, Lo YC, Durant J, Dargan PI, Swarthout T, et al. Outbreak of fatal childhood lead poisoning related to artisanal gold mining in northwestern Nigeria, 2010. Environ Health Perspect 2011;120(4):601–7.

Garza A, Vega R, Soto E. Cellular mechanisms of lead neurotoxicity. Med Sci Monit 2006;12(3):RA57–65.

Greig J, Thurtle N, Cooney L, Ariti C, Ahmed AO, Ashagre T, et al. Association of blood lead level with neurological features in 972 children affected by an acute severe lead poisoning outbreak in Zamfara state, northern Nigeria. PLoS One 2014;9(4), e93716.

Kaufman JA, Brown MJ, Umar-Tsafe NT, Adbullahi MB, Getso KI, Kaita IM, et al. Prevalence and risk factors of elevated blood Lead in children in gold ore processing communities, Zamfara, Nigeria, 2012. J Health Pollut 2016;6(11):2–8.

Lo YC, Dooyema CA, Neri A, Durant J, Jeffries T, Medina-Marino A, et al. Childhood lead poisoning associated with gold ore processing: a village-level investigation-Zamfara state, Nigeria, October-November 2010. Environ Health Perspect 2012;120(10):1450–5.

Macrotrends. Historical gold prices over the past 100 years, https://www.macrotrends.net/1333/historical-gold-prices-100-year-chart; 2020. [Accessed 26 March 2020].

National Toxicology Program (NTP), National Institute of Environmental Health Sciences (NIEHS), National Institutes of Health (NIH). NTP monograph on health effects of low-level lead. Washington, DC: U.S. Department of Health & Human Services; 2012.

Anon. Nigeria Demographic and Health Survey (NDHS). Abuja, Nigeria: National Population Commission of Nigeria and ICF Macro; 2008. 2009.

Orfila MP. A general system toxicology or, a treatise on poisons found in the mineral, vegetable and animal kingdoms [electronic resource]: considered in their relations with physiology, pathology and medical jurisprudence. Philadelphia, Pennsylvania: M. Carey; 1817.

Plumlee GS, Durant JT, Morman SA, Neri A, Wolf RE, Dooyema CA, et al. Linking geological and health sciences to assess childhood lead poisoning from artisanal gold mining in Nigeria. Environ Health Perspect 2013;121(6):744–50.

Smith D, Strupp BJ. The scientific basis for chelation: animal studies and lead chelation. J Med Toxicol 2013;9:326–8.

Stansfield KH, Pilsner R, Lu Q, Wright RO, Guilarte TR. Dysregulation of BDNF-TrkB signaling in developing hippocampal neurons by Pb^{+2}: implications for an environmental basis of neurodevelopmental disorders. Toxicol Sci 2012;127(1):277–95.

Thurtle N, Greig J, Cooney L, Amitai Y, Ariti C, Brown MJ, et al. Description of 3,180 courses of chelation with dimercaptosuccinic acid in children <5 years with severe lead poisoning in Zamfara northern Nigeria: a retrospective analysis of programme data. PLoS Med 2014;11(10):1–18.

Tirima S, Bartrem C, von Lindern I, et al. Environmental remediation to address childhood lead poisoning epidemic due to artisanal gold mining in Zamfara, Nigeria. Environ Heal Perspect 2016;124(9):1471–8.

Tirima S, Bartrem C, von Lindern I, et al. Food contamination as a pathway for lead exposure in children during the 2010–2013 lead poisoning epidemic in Zamfara, Nigeria. J Environ Sci (China) 2018;67:260–72.

Chapter 1.9

Itai-Itai disease—Japan, 1955

Alan D. Woolf

Boston Children's Hospital & Harvard Medical School, Boston, Massachusetts, United States

The tragic story of industrial pollution in Toyama, Japan, is the story of a silent epidemic that evolved over more than half a century into the worst cadmium poisoning of a population that the world has ever known. The Toyama Prefecture is a rural plain in the northwest coastal area of central Japan on the banks of the fast-moving Jinzugawa (Jinzu) River (Figs. 1.9.1 and 1.9.2). The Jinzu River, fed by two mountain streams: the Miya and Takahara Rivers, runs 126 km northward from mountains with peaks as high as 3000 m (Aoshima, 2016). At the second Jinzu dam, the waters flow more gently fanning out into

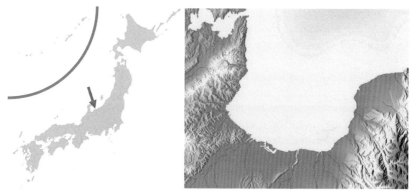

FIG. 1.9.1   (A) Map of Japan with arrow indicating vicinity of Toyama Prefecture. (B) Toyama Bay. *((A) from https://commons.wikimedia.org/w/index.php?title=Special:Search&limit=20&offset=60&profile=default&search=Map+of+Japan&advancedSearch-current=%7b%7d&ns0=1&ns6=1&ns12=1&ns14=1&ns100=1&ns106=1#/media/File:Blank_map_of_Japan.svg" https://commons.wikimedia.org/w/index.php?title=Special:Search&limit=20&offset=60&profile=default&search=Map+of+Japan&advancedSearch-current={}&ns0=1&ns6=1&ns12=1&ns14=1&ns100=1&ns106=1#/media/File:Blank_map_of_Japan.svg. (B) from https://commons.wikimedia.org/w/index.php?search=Toyama+Bay&title=Special%3ASearch&go=Go&ns0=1&ns6=1&ns12=1&ns14=1&ns100=1&ns106=1#/media/File:Toyama_Bay.png.)*

History of Modern Clinical Toxicology. https://doi.org/10.1016/B978-0-12-822218-8.00024-7
109

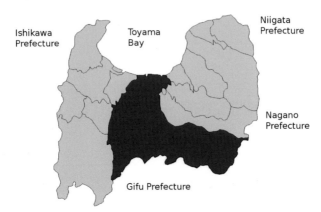

FIG. 1.9.2 Detail of Toyama Prefecture. *Source: https://commons.wikimedia.org/w/index. php?search=Toyama%20prefecture&title=Special%3ASearch&ns0=1&ns6=1&ns12=1&ns14=1& ns100=1&ns106=1#/media/File:Toyama_in_Toyama_Prefecture.png, Author: Krisgrotius.*

the Jinzu River basin and depositing sediments in the delta region before empty-ing into the Japan Sea. In the 1960s the basin was home to more than 1 million people, including farmers growing rice, soybeans, and other vegetables on land fed by irrigation from the river basin. Fishermen fished the river to supply an-other staple in the Japanese diet. The populace also used river water for drinking and other household purposes.

Mining for gold and silver in this mountainous region of Japan began as early as the 16th century. Later in the 20th century, the Kamioka Mine, owned by the Mitsui Mining & Smelting Company Ltd. (Mitsui Kinzoku), operated in the mountains about 30 km upstream from Toyama City (Kaji, 2012). Until the 1940s the mine produced mainly lead, which was distributed throughout Japan and used in the fabrication of a variety of commercial products, machinery, and military supplies. The mine was one of the richest sources of zinc in all of Japan and beginning in the 1940s was almost exclusively producing lead and zinc to meet the country's wartime demands. In geological formations, cad-mium runs in the same ores as copper and zinc (e.g., sphalerite ore) and so is present as a by-product in mining operations aimed at extracting these metals (Kaji, 2012).

Industrial-scale zinc mining operations at the Kamioka mine inevitably produced cadmium-containing slag and liquid sludge beginning in 1905. The tailings contaminated the river bed and the soil of lands fed by river tributar-ies downstream. Retention settling pools and other methods implemented as early as 1916 by the mining company to reduce the waste effluent were in-adequate to prevent the finely powdered cadmium-containing particles from entering the waste stream. These pollutants were discharged into the Takahara River where the river merges with the Jinzu. Rivers can carry such metals as contaminated particulates for considerable distances, as far as 80 km from the source.

Mining operations at the Mitsui plant increased during both World Wars I and II. The military demands for raw metals required maximum production efforts during the second Sino-Japanese War (1937–45). Cadmium-containing wastes had polluted the river waters and settled into riverbed sediments for more than 50 years before adverse health effects associated with the pollution began to be suspected in the 1950s. By 1977 an estimated 3000 tons of cadmium had been distributed into the agricultural plain downstream (Kasuya et al., 1992). Even as late as 1982, 80 kg/year of cadmium was being discharged into the river. Studies of cadmium content of paddy field soils around Toyama as early as 1967 showed elevated concentrations of cadmium greater than 1 ppm and as high as 8 ppm. Even as late as 1984–85, samples of irrigated soils near the river in areas marked as polluted had mean cadmium levels of 1.13 ppm (Kasuya et al., 1992).

Cadmium in fish, rice, and vegetables

Not only did cadmium from the industrial waste contaminate the water and river bed downstream from the mining concern but it also concentrated in the tissues of fish caught from the river and in foodstuffs grown in the contaminated soil and paddy fields fed by river water. The fine particles containing cadmium were oxidized, releasing toxic ions easily absorbed into crops, fish, and people. By the 1950s, farmers and fishermen in the Jinzu River basin noted that crop yields were down and there were not as many fish to catch. Rice is a particularly efficient accumulator of metal contaminants such as arsenic and cadmium. There were elevated cadmium levels in staples of the Japanese diet such as fish, rice, and soybeans. About 40% of unpolished rice grown in polluted areas harvested in 1971–76 had elevated cadmium concentrations exceeding the 0.4 ppm threshold above which it was not advisable to be eaten, and 9% had cadmium levels exceeding 1 ppm (Aoshima, 1987; Kasuya et al., 1992). Although rice production in paddies heavily polluted with cadmium had been prohibited by law in the 1970s, it was still widely grown in polluted areas for private consumption. Even as late as 1983–84, rice harvests in the Toyama prefecture had some measured cadmium levels over 0.4 ppm (Aoshima, 1987; Kasuya et al., 1992). The Jinzu River basin included the towns of Fuchu-machi, Ohsawano, Yatsuo, and Toyama City, whose people were served by agricultural lands irrigated by the river; these were the areas where Itai-Itai disease was later found to be endemic.

Discovery of Itai-Itai disease

The poisoning got its name, *Itai Itai Byō disease* (Japanese for "ouch ouch" or "it hurts it hurts" disease) referring to the common severe bone pain associated with elevated body burdens of cadmium from chronic environmental exposures. Victims with advanced disease also suffered the intense, incapacitating pain of the many fractures experienced after only seemingly minor trauma. For a long time, people living along the Jinzu River had suffered medical ills, but attributed them to some unknown sort of infection or just a natural infirmity. A local physician, Dr. Shigejiro Hagino identified the disease among his patients as early as 1935 (Kaji, 2012). Although mining activities had been ongoing in the mountains for centuries, it was not until 1955 that his son, Dr. Noboru Hagino, a physician living in Fuchu, described symptoms of bone and joint pain, especially in the pelvis and legs, occurring in some of his patients too. The local newspaper, the *Toyama Shinbun,* first coined the term: "Itai Itai disease" "it hurts it hurts" as describing the exclamations of patients suffering the bone and joint pain (Kaji, 2012). The younger Dr. Hagino, as well as his father, suspected that the cause of the disease was due to wastes coming from the mine. Informal records from previous decades suggested that the syndrome had been endemic to the local inhabitants of the Jinzu River basin at least since the 1930s and possibly before that (Tsuchiya, 1969a). Dr. Noboru Hagino and others presented their clinical findings at medical meetings; osteomalacia seemed to be the cardinal feature of the condition. The incidence of the disease was disproportionately high in women over the age of 40 years. Dr. Hagino's theory that the mining was responsible was heavily criticized by others, who claimed the disease was caused by poor diet, too strenuous work, or too much sunshine.

Early epidemiologic investigations

Two study groups were subsequently formed in 1961, one by the Japanese Ministry of Health and Welfare, the Ministry of Education and health authorities of the local prefecture. A second "Inspection Board of Ouch-Ouch Disease" was also charged with investigating the cause of Itai-Itai disease (Kaji, 2012). One group included medical faculty and epidemiologists from the nearby Kanazawa University School of Medicine. These two groups merged their efforts. They studied clinical characteristics of nine middle-aged female patients admitted to Kanazawa University Hospital for treatment of Itai-Itai disease, comparing them to eight patients suffering from other bone disease and four healthy, younger persons (Tsuchiya, 1969a; Tsuchiya, 1969b). The patients had increased excretion of cadmium in their urine, but no elevations in the urinary levels of lead or zinc.

Governmental and prefecture health authorities subsequently began mass surveys of people living in the prefecture over the next several years in the 1960s. They developed clinical criteria (e.g., bone pain, shortened height, and gait disturbances) and radiological measures (e.g., bone cortex thinning and decalcification, healing zones, and multiple fractures) for the diagnosis of Itai-Itai disease, including blood (i.e., alkaline phosphatase and phosphorus) and urine (i.e., protein and glucose) tests. A total of 223 cases of Itai-Itai disease were identified by the study group; and it attributed 56 previous deaths to the disease (Tsuchiya, 1969a, b). Meanwhile, three different institutes (the Okayama Agricultural Institute, Toyama Prefecture Health Institute and Kanazawa University) began to take samples from different layers of the waste piles of the Kamioka Mine, as well as soil and water samples downstream. The cadmium measured in the slag and the river sediments and paddy soil samples was found to be quite elevated.

The results of the study group's investigations confirmed that the health problems experienced by people living in the Toyama Prefecture were not caused by lead poisoning, malnutrition, hard labor, "senile osteomalacia," excessive vitamin D intake, infections, or any of the other explanations offered by some researchers and mining company officials. The study group concluded that Itai-Itai disease was confined to the Jinzu River basin, was manifest early as proximal tubular dysfunction discovered in the kidney function of many of the local people, and was caused by cadmium coming from the Kamioka mine.

Formal recognition of Itai-Itai disease by Japanese government

Notably the Ministry of Health & Welfare in Japan recognized that a new approach to address industrial impacts on the environment was needed, and in 1964 a pollution department was established within the ministry (Kaji, 2012). The Toyama Prefecture health authorities began conducting formal health surveys for adult residents in the Jinzu River basin in 1967, with record-keeping used in follow-up studies of the natural history of the disease for decades. In 1968, the Ministry of Health and Welfare in Japan made a formal statement that the cause of Itai-Itai disease was due to cadmium pollution. This recognition was unfortunately much too late for those who had died of Itai-Itai disease in the 1940s and 1950s. It has been estimated that more than 7000 people living in the Toyama Prefecture suffered health effects related to Itai-Itai disease, let alone hundreds more victims who went undiagnosed and undiscovered during mining operations dating back to the 1930s and before.

Subsequently, prefecture authorities surveyed the rice paddies in the 1970s and found soil cadmium levels four times higher than paddies in unpolluted areas, and cadmium levels 2.5 times higher in rice grown in those contaminated sites (Aoshima, 2016). Soil replacement in the agricultural plain was undertaken by the Japanese government from 1980 to 2012, reclaiming some formerly polluted paddies that now grew rice with much safer cadmium levels of ≤ 0.1 ppm.

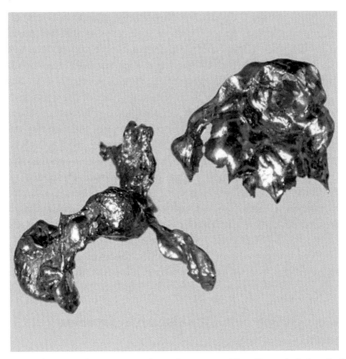

FIG. 1.9.3 Cadmium pieces. *(From https://commons.wikimedia.org/w/index.php?search=cadmium&title=Special%3ASearch&profile=advanced&fulltext=1&advancedSearch-current=%7B%7D&ns0=1&ns6=1&ns12=1&ns14=1&ns100=1&ns106=1#/media/File:Cadmium-pieces.jpg)*

Toxicology

Cadmium has a variety of industrial and commercial uses, including the manufacture of plastics, alloys, pigments, rechargeable batteries, and other products (Fig. 1.9.3). A common source of cadmium exposure generally is cigarette smoking. Blood cadmium levels in smokers are higher than nonsmokers. About 5% of ingested cadmium is absorbed via the gastrointestinal tract, although as much as 20% may be absorbed by individuals deficient in iron or calcium (Friberg, 1984). After absorption, cadmium is transported to the liver by albumen, where it induces production of the protein, metallothionein, to which it is bound tightly (Fig. 1.9.4). Normal whole blood concentrations of cadmium are less than 5 mcg/L and normal urinary excretion is < 2 mcg/day (< 1 mcg/g creatinine). Cadmium concentrations in segmental hair samples are also useful biomarkers of an accumulating body burden of the metal over time.

The nephrotoxic Cd-thionein complex accumulates in proximal renal tubules, where Cd is released intracellularly, damaging proximal tubular cells (Fig. 1.9.4). The metal then is released and bound again to metallothionein, leading to its prolonged retention in the glomerulus. As the binding capacity

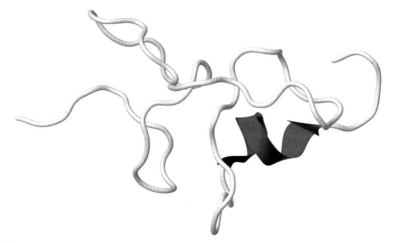

FIG. 1.9.4 Cartoon of metallothionein with red areas showing metal binding sites. *(From https://commons.wikimedia.org/wiki/Category:Metallothionein#/media/File:Metallothionein. png) Author: Jmol software developing team.)*

of metallothiolein is exceeded, newly freed cadmium ions continue to damage tubular cells. The body has no physiological mechanism to enhance elimination of cadmium; cadmium urinary excretion is a good measure of body burden (Friberg, 1984). As much as one-third of the total body burden of Cd is deposited either in the liver or the kidneys, where it is stored with a biological half-life as long as 30 years. With continued dietary exposures, ingested cadmium progressively accumulates in the body over time and contributes to the progressive nature of Itai-Itai disease over time. As renal damage progresses, the kidney is able to store less and less cadmium and its excretion into urine increases as the levels in the renal cortex itself go down (Friberg, 1984). At autopsy, cadmium concentrations in the liver, pancreas, and thyroid were 5 times higher in patients with Ita-Itai disease than in those of uncontaminated controls (Aoshima, 2016).

Health effects

Itai-Itai disease is most common in menopausal, multiparous women, especially those who have diets deficient in calcium and vitamin D. Other dietary deficiencies, including iron and protein, enhance cadmium absorption. Cadmium itself also inhibits vitamin D hydroxylation, which contributes to low vitamin D activity. Derangements in calcium/phosphorus metabolism contribute to more severe osteomalacia. Severe Itai-Itai disease presents initially as a dull pain over the shoulders, spine, lower back, and knees, with spreading discomfort to the arms and legs over time. Multiple pseudofractures heal with noncalcified osteoid formation. Some such fractures can remain nonunited, eventually leading to bony abnormalities and distortions, with curvatures, loss of body length, and increasing disability (Blainey et al., 1980). Patients developed a hunched over appearance, a loss of stature, and a slow, waddling-like gait, with progressive impairment of their everyday functioning.

Serum alkaline phosphate levels rise over time and the bones become malformed, brittle, and fragile. The osteomalacia becomes so severe that spontaneous fractures are possible with changes in position, sneezing, or other seemingly minor precipitants. Pathology shows a softening of the bones with "loose zones" of matrix disruption, bone remodeling, and osteoid formation. One autopsy study (Baba et al., 2014) of 61 women who had died from Itai-Itai disease showed that the severity of their osteomalacia correlated with the severity of their renal tubulopathy.

Renal damage in Itai-Itai disease

Patients with significant cadmium body burdens develop progressive impairment of renal function with decreasing glomerular filtration rates, proximal tubular injury, and metabolic acidosis. Increased chloride concentrations and renal calcium wasting contribute to urinary tract stone formation in some patients. One 1983–84 study of 158 middle-aged women living in the Jinzu River basin found elevated urinary levels of beta-2 microglobulin, alpha-1 microglobulin, amino acids, glucose, phosphorus, and cadmium compared with controls living in unpolluted areas (Aoshima, 1987). This study confirmed dysfunction in proximal tubular reabsorption in the kidneys of women living in a cadmium-contaminated environment.

Urinary excretion of the low molecular-weight protein, beta-2 microglobulin, is a very sensitive biomarker of cadmium-related renal injury (Nogawa et al., 1983; Aoshima, 1987). Those patients with Itai-Itai disease had renal damage, the severity of which correlated with both the amount of beta-2 microglobulin excretion and their blood cadmium levels. Beta-2 microglobulinuria > 1000 µg per gram creatinine indicated advanced, irreversible tubulopathy. Not only is there tubular dysfunction but the entire glomerulus becomes involved in the progression of renal failure typical of severe Itai-Itai disease (Friberg, 1984). Patients with advanced Itai-Itai disease and renal dysfunction experienced in parallel generalized amino aciduria, hypercalciuria, phosphaturia, generalized proteinuria, and glycosuria characteristic of a full-blown Fanconi Syndrome (Nogawa et al., 1983). Even years later, follow-up measurements of renal function in women with advanced Itai-Itai disease showed continued deterioration.

In addition, the tubular damage interfered with the usual renal conversion of vitamin D to its 1,25 dihydroxy cholecalciferol active metabolite. This chronic deficiency of vitamin D exacerbated the osteomalacia and osteoporosis seen in the disease and could be reversed somewhat when victims were given supplemental calcium and vitamin D in their diets (Blainey et al., 1980). The anemia of chronic disease seen in Itai-Itai disease was attributed to the progressive renal damage, with reductions in the production of erythropoietin and corresponding reductions in red blood mass (Table 1.9.1).

TABLE 1.9.1 Adverse health effects from chronic cadmium poisoning.

Anemia
Cancer (renal, urinary tract, and possibly others)
Bone deformities
Bone pain, severe
Bone fractures
Metabolic acidosis
Nephrolithiasis
Osteomalacia, osteoporosis (increased alkaline phosphatase)
Pseudofractures
Renal disease—tubulointerstitial nephritis
Renal tubular dysfunction (in an advanced state: Fanconi syndrome)
Amino aciduria
Low molecular weight (MW < 40,000) proteinuria
Glucosuria
Hypercalciuria
Phosphaturia
Renal failure
Table created by author.

Long-term clinical toxicity

Victims of Itai-Itai disease originally identified by health surveys in the 1960s have been followed for years. Health consequences of long-term exposure included severe disabilities due to the continued toxic effects of cadmium, especially on the skeleton and kidneys. While supplemental vitamin D and calcium could ameliorate some of the symptoms, other therapies, including chelation, were ineffective. Supportive care, more nutritious uncontaminated food and water, and long-term rehabilitation were all that could be offered to victims.

Long-term follow-up studies used data from health impact surveys originally performed on 7529 residents of the polluted Jinzu River basin by the Ministry of Health and Welfare in the 1970s and 1980s and compared mortality rates with 2149 controls living in areas unpolluted by cadmium (Nishijo et al., 2018). Researchers identified increased mortality from renal and uterine cancers in women with a history of proteinuria and/or glucosuria linked to elevated cadmium body burdens and a previous diagnosis of Itai-Itai disease. Besides cancer, women with Itai-Itai disease were also more likely to die from pneumonia and renal disease (Nishijo et al., 2017). Other studies confirmed lowered life expectancies for both men and women suffering from Itai-Itai disease in the Jinzu River basin, with increased mortality from cancers, ischemic heart disease, and renal disorders (Maruzeni et al., 2014). Mortality rates were highest in the populations that lived closest to the polluted river areas and lower in areas of low pollution further away. Other factors, such as hard agricultural labor or, in women, the number of pregnancies/deliveries did not contribute to the observed higher mortality rate attributable to Itai-Itai disease (Kobayashi et al., 2002).

Aftermath and government restitution

The "Itai-Itai Disease Residents' Association" was established in Fuchu-machi by victims and activists (including Dr. Hagino) in 1966 with aims to provide relief to victims, free water supplies, remediation of soil in the agricultural paddies, and acknowledgment of corporate responsibility (Kaji, 2012). The first lawsuit against both the government and the mining company was filed in 1968 for 61 million yen by young lawyers representing 14 victims of Itai-Itai disease and their families (Kaji, 2012). After much testimony, onsite verifications and pleadings, the court verdict came down in favor of the plaintiffs in 1971. An appeal by the Mitsui Mining Company was dismissed a year later; and the company was held responsible for compensating victims for all damages and for remediating contaminated soils.

A restitution program had been proposed by the Japanese government to provide compensation from the mining company to patients suffering from advanced Itai-Itai disease. For purposes of relief, victims were registered, using government-derived definitions:

1. by geography (living in a polluted locale),
2. symptoms beginning in adulthood (ruling out congenital disease),
3. evidence of renal tubulopathy by virtue of proteinuria and/or glucosuria, and
4. the presence of clinically evident osteomalacia and osteoporosis.

While over 400 patients were estimated to have been afflicted with Itai-Itai disease between 1910 and 2007 (Kaji, 2012), as of 2015, only 200 patients had been officially certified with the disease for compensation by the company (Aoshima, 2016). And there were many other inhabitants of the Jinzu River basin who were not diagnosed and were not counted, but who suffered and died from cadmium toxicity-related causes.

Company officials and the victims' association together hammered out the "Pollution Control Agreement" to implement the court's findings, including the right of community representatives to inspect the factory at any time of their choosing. Regular inspections with community participation started in 1972 and slowly a more productive, collaborative relationship with company leaders was forged (Kaji, 2012). Over the next 40 years, the company reduced the cadmium content in the factory's effluent dramatically, so that there was no further pollution of the restored agricultural lands downstream in the river basin. The Mitsui

Company paid some 280 million yen for inspections and more research between 1972 and 2010, and invested 21.3 billion yen in pollution control strategies, based on advice from experts within the Association (Kaji, 2012).

The Mitsui Mining & Smelting Company Ltd. closed the Kamioka Mine in June 2001, and there are no more mining operations on the mountain today, although refining and smelting of imported ore continues, using the present facilities (Kaji, 2012). There is today a museum dedicated to the people living along the Jinzu River who have suffered from Itai-Itai disease (Toyama Prefecture Itai Itai Museum, 2019).

Lessons learned

Lessons learned from the Jinzu River cadmium pollution tragedy include the realization that once the contamination of an ecosystem occurs, the consequences to the environment and the people living there are much longer lasting than anyone could have imagined. Many of the effects on the health of the population were a legacy that claimed an entire generation.

It was demonstrated that a "wait-and-see" scientific approach to community health concerns was not good enough—aggressive remediation and health-promoting public policies could and should be enacted using the guidance of available scientific studies rather than waiting years for conclusive evidence. Waiting for definitive studies would risk further cases of illness due to suspected environmental pollution—a "precautionary principle" was shown in Toyama to be the correct administrative rationale for action (Kaji, 2012).

The legal remedies consequent to this industrial catastrophe also modeled how long-term solutions could be pursued. The affected communities were involved in monitoring of compliance, factory inspections, and decision-making regarding environmental pollution control and prevention. Public participation reduced the potential risk for further pollution of the community by industrial mining operations.

Cadmium contamination in other Japanese prefectures

Chronic cadmium poisoning from environmental sources was eventually recognized in other locales in Japan besides the Toyama Prefecture. For example, health authorities in Kosaka and Odate, towns in the Akita Prefecture that are near several satellite mines and smelting operations, recently performed hospital-based screenings of patients with unexplained declining renal function. They reported evidence of cadmium-related nephrotoxicity in 10% of 57 older patients, as evidenced by increased blood and urine cadmium levels and increased urinary excretion of beta-2 microglobulin protein (Sasaki et al., 2019). Cases were also reported among people living in the Kakebashi river basin in the Ishikawa Prefecture, people living in the Ichi River Basin in the Ilyuogo Prefecture, people in Annaka City in the Gumma Prefecture, and people living in the Sasu area and Izuhara town in the Nagasaki Prefecture (Kanazawa University, 2019).

References

Aoshima K. Epidemiology of renal tubular dysfunction in the inhabitants of a cádmium-pollluted área of the Jinzu River basin in Toyama prefecture. Tohoku J Exp Med 1987;152:151–72.

Aoshima K. *Itai-itai* disease: renal tubular osteomalacia induced by environmental exposure to cádmium - historical review and perspectives. Soil Sci Plant Nutrition 2016;62(4):319–26.

Baba H, Tsuneyama K, Kumada T, Aoshima K, Imura J. Histopathological analysis for osteomalacia and tubulopathy in ita-itai disease. J Toxicol Sci 2014;39(1):91–6.

Blainey JD, Adams RG, Brewer DB, Harvey TC. Cadmium-induced osteomalacia. Br J Ind Med 1980;37:278–84.

Friberg L. Cadmium and the kidney. Environ Health Perspect 1984;54:1–11.

Kaji M. Role of experts and public participation in pollution control: the case of Itai-itai disease in Japan. Ethics Sci Environ Politics 2012;12:99–111.

Kasuya M, Teranishi H, Aoshima K, Katoh T, Horiguchi H, Morikawa Y, Nishijo M, Iwata K. Water pollution by cadmium and the onset of itai-itai disease. Water Sci Technol 1992;25(11):149–56.

Kobayashi E, Okubo Y, Kido T, Nishijo M, Nakagawa H, Nogawa K. Influence of years engaged in agriculture and number of pregnancies and deliveries on mortality in inhabitants of ther Jinzu River basin area, Japan. Occup Environ Med 2002;59:847–50.

Kanazawa University. Itai Itai Disease 2019, http://www.kanazawa-med.ac.jp/~pubhealt/cadmium2/cadmium02.html.

Maruzeni S, Nishijo M, Nakamura K, Morikawa Y, Sakurai M, Nakashima M, et al. Mortality and causes of death of inhabitants with renal dysfunction induced by cadmium exposure of the polluted Jinzu River basin, Toyama Japan: a 26-year follow-up. Environ Health 2014;13:18–30.

Nishijo M, Nakagawa H, Suwazono Y, Nogawa K, Kido T. Causes of death in patients with Itai-itai disease suffering from severe chronic cadmium poisoning: a nested case-control analysis of a follow-up study in Japan. BMJ Open 2017;7(7), e015694.

Nishijo M, Nakagawa H, Suwazono Y, Nogawa K, Sakurai M, Ishizaki M, Kdo T. Cancer mortality in residents of the cadmium-polluted Jinzu River basin in Toyama, Japan. Toxics 2018;6:23–34.

Nogawa K, Yamada Y, Honda R, Ishizaki M, Tsuritani I, Kawano S, Kato T. The relationship between itai-itai disease among inhabitants of the Jinzu river basin and cadmium in rice. Toxicol Lett 1983;17(3–4):263–6.

Sasaki T, Horiguchi H, Arakawa A, Oguma E, Komatsuda A, Sawada K, et al. Hospital-based screening to detect patients with cadmium nephropathy in cadmium-polluted areas in Japan. Environ Health Prev Med 2019;24(8):1–8.

Toyama Prefecture Itai Itai Museum. Toyama Prefectural Ita Itai Disease Museum, http://itaiitai-dis.jp/lang/english/disease/02.html; 2019. [Accessed 30 December 2019].

Tsuchiya K. Causation of ouch-ouch disease (Itai-Itai Byō)—an introductory review. I. Nature of the disease. Keio J Med 1969a;18(4):181–94.

Tsuchiya K. Causation of ouch-ouch disease (Itai-Itai Byō)—an introductory review. II. Epidemiology and evaluation. Keio J Med 1969b;18(4):195–211.

Chapter 1.10

Japan "Yusho" poisoning, 1968 and Taiwan "Yucheng" poisoning, 1979

Alan D. Woolf
Boston Children's Hospital & Harvard Medical School, Boston, Massachusetts, United States

Rice and rice oil used in cooking are food staples in Japan. In 1968 in the western region of Japan, the rice oil used in everyday cooking was contaminated with heated Kanechlor 400, a mixture of polychlorinated biphenyls (PCBs), polychlorinated quarterphenyls (PCQs), and polychlorinated dibenzofurans (PCDFs). These man-made chemicals have great potential for toxicity, including skin eruptions, disturbed growth in children, lipid metabolic changes, endocrine and immune disturbances, cancer induction and neurotoxicity.

Yusho discovery

The first victim of Yusho was a 3-year old girl evaluated at the Kyushu University Hospital clinic for an unusual, acne-like facial rash in June 1968. By August 13, patients from four families had been referred to the same clinic with similar symptoms (Yoshimura, 2003). By October, still others were found to be afflicted with the mysterious disease. Symptoms included increased eye discharge, pigmentation of the skin, and acneiform skin rashes. Newspaper reports linked the symptoms to ingestion of a particular rice oil, and so the illness was named using the Japanese word "Yusho" or "oil disease."

Epidemiology

A government-sponsored Study Group for Yusho was established at Kyushu University in October 1968. It first described the clinical manifestations in 325 Yusho patients and then constructed a survey of people living in the Fukuoka and Nagasaki Prefectures using defined criteria for inclusion in a case-control study. Consuming rice bran oil contaminated by Kanechlor 400 (chlorine content: 48%) manufactured by the Kanemi Company (K-oil) and produced in Kitakyushu City on or about February 5–6, 1968, was quickly identified as the key feature distinguishing the difference between cases and controls (Kuratsune et al., 1972;

History of Modern Clinical Toxicology. https://doi.org/10.1016/B978-0-12-822218-8.00041-7

121

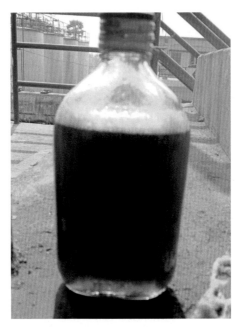

FIG. 1.10.1   Crude rice-bran oil. *(Source: wikimedia commons, https://commons.wikimedia.org/w/index. php?search=crude+rice+bran+oil&title=Special:MediaSearch&go=Go&type=image Author: Palajiri)*

Yoshimura, 2003). Lots of both bottled and canned oil shipped between February 5 and 15 were the only products implicated; oil produced outside that time period was not contaminated (Fig. 1.10.1).

A subsequent prospective investigation by the Yusho Study Group established an attack rate of 64% among exposed people, and correlated the severity of symptoms to the estimated dose of oil intake (Yoshimura, 2003). The case-control study confirmed two significant associations: using rice-bran oil and eating fried foods or tempura every day and the development of Yusho (Kuratsune et al., 1972). Analysis of the suspected rice oil products revealed dioxins present at levels of 2000–3000 ppm. From people's estimates of 800 mL K-oil consumed during February 5 and 6, 1968, investigators calculated the average amount of Kanechlor ingested by Yusho victims to be between 0.5 and 2.0 g.

The outbreak of Yusho involved not only Fukuoka and Nagaski Prefectures but also spread to 20 other prefectures in Western Japan. It peaked in July 1968 and was thought to be over by the end of the year. More than 1961 people had been certified as exposed by government officials by the end of March 2011 and 539 had died—43 years after the original mass exposure (Yoshimura, 2012).

Identifying the chemical poisons

Initially the oil implicated in Yusho was tested for a range of contaminants including pentachlorophenol, naphthalene, machine oil, and pesticides (organochlorines) but none were found. Professor Inagami, on the Faculty of Agriculture at Kyushu University, studied the rice bran oil refining process, especially a deodorization step wherein the oil was heated to 200°C under low atmospheric pressure, using a sealed pump heater containing a heat exchange matrix using Kanechlor 400, a PCB. He found PCBs in samples of the oil consumed by victims of Yusho which he suspected originated from the leaking pump heater. Later, small holes were discovered in the old heating pipe used in the heat exchanger for the deodorization process.

Fresh bottles of the K-oil produced in February were also tested and found to have high chlorine content compared with oil produced at other times (Yoshimura, 2003). Later, analysis of a fatty tissue biopsy from one of the victims also showed increased PCBs. However, doubts continued since PCB levels in the blood of Yusho patients were low and the symptoms could not be reproduced in animal models. It was later discovered that Kanechlor 400 also contained polychlorinated quaterphenyls (PCQs), PCDFs, and polychlorinated dibenzodioxins (PCDDs), in addition to PCBs, all of which are included in the class of compounds termed 'dioxin'. When Kanechlor 400, used as the medium in a heat exchanger, is heated to temperatures greater than 200°C, PCQs and PCDFs are thermochemically created from PCBs. About 20 different PCQ congeners were leaking into the processed cooking oil (Miyata et al., 1985). As a result, the dioxins in the contaminated oil were not the same as those from other known sources of PCBs. Blood of both Yusho and Yu-Cheng (Yu-Cheng to be described later in this chapter) victims also contained, in addition to PCBs, other chemicals—PCQs and PCDFs—that were not detected in the blood of either workers exposed to PCBs or unaffected controls (Kashimoto et al., 1985). Yusho patients still had elevated PCQ levels measured in their blood 11 years after the incident. A supplement to the diagnostic criteria for Yusho was revised on June 14, 1976, to include "unusual composition and concentration of polychlorinated quarterphenyls (PCQs) in the blood" (Furue et al., 2005):

≥ 0.1 ppb—abnormally high
0.03–0.09 ppb—boundary
≤ 0.02 ppb (detection limit)—normal

It has been suggested that the contaminant most responsible for the health issues in Yusho patients was the dioxin-like furan compound: 2,3,4,7,8-pentachlorodibenzofuran (PeCDF) (Matsumoto et al., 2015). Follow-up check-ups of Yusho patients in 2003 continued to show a profile of high levels of dioxins and 2,3,4,7,8-PeCDF in their blood (Furue et al., 2005):

	Yusho patients $N = 269$	Controls $N = 52$
Blood dioxins (pg TEQ/g lipid)	125 (range: 5.5–1176.6)	37 (8.5–85.4)
2,3,4,7,8-PeCDF (pg/g lipid)	176.2 (2.6–1953.5)	15.2 (3.5–41.7)

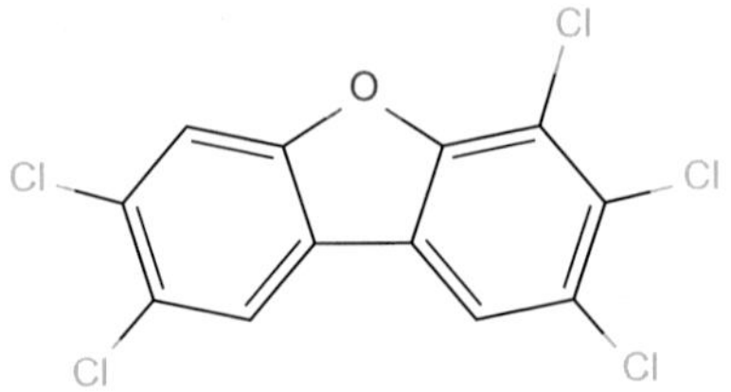

FIG. 1.10.2   Chemical structure of 2,3,4,7,8-pentachlorodibenzofuran (2,3,4,7,8-PeCDF).

It has been estimated that PCDFs contributed about 65% of the TEQ (Toxic Equivalency) in the blood of Yusho victims (Mitoma et al., 2018). The chemical structure of the PCDF is shown in Fig. 1.10.2.

Dioxin background

Dioxins are manmade chemicals produced as a by-product of waste incineration and in the manufacture of paper and pulp bleaching and the synthesis of some chlorine-containing organic chemicals, such as herbicides, pesticides, and fungicides. PCBs were formerly used as dielectric liquids in transformers, as industrial lubricants, and for other industrial and manufacturing purposes. They are environmentally persistent, lipophilic, bio-accumulative pollutants. TCDD (2,3,7,8 tetrachlorodibenzodioxin) was the chemical found in trace amounts as a by-product in the "Agent Orange" chemicals: 2,4 dichlorophenoxtacetic acid (2,4 D) and 2,4,5 trichlorophenoxyacetic acid (2,4,5 T) used as defoliant herbicides delivered by airplanes over large swaths of land during the Vietnam War, which sickened thousands of Vietnamese, as well as American troops. Much of what we know about the toxic effects of dioxins in humans has been learned from occupational exposures of workers in electrical and other industries. Accidental exposures of the public, such as those seen at the chemical explosion at Seveso Italy and in the Yusho and Yu-Cheng oil contamination incidents in Japan and Taiwan, and follow-up studies of veterans of the Vietnam War have provided additional data on toxicity. The reader will find details on the Seveso disaster in Chapter 1.3 of this book. The poisoning of a Ukrainian politician, Viktor Yushchenko, in which pure TCDD was used, is described in Chapter 2.6.

Symptoms and signs of Yusho

Symptoms and signs of Yusho are shown in Table 1.10.1.

Reproductive effects in Yusho patients

Exposure to dioxins has been associated with adverse reproductive effects as well as adverse health effects in children, who are perhaps more vulnerable than adults due to their smaller size, longer life spans, and still developing

TABLE 1.10.1 Clinical findings in Yusho and Yu-Cheng poisoning.

General

Fatigue

Lassitude

Weight loss

Anorexia

Gastrointestinal

Abdominal pain

Diarrhea

Constipation

Integument

Pruritus

Chloracne

Increased sebum

Sebaceous cysts

Face and truncal comedones

Black comedones

Scar formation

Increased sweating

Gingival pigmentation, gingivitis

Nail deformities

Natal teeth

Deformed or missing teeth

Hair follicle accentuation

Hyperpigmentation

Eye

Eye discharge

Meibomian gland cysts or discharge

Liver

Hepatomegaly

Continued

TABLE 1.10.1 Clinical findings in Yusho and Yu-Cheng poisoning—cont'd

Pulmonary
Cough
Increased sputum
Bronchitis
Musculoskeletal
Joint aches and pains
Arthralgia
Weakness
Bursitis
Neurological
Headache
Extremity paresthesias or numbness
Anxiety, depression
Pediatric
Delayed developmental milestones
Cognitive deficits
Learning disabilities
Behavioral issues
Interference with growth
Increased infections
Reproductive
Menstrual difficulties
Increased spontaneous abortion
Hyperpigmented newborns
Low birth weight
Late findings
Chronic liver disease
Cirrhosis
Acute myocardial infarction and heart disease
Liver cancer
Lung cancer (males)

Table created by author using references: Guo 2004, Yoshimura 2003, Yoshimura 2012, Mitoma 2015, Imamura 2007, Furue 2005, Kuratsune 1972.

organ systems. Passage of dioxin-like chemicals and PCBs via the placenta and during breast feeding has been well-established by multiple research studies. Dioxins have endocrine disruption potential: some dioxin-like chemicals have both estrogenic and antiestrogenic effects, while others have androgenic and antiandrogenic effects. Animal and human studies have shown associations with increased rates of stillbirth and spontaneous abortion. Reproductive difficulties in women diagnosed with Yusho were reported, with increased rates of preterm delivery and induced abortions, changes in the sex ratio of births and low birth weight for gestational age (Tsukimori et al., 2008). Some infants—both still-births and live births—of mothers with Yusho or Yu-Cheng oil poisoning were born with unusually dark grayish-brown pigmentation (so-called "cola-colored" or "black" babies) which gradually faded over time (Hsu et al., 1985).

Studies of children born to Taiwanese women suffering from Yu-Cheng poisoning documented increased delays in reaching developmental milestones, lower cognitive scores, higher rates of learning disabilities, and increased behavioral concerns relative to controls (Guo et al., 2004). Other findings of the same study included increased frequencies of natal teeth and deformed or missing teeth, as well as more instances of otitis media, bronchitis, and respiratory infections in children of Yu-Cheng mothers compared with controls.

Long-term clinical effects in patients

Many Yusho patients had a variety of subjective complaints that continued after 1968. They complained of weakness, lassitude, swelling of the upper eyelids, increased secretion from Meibomian glands, excessive sweating, itching, swelling and numbness of the limbs, headaches, cough, altered menstruation, cough, difficulty hearing, reddish skin plaques, pigmented gingiva and mucous membranes, accentuated hair follicles, and eye discharge (Kuratsune et al., 1972; Furue et al., 2005). In a study of 359 Yusho patients in 2001–03, more than 30 years after the incident, the mean blood level of 2,3,4,7,8-pentachlorodibenzofuran (PeCDF) was measured at 177.50 pg/g lipids, much higher than that of normal controls (15.2 ± 8.9 pg/g lipids) (Imamura et al., 2007). In follow-up cohort studies of both Yusho and Yu-Cheng patients, increased mortality from cancers (all categories) was noted (Hsu et al., 1985; Steenland et al., 2004). In particular, death rates due to hepatocellular carcinoma and liver cirrhosis were elevated (Hsu et al., 1985).

Even 35–40 years after the Yusho outbreak, survivors had higher rates of medical conditions and lingering symptoms than did the general Japanese population (Kanagawa et al., 2008; Akahane et al., 2018). After adjusting for confounders such as age, cigarette smoking etc., skin conditions such as hyperpigmentation and acneiform eruptions were more prevalent among Yusho victims, along with such findings as weight loss, headache, cough, abdominal pain, diarrhea or constipation, fatigue, arthralgias, extremity numbness, orthostatic hypotension, hypohidrosis, hoarseness, cardiac insufficiency, tachycardia, eczema, osteoporosis, and hair loss. Serum concentrations of 2,3,4,7,8 PeCDF still correlated with arthralgias; serum PCB levels correlated with ophthalmologic symptoms; and PCQ levels correlated with total cholesterol (Kanagawa et al., 2008). Fifty years after the incident, differences in neuromuscular function such as hand-grip strength and functional reach could be discerned among men who were Yusho incident survivors, based on the TEQ of dioxins measured in their blood (Fukushi et al., 2019). Overall, net survival was found to be lower among older male Yusho patients (Onozuka et al., 2014).

Carcinogenicity

Polychlorinated dibenzo-*p*-dioxins (PCDDs) and PCDFs were declared Class 1 carcinogens by the International Agency for Research on Cancer (IARC) in 1997, based on animal studies, occupational data, and follow-up studies of the 1976 Seveso, Italy disaster. 2,3,7,8-tetrachlorodibenzo-*p*-dioxin (TCDD) was unique in that it was considered by IARC as a cause of all cancers at all sites, rather than cancers associated with a few specific organ types (Steenland et al, 2004). Follow-up studies of Yusho and Yu-Cheng victims have shown higher rates of lung and liver cancers, as well as concerns about a more frequent occurrence of malignant neoplasms of the stomach and both the lymphatic and hematopoietic systems (Mitoma et al., 2015).

Autopsy findings

The toxic effects of some of the isomers of PCDFs, such as 2,3,7,8-tetrachlorodibenzofurans (TCDF), 2,3,4,7,8-pentachlorobenzofurans (PCDF), and 1,2,3,4,7,8-hexachlorinated dibenzofurans (HCDF) are hundreds to thousands of times more potent than PCBs. At autopsy, liver, adipose tissue, and intestinal concentrations of PCDFs, and PCQs were all 100–1000s times higher than those in either PCB-exposed workers or unexposed individuals (Miyata et al., 1985). Thus Yusho and Yu-Cheng were both illnesses that were different than either occupational exposures to PCBs in the workplace or effects associated with other known environmental background sources of PCBs. They were different both in the types of the chemicals involved as well as the dose and body burden.

Therapies for dioxin poisoning

A number of different treatments were offered to patients with Yusho, although none could be shown to alleviate all of their subjective complaints (Furue et al., 2005). A diet high in fiber and supplemented with cholestyramine seemed to increase the fecal excretion of some dioxins. Antioxidants such as vitamin B, hormone therapy, and plastic surgery for skin lesions were also pursued by some patients. Phytochemicals and herbal remedies have also been advised for their antioxidant properties, but are without any known effectiveness in alleviating symptoms or reducing the body burden of dioxins. Fasting therapy seemed to mobilize dioxins from adipose tissue in animal studies, and redistribute the chemicals to other target organs such as brain, liver blood, lungs, and muscle. "Kampo," a traditional herbal medicine from China, is composed with a variety of herbs thought to benefit health. One specific form of Kampo made with *Keishibukuryogan*, was shown to have some effect on inhibiting AhR signaling and is a popular Kampo treatment in Japan (Mitoma et al., 2018). It was investigated as a treatment for Yusho in an open-label, one-armed clinical trial in 2015 and, although 10 of the 52 patients enrolled dropped out of the study due to gastrointestinal side-effects, the rest experienced some subjective relief from skin and respiratory symptoms, improved alertness, and reduced fatigue (Mitoma et al., 2018).

Toxicology of dioxins and dioxin-like chemicals

Dioxins are a class of over 400 chemicals that have similar chemical structures—chlorinated dibenzo-*p*-dioxins, PCBs, and PCDF congeners, of which about 30 (7 dioxins, 10 PCDFs, and 12 dioxin-like PCBs) have been shown to have toxicity in humans (Schecter et al., 2006). PCBs and PCDFs are similar compounds in chemical structures and also their biological and toxicological properties, although they can show extreme differences in toxic potency. The toxicity of TCDD is mediated in part by its ability to induce the aromatic hydrocarbon receptor (AhR), which is a nuclear receptor and transcription factor conserved in most animal and human cells. TCDD forms a heterodimer with AhR inducing or suppressing the transcription of numerous genes (Sorg, 2014). Downstream, this toxic effect produces many cellular changes in functionality. For all of the 30 chemicals in the dioxin series of interest for their human toxicity, their "total dioxin toxic equivalency" or TEQ expresses the potency of each chemical in its ability to activate the AhR receptor, compared with the standard of 2,3,7,8-tetrachlorodibenzodioxin (TCDD) (Schecter et al., 2006). Table 1.10.2 presents the TEQ (also displayed as 'toxic equivalency factor' or TEF) of different dioxins and dioxin-like compounds.

A cardinal feature of Yusho was chloracne and other skin lesions: cysts, inflammation, comedones, accentuation of hair follicles, and changes in skin pigmentation. Research has shown that these skin manifestations are the result of dioxin's concentration in the skin as a target organ: in epidermis, sebaceous glands, and hair follicles. There, dioxin compounds induce AhR and CYP1A1, CYP1A2, and CYP1B1 enzymes. A cascade of subcellular effects can produce exaggerated changes in melanocytes, keratinocytes, and sebocytes, as well as an intense inflammatory response (Furue and Tsuji, 2019). Acceleration of epidermal differentiation results in the chloracne seen clinically, and upregulation of melanocytes releases large amounts of melanin, accounting for pigment changes (Furue and Tsuji, 2019).

These chemicals are potent inducers of hepatic microsomal P-450 mixed function oxidases (MFO) in animals (Kunita et al., 1985). Such enzyme

TABLE 1.10.2 Toxicity equivalence factors for dioxins and dioxin-like compounds.*

Recommended toxicity equivalence factors (TEFs) for human health risk assessment of polychlorinated dibenzo-p-dioxins, dibenzofurans, and dioxin-like polychlorinated biphenyls compound	TEF
Polychlorinated dibenzo-p-dioxins (*PCDDs*)	
2,3,7,8-TCDD	1
1,2,3,7,8-PeCDD	1
1,2,3,4,7,8-HxCDD	0.1
1,2,3,6,7,8-HxCDD	0.1
1,2,3,7,8,9-HxCDD	0.1
1,2,3,4,6,7,8-HpCDD	0.01
OCDD	0.0003
Polychlorinated dibenzofurans (PCDFs)	
2,3,7,8-TCDF	0.1
1,2,3,7,8-PeCDF	0.03
2,3,4,7,8-PeCDF	0.3
1,2,3,4,7,8-HxCDF	0.1
1,2,3,6,7,8-HxCDF	0.1
1,2,3,7,8,9-HxCDF	0.1
2,3,4,6,7,8-HxCDF	0.1
1,2,3,4,6,7,8-HpCDF	0.01
1,2,3,4,7,8,9-HpCDF	0.01
OCDF	0.0003
Polychlorinated biphenyls (PCBs)	
3,3',4,4'-TCB (77)	0.0001
3,4,4',5-TCB (81)	0.0003
3,3',4,4',5-PeCB (126)	0.1
3,3',4,4',5,5'-HxCB (169)	0.03
2,3,3',4,4'-PeCB (105)	0.00003

TABLE 1.10.2 Toxicity equivalence factors for dioxins and dioxin-like compounds—cont'd

Recommended toxicity equivalence factors (TEFs) for human health risk assessment of polychlorinated dibenzo-*p*-dioxins, dibenzofurans, and dioxin-like polychlorinated biphenyls compound	TEF
2,3,4,4′,5-PeCB (114)	0.00003
2,3′,4,4′,5-PeCB (118)	0.00003
2′,3,4,4′,5-PeCB (123)	0.00003

* Table modified from Table 2 (pages 12 and 13) US EPA Recommended Toxicity Equivalence Factors (TEFS) for Human Health Risk Assessments of 2,3,7,8-Tetrachloro-p-dioxin and Dioxin-like Compounds. EPA/100/R 10/005 December 2010. www.epa.gov/osa

induction can disrupt endocrine functions and may be related to dioxins as possible carcinogens. In animal experiments using cynomolgus monkeys, Kunita et al. (1985) demonstrated that PCB-treated animals showed no dermal lesions, whereas those given PCDFs or mixtures of PCBs, PCQs, and PCDFs all developed skin lesions. Animals in this study also showed evidence of the liver hypertrophy, hepatic cytochrome enzyme induction, thymic atrophy, and immunosuppression seen with PCBs alone (Kunita et al., 1985). Authors concluded that PCDFs were the primary causative agent in producing Yusho symptomatology.

Half-life of dioxins

TCDD itself is a lipophilic chemical that easily traverses cell membranes and is stored in fat. In Yusho patients, dioxin levels were generally higher in women than men, perhaps related to differences in adiposity and sebum excretion, among other factors. Lactation reduces blood levels in the breast-feeding mother, but the dioxins in breast milk increase levels in the blood of the infant. In humans, dioxins and dioxin-like compounds have long half-lives of about 7–15 years. One of the main sources of excretion and elimination of dioxin-like compounds besides in feces is through sebum formation in the skin. For that reason, as sebum secretion decreases during aging, the projected half-life of some persistent dioxin-like compounds, such as 2,3,4,7,8-PeCDF, one of the major contaminants in Yusho, increases. It has become clear from follow-up studies that the elimination of dioxin-like chemicals is concentration dependent. For some Yusho patients in whom it was measured, the half-life of PeCDF was calculated to be less than 13.3 years; but for others who started with higher blood concentrations, it approached infinity (Matsumoto et al., 2015). Even 50 years after the event, dioxin concentrations in Yusho victims have remained much higher than predicted (Mitoma et al., 2018).

Chick edema disease

In the aftermath of the Yusho epidemic, it was learned that a zoo-epidemic of "chick edema disease" had taken place in western Japan, affecting about 2 million chickens and killing more than 400,000 of them. This epidemic occurred during the same period as Yusho: February to March 1968. At autopsy, the chickens had a yellowish mottled liver, subcutaneous edema, and pulmonary edema. It was discovered that the manufacturers of chicken feed had used "dark oil" produced by the K company purchased between February 6–27, 1968, as an ingredient in the feed (Kuratsune et al., 1972). The investigation of the chicken disease unfortunately was undertaken too late to prevent the distribution of the contaminated cooking oil in Japan and the resultant outbreak of Yusho in humans.

Yu-Cheng poisoning—Taiwan

A second, similar poisoning event involving PCB-containing rice oil occurred in Taiwan in 1979. During the processing of rice oil in central Taiwan to remove color and odor, the oil underwent a heat transfer using a PCB mixture (Kanechlor 400, 500) manufactured in Japan. Unfortunately a leakage occurred in the sealed process. PCBs and related dioxin-like chemicals were produced by heat degradation. Polychlorinated dibenzofurans (PCDFs) and ter- and quaterphenyl (PCTs and PCQs) compounds, in addition to PCBs, contaminated the rice-bran oil that was subsequently distributed to the general population. The syndrome of related health effects, which were similar to those see in the Yusho and Seveso dioxin epidemics (and the poisoning of Viktor Yushchenko), were termed "Yu Cheng Syndrome," Taiwanese for "oil disease." Samples of the cooking oil from the homes of victims in Taiwan were heavily contaminated with PCBs, PCQs, and PCDFs at average levels of 62, 20, and 0.14 ppm, respectively (Miyata et al., 1985). These levels were only about one-tenth those reported in the Yusho outbreak. By 1980, 2061 people were registered with the health department of the Taiwanese Provincial Government and determined to be Yu-Cheng victims (Hsu et al., 1985).

The daily intake of PCBs over the course of a few years was estimated at 7.9 mg in Yusho patients and 4–12 mg in Yu-Cheng patients; their daily intake of PCDFs was estimated to be 3.4 mg in Yusho and 3.84 mg in Yu-Cheng, respectively (Kashimoto et al., 1985). Later studies and comparisons with occupational exposures led researchers to conclude that Yusho and Yu-Cheng illnesses were most likely related specifically to ingestion of PCDFs and PCQs rather than PCBs themselves (Miyata et al., 1985).

Dioxins are persistent and accumulate in adipose fat and other tissues where they are stored for years. Measurements of dioxin levels in the tissues of Yu-Cheng victims at autopsy 10 years later were still very elevated. For example, one patient who died 9 years after the incident still had in his liver a PCDF level 1016 times higher and a PCQ level 15 times higher than that in the livers of unexposed controls (Miyata et al., 1985). Consequences of Yu-Cheng in a 13-year follow-up study included higher rates of liver disease, including cirrhosis, and increased mortality rates from liver-related disease (Yu et al., 1997).

Lessons learned

The Yusho and Yu-Cheng poisoning episodes again pointed out several enduring lessons to be learned by clinical toxicologists, public health agencies, governmental health officials, and others with accountability for a population's protection from chemical toxic events.

- *Delayed Symptoms*—Some highly toxic substances, such as the compounds included in the dioxin class of chemicals, have delayed onset of adverse effects. These effects may include only subtle clinical symptoms, physical findings and/or only changes in laboratory measures of early dysfunction involving the body's organ systems. This delay challenges the detection of the threat to the public's health and safety. Large numbers of people can be affected before the hazard is recognized; health care resources are subsequently easily overwhelmed.
- *Environmental Persistence*—The persistence of some chemicals in the environment, with long half-lives and resistance to natural degradation, prolongs, and complicates the threat to the public's health.
- *GMP*—The lack of standardized good manufacturing practices (GMPs) and regulatory policies by governmental agencies risk mass poisoning disaster events involving the general public that we have described elsewhere in this Section. When GMPs are not created, implemented, monitored, and enforced, tainted products can reach the commercial stream available for purchase by unwary consumers, with untoward health consequences.
- *Enduring Psychosocial Impact*—Such poisoning episodes can have subtle long-term psychosocial impacts. Environmental incidents of contamination of drinking water or foodstuffs can impact the population for months to years after the event. Continuing uncertainty regarding the possible impacts on their future health and that of their children can result in under-recognized mental health effects on the populace, engendering stress-induced emotions such as anxiety, fear, anger, resentment, and clinical depression.

References

Akahane M, Matsumoto S, Kanagawa Y, Mitoma C, Uchi H, Yoshimura T, Furue M, Imamura T. Long-term health effects of PCBs and related compounds: a comparative analysis of patients suffering from Yusho and the general population. Arch Environ Contam Toxicol 2018;74:203–17.

Fukushi J, Tsushima H, Matsumoto Y, Mitoma C, Furue M, Miyahara H, Nakashima Y. Influence of dioxin-related compounds on physical function in Yusho incident victims. Heliyon 2019;5, e02702.

Furue M, Tsuji G. Chloracne and hyperpigmentation caused by exposure to hazardous aryl hydrocarbon receptor ligands. Int J Environ Res Public Health 2019;16:4864.

Furue M, Uenotsuchi T, Urabe K, Ishiokawa T, Kuwabara M, Yusdho SG. Overview of Yusho. J Dermatol Sci Suppl 2005;1(1):S3–S10.

Guo YL, Lambert GH, Hsu CC, Hsu MM. Yucheng: health effects of prenatal exposure to polychlorinated biphenyls and dibenzofurans. Int Arch Occup Environ Health 2004;77(3):153–8.

Hsu ST, Ma CI, Hsu SK, Wu SS, Hsu NH, Yeh CC, Wu SB. Discovery and epidemiology of PCB poisoning in Taiwan: a four-year follow-up. Environ Health Perspect 1985;59:5–10.

Imamura M, Kanagawa Y, Martcumoto S, Tajima B, Uenotsuchi T, Shibata S, Furue M. Relationship between clinical features and blood levels of pentachlorodibenzofuran in patients with Yusho. Environ Toxicol 2007;22(2):124–31.

Kanagawa Y, Matsumoto S, Koike S, Tajima B, Fukiwake N, Shibata S, et al. Association of clinical findings in Yusho patients with serum concentrations of polychlorinated biphenyls, polychlorinated quaterphenyls, and 2,3,7,8 pentachlorodibenzofuran more than 30 years after the poisoning event. Environ Health 2008;7:47.

Kashimoto T, Miyata H, Fukushima S, Kunita N, Ohi G, Tung T-C. PCBs, PCQs, and PCDFs in blood of Yusho and Yu-Cheng patients. Environ Health Perspect 1985;59:72–8.

Kunita N, Hori S, Obana H, Otake T, Nishimura H, Kashimoto T, Ikegami N. Biological effect of PCBs, PCQs, and PCDFs present in the oil causing Yusho and Yu-Cheng. Environ Health Perspect 1985;59:79–84.

Kuratsune M, Yoshimura T, Matsuzaka J, Yamaguchi A. Epidemiologic study on Yusho, a poisoning caused by ingestion of rice oil contaminated with a commercial brand of polychlorinated biphenyls. Environ Health Perspect 1972;1:119–28.

Matsumoto S, Akahane M, Kanagawa Y, Kajiwara J, Mitoma C, Uchi H, et al. Unexpectedly long half-lives of blood 2,3,7,8 pentachlorobenzofuran (PeCDF) levels in Yusho patients. Environ Health 2015;14:76.

Mitoma C, Uchi H, Tsukimori K, Yamada H, Akahane M, Imamura T, Utani A, Furue M. Yusho and its latest findings—a review in studies conducted by the Yusho group. Environ Int 2015;82:41–8.

Mitoma C, Uchi H, Tsukimori K, Todaka T, Kajiwara J, Shimose T, Akahane M, Imamura T, Furue M. Current state of yusho and prospects for therapeutic strategies. Environ Sci Pollut Res Int 2018;25(17):16472–80.

Miyata H, Fukushima S, Kashimoto T, Kunita N. OCBs, PCQs, and PCDFs in tissues of Yusho and Yu-Cheng patients. Environ Health Perspect 1985;59:67–72.

Onozuka D, Hirata T, Furue M. Net survival after exposure to polychlorinated biphenyls and dioxins: the Yusho study. Environ Int 2014;73:28–32.

Schecter A, Birnbaum L, Ryan JJ, Constable JD. Dioxins: an overview. Environ Res 2006;101(3):419–28.

Sorg O. AhR signaling and dioxin toxicity. Toxicol Lett 2014;230(2):225–33.

Steenland K, Bertazzi P, Baccarelli A, Kogevinas M. Dioxin revisited: developments since the 1997 IARC classification of dioxin as a human carcinogen. Environ Health Perspect 2004;112(13):1265–8.

Tsukimori K, Takunaga S, Shibata S, Uchi H, Nakayama D, Ishimaru T, et al. Long-term effects of polychlorinated biphenyls and dioxins on pregnancy outcomes in women affected by the Yusgho incident. Environ Health Perspect 2008;116(5):626–30.

Yoshimura T. Yusho in Japan. Ind Health 2003;41:139–48.

Yoshimura T. Yusho: 43 years later. Kaohsiung J Med Sci 2012;28(7 Suppl):S49–52.

Yu ML, Guo YL, Hsu CC, Rogan WJ. Increased mortality from chronic liver disease and cirrhosis 13 years after the Taiwan "Yucheng" ("oil disease") incident. Am J Ind Med 1997;31(2):172–5.

Section 2

Notable pharmaceutical poisoning incidents and poisoned people

Alan D. Woolf
Boston Children's Hospital & Harvard Medical School, Boston, Massachusetts, United States

In this section we describe examples of pharmaceutical poisonings in the annals of clinical toxicology. These episodes gained considerable international publicity at the time and included 'lessons learned' for clinical toxicologists and public health officials alike. Instances of both intentional and inadvertent incidents are included. Culpability for such intentional events as the sulfanilamide disaster of the 1930s involved unscrupulous businessmen, drug wholesalers, and pharmacists. The Tylenol murders, another intentional adulteration, resulted in lasting product changes: improved manufacturing operations and advancements in product design and packaging to insure the safety of over-the-counter drugs. The sulfanilamide disaster led to new governmental public health policies involving mandated pre-market testing, manufacturing, sale, and distribution of pharmaceuticals. Such governmental policies were again strengthened around the world after the thalidomide tragedy that unfolded in the 1950s.

The "gasping baby syndrome" involved an excipient, benzyl alcohol, commonly found in pharmaceuticals administered parenterally that proved toxic to a vulnerable population: premature infants. The syndrome, discovered by astute clinicians, reinforced the teaching that important differences exist in how people of different ages metabolize and react to chemicals, toxins and xenobiotics.

Included in this section is the tragic story of Dr. Karen Wetterhahn, a Dartmouth chemist specializing in the investigation of properties of metals, who died of dimethylmercury poisoning. From her death, new lessons were learned about unrecognized gaps in the safety of people working in toxicology laboratories, and changes in policies and practices were made.

The poisoning of individuals or groups of individuals for personal or political reasons has a long history dating back to ancient times (see other Book Titles in this Series). Because of space limitations, other recent terrorist incidents are not included, such as the Tokyo subway attack with nerve gas or the newer political assassination attempts using neurotoxic poisons. The use of poisonous chemicals in warfare throughout modern history is also beyond the scope of the book. A chapter is devoted in this section to the stories of two recent notorious poisonings that gained wide publicity. Two prominent individuals, a Ukrainian and a Bulgarian, were poisoned for political purposes. In both of those cases, lessons were learned about the actions of exotic poisons, dioxin and ricin respectively, and new information about how they affected people. A timeline of the events described in the chapters of this section is shown below (Fig. 1).

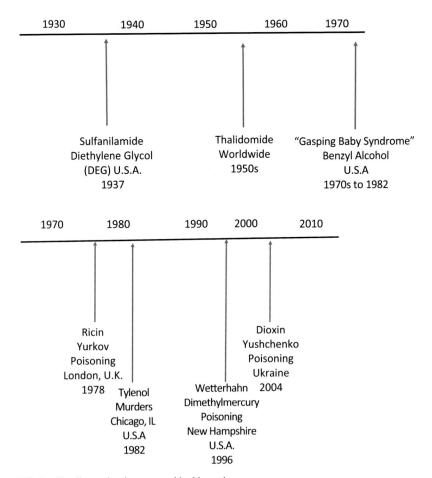

FIG. 1 Timeline: poisonings covered in this section.

Chapter 2.1

Sulfanilamide (diethylene glycol) disaster—United States, 1937

Alan D. Woolf

Boston Children's Hospital & Harvard Medical School, Boston, Massachusetts, United States

It was a brilliant German chemist and pathologist, Dr. Gerhard Domagk, who in 1932 discovered that a sulfur-containing red dye, Prontosil, first synthesized in the early 1900s, had antibacterial properties against *Streptococcus* when injected into mice. He won the Nobel Prize for Physiology and Medicine in 1939 for this discovery of the first in the class of sulfonamide compounds. The advent of this first antibiotic, sulfanilamide, was heralded as a new age of "miracle" drugs, effective in curing a variety of common, sometimes deadly, infections (Fig. 2.1.1). Sulfanilamide was used to treat maladies such as sore throats caused by *Streptococcus,* abscesses, pyelitis, prostatitis, diphtheria, cystitis, gonorrhea, and syphilis (Calvery and Klumpp, 1939). Manufacturers enthusiastically embraced sulfanilamide and rushed to produce thousands of bottles of the new drug to distribute to markets around the country. The use of this new antibiotic spread so rapidly in the United States that the supply could not keep pace with the demand. However, the only applicable Federal legislation, the Pure Food & Drug Act of 1906, was intended to address mainly the adulteration of food; it did not provide a regulatory structure covering the safety or effectiveness of new drugs. The 1906 regulations, inadequate as they were, were enforced by the Bureau of Chemistry of the Department of Agriculture, the forerunner of the FDA, which was founded in 1930.

As a result, without any regulatory constraints or oversight, short-cuts were taken to bring the agent to market. Thus the manufacture of a batch of a new "elixir" (even though it contained no ethanol) of sulfanilamide by S.E. Massengill Co. manufacturing pharmacists in Bristol Tennessee was made to meet the demand for a liquid product. The Massengill chief chemist, Mr. Harold Watkins, used diethylene glycol (DEG), a cheap sweet-tasting solvent, and raspberry extract to formulate a preparation more agreeable, especially for children, who could not or would not take tablets or capsules of the drug (Federal Register, 1937). The "elixir" was manufactured quickly to take advantage of the growing southern market for the drug and the final product contained about

History of Modern Clinical Toxicology. https://doi.org/10.1016/B978-0-12-822218-8.00045-4
139

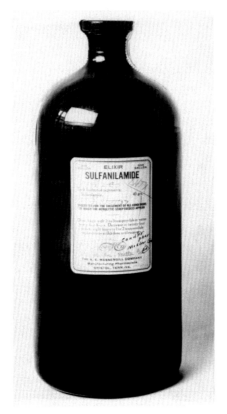

FIG. 2.1.1 Elixir of sulfanilamide. *(From https://en.wikipedia.org/wiki/Elixir_sulfanilamide#/media/File:Elixir_Sulfanilamide.jpg.)*

72% DEG by volume. Without the need for premarketing animal or other studies, none was undertaken. It was not appreciated that DEG is a potent renal and liver toxin, as well as a neurotoxin.

Toxicity of diethylene glycol

DEG is a commercial antifreeze and solvent whose properties make it attractive for a variety of uses, such as in refrigeration or in the production of resins or as a substitute for glycerine. DEG (CAS 111-46-6; MW 106) is a condensation product of two moieties of ethylene glycol joined by an ether bond to form the DEG molecule (Fig. 2.1.2). Although there were only two toxicity studies of DEG prior to 1937, animal studies after the sulfanilamide tragedy had confirmed the toxicity of the sulfanilamide elixir containing the solvent. The kidneys and liver were reported to be the two main target organs in a variety of animals, including rats, dogs, and rabbits (AMA Part I, 1937a; Geiling and Cannon, 1938; Weatherby and Williams, 1939). However, it is clear that there is inter-species variation in how DEG is metabolized. Unlike the rat, man does not

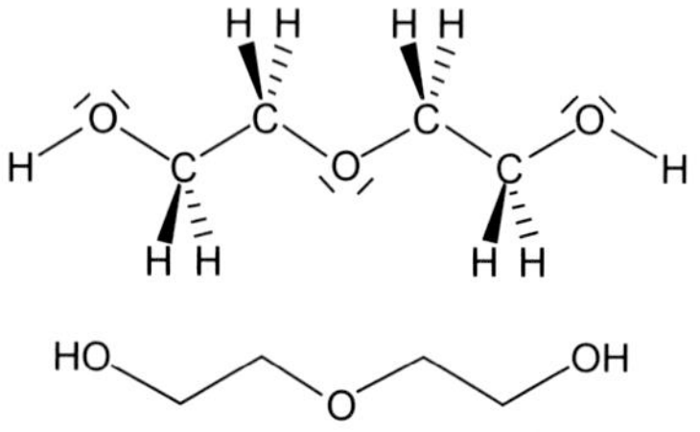

FIG. 2.1.2 Diethylene glycol. *(From https://commons.wikimedia.org/wiki/File:Diethylene-glycol-chemical.png.)*

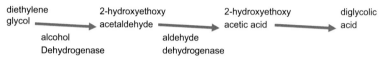

FIG. 2.1.3 Metabolism of diethylene glycol in humans.

metabolize DEG by breaking the ether bond releasing nephrotoxic ethylene glycol. Instead 2-hydroxyethoxyacetic acid (HEAA) is produced by the enzymes: alcohol dehydrogenase and aldehyde dehydrogenase in the liver, as the metabolite (Fig. 2.1.3). Victims of DEG poisoning showed widespread pathology of both the liver and kidneys at autopsy (Geiling and Cannon, 1938; Lynch, 1938; Bowie and McKenzie, 1972). Histology of the enlarged liver showed centrilobular hydropic degeneration. Swollen kidneys showed sparing of the glomerulus, but extensive tubular necrosis with luminal proteinaceous casts. There was cortical necrosis, renal tissue anoxia and infarction, and hemorrhage, but no evidence of the calcium oxalate crystals in the tubular lumens, as is commonly seen in ethylene glycol poisoning. There was also neurological toxicity, since DEG easily passed the blood-brain barrier and disrupted neural functioning.

The mechanism of toxicity of DEG and its biological fate in humans has only recently been further clarified. Schier et al. (2013) analyzed samples of blood, urine, and cerebrospinal fluid frozen and archived from victims of the 2006 Panama DEG poisoning episode (discussed later) and found both HEAA and diglycolic acid in all three body fluids, suggesting that these two metabolites play a major role in the toxicity seen after DEG ingestion. Animal models have confirmed the nephrotoxic and hepatotoxic effects of diglycolic acid, which accumulates inside renal tubular cells (Robinson et al., 2017).

Clinical toxicology

Victims of DEG poisoning often present with vomiting, fever, abdominal pain, and diarrhea. They manifest the tachypnea, acidotic breathing, and dehydration seen in patients with underlying severe metabolic acidosis (Bowie and McKenzie, 1972; Okuonghae et al., 1992). On examination, there is evidence of hepatomegaly, splenomegaly, skin pallor, sometimes jaundice, and tenderness in the vicinity of the kidneys. Patients often are irritable upon presentation or complain of headache. They may have tremors or signs of a peripheral neuropathy (Rentz et al., 2008). Neurological symptoms often progress to a depressed consciousness or patients may lapse into coma, with positive meningeal signs and sometimes seizure activity. Cerebrospinal fluid may reveal pleiocytosis and elevated protein (Bowie and McKenzie, 1972). Peripheral blood counts show a leukocytosis. There can be evolving osmolar and anion gaps and a rise in both the blood urea nitrogen (BUN) and creatinine, seen in impaired renal function. Urine obtained from patients shows an active sediment with casts. Many patients progress to life-threatening, anuric renal failure, encephalopathy, coma, and hepatorenal syndrome. The differential diagnosis often considered before DEG poisoning is suspected includes gastroenteritis, sepsis, acute renal failure of infectious or other causes, meningitis, Guillain-Barre Syndrome, or poisoning with another chemical, such as ethylene glycol.

Patients can survive DEG poisoning if they are treated early in their course with aggressive management, including: intensive care, ventilatory support, parenteral nutrition, attention to acid-base, fluid and electrolyte balance, and hemodialysis. While the antidote, fomepizole, which blocks alcohol dehydrogenase and would prevent formation of the toxic metabolites, might prevent toxicity if administered early in an acute DEG poisoning, its benefit has not yet been demonstrated clinically.

Timeline of the tragedy

During September and October, 1937, the elixir was distributed mostly from Bristol Tennessee and Kansas City Missouri, although small amounts were also shipped from San Francisco and New York. Most of the supplies were destined for southern states, including Texas, Missouri, Oklahoma, Mississippi, Arkansas, Tennessee, Alabama, Georgia, and the Carolinas. In 1937–38, physicians began to document cases. Patients, including children, who were treated with the apparently tainted sulfanilamide showed early symptoms of "heartburn", headaches, dizziness, malaise, back and abdominal pain, vomiting, anorexia and occasionally diarrhea. They later developed anuric renal failure, experienced seizures, lapsed into coma, and died (Lynch, 1938). Autopsies showed evidence of destruction of the renal cortex and tubular cells, along with evidence of infarction (Lynch, 1938). There was also evidence of gastritis and centrilobular necrosis of the liver. Of an estimated 240 gal of the poisonous drug manufactured and distributed (Calvery and Klumpp, 1939), over 234 gal were subsequently retrieved during the extraordinary recall effort to locate suppliers and salesmen and confiscate supplies. It was estimated if all 240 gal had been consumed, there would have been over 4000 deaths (Wax, 1995).

An estimated 365 people were sickened over a 4-week period, including young children, and there were 105 deaths (34 children and 71 adults), before the discovery of the toxic glycol additive was made. Laboratory studies of the elixir and DEG itself subsequently confirmed the same pathological lesions were seen in the kidneys and liver in dogs and rabbits as were evident in human autopsies. Researchers also noted cumulative toxic effects following repeated dosing (Geiling and Cannon, 1938). The mean fatal dose of DEG was 38 g in children (about 10 teaspoons of the cumulative dosing) of the elixir and 71 g in adults, with a survival of 9.4 days after ingestion of the first dose (range: 2–22 days). The American Medical Association (AMA) Chemical Laboratory commissioned these studies and performed analyses of the elixir itself, which it reported out in special articles in the scientific literature as early as November 1937 to alert practitioners to the danger (AMA Part I, 1937a; AMA Part II, 1937b).

Congressional remedies

Reports from the AMA Chemical Laboratory in 1937 point out that "Under the present Food and Drugs Act or even under any of the food and drug bills now before Congress, there seems to be no provision which would prevent a repetition of this tragedy" (AMA Part II, 1937b). This sentinel poisoning event was reported out to Congress in the Federal Register by the Secretary of Agriculture in 1937 (Federal Register, 1937). In his Letter to Congress, the Secretary noted that a "few simple tests on experimental animals would have demonstrated the lethal properties of the elixir" and the entire tragedy averted. His recommendations for legislation to Congress included:

1. License control of new drugs.
2. Prohibition of drugs which are dangerous to health.
3. Requirement that drug labels bear appropriate directions for use and warnings against probable misuse.
4. Prohibition of secret remedies by requiring that labels disclose fully the composition of drugs.

The shortcomings in the labeling of drugs and the premarket testing of drugs prior to their release for public consumption, as painfully revealed by the sulfanilamide disaster, led to the passage of the Food, Drug & Cosmetic Act of 1938.

Aftermath

In the tragedy's aftermath, Dr. Samuel E. Massengill pleaded guilty to adulteration and misbranding (including an ingredient not listed on the label) and paid the largest fine ever imposed for violations of the 1906 Pure Food & Drug Act, about $26,100 (The $26,100 in 1937 dollars is equivalent to about $484,000 in 2021 dollars.). Dr. Watkins, the Massengill chemist implicated in the adulteration, committed suicide.

The sulfanilamide disaster in the United States led to the passage of the 1938 Federal Food, Drug and Cosmetic Act. This complex legislation mandated a complete overhaul of the regulation and oversight of the premarket testing, development, and licensing of pharmaceuticals in the United States. It provided the regulatory structure to give the Food & Drug Administration its oversight authority to require that pharmaceutical manufacturers demonstrate a drug's safety before distributing and marketing it to the public. The accompanying New Drug Application Standard, which was greatly strengthened after the thalidomide tragedy 20 years later (see Chapter 2.4), was implemented for the regulation of proposed new drugs prior to marketing. This model legislation was adopted elsewhere in the world with the goal of assuring the safety of medications sold to the public. It remains in effect in the United States today.

Diethylene glycol adulterant tragedies around the world

Unfortunately, there have continued to be episodes around the world in which DEG was substituted as a solvent in a medicinal product. In 1969, seven children in the Cape Town area of South Africa died of renal and liver failure. It was later discovered that all had been given one of two sedative medications (known as Pronap or Plaxim) prepared with DEG as the diluent (Bowie and McKenzie, 1972).

In January, 1986, at the JJ Hospital in central India, 14 patients ranging in age from 10 to 76 years died of unnatural causes. Another 7 adult patients being treated for cataracts at Patna Medical College and Hospital also unexpectedly died. Investigation revealed all of these patients had been administered glycerine (glycerol) tainted with 18.5% DEG when an industrial grade chemical was mistakenly substituted for the medicinal grade product (Pandya, 1988).

Again, at the Jos University Teaching Hospital (JUTH) in Nigeria in 1990, 47 children were admitted with acute renal failure and died due to ingestion of a medicinal paracetamol syrup adulterated with DEG (Okuonghae et al., 1992). Traders and wholesalers in East Nigeria sold the DEG to local pharmacists mislabeled as propylene glycol. The pharmacists then used it as the solvent in preparing the drug locally for parents to use to treat their children's fevers. Autopsies of the poisoned children showed extensive renal cortical necrosis, central hepatic degeneration, adrenal hemorrhages, cerebral edema, and congestion of the lungs.

Also, a children's hospital in Dhaka, Bangladesh, investigated 339 child patients admitted with renal failure of unknown cause (and a 70% mortality rate) during the years 1990–93 and compared their features with 90 children with a known cause of renal failure (Hanif et al., 1995). Researchers discovered that 19 of 69 paracetamol elixirs administered to the cases had been prepared with DEG as the sole diluent, which accounted for many of the patients presenting with renal failure. A broader investigation by WHO revealed that 5 of 104 different brands of paracetamol produced by more than 100 licensed Bangladeshi manufacturers contained DEG. The Bangladesh government belatedly banned all paracetamol sales in December of 1992 until their safety could be assured.

Subsequently over the next 12 months, total admissions to the children's hospital for renal failure declined by 53% and renal failure from unexplained causes declined by 84% (Hanif et al., 1995).

Later, in 1996, a Haitian poisoning disaster occurred in which DEG was present in a mislabeled glycerin solvent imported from China. The tainted glycerin was used in the local formulation of two liquid acetaminophen-containing antipyretic medicines, "Afebril" and "Valodon." These two drugs were marketed by a local pharmaceutical company, Pharval, and intended for both children and adults. As many as 15,000 bottles of DEG-tainted acetaminophen were produced; about 40% of the bottles on the market were from contaminated lots (O'Brien, 1998). Although the first case was subsequently identified as occurring in November 1995, by July 3, 1996, over 86 childhood cases were reported, with 80 deaths (McCarthy, 1996). Eleven Haitian children were flown to hospitals in the United States for hemodialysis (Scalzo, 1996). Significantly there was no FDA-equivalent governmental agency in Haiti to provide oversight of pharmaceutical manufacturing practices, a situation lamented at the time in medical commentaries (Wax, 1996; Woolf, 1998).

The Pan-American Health Organization, a regional office of WHO, and the US CDC conducted the investigation and testing of drug samples (PAHO, 1996). A follow-up study of 109 cases of acute renal failure found that of 89 children who remained in Haiti, 87 (98%) died, whereas 3 of 11 (27%) children flown to the United States for treatment died before intensive medical management could be initiated. The estimated toxic dose of DEG was 1.34 mL/kg (range: 0.22–4.22 mL/kg) (O'Brien et al., 1998).

Again, in Panama in September 2006, a physician noticed an unusual cluster of cases of acute renal failure. A case-control study identified an erroneous substitution of DEG as a solvent in specific lots of two prescription cough syrups. This led to another epidemic of poisoning of both adults and children resulting in at least 78 deaths in Panama (Rentz et al., 2008). The glycerin solvent imported from China had 22% by volume of DEG; after preparation, the cough syrup contained a final concentration of 8.1% DEG. Patients with respiratory complaints had been instructed to take the tainted cough syrup up to three times daily. Severely affected victims developed abdominal complaints, acute renal failure, cranial and somatic peripheral neuropathies, and encephalopathy. The magnitude of the epidemic was never fully documented: more than 60,000 bottles of cough syrup had been distributed and then later recalled. The Panamanian government registered only 119 official cases.

Table 2.1.1 illustrates mass poisonings involving DEG used as an inappropriate ingredient in a variety of pharmaceuticals from around the world. In most instances, the DEG was mistakenly or intentionally added as a cheaper substitute for other nontoxic solvents such as glycerol or propylene glycol. All of these drugs were manufactured without adequate testing and were distributed to the public without any premarketing governmental and industry oversight.

TABLE 2.1.1 Worldwide mass diethylene glycol poisonings.

Year	Country	Vehicle	DEG	# People	Deaths	References
1937	USA	Sulfanilamide	72%	353	105	Geiling and Cannon (1938) and Calvery and Klumpp (1939)
1969	South Africa	Sedatives	Unknown	7	7	Bowie and McKenzie (1972)
1985	Spain	Topical cream	6.2–7.1g/kg	5	5	Cantarell et al. (1987)
1986	India	Glycerine	18.5%	21	21	Pandya (1988)
1990	Nigeria	Acetaminophen	Unknown	47	47	Okuonghae et al. (1992)
1990	Bangladesh	Acetaminophen	Unknown	339	236	Hanif et al. (1995)
1992	Argentina	Respiratory syrup	65%	29	15	Ferrari and Giannuzzi (2005)
1996	Haiti	Acetaminophen	14.4%	109	88	O'Brien et al. (1998)
1998	India	Cough syrup	17.5%	36	33	Singh et al. (2001)
		Acetaminophen	15.4%[a]	11	8	Hari et al. (2006)
2006	Panama	Cough syrup	8%	119	78	Rentz et al. (2008)
2009	Nigeria	Teething Powder	Unknown	84	84	NY Times[b]

[a]Range 2.3%–22.3% median 15.4%.
[b]http://www.nytimes.com/2009/02/07/world/africa/07nigeria.html.

All of these episodes occurring globally illustrated the woeful inadequacy of drug safety monitoring, especially by underfunded, understaffed, and overwhelmed governmental agencies in economically disadvantaged, developing countries. They all clearly point to the necessity for requiring and enforcing good manufacturing practices for all pharmaceuticals produced worldwide.

References

American Medical Association Chemical Laboratory. Elixir of sulfanilamide-Massengill Part I. JAMA 1937a;109(19):1531–9.

American Medical Association Chemical Laboratory. Elixir of sulfanilamide-Massengill Part II. JAMA 1937b;109(21):1724–7.

Bowie MD, McKenzie D. Diethylene glycol poisoning in children. S Afr Med J 1972;46:931–4.

Calvery HO, Klumpp TG. The toxicity for human beings of diethylene glycol with sulfanilamide. South Med J 1939;32(11):1105–9.

Cantarell MC, Fort J, Camps J, Sans M, Piera L. Acute intoxication due to topical application of diethylene glycol. Ann Intern Med 1987;106:478–9.

Federal Register. U.S. Senate. Report of the Secretary of Agriculture on deaths due to elixir sulfanilamide—Massengill. Document #124, 75th Congress 2nd Session. November 16, 1937; 1937.

Ferrari LA, Giannuzzi L. Clinical parameters of postmortem analysis and estimation of the lethal dose in victims of massive intoxication with diethylene glycol. Forensic Sci Int 2005;153:45–51.

Geiling EMK, Cannon PR. Pathologic effects of elixir of sulfanilamide (diethylene glycol) poisoning. JAMA 1938;111(10):919–27.

Hanif M, Mobarak MR, Ronan A, Rahman D, Donovan JJ, Bennish ML. Fatal renal failure caused by diethylene glycol in paracetamol elixir: the Bangladesh epidemic. Br Med J 1995;311:88–91.

Hari P, Jain Y, Kabra SK. Fatal encephalopathy and renal failure caused by diethylene glycol poisoning. J Trop Pediatr 2006;52:442–4.

Lynch KM. Diethylene glycol poisoning in the human. South Med J 1938;31(2):134–8.

McCarthy M. Syrup contamination linked to Haitian child deaths. Lancet 1996;348(9024):394.

O'Brien KL, Selanikio JD, Hecdivert C, Placide MF, Louis M, Barr DB, et al. Epidemic of pediatric deaths from acute renal failure caused by diethylene glycol poisoning. JAMA 1998;279(15):1175–80.

Okuonghae HO, Ighogboja IS, Lawson JO, Nwana JC. Diethylene glycol poisoning in Nigerian children. Ann Trop Paediatr 1992;12:235–8.

Pan American Health Organization. Deaths in Haiti renal failure epidemic rise to 49. Update issued in Washington DC, July 3; 1996.

Pandya SK. An unmitigated tragedy. Br Med J 1988;297:177–9.

Rentz ED, Lewis L, Mujica OJ, Barr DB, Schier JG, Weerasekera G, et al. Outbreak of acute renal failure in Panama in 2006: a case-control study. Bull World Health Organ 2008;86:749–56.

Robinson CN, Latimer B, Abreo F, Broussard K, McMartin KE. In vitro evidence of nephrotoxicity and altered hepatic function in rats following administration of diglycolic acid, a metabolite of diethylene glycol. Clin Toxicol 2017;55(3):196–205.

Scalzo AJ. Diethylene glycol toxicity revisited: the 1996 Haitian epidemic. Clin Toxicol 1996;34(5):513–6.

Schier JG, Hunt DR, Perala A, McMartin AKE, Bartels MJ, Lewis LS, McGeehin MA, Flanders WD. Characterizing concentrations of diethylene glycol and suspected metabolites in human serum, urine, and cerebrospinal fluid samples from the Panama DEG mass poisoning. Clin Toxicol 2013;51(10):923–9.

Singh J, Dutta AK, Khare S, Dubey NK, Harit AK, Jain NK, Wadhwa TC, et al. Diethylene glycol poisoning in Gurgaon India, 1998. Bull World Health Organ 2001;79:88–95.

Wax P. Elixirs, diluents, and the passage of the 1938 federal food, drug, and cosmetic act. Ann Intern Med 1995;122(6):456–61.

Wax P. It's happening again—another diethylene glycol mass poisoning. Clin Toxicol 1996;34(5):517–20.

Weatherby JH, Williams GZ. Studies on the toxicity of diethylene glycol elixir of sulfanilamide-Massengill and a synthetic elixir. JAMA 1939;28(1):12–7.

Woolf AD. A dark wood revisited—the Haitian diethylene glycol poisoning tragedy. JAMA 1998;279:1215–6.

Chapter 2.2

Gasping syndrome, 1982

Alan D. Woolf
Boston Children's Hospital & Harvard Medical School, Boston, Massachusetts, United States

Neonatologists in the 1970s and early 1980s were making tremendous advances in their ability to rescue and sustain extremely immature infants, some as early as 25–26 weeks of gestation, weighing no more than 650–750 g at birth. Using advanced technologies such as ventilator support, airway management, total parenteral nutrition, and new antibiotic regimens, the survival of such infants, though slim, was improving. Access was secured by the catheterization of umbilical arteries and veins, although this route had complications of its own, including hemorrhage, thrombosis, and infection. Such access afforded clinicians the ability to give these complex infants carefully controlled amounts of fluid, electrolytes, nutrients, lipid supplements, antibiotics, vasopressors, and other life-saving therapeutics.

Benzyl alcohol preservative

Benzyl alcohol ($C_6H_5CH_2OH$) was and is commonly used as a preservative for pharmaceuticals and other medical products. It is bacteriostatic to gram-positive bacteria and is an effective antiseptic agent (Fig. 2.2.1).

In small concentrations (0.9%), benzyl alcohol is present in many pharmaceutical solutions. All medications are required to include an antimicrobial preservative in multiuse vials containing common agents, such as bacteriostatic sterile water, 5% dextrose in water, and sterile isotonic saline, used as flushing solutions for intra-arterial and intravenous lines. Such flushing solutions containing benzyl alcohol were used liberally in neonatal intensive care units. Isotonic saline was used as a flush for intra-tracheal tubes for those infants on ventilator support. Notably the frequency or volume of such flushes was not routinely recorded or counted during the care of the infant in neonatal intensive care nurseries. Also, with each flush, infants received a high dose of benzyl alcohol preservative relative to their body weight, in comparison with older children or adults in whom such flushing solutions were also commonly used.

History of Modern Clinical Toxicology. https://doi.org/10.1016/B978-0-12-822218-8.00038-7

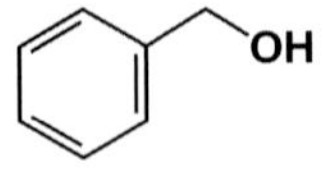

FIG. 2.2.1   Chemical formula of benzyl alcohol.

Poisoning epidemic discovered

Owing to their complex medical problems, many extremely premature infants died from such causes as infection, respiratory distress syndrome, intracranial hemorrhages or strokes, cardiovascular failure, renal or hepatic failure, or a myriad of other complications. It was unfortunately a commonplace but faulty assumption that children (and, in this case, specifically premature infants) would detoxify pharmaceuticals given parenterally in the same manner as would older infants, children, and adults. However, two teams of astute neonatology specialists, working independent of each other in New Orleans (Gershanik et al., 1982) and Portland (Brown et al., 1982), were perplexed by 16 deaths of premature infants under their care. These deaths were preceded by the onset of a progressive encephalopathy, hypotension, bradycardia, severe refractory metabolic acidosis, high anion gap, respiratory depression, and a characteristic breathing pattern that was more like gasping. Preterminal events often included intracranial hemorrhage, seizures, and cardiovascular collapse (Table 2.2.1).

Toxicity studies of benzyl alcohol

Benzyl alcohol toxicity was the subject of many animal studies where, in very high concentrations, it could produce encephalopathy, vasodilation, respiratory depression and failure, seizures, paralysis, and acidosis. Rodent studies reported an LD50 for 0.9% benzyl alcohol of approximately 33 mL/kg (300 mg/kg) by rapid and 40 mL/kg (360 mg/kg) by slow intravenous infusion (Kimura et al., 1971). On the basis of these and other animal studies, rapid intravenous infusion of adult humans with as much as 30 mL of 0.9% benzyl alcohol (approximately 4.5 mg/kg) in saline was thought to be safe for use as a preservative in medications. What was missing was research into its safety when given parenterally to premature infants who developmentally have very immature liver and kidney functions.

Toxicity of benzyl alcohol in premature newborns

Benzyl alcohol is oxidized in the body first to benzaldehyde by alcohol dehydrogenase and then to benzoic acid by aldehyde dehydrogenase, and then the benzoic acid is conjugated with glycine in the liver, and excreted as hippuric acid in the urine. However, newborns lack the enzymatic ability to conjugate the intermediary molecule, using glycine, in an immature liver. Thus the much less toxic metabolite, hippuric acid, which is normally excreted into urine, is found

TABLE 2.2.1 Clinical characteristics of "Gasping syndrome."

Vulnerable patients

Extremely premature infants

Dependence on invasive support (e.g., umbilical artery catheterization, intubation and ventilation)

Clinical manifestations

Pulmonary: gasping respirations, respiratory distress, respiratory depression

Cardiovascular: hypotension, tachycardia, cardiovascular collapse

Neurological: decreased activity, intraventricular hemorrhage, kernicterus, seizures, progressive unresponsiveness (encephalopathy)

Hepatic failure

Renal failure

Laboratory abnormalities

Refractory metabolic acidosis

Increased urinary excretion: benzyl alcohol, benzoic acid, hippuric acid

Increased anion gap

Increased osmolar gap

Thrombocytopenia

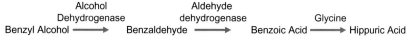

FIG. 2.2.2   Metabolism of benzyl alcohol to hippuric acid.

only in limited amounts. Most of the benzyl alcohol and benzoic acid remains in the blood, contributing not only to a metabolic acidosis but also to elevated anion and osmolar gaps (Fig. 2.2.2).

Neonatologists in the neonatal intensive care unit at Southern Baptist Hospital in New Orleans, Louisiana, studied 10 premature infants with "gasping syndrome" (they coined the term) all of whom had umbilical arterial lines and required ventilator support (and frequent arterial blood gases monitoring) (Gershanik et al., 1982). They compared them with eight matched control infants in their unit who did not develop gasping syndrome and did not require umbilical artery catheters for longer than a week and another five premature infants who were ventilated and had umbilical arterial catheters but did not receive either bacteriostatic water or sodium chloride. Investigators determined approximate benzyl alcohol intake and measured it in blood and urine of the infants. They found that elevated levels of benzyl alcohol had accumulated in the blood of gasping syndrome babies, likely reflecting the immature liver's inability to keep up with conjugating and detoxifying the overload. A relative glycine deficiency could also reduce the conjugation to the safer hippuric acid for excretion. Gasping syndrome infants had comparatively elevated urinary levels of both benzoic and hippuric acids. The researchers' calculation of the apparent dose of benzyl alcohol given parenterally to the gasping syndrome infants during routine umbilical artery catheter flushing was as much as 20–50 times higher on a daily basis than what was considered the safe dose of 0.9% benzyl alcohol for adults (Gershanik et al., 1982). Subsequently, others reported cases of gasping syndrome affected premature infants in other neonatal intensive care units around the country and reported on the epidemiology and natural history of the illness (Anderson et al., 1984). Menon et al. (1984) screened infants with benzyl alcohol levels and found, in comparison with unexposed controls, increased rates of metabolic acidosis, intraventicular hemorrhage, and mortality, although the affected infants did not necessarily have gasping respirations and did not develop kernicterus.

Brown et al. (1982) noted that 10 of 16 babies weighing less than 1250 g admitted to their unit between August 1981 and January 1982 died of the gasping syndrome and, on the basis of assays of urinary organic acids by gas chromatography/mass spectrometry found excessive excretion of both hippuric and benzoic acids, which could largely explain the characteristic high anion gap found in the affected infants. They measured the volume and frequency of typical flushes for these extremely premature babies in their unit, nine of whom were on ventilator support and all of whom had central catheters. They found the average volume to be about 21.2 mL/kg/day, delivering 191 mg/kg/day of benzyl alcohol—but it ranged up to 45 mL/kg or 405 mg/kg of benzyl alcohol dosed in a single day, which approached the LD_{50} previously calculated in animal studies. They concluded with advice that the use of benzyl alcohol as a preservative be discontinued in neonatal intensive care units.

FDA issues benzyl alcohol warning

As a result, in 1982 the FDA (FDA, 1982) issued a general warning applied to all benzyl alcohol containing medical products that they were not intended for use in newborn infants. More than 50,000 letters were mailed to pediatricians, pharmacists, and hospital administrators advising them of the new directive (Lovejoy Jr., 1982). The United States Pharmacopoeia (USP) also advised against the use of such multivial packages of isotonic saline or 5% dextrose in water solutions in newborns. The American Academy of Pediatrics' Committee the Fetus and Newborn and Committee on Drugs, in a joint communication (AAP, 1983), suggested single unit use of non-preserved solutions or single use syringes filled with nonpreservative containing flushes prepared in hospital pharmacies.

It is likely that clinicians in other neonatal intensive care units did not recognize the threat of such standard flush procedures. Since premature infants died for a variety of other reasons, this iatrogenic cause of death was likely never considered in other probable cases. Thus the total death toll among premature infants attributable to benzyl alcohol poisoning and gasping syndrome will never be known. Subsequent studies of premature infants suggested that the discontinuing of the use of benzyl alcohol in those neonatal intensive care units cut the rate of intraventricular hemorrhage in half (Hiller et al., 1986) and reduced the incidence of kernicterus and intraventricular bleeding to zero (Jardine and Rogers, 1989). Benda et al. (1986) reviewed records of all NICU infants weighing < 1250 g for 13 months before and after the use of solutions containing benzyl alcohol was stopped. They found reductions in both mortality rate (from 80.7% to 45.7%) and incidence of grade III/IV intraventricular hemorrhage (from 46% to 19%) among infants < 1000 g birth weight who did not receive the preservative compared with those who did.

Lessons learned

The gasping syndrome illustrated the danger of extrapolating chemical safety data collected on older infants, children, adolescents, or adults to the potential risks such chemicals might pose to newborns and premature infants.

It also demonstrated the need to investigate and test the safety of excipients (so-called "inactive ingredients") such as flavorings, colorings, stabilizers, preservatives, anticaking compounds and others "generally recognized as safe" (GRAS) in especially vulnerable populations, such as premature infants and newborns.

Aftermath — Hospital pharmacy changes

After the FDA's warning in 1982, neonatal units around the country switched to sterile but nonpreservative containing dextrose in water and saline solutions for flushing (Jarvis and Sikes, 1983). Flushing solutions were not the only medications containing benzyl alcohol as a preservative. For example, heparin, used to keep central lines open, also contained benzyl alcohol. However, it was thought that the amount of such medications used was small compared with the frequency of flushing of umbilical catheters, and the dose of preservative received would be negligible, even in premature infants. Still, clinicians were thereafter advised to use preservative-free sodium heparin for injection in newborns and young infants. Since the *minimum* dose of benzyl alcohol associated with gasping syndrome was never established, health care providers were subsequently urged to be cautious when using any pharmaceuticals containing it in premature infants and newborns.

References

American Academy of Pediatrics. Benzyl alcohol: toxic agent in neonatal units. Pediatrics 1983;72(3):356–8.

Anderson CW, Ng KJ, Andresen B, Cordero L. Benzyl alcohol poisoning in a premature newborn infant. Am J Obstet Gynecol 1984;148(3):344–6.

Benda GI, Hiller JL, Reynolds JW. Benzyl alcohol toxicity: impact on neurologic handicaps among surviving very low birth weight infants. Pediatrics 1986;77(4):507–12.

Brown WJ, Buist NRM, Gipson HTC, Huston RK, Kennaway NG. Fatal benzyl alcohol poisoning in a neonatal intensive care unit. Lancet 1982;1:1250.

FDA. Benzyl alcohol may be toxic to newborns. FDA Drug Bull 1982;12:10–1.

Gershanik J, Boecler B, Ensley H, McCloskey S, George W. The gasping syndrome and benzyl alcohol poisoning. N Engl J Med 1982;307(22):1384–8.

Hiller JL, Benda GI, Rahatzad M, Allen JR, Culver DH, Carlson CV, Reynolds JW. Benzyl alcohol toxicity: impact on mortality and intraventricular hemorrhage among very low birth weight infants. Pediatrics 1986;77(4):500–6.

Jardine DS, Rogers K. Relationship of benzyl alcohol to kernicterus, intraventricular hemorrhage, and mortality in preterm infants. Pediatrics 1989;83(2):153–60.

Jarvis WR, Sikes RK. Changing practices in the use of benzyl alcohol-preserved solutions in neonatal intensive care units in Georgia. J Med Assoc Ga 1983;72(10):707–8.

Kimura ET, Darby TD, Krause RA, Brondyk HD. Parenteral toxicity studies with benzyl alcohol. Toxicol Appl Pharmacol 1971;18:60.

Lovejoy Jr FH. Fatal benzyl alcohol poisoning in neonatal intensive care units. A new concern for pediatricians. Am J Dis Child 1982;136(11):974–5.

Menon PA, Thach BT, Smith CH, Landt M, Roberts JL, Hillman RE, Hillman LS. Benzyl alcohol toxicity in a neonatal intensive care unit. Incidence, symptomatology, and mortality. Am J Perinatol 1984;1(4):288–92.

Chapter 2.3

Tylenol cyanide poisoning in United States, 1982

Alan D. Woolf

Boston Children's Hospital & Harvard Medical School, Boston, Massachusetts, United States

Cyanide-containing compounds have many industrial and commercial uses, and they have been readily available from chemical supply houses and other sources. Cyanide also has a notorious history of use as an instrument of murder and suicide dating back to ancient times. Modern-day catastrophic tragedies involving cyanide include its use by Nazi Germany as an agent (hydrogen cyanide as Zyklon B) for killing millions of people in gas chambers during the Holocaust in World War II. Cyanide was again used as an agent of both murder and suicide in the disaster occurring at the People's Temple cult of leader Jim Jones in Jonestown in the northwest part of Guyana. Some 918 people died there on November 19, 1978 as a consequence of the fanatical beliefs of their charismatic leader. Neither of these historical cyanide-associated disasters will be detailed further in this book, since there are so many excellent accounts elsewhere.

However, a poisoning involving cyanide was a sentinel event in clinical toxicology that is sometimes overlooked. It changed forever how over-the-counter consumer products are packaged and distributed to stores for retail sales. The Tylenol murders in the Chicagoland area in October 1982 shocked the nation, with tremors felt around the world. A young girl, Mary Kellerman, living with her family in Elk Grove Village, IL, awoke with a sore throat and fever in the early morning of Wednesday October 6, was given an Extra-Strength Tylenol (ES-TYLENOL) capsule by her mother, and was dead within hours. Physicians at first attributed her death to a rarity—a stroke in childhood (Beck et al., 1982) (Fig. 2.3.1).

Not long after, Mary Reiner, a 27-year-old Winfield, IL native, took two capsules for a headache and died (Beck et al., 1982). Within a day several more unexplained deaths were reported in the Chicagoland area. Adam Janus, a 27-year-old, collapsed in his home in Arlington Heights, IL, and died within hours. He was thought to have suffered a heart attack. Grieving relatives—his 25-year-old

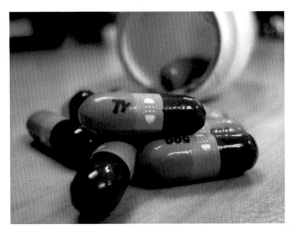

FIG. 2.3.1 Extra-Strength Tylenol capsules. *(From https://en.wikipedia.org/wiki/File:Tylenol_rapid_release_pills.jpg.)*

brother, Stanley, and pregnant 19-year-old sister-in-law, Theresa, both from Lisle, IL—who took ES-Tylenol from the same bottle that Adam had used the same day for their stress-induced headaches—also collapsed and died within the next 48 h (Markel, 2014). That night, two first responder firemen, Philip Cappitelli and Richard Keyworth, in reviewing the bizarre events of the day, realized that all three victims had taken ES-Tylenol (Beck et al., 1982). Later the next day, Mary McFarland, a 31-year-old from Elmhurst, IL, died suddenly and ES-Tylenol (Lot No. 1910MD) was found in her purse. On Friday of the same week, a 35-year-old flight attendant Paula Prince was found dead in her apartment in Chicago; her body was not far away from a bottle of ES-Tylenol (Beck et al., 1982). Thus within a few days, seven unexpected deaths in Chicago and its suburbs were linked to a common point source: the purchase and use of ES-Tylenol products.

Cyanide identified

The physician of one of the patients who died had called the Rocky Mountain Poison Center for advice. The clinical toxicologist there queried whether the victim had been exposed somehow to hydrogen sulfide, which can be lethal. When that possibility was denied, the clinical toxicologist offered cyanide poisoning as the other likely explanation. Early on, public health officials in Chicago independently suspected cyanide poisoning as the cause of death. The symptoms were typical, and there was a "bitter almond" aroma off-gassing from the capsules. Cyanide is known for its quick "knock down" lethality—with a high enough dose, people collapse almost instantaneously. That cyanide poisoning was the cause was confirmed by laboratory testing of blood of the victims and also analysis of the capsules of the ES-Tylenol taken from the murder scenes. Some capsules had been adulterated with as much as 500–600 mg potassium cyanide (KCN; in humans LD50=140 mg; LD100=200-300 mg) (Wolnik et al., 1984).

Toxicology of cyanide

Cyanide prevents the extraction of oxygen from the blood at the tissue level. It binds to iron, inactivating mitochondrial cytochrome oxidase a3, an enzyme critical to aerobic cellular metabolism. This disrupts the electron transport chain and prevents the continuous generation of adenosine triphosphate (ATP), which is necessary for cellular respiration. Oxidative phosphorylation is uncoupled, ATP cannot be regenerated, and normal aerobic cellular function is incapacitated despite adequate oxygen availability to the cell. With rapidly diminishing energy stores, the cell resorts to anaerobic metabolism, resulting in lactic acid formation.

While this is the major mechanism of cyanide's cellular level toxicity, cyanide also disrupts cytosolic calcium homeostasis and has other enzymatic inhibitory actions. Cell death can occur quickly, especially in sensitive body organs such as the central nervous system. Neurons in the brainstem respiratory center, for example, are quickly killed by cyanide's actions, leading to respiratory arrest. The endogenous enzyme, rhodanase, can metabolize small amounts of cyanide ion by conjugating it to the body's limited supplies of thiol moieties, resulting in the less toxic metabolite, thiocyanate. Small amounts of cyanide can also be detoxified by its binding to the endogenous vitamin B12 precursor, hydroxycobalamin, to form the less toxic conjugate, cyanocobalamin. The oral lethal dose (LD50) of potassium cyanide in mouse models is 9.9–11.8 mg/kg, depending on the age of the animal (Sabourin et al., 2016). The lethal dose in human adults is about 200–300 mg.

Clinical toxicity

Cyanide poisoning can occur by ingestion, inhalation, dermal or mucous membrane exposure, or from parenteral injection. Many victims of poisoning with potassium cyanide rapidly become comatose and suffer seizures and circulatory collapse. Some may develop noncardiogenic pulmonary edema, a variety of cardiac dysrhythmias, and/or anoxic encephalopathy. Metabolically, cyanide poisoning produces a high anion gap, lactic acidosis. One recent review of published cases and case series describing 102 patients of acute cyanide poisoning found that patients were unresponsive (78%), hypotensive (54%), or had respiratory failure (73%) (Parker-Cote et al., 2018). Physical findings of patients in that series included cardiac arrest (20%), seizures (20%), cyanosis (15%), and a "cherry red" skin coloration (11%). In 15% of cases, an almond-like odor was present, although that is considered an unreliable sign of the presence of cyanide. In that review, 26 of the 102 patients died, most from respiratory failure, refractory hypotension, and cardiac arrest (Parker-Cote et al., 2018). There are cyanide antidotes used in the management of poisoning that can reverse cyanide's toxic effects if given soon enough after exposure. Details of the history of cyanide antidotes are presented in Chapters 3.3 and 3.8 of this book.

Aftermath of the murders

The trust that people had in the safety of nonprescription drugs and other products intended to be swallowed orally was suddenly broken. A subsidiary of the Johnson & Johnson Company, the McNeil Consumer Products Co., manufacturer of the Tylenol brand, immediately recalled two batches of all of its over-the-counter capsule-containing products—more than 264,000 bottles and over a million capsules—and it stopped all advertising of those products. The company eventually destroyed more than 31 million capsules valued at $100 million (Haberman, 2018). Some state health departments banned all Tylenol products; many pharmacies pulled all Tylenol products from their shelves. At the same time the Food & Drug Administration (FDA) launched a massive education campaign, warning Americans not to take any Tylenol capsules. Poison control centers across the country faced a surge of calls from worried consumers, some of whom were bringing their Tylenol back to pharmacies for a refund and others abstaining from the use of all analgesics. While symptoms of cyanide toxicity include headache, vomiting, agitation, and lethargy, the situation was confused by the fact that people were taking Tylenol products precisely because they had been feeling ill. People were told to refrain from even touching suspect bottles and capsules, since cyanide can be absorbed through the skin.

A total of 15 law enforcement agencies, including more than 100 local police detectives, the Illinois Bureau of Law Enforcement, and the Federal Bureau of Investigation (FBI), were all involved in the forensics assessments, the search for clues, and the pursuit of who might have committed these crimes. There were two lots of ES-Tylenol found at the scenes of the homicides that were identified as containing contaminated capsules—lot MC2880 (produced in Fort Washington PA) and 1910MD (produced in Round Rock, Texas) (Beck et al., 1982). The fact that boxes of ES-Tylenol were manufactured by separate plants in Texas and Pennsylvania—and a detailed review of manufacturing practices and quality control—ruled out the possibility of an unintentional error at the point of manufacture or shipping. This made much more likely the circumstance that capsules were purposefully adulterated once the products had reached Illinois.

More than 300 samples of adulterated capsules were sent to the FDA's Elemental Analysis Research Center (EARC) for analysis using inductively coupled plasma atomic-emissions spectrometry (ICP-AES) to quantitate trace element contaminants (down to ppb) accompanying the almost-pure KCN. There were three unopened bottles of capsules that were confiscated during the recall from drugstores that contained adulterated capsules and were sent to EARC for analysis (Wolnik et al., 1984). There, analyses of over 30 distinctive trace elements, such as calcium, barium, sodium, iron, and magnesium, allowed researchers to "chemically fingerprint" the KCN powder used in the murders. Capsules from different bottles had close to the same quantities, in mcg/g, of these profiled elements. There were only three sources of KCN used by commercial entities in the United States—and sources in Germany and England were quickly ruled out because the trace element signature did not match what was found in the adulterated capsules. Thus the KCN manufacturer was narrowed down to the DuPont Company (Wolnik et al., 1984), although that knowledge did not help detectives much in their search. KCN was generally available in the United States commercially for use in the manufacturing industries, galvanizing and metallurgy, plastics, pesticides, and pharmaceuticals production. Commercial cyanide also had uses in hospital laboratories and other outlets. There were more than 65 sources of KCN in the Chicago area; so that it was easily obtained by the perpetrator for this nefarious purpose (Wolnik et al., 1984).

While it was determined that these deaths were random, intentional, and attributable to product tampering, no perpetrator was ever identified. While there were a few "persons of interest," detectives could not obtain usable fingerprints off the capsules. No individual was criminally charged, and all leads went cold. Was it a disgruntled employee or a competitor resenting Tylenol's increased market share throughout the 1970s over aspirin and other types of analgesics? The event seemed confined to ES-Tylenol lots distributed in the Chicago area only, without an explanation. Both media and public health officials referred to the widespread panic as akin to "pharmaceutical terrorism." (Table 2.3.1).

TABLE 2.3.1 Tips against tampering.

Tablets

- Has their appearance changed? Is the color different? Do they have unusual spots?
- Do the tablets have a different odor or taste?
- Are the tablets moist instead of dry?
- Do the tablets differ in size or thickness?
- If imprinted, is the imprint missing on some or different on others?

Capsules

- Are they cracked or dented?
- Do they have their normal shiny appearance or are some dull or show signs they have been tampered with?
- If imprinted, is the imprint missing from some?
- Are any of a different size and color?
- Do the capsule contents appear to be of differing amounts? Are the capsules of differing lengths?
- Do they have an unexpected or unusual odor?

From the November–December issue of "About Your Medicines," a newsletter for consumers about medicines and their use. Copyright, The United States Pharmacopeial Convention.

Changes in product design and packaging

The lesson was well-learned by those businesses whose success depended on manufacturing safe and pure products intended for use by the public. In the aftermath of the Tylenol murders, new packaging standards and policies were adopted nationwide. Some manufacturers abandoned capsules altogether, and switched to tablets. But capsules are a more suitable vehicle for certain types of pharmaceuticals. Drug companies retooled their packaging to include plastic and metallic foil seals, individual capsule blister packs, and other barriers. Consumers were warned how to inspect products for possible tampering by the U.S. Pharmacopeial Convention (Murphy, 1986) (Fig. 2.3.2).

At the time of the poisonings, McNeil Consumer Products suffered an enormous blow to its brand and its image, let alone substantial financial losses, and its share of the analgesic market declined from 37% to 7% in the short term (Dunea, 1983). Subsequently the company invested over $100 million in new packaging featuring cotton wads, seals, and barrier tabs. It also developed an alternative pill technology—the "caplet"—and introduced it to consumers in many OTC products. The caplet had a single intact, smooth, hard surface which was much more difficult to alter and taint than a two-piece gelatin pill that could be opened, filled with an adulterant, and then re-assembled. McNeil gave out thousands of free samples of bottles of Tylenol with the new safety features to win back the trust of consumers. A survey given to 300 parents a year or two after the Tylenol murders found that, while all participants reported increased anxiety about the use of OTC drugs, few had changed their behaviors or practices in the way they used these

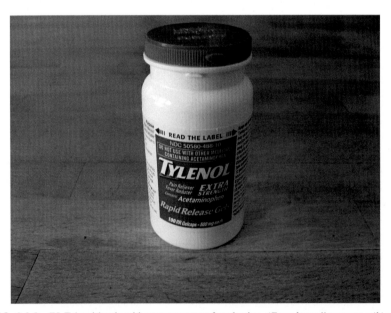

FIG. 2.3.2 ES Tylenol bottle without tamper-proof packaging. *(From https://commons.wikimedia.org/wiki/File:Tylenol_bottle_closeup_crop.jpg.)*

pharmaceuticals (Dershewitz and Levin, 1984). The sales of Tylenol rose from 4% to 30% market share within 12 months after the murders, only 5% below its market share prior to the tampering incidents (Dershewitz and Levin, 1984). It remains one of the most remarkable stories of the recovery of a company's image and brand name by its response to a calamity (Haberman, 2018).

Copycat incidents

In 1983, a year after the seven Chicago murders, Congress passed legislation (the Tylenol Bill) making it a Federal crime to tamper with a product knowing that it would cause bodily harm. It also made it a Federal crime to falsely threaten that products had been or would be tainted (https://www.upi.com/Archives/1983/05/10/Congress-passes-anti-tampering-bill/3638421387200/). However, as noted at the time by public health officials, no product is guaranteed to be 100% tamper proof. Other copycat poisoning incidents involving nonprescription drugs continued to be reported after the Tylenol murders (Dunea, 1983). Incidents have been recorded since then; examples include hydrochloric acid in eye-drops, rat poison or cyanide in analgesic products, insecticide in orange juice, and sodium hydroxide and mercuric chloride placed in capsules in separate incidents.

In 1991 the CDC reported a contamination incident in Washington state involving three adults sickened (two of whom died) by cyanide placed in Sudafed-R 12-Hour capsules (a nonprescription decongestant containing 120 mg pseudoephedrine hydrochloride) (Howard et al., 1991). All three had detectable levels of cyanide in their blood. The manufacturer: Burroughs-Wellcome Company, recalled all Sudafed-R 12-Hour products in the United States and warned consumers. In that episode, packaging of the Sudafed-R capsules included four tamper-resistant features: a two-part plastic capsule sealed with a band, encasement of capsules in a blister-pack with a foil-backed clear plastic film, containment in a box with a safety tab which must be broken to open the box, and labeling of both the box and the packs with matching code numbers. In 3 of the 4 packages, the tamper resistant features had been compromised—look-alike capsules had been substituted in altered blister packs with different code numbers than the boxes. The contaminated blister packs had been substituted, then the box was reconstructed and the outer packaging resealed (Howard et al., 1991).

U.S. packaging and labeling regulation reforms

In the U.S., labeling and packaging of medications are regulated by Federal laws and state statutes to assure the public of the medication's identity, purity, product quality and consistency, and strength. The FDA's laws are intended to assure the public that the product has no adulteration or contamination and is tamper-proof. The Federal Poison Prevention Packaging Act of 1970 (https://www.cpsc.gov/Regulations-Laws--Standards/Statutes/Poison-Prevention-Packaging-Act) (accessed on January 8, 2020) is officially known as Title 16

Code of Federal Regulations (CFR) 1700–1702. It was originally enacted as a response to accidental childhood poisonings involving medications, especially poisonings and deaths associated with aspirin. Child-resistant closures (CRC) have since been a remarkably effective strategy for poisoning prevention among children under the age of 5 years; childhood deaths from accidental poisonings in the United States have declined to very low levels (See chapters in Section 4 of this book that describe in detail such poisoning prevention measures.).

Since 1982 and in response to the Tylenol murders, the FDA issued new regulations concerning how medications should be labeled and packaged. Changes in Title 21 CFR 211 of the Federal Code were enacted. Subpart G of 21 CFR 211 includes materials examination and usage criteria (211.122), labeling issuance (211.125), packaging and labeling (P&L) operations (211.130), tamper-evident packaging requirements for over-the-counter (OTC) human drug products (211.132), drug product inspection (211.134) and expiration dating (211.137). Section CFR 211.132 requires that any two-piece hard gelatin capsule must be sealed using tamper-evident technology. Labeling on all OTC medication products was required to include identification of all tamper-evident features and capsule sealing technology. This information was mandated to be prominently displayed on the label, alerting consumers as to what to look for and how to tell if the barriers had been breached.

The law also requires a robust process of traceability of individual lots of a product should there be an incident or another reason for an investigation or product recall. Details of various aspects of the regulations can be found at the FDA's website (https://www.accessdata.fda.gov/scripts/cdrh/cfdocs/cfcfr/CFRSearch.cfm?CFRPart=211&showFR=1&subpartNode=21:4.0.1.1.11.7 accessed on January 8, 2020).

These industry-wide practices in the United States have not necessarily been adopted elsewhere in the world. The safety of Internet-accessed purchases of pharmaceutical products from international pharmacies is not within the scope of regulation by the FDA. One 2011 report (Veronin, 2011) investigated the availability of products for purchase over the Internet that did not meet such tamper-resistant safeguards or were not sold in child-resistant containers. Of 41 generic medicines purchased, only 1 would have met the requirements of the US laws.

References

Markel H. How the Tylenol murders of 1982 changed the way we consume medication. PBS News-Hour; 2014. https://www.pbs.org/newshour/health/tylenol-murders-1982. [Accessed 8 January 2020].

Beck M, Monroe S, Prout LR, Hager M, LaBreque R. The Tylenol scare: the death of seven people who took the drug triggers a nationwide alert—and a hunt for a madman. Newsweek 1982;100(15):32–6.

Dershewitz RA, Levin GS. The effect of the Tylenol scare on parent's use of over-the-counter drugs. Clin Pediatr (Phila) 1984;23(8):445–8.

Dunea G. Death over the counter. Br Med J 1983;296:211–2.

Haberman C. How an unsolved mystery changed the way we take pills. N Y Times Mag 2018. https://www.nytimes.com/2018/09/16/us/tylenol-acetaminophen-deaths.html. [Accessed 1 January 2020].

Howard J, Pouw TH, Arnold J, Logan B, Kobayashi JM, Davis J. Epidemiologic notes and cyanide poisonings associated with over-the-counter medication—Washington State 1991. MMWR Morb Mortal Wkly Rep 1991;40:161–8.

Murphy DH. Cyanide-tainted Tylenol: what pharmacists can learn. Am Pharm 1986;NS26(5):19–23.

Parker-Cote JL, Rizer J, Vakkalanka JP, Rege SV, Holstege CP. Challenges in the diagnosis of acute cyanide poisoning. Clin Toxicol 2018;56(7):609–17.

Sabourin PJ, Kobs CL, Gibbs ST, Hong P, Matthews CM, Patton KM, et al. Characteristics of a mouse model of oral potassium cyanide intoxication. Int J Toxicol 2016;35(5):584–603.

Veronin M. Packaging and labeling of pharmaceutical products obtained from the internet. J Med Internet Res 2011;13(1), e22.

Wolnik KA, Fricke FL, Bonnin E, Gaston CM, Satzger RD. The Tylenol tampering incident— tracing the source. Anal Chem 1984;56(3):466A–70A. 474A.

Chapter 2.4

Thalidomide tragedy, 1950s

Alan D. Woolf

Boston Children's Hospital & Harvard Medical School, Boston, Massachusetts, United States

The 1940s and 1950s saw remarkable advances in the introduction of new and effective pharmaceuticals, such as isoniazid—the tuberculosis-fighting antimicrobial. The first clinical trials proving isoniazid's effectiveness for TB were carried out at Sea View Hospital in Staten Island, NY, and the successful results were made public in 1952. Penicillin was first discovered in mold by Alexander Fleming in 1928, but it was not mass produced as one of the most effective antibiotics ever known until the World War II era. The antibiotic, sulfanilamide, was introduced in the 1930s (see Chapter 2.1). Oxytetracycline was first mass produced by Pfizer Corporation in the early 1950s. In 1953, Jonas Salk administered his invention—the first parenteral killed polio vaccine—to himself, his wife, and sons. That vaccine proved to be instrumental in curbing the worldwide polio epidemics that had handicapped and killed thousands of victims, many of them children, since the 1890s. And so, newspapers, magazines, radio, and other media touted these as remarkable times of the discovery of "wonder drugs." The advent of a new medicine—thalidomide—in the 1950s as an anti-convulsant, anxiolytic, antispasmodic, anti-emetic, and mild sedative was welcomed enthusiastically by the general public and medical practitioners alike (Fig. 2.4.1).

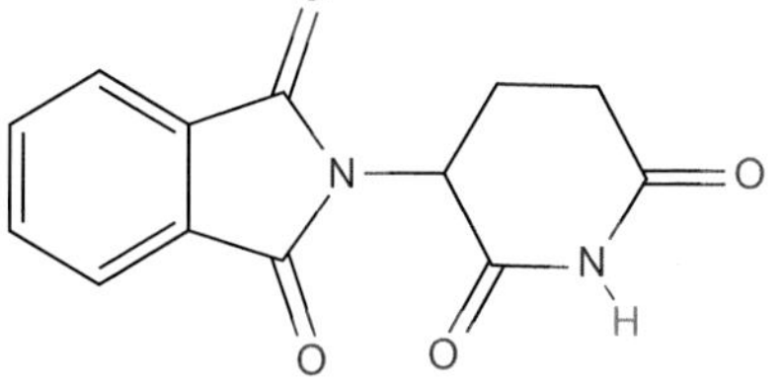

FIG. 2.4.1 Chemical structure of thalidomide.

History of Modern Clinical Toxicology. https://doi.org/10.1016/B978-0-12-822218-8.00058-2

Thalidomide's insufficient premarketing testing

Thalidomide (Thalomid; alpha-(*N*-phthalimido)-glutarimide), a racemic glutamic acid derivative, was originally discovered by the Swiss pharmaceutical company CIBA AG in 1952 and intended for use as a tranquilizer and an anticonvulsant (Rehman et al., 2011). However, work by Herbert Keller demonstrated that it also helped to sedate people suffering from insomnia and make them relaxed. It was also remarkably free of measurable adverse effects during limited testing in experimental animals. A crystalline white, tasteless powder, it was tolerated in such high doses that an LD50 was difficult to calculate and the drug was deemed nontoxic. Since at the time it was not believed that drugs could pass the placental barrier, it was not tested in pregnant animals in premarketing studies.

In Germany, Chemie Grunenthal Pharmaceuticals first synthesized thalidomide, obtained a 20-year patent, and undertook clinical trials in 1954 (Shafique, 2019). It then mass-produced thalidomide for over-the-counter sales as a cough and cold remedy under the trade name: *Grippex*. It was also marketed under the trade names: *Contergan* and *Distaval*, as an effective and inexpensive hypnotic-sedative for inducing deep sleep. Distaval was welcomed as one of the fashionable anti-anxiety sedatives that were popularized in the 1950s. Since thalidomide's anti-emetic action was also found to relieve the nausea and vomiting associated with "morning sickness" in pregnancy, it was introduced into obstetrical practice and was greeted with great enthusiasm by pregnant women in more than 40 countries throughout Europe, Asia, Canada, Australia, and South America during the post-World War II baby boom in the 1950s. By the mid-1950s, thalidomide was marketed by 14 pharmaceutical companies under more than 37 trade names and sales were brisk following intense marketing campaigns (Shafique, 2019). In its first year of production, Grunenthal was selling more than 90,000 units per month (Moro and Invernizzi, 2017). By 1956, the drug was being distributed in more than 20 countries worldwide. An estimated 14.6 t of the drug were sold in 1960 alone (Rehman et al., 2011).

Blocked in America

The William S. Merrrell Company, a pharmaceuticals distributor, petitioned the FDA for permission to introduce thalidomide into the American market under the trade name: Kevadon (Fig. 2.4.2). It also commenced clinical trials in the United States, over which the FDA had no control, and distributed thalidomide directly to thousands of participants. However, most pregnant women in the United States who participated in the clinical trials took the drug in their third trimester of pregnancy, thus escaping the window of vulnerability to its teratogenic effects (Moro and Invernizzi, 2017). Dr. Frances Oldham Kelsey, newly employed by the FDA in 1960, was charged with reviewing the scientific data for thalidomide during the new drug approval process. Her superiors had assigned her to the application because they considered it a rather easy task for an entry-level worker. However, Dr. Kelsey brought a thoroughness to her new job and assignment that caused her to worry about the lack of rigorous scientific evidence of the safety of thalidomide in humans, especially with respect to its association with irreversible peripheral neuropathies as a side-effect. She felt that the production of the drug had been rushed without sufficient animal testing; for example, there had been no testing of thalidomide in pregnant animals. She would not approve the application and thereby delayed its introduction into the United States, effectively blocking its distribution (Fig. 2.4.3).

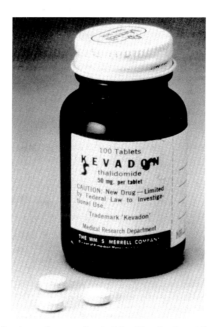

FIG. 2.4.2 "Kevadon"—the trade name for thalidomide, distributed by the William S. Merrill Company. *(From https://commons.wikimedia.org/wiki/File:FDA_History_-_Thalidomide_ (4,901,386,994).jpg.)*

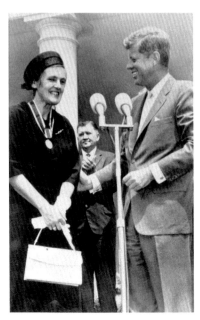

FIG. 2.4.3 President John F. Kennedy presents the President's Award for Distinguished Federal Civilian Service to Dr. Frances Oldham Kelsey in August, 1962, for her role at the FDA in denying approval of the drug: Thalidomide. *(From https://commons.wikimedia.org/wiki/File:Frances_Oldham_Kelsey_and_John_F._Kennedy.jpg.)*

Birth defects linked to thalidomide use in pregnancy

The first known case of thalidomide teratogenicity was a girl born on December 25, 1956, in Stolberg Germany—home to the manufacturer, Chemie Grunenthal. The infant was born without ears to a woman whose husband worked for Grunenthal and had given his wife samples of the drug (Lenz, 1988). Cases of birth defects began to be reported in Great Britain and throughout Europe a year later, when the epidemic became more widespread and noticeable. It certainly was not appreciated by physicians during its widespread marketing that thalidomide is a potent teratogen; they promoted its use by their patients for a variety of ailments. The defects most commonly included limb "flipper-like" deformities known as phocomelia. Infants were also born with missing or malformed eyes or ears or foreshortened limbs and severely deformed hands and feet or complete absence of limbs (amelia). As many as 25% of children also had eye damage and 33% had some hearing impairments (Newbronner and Atkin, 2018). Less common defects involved the heart, kidneys, gallbladder, and genitalia. Thalidomide use was also associated with increased rates of miscarriage, stillbirth, and infant mortality.

Other malformations included those of the head, face, tongue, and teeth. Body systems, including the gastrointestinal, cardiovascular and neurological systems, could be affected. Other complications included behavioral and learning disabilities. Dr. William McBride (1961), an Australian obstetrician, and Dr. Widukind Lenz (Lenz, 1962; Lenz and Knapp, 1962), a German pediatrician and geneticist, made independent observations linking cases of congenital defects to the use of thalidomide and published their findings in the journal, *Lancet* (Lenz et al., 1962). Others confirmed the association in the growing number of cases and the drug was subsequently withdrawn in Germany in November 1961, unfortunately much too late for thousands of victims who were never compensated. Soon thereafter, experiments in chick embryos and pregnant rabbits confirmed in laboratory animals the drug's teratogenicity (Kemper, 1962; Cameron and Chrislie, 1962; Boylen et al., 1963; Yang et al., 1963).

Poor communications to other countries of the drug's toxicity and ban in Germany unfortunately led to its continued marketing and use in Japan, Brazil, Sweden and other countries into 1962 and even into 1963 before thalidomide was withdrawn. This resulted in continued births of malformed children (Lenz, 1988). An estimated 10,000 children in Britain, Canada, Germany, Japan, Brazil, Australia, and 40 other countries were born with thalidomide-induced deformities (Fig. 2.4.4).

Families were devastated by the spreading epidemic of birth defects. Mothers, guilt-ridden about their use of thalidomide, could not tell their husbands or family or friends. This hampered public health authorities seeking to

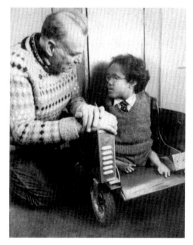

FIG. 2.4.4   Photograph of Terry Wiles (right) who was born with phocomelia due to thalidomide. *(From https://commons.wikimedia.org/wiki/File:Len-terry-wiles.jpg.)*

identify possible new cases when pursuing their investigation of the outbreak. Some pregnant women responded by seeking out abortions, regardless of their religious beliefs or its legality. There were even cases of infanticide committed by distraught parents.

Thalidomide toxicology and clinical toxicology

Very little of the parent compound—thalidomide—is excreted unchanged in urine (Schumacher et al., 1965). It undergoes spontaneous hydrolysis and non-enzymatic metabolism, with the production of more than 100 active metabolites, many of which are thought to be responsible for both its therapeutic and adverse effects, including its teratogenicity (Schumacher et al., 1965). Animals also vary in how they metabolize thalidomide and the metabolites are species-specific; thus, errors could easily be made in extrapolating results from animal experiments to humans. The malformations seen in humans after exposure to thalidomide in pregnancy were not seen in all animal species (e.g., rodent models).

The effects on embryogenesis were dependent on exposure to the drug in the first trimester, during organogenesis. The susceptible period was days 20–34 after fertilization (35–50 days after the last menstrual period). Upper limb malformations occurred at days 24–32, lower limbs at days 27–34; external ear malformations at days 20–24, inner ear at days 24–34, and thumb hypoplasia at days 21–28 (Kim and Scialli, 2011). Pregnant women taking the drug later in pregnancy gave birth to infants without evidence of congenital defects.

For many years, it was not known how thalidomide caused birth defects. Over 30 hypotheses have been posited over the years, from induction of oxidative stress to interference with folate or glutamate metabolism to inhibition of DNA synthesis. The parent compound is rapidly broken down in the liver to more than 100 metabolites. However, research has isolated at least one of those compounds capable of antiangiogenesis-inhibiting vascular growth. This interference with the branching, developing blood vessels needed to nourish the growing skeletal system or eyes or ears or other systems during that very sensitive time of organogenesis during the first trimester of pregnancy may explain how the irreversible organ or limb damage occurs. Most recently, research has shown that thalidomide causes limb defects by preventing angiogenic outgrowth from limb buds. Using a tetrafluorinated analog of thalidomide (CPS49), Therapontos and colleagues showed that the loss of immature blood vessels upstream during embryogenesis explains both the timing (drug effect only during early fetal growth) and its relative tissue specificity (limb morphogenesis) (Therapontos et al., 2009). They showed that CPS49 inhibited endothelial cell proliferation and migration at critical junctures of development, preventing cellular formation of vascular tubes into immature blood vessels essential to limb development.

Besides its teratogenic potential, thalidomide's toxicity commonly includes fatigue, weakness, tremors, rashes, neutropenia, xerostomia, constipation, ataxia, mild bradycardia, mild peripheral edema, hearing loss, venous thromboembolism, and somnolence (Ghobrial and Rajkumar, 2003). Peripheral sensorimotor neuropathies are a risk; nerve damage can be permanent. Thalidomide also can rarely cause menstrual irregularities, seizures, Stevens-Johnson syndrome, endocrine disturbances, impotence, elevated liver function tests, and toxic epidermal necrolysis (Ghobrial and Rajkumar, 2003).

Corporate responsibility

Public health authorities in Germany were slow to react to warnings from scientists that thalidomide was responsible for the many malformations being reported. Grunenthal Company reportedly knew of thalidomide's suspected neurological side-effects as early as 1957. However, the drug continued to be manufactured, promoted and sold by pharmaceutical distributors up until the global ban in 1962, and even after that in some locales around the world.

The consequences of the thalidomide tragedy reverberated throughout Europe and the United States. Dr. Kelsey was hailed as a hero in the United States for blocking the sales of the drug. The company, Grunenthal, at first denied any responsibility and blamed the deformities on everything from infectious causes to new chemical cleaners to nuclear fallout. However, it became apparent that the drug was responsible. Corporate leaders of the pharmaceutical company were arraigned in criminal courts in 1968 in West Germany.

Companies were sued in different countries by the thousands of victims for damages associated with thalidomide's use. Still, the powerful pharmaceutical companies responsible for its distribution and marketing in different countries had previously obtained indemnity agreements with distributors, limiting their liability and avoiding criminal prosecution (Moro and Invernizzi, 2017). The Grunenthal Company finally issued an apology for its role in the thalidomide tragedy in 2012, almost 50 years too late.

Families with affected children joined together to advocate for the rights of the victims for compensation from the companies and/or the governments themselves and multiple lawsuits were filed in many countries. After all, it was the absence of effective governmental agency oversight that allowed a dangerous drug to be distributed to the public. Some countries responded belatedly with compensation, acknowledging victims' rights. Still, some governmental agencies would not verify the status of a victim as qualifying for compensation without the provision of a previous prescription for thalidomide, which might have been written months to years previously. The judicial process itself was so slow and deliberate as to delay the consideration of cases for years. In Britain, one thalidomide distributor, the Distillers Corporation, was required eventually to paid 20 million British pounds to victims and their families. In Japan, the government allocated 28–40 million Yen to the victims (Moro and Invernizzi, 2017). However many, if not most, children deformed by thalidomide suffered enormous physical limitations and emotional and social consequences for their entire lives, and were never fully compensated for the ensuing struggles they experienced. Their medical and rehabilitation costs were never recovered from the company, whose profit motive outweighed considerations of the safety of the public.

Rehabilitation services

One of the consequences of the thalidomide-related epidemic of congenital defects was the need to expand rehabilitation and support services for those affected children and their families. New types of artificial limbs were developed in the 1960s to improve their functionality and quality of life. It was learned that the physical deformities in most cases did not affect the mental abilities of the children; they often only needed special educational services adapted to meet their physical limitations (Fig. 2.4.5).

Changing social mores recognized the rights of victims to governmental investments and assistance so as to achieve an acceptable quality of life. Promising medical advances and the provision of a network of professional

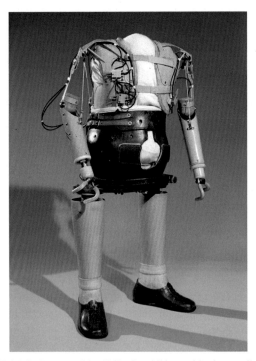

FIG. 2.4.5 Artificial limbs created in 1960s for children with phocomelia, which often included absence of the upper and lower limbs. *(From https://commons.wikimedia.org/wiki/File:Artificial_limbs_for_a_thalidomide_child,_1961-1965_(9660575567).jpg. Source: Science Museum London/Science and Society Picture Library. Uploaded by Mr. John Cummings)*

support services to their families would enable some thalidomide victims to develop and adapt so as to achieve independence and productive lives. However, a review of 25 follow-up studies (Newbronner and Atkin, 2018) documented the continuing primary and secondary complex health problems and the consequences of the discriminatory social context that survivors with thalidomide embryopathy have endured throughout their lives.

Historical context

The thalidomide tragedy unfolded within the historical context of dynamic economic, cultural, and social changes:

- The unchecked growth of politically and economically powerful, multinational pharmaceutical companies who self-monitored drug development and clinical trials
- Lax governmental regulatory oversight and premarketing testing of drugs
- The globalization of pharmaceutical products
- Increasing role of the media in healthcare-related educational outreach
- The postwar "Baby Boom"
- The rapid postwar rise of consumerism and consumer demands responsive to aggressive advertising
- The era of the discovery and promotion of "wonder drugs"

Reform: Regulation of new pharmaceuticals

The tragedy led to important and comprehensive pharmaceutical regulatory reforms and drug controls in the United States, Great Britain, Brazil, and other countries. The mandatory provision of rigorous scientific evidence of efficacy and safety of an experimental new drug employing in vitro and animal studies, including developmental studies, before proceeding to clinical trials was implemented. Many of the provisions in today's regulations of investigational new drugs stem from the catastrophic thalidomide experience.

The thalidomide tragedy revealed the need to perform developmental testing of all pharmaceutical products prior to licensing, to include effects on fertility and reproduction, teratogenicity, and perinatal effects (Kim and Scialli, 2011).

Thalidomide research demonstrated the potential for error in extrapolating from experiments in one species of animals to determine adverse health effects in humans. It revealed the need to investigate drug effects in more than one animal species, since interspecies differences exist in the pharmacokinetics and metabolism of drugs and in differential sensitivities of animals to their adverse effects. In the United States, the infrastructure of the FDA was overhauled to improve its ability to manage a new, more rigorous application process and to provide appropriate oversight of the development of new drugs, termed the Investigational New Drug (IND) protocol still in effect today. Curiously, thalidomide is also used now as a "model" teratogen in the investigation of effective alternatives to developmental testing in animals, such as cell culture and other in vitro methodologies.

Rebirth of thalidomide

The worldwide ban on thalidomide in 1962 was not the end of the story for this drug. Despite its notorious origins, thalidomide later emerged as an effective drug for treating some inflammatory conditions and certain types of cancer. Further testing of thalidomide in the 1970s and 1980s focused on aspects of its unusual pharmacology, including its antiangiogenic and antiinflammatory effects. It also potently activates subsets of T cells, shifts cytokine production, blocks tumor necrosis factor-alpha, and has other immunomodulary properties (Rehman et al., 2011). It has shown some benefit in the treatment of patients with leprosy, preventing the skin lesions of the associated erythema nodosum leprosum (ENL) (Kim and Scialli, 2011). It has also been used in clinical trials for the treatment of multiple myeloma and other cancers, such as renal cell carcinoma, Kaposi's sarcoma, prostate cancer, and myelofibrosis (Shafique, 2019). It has been used to treat vascular malformations and ophthalmologic diseases of the retina and has shown promise in the treatment of HIV wasting syndrome and as a palliative measure in cancer cachexia syndrome (Rehman et al., 2011).

Thalidomide was subsequently approved by the FDA in 1998 for use in the treatment of ENL. At that time, the FDA mandated extensive precautions and contraindications related to thalidomide's potent teratogenicity. In 2006, the FDA approved thalidomide through its accelerated track for use as a first-line agent in the treatment of multiple myeloma (Shafique, 2019). More than 118 analogs of the drug have been synthesized and investigated for their antiangiogenic and antiinflammatory effects, immune modulating activity, and other pharmacological properties that might yield potential therapeutic benefits (Franks, 2004).

The current maker of thalidomide, Celgene Corporation, has implemented the System for Thalidomide Education and Prescribing Safety (STEPS) to monitor physician prescribing of the drug and safeguard against exposure of pregnant women or women of childbearing age (Ghobrial and Rajkumar, 2003) (Kim and Scialli, 2011). Before being prescribed the drug, women must receive negative pregnancy tests and because it is passed via semen, men must use a condom or abstain from sexual intercourse altogether. Contraception is begun 4 weeks prior to starting the drug. If a woman misses a menstrual period, then thalidomide use must be discontinued immediately. Only 4-week supplies of drug are dispensed and there are no automatic prescription refills. Still, the black-market, unapproved, and unsupervised use of the drug in some countries has been associated with the births of additional children with severe malformations.

Aftermath

The thalidomide tragedy brought to light societal level public health, ethical and human rights issues, some of which are still controversial and/or evolving today.

- Ethical issues related to conflicts of interest in medical science, medical practice, and the pharmaceutical industry
- Ethical issues regarding the right to life
- Basic human rights to health and drug safety
- Need to protect and compensate victims of the pharmaceutical industry
- Needs of people with disabilities
- Protection of patient rights
- Role of the media in helping to publicize public health issues
- Advocacy for victims of medicine-related injury

References

Boylen JB, Horne HH, Johnson WJ. Teratogenic effects of thalidomide and related substances. Lancet 1963;1:552.

Cameron JM, Chrislie GA. Thalidomide and congenital abnormalities. Lancet 1962;280(7262):937.

Franks ME, Macpherson GR, Figg WS. Thalidomide. The Lancet 2004;363:1802–11.

Ghobrial IM, Rajkumar SV. Management of thalidomide toxicity. J Support Oncol 2003;1(3):194–205.

Kemper F. Thalidomide and congenital abnormalities. Lancet 1962;ii:836.

Kim JH, Scialli AR. Thalidomide: the tragedy of birth defects and the effective treatment of disease. Toxicol Sci 2011;122(1):1–6.

Lenz W, Pfeiffer RA, Kosenow W, Hayman DJ. Thalidomide and congenital abnormalities. The Lancet 1962;279(7219):45–6.

Lenz W, Knapp K. Foetal malformations due to thalidomide. Ger Med Mon 1962;7:253–8.

Lenz WA. A short history of thalidomide embryopathy. Teratology 1988;38:203–15.

McBride WG. Thalidomide and congenital abnormalities. Lancet 1961;2:1358.

Moro A, Invernizzi N. The thalidomide tragedy: the struggle for victims' rights and improved pharmaceutical regulation. Hist Cienc Saude Manguinhos. 2017; 24 (3). https://doi.org/10.1590/s0104-59702017000300004, [Accessed 9 October 2019].

Newbronner E, Atkin K. The changing health of thalidomide survivors as they age: a scoping review. Disabil Health J 2018;11(2):184–91.

Rehman W, Arfons LM, Lazarus HM. The rise, fall, and subsequent triumph of thalidomide: lessons learned in drug development. Ther Adv Hematol 2011;2(5):291–308.

Schumacher H, Smith RL, Williams RT. The metabolism of thalidomide: the fate of thalidomide and some of its hydrolysis products in various species. Br J Pharmacol 1965;25:338–51.

Shafique A. Thalidomide—an overview and the species-specific teratogenicity. Res J Congenital Dis 2019;2(1):1–10.

Therapontos C, Erskine L, Gardner ER, Figg WD, Vargesson N. Thalidomide induces limb defects by preventing angiogenic outgrowth during early limb development. PNAS 2009. www.pnas.orgcgidoi10.1073pnas.0901505106.

Yang TJ, Yang TS, Liang HM. Thalidomide and congenital abnormalities. Lancet 1963;1:552–3.

Chapter 2.5

Dimethylmercury death— Professor Wetterhahn, 1996

Alan D. Woolf
Boston Children's Hospital & Harvard Medical School, Boston, Massachusetts, United States

There is no more tragic story of accidental poisoning than the occupational mishap, originally thought to be trivial, which led to the death of a chemist of international stature. Dr. Karen Wetterhahn was a brilliant chemist at Dartmouth College who studied the chemical characteristics of heavy metals. She graduated from St. Lawrence University in 1970 and earned her doctorate at Columbia University (Karen, 2017). She worked at Columbia's Institute for Cancer Research, sponsored by the National Institutes of Health (NIH), before she was recruited in 1976 to come to Dartmouth as its first female chemistry professor. She loved teaching and was an accomplished cancer investigator, specializing in the oncogenic properties of toxic metals such as chromium and nickel. She was interested in studying health effects of metals that are common environmental contaminants, for example, at toxic waste sites. Dr. Wetterhahn had achieved international renown for her accomplishments in scientific research in the field of chemistry (Fig. 2.5.1).

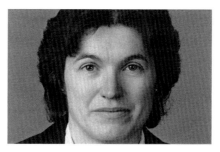

FIG. 2.5.1   The late Dr. Karen Wetterhahn: a distinguished Dartmouth University chemist *(Source: Courtesy of Dartmouth College Library).*

History of Modern Clinical Toxicology. https://doi.org/10.1016/B978-0-12-822218-8.00054-5

Professor of chemistry on Dartmouth Faculty

Dr. Wetterhahn thrived at Dartmouth. She served as a role model and mentor to young women student scientists at every stage of their careers. A prominent cancer researcher, she was a co-founder of Dartmouth's Women in Science Project and was a past-officer of the American Association for Cancer Research (Karen, 2017). She was promoted to Dean of Graduate Studies (1990), Associate Dean of the Faculty for the Sciences (1990–94), and Acting Dean of the Faculty of Arts and Sciences (1995). She was awarded a $7 million grant from the National Institute for Environmental Health Sciences (NIEHS) in 1995 to establish an interdisciplinary Toxic Metals Superfund Research Program at Dartmouth (see Dartmouth Toxic Metals Superfund Research Program http://www.dartmouth.edu/~toxmetal/TXQAcr.shtml). This program continues to draw together scientists from Dartmouth College and the Geisel School of Medicine at Dartmouth, as well as collaborators and co-leaders from other academic institutions.

August 14, 1996, laboratory incident

On August 14, 1996, she was working with dimethylmercury, a dense, viscous, colorless solution readily absorbed through skin. Dimethylmercury is a potent neurotoxin; a lethal dose is about 5 mg/kg. She was attempting to use it to calibrate a nuclear magnetic resonance (NMR) instrument, since she was skeptical about the accuracy of the other commonly used standard, mercuric chloride. Dimethylmercury is used by some scientists as a standard for calibrating the NMR spectrometers prior to scanning new chemicals for their atomic "signatures." Dimethylmercury is used as a standard rather than other chemicals because it is pure, not affected by pH or concentration, and requires no dilution (Endicott, 1998). Because of its extreme toxicity, Dr. Wetterhahn was working under a laminar flow, reverse ventilation fume hood and wearing a protective laboratory coat, face shield, and latex gloves. As she was pipetting the dimethylmercury, one or two drops of the fluid accidentally fell onto her left latex glove. She ended her experiments for the day, threw away the gloves, entered her records of work for the day in the lab book, went home, and thought nothing more of it.

Signs of illness

She was apparently healthy after the episode. She worked as usual each day; she participated in a scientific meeting several months after the incident. But dimethylmercury begins to penetrate brain tissue and cause progressive damage even before clinical symptoms become apparent. She began to experience some subtle neurological symptoms of poisoning about 3 months after the exposure, with a few episodes of nausea and vomiting some weeks apart. Soon she experienced more pronounced symptoms: slurred speech, altered handwriting, and a stumbling, unsteady gait. She needed her husband to pick her up at work because she was not well enough to drive herself home (Endicott, 1998). However, no connection with the spilled dimethylmercury was made until about 5 months after the exposure, when she developed more pronounced neurological symptoms including paresthesias, ataxic gait, dysarthria, high-pitched tinnitus, and both hearing and vision loss.

She sought medical advice from a neurologist. She was noted to have a wide-based gait and some "scanning speech" and to have lost 6.8 kg of her body weight over several months. It was at that time that she recalled the incidental exposure to at most a few drops (0.1–0.5 cc's) of the liquid dimethylmercury.

Toxicology of dimethylmercury

Mercury is neurotoxic and has no physiological role in the body. It exists in three forms: as the liquid element and as inorganic salts and organic compounds; of the three, organic forms are thought to be the most toxic. Historically, mercury had many uses in medicine as an antiseptic and antifungal preservative, as an antisyphilitic agent, as a laxative, as a diuretic, in dental amalgams, in medical devices and in the processing of radiographic film, although it is no longer used for any of these purposes. Mercury is still present in some batteries, electronics, and other products. It has uses in commercial, mining, and manufacturing industries. Mercury is also a widespread environmental pollutant, from sources such as sewage, coal-fired generating plants, mining and smelting effluents, and others sources (see Chapter 1.2). It contaminates lakes, rivers, and even oceans; and it is present in some common types of seafood, especially in predator fishes.

Dimethylmercury was first synthesized in 1865. It is rapidly converted to methylmercury in the body with a half-life of uptake into hair of about 5.6 days and some immediate excretion through exhaled breath (Nierenberg et al., 1998). Thereafter the organic molecule, methylmercury, has a prolonged half-life in blood of about 74.6 days (Nierenberg et al., 1998). Toxicity is thought to be mediated by the slow conversion of methylmercury to divalent inorganic mercury metabolites. In a dose-dependent, rate-limited, ageing process, there is slow neuronal cell death and gliosis, until enough time has elapsed so that the number of viable cells is diminished enough to result in marked brain degeneration and in overt symptoms, as was the case in this poisoning (Weiss et al., 2002). Mercury specifically targets small granule cells of the cerebellum and neurons in the visual cortex, as well as other sites in the central nervous system, while sparing other cell types such as Purkinje cells. This variable distribution into susceptible cells may also explain the long latency period before the onset of overt symptoms of toxicity (Weiss et al., 2002). Another possibility explaining a long latency period is that of low level, chronic environmental exposures requiring slow accumulation of toxic metabolites, such as that seen in the Japanese Minamata and Niigata epidemics described in Chapter 1.2 of this text.

January 1997—Dr. Wetterhahn hospitalized

Dr. Wetterhahn was hospitalized with a diagnosis of mercury poisoning in January 1997. Chelation therapy was started with dimercaptosuccinic acid (DMSA) which effected, at first, a moderate urinary mercury diuresis (Nierenberg et al., 1998). Despite aggressive therapy, including exchange blood transfusion and multiple rounds of chelation, the illness continued its progressive worsening. She had restricted visual fields and reported flashes of light. She became deaf and had peripheral neuropathy. Her body burden of mercury was much too high for that treatment to be effective, like chipping slivers of ice off a glacier. Her whole blood mercury concentration was 4000 mcg/L, about 800 times higher than the reference level (50 mcg/L) for toxicity. Her total body burden of mercury, calculated using hair, blood, and urine concentrations, was about 1344 mg of mercury, the amount contained in about 0.44 mL of dimethylmercury solution (Nierenberg et al., 1998; Siegler et al., 1999). The serial measurements of mercury in hair samples showed the kinetics of the metal's distribution in her body over time. Within weeks of hospitalization, she suffered halting speech, a shrinking field of vision, further memory loss, and cognitive decline to the point of only spontaneous eye opening without signs of awareness. She became decorticate and decerebrate, slipping into a coma in February from which she never recovered. She lapsed into a vegetative state in the ensuing months, and died at the age of 48 years on June 8, 1997, 298 days after the original exposure.

Mercury pathology

Dr. Wetterhahn encouraged the publishing of details of Her illness as a warning to other scientists not to repeat her mistake and to learn safer methods of handling highly toxic compounds such a dimethylmercury. Her case was published in the *New England Journal of Medicine* in 1998 (Nierenberg et al., 1998). Scientists were shocked by the case. Most had little idea of the inherent danger posed by dimethylmercury, when mercury in its various forms is such a ubiquitous contaminant in the environment (Kulig, 1998). Autopsy results showed extreme thinning of the cerebellum, with shrinkage and atrophy of the folia, gliosis, and extensive cell loss there and in the cerebral cortex (Siegler et al., 1999). Mercury tissue levels in the frontal lobe and visual cortex averaged 3.1 μg/g of tissue (3100 ppb), more than six times the concentration in blood at the time of death and many times higher than the amount of mercury usually found in the brains of individuals unexposed to specific sources of contamination by the metal (2–50 ppb) (Nierenberg et al., 1998) (Fig. 2.5.2).

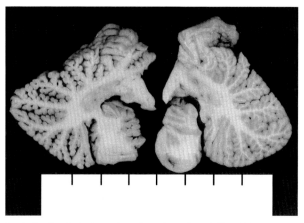

FIG. 2.5.2 Cerebellar hemispheric sections from the patient (left) and from a woman of approximately the same age without neurologic disease (right). *(Source: Figure taken from Figure 3 in Nierenberg et al. NEJM1998; 338(23): page 1674 with permission)*

What was not appreciated prior to this incident was the extreme potency of dimethylmercury in comparison with methylmercury on an equimolar basis. The fact that the liquid metal could penetrate so quickly through a glove barrier and be so quickly and completely absorbed after a dermal exposure also was not known. In the aftermath of this tragedy, scientists tested the permeability of latex glove material. Their studies revealed that liquid dimethylmercury could penetrate those gloves to skin within 15 s and perhaps instantaneously, so that they provided no barrier protection at all (Blayney et al., 1997). The authors confirmed that Dr. Wetterhahn had suffered only a transdermal exposure, not including an inhalational route, since she was working under a fume hood at the time of the accident. They recommended a change in laboratory operating procedures to include a safer laminate glove (e.g., SilverShield) be worn under neoprene, nitrile, or similar long-cuffed barrier gloves when handling aggressive, highly toxic chemicals. The authors also urged scientists to substitute a safer standard compound for NMR calibration measurements than dimethylmercury because of its inherent hazard.

Aftermath—Laboratory standard operating procedures changed

Dr. Wetterhahn's intent to change laboratory standards of safety was realized. the US Occupational Safety & Health Administration (OSHA) issued an advisory regarding revisions to its safe laboratory procedures. The inadequacy of the Material Data Safety Sheet (MSDS) on dimethylmercury at the time, recommending only chemically resistant gloves, was noted. After OSHA investigated this tragedy, the agency issued new guidance to scientists and others working with extremely toxic chemicals, including dimethyl mercury (OSHA, 1998). The agency fined Dartmouth $9000 for inadequate precautions and required the university to hire a chemical safety officer, improve signage, require use of appropriate chemical resistant gloves, and revise their safety practices. Other scientists have subsequently changed their standard operating procedures, with guidance from OSHA and other health agencies. OSHA, the NIH, and other agencies have discouraged the routine use of supertoxic metals, such as dimethylmercury, in calibration techniques and other research methodologies. All acknowledge the inherent risks of working with supertoxic metals and highly volatile chemicals. In addition, scientists are creating new chemicals with an unknown hazard all the time; they cannot let down their guard (Goldberg, 1997; Blayney et al., 1997; Endicott, 1998).

Wetterhahn awards

The NIEHS created the "Karen Wetterhahn Memorial Award" in her honor shortly after her death. In recognition of her leadership in the Superfund Research Program, the award stipulates that potential applicants, graduate students or postdoctoral researchers, must be involved with Superfund Research Program grants.

Dartmouth established several memorials in her honor, including a graduate fellowship in chemistry and an annual faculty award for distinguished creative or scholarly achievement.

A Dartmouth library reading room and the annual undergraduate science symposium have also been named in her honor and her portrait now hangs in Dartmouth's Baker-Berry Library.

References

Blayney MB, Winn JS, Nierenberg DW. Handling methylmercury. Chem Eng News 1997;75(19):7.
Endicott K. The trembling edge of science. Dartmouth Alumni Magazine; 1998.
Goldberg C. Colleagues vow to learn from chemist's death. New York Times; October 1997.
Karen RS. Wetterhahn, the chemist whose poisoning death changed safety standards. Dartmouth Alumni Magazine; 2017.
Kulig K. A tragic reminder about organic mercury. N Engl J Med 1998;338:1692–4.
Nierenberg DW, Nordgren RE, Chang MB, Siegler RW, Blayney MB, Hochberg F, Toribara TY, Cernichiari E, Clarkson T. Delayed cerebellar disease and death after accidental exposure to dimethylmercury. N Engl J Med 1998;338(23):1672–6.
OSHA. Dimethylmercury. Safety Health Bull 1998.
Siegler RW, Nierenberg DW, Hickey WF. Fatal poisoning from liquid dimethylmercury: a neuropathologic study. Hum Pathol 1999 Jun;30(6):720–3.
Weiss B, Clarkson TW, Simon W. Silent latency periods in methylmercury poisoning and in neurodegenerative disease. Environ Health Perspect 2002;110(Suppl 5):851–4.

Chapter 2.6

Yushchenko (dioxin), 2004 and Markov (ricin), 1978: Two political poisonings

Alan D. Woolf
Boston Children's Hospital & Harvard Medical School, Boston, Massachusetts, United States

Chapter 2.6.1

Viktor Yushchenko

The Ukraine has always been a country with sharp political divisions. Since the downfall of the Soviet Union and Ukraine's declaration of its independence in August 1991, these divisions have only grown more intense. Its eastern region is dominated by ethnic Russians closely aligned with Russian values and interests. The western section has been more independent and aligned with the West (Fig. 2.6.1).

Viktor Yushchenko, a prominent political figure in the Ukraine in the 1990s, was poisoned with a dioxin-containing substance probably in his food, during an election campaign in 2004. Yushchenko, who had been president of the Ukraine in 2001 and favored economic ties with the European Union and membership in NATO, was ousted by a no confidence vote of the eastern oligarchy-dominated parliament. He then formed a new political party: "Now Ukraine" which advocated for closer ties with the West and subsequently attained a majority in the parliament (McKee, 2009). The ruling party was more aligned with Russia and the ethnic Russian population in the eastern Ukraine. Its pro-Russian president had finished his two terms in office, and a new election in 2004 saw two candidates emerge from more than 26 who were originally running for the office. Viktor Yushchenko was one of those candidates and the campaign was marked by vicious attacks and a popular struggle, with a vote scheduled in October 2004.

History of Modern Clinical Toxicology. https://doi.org/10.1016/B978-0-12-822218-8.00016-8

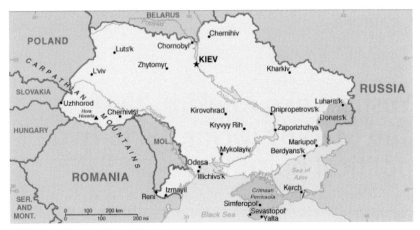

FIG. 2.6.1 Map of Ukraine. *(From https://www.cia.gov/library/publications/the-world-factbook/geos/up.html. Author: Directorate of Intelligence, Central Intelligence Agency, USA.)*

Shortly after dining in Kiev at a formal dinner with security forces on September 5, 2004, Yushchenko developed a headache and abdominal discomfort. He rapidly became seriously ill and was hospitalized. At first, his diagnosis was thought to be acute pancreatitis; he was given supportive care, the symptoms abated, and he was discharged from the hospital. However, 3–4 weeks later he developed a mysterious, life-threatening, multisystem illness, including a severely disfiguring facial rash. A British clinical toxicologist, Dr. John Henry, postulated at the time that this was likely a case of intentional dioxin poisoning. Yushchenko went back on the campaign trail despite his illness and lost a close election reportedly marked by electoral fraud (McKee, 2009) (Fig. 2.6.2).

Yushchenko's dose of TCDD

A detailed study of his medical condition was subsequently published in *The Lancet* in 2009 (Sorg et al., 2009). Mr. Yushchenko gave permission for the toxicologists to reveal his medical results, "to further medical science." As opposed to previous human exposures to dioxins, such as dioxins released in the Seveso Italy explosion or contaminating cooking oil in the Yusho disaster (see Chapters 1.3 and 1.10), where the populace was exposed to a mixture of the dioxin or dioxin-like family of chemicals, this poisoning was carried out with a single chemical. The most lethal of the dioxins: 2,3,7,8-tetrachlorodibenzo-*p*-dioxin (TCDD) used in this poisoning was pure; it must have been prepared in a laboratory. Although the daily dose of dioxins in humans (mostly contained in food) is estimated at 4 pg/kg, Yushchenko's one-time dose was estimated at about 20 mcg/kg—about 5 million-fold higher than the maximum accepted daily dose for the population (Saurat et al., 2012). Measurements of his serum TCDD levels taken after he became sick exceeded 108,000 pg/gm lipid weight, approximately 50,000 times higher than the value found in a general populace

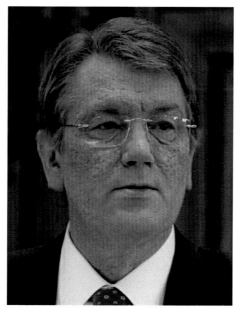

FIG. 2.6.2   Viktor Yushchenko: before and after pure dioxin poisoning. *(From https://commons.wikimedia.org/wiki/File:Viktor_Yuschenko.jpg.)*

(Sorg et al., 2009). This level translates to a body burden of more than 1 mg of dioxin. At the same time, measurements of the concentration of 17 other chemicals in the dioxin class did not reveal any levels above those found in the general Ukrainian population, confirming this incident as an intentional poisoning with TCDD alone. The half-life of TCDD in Yushchenko's case was calculated to be 15.4 months (Sorg et al., 2009). The skin, adipose cells, and the blood were tissues containing large amounts of TCDD.

Toxicology of dioxins

Dioxins are a class of over 400 chemicals that have similar chemical structures—chlorinated dibenzo-*p*-dioxins, polychlorinated biphenyls (PCB), and polychlorinated dibenzofuran (PCDF) congeners, of which about 30 (7 dioxins, 10 PCDFs, and 12 dioxin-like PCBs) have been shown to have toxicity in humans (Piérard et al., 2005; Schecter et al., 2006). They are environmentally persistent, lipophilic, bio-accumulative pollutants. Dioxins are produced as a by-product of waste incineration and in the manufacture of paper and pulp bleaching and the synthesis of some chlorine-containing organic chemicals, such as herbicides, pesticides, and fungicides. In the Yushchenko poisoning, a single dioxin chemical, TCDD, was weaponized as an ingested poison.

TCDD was the chemical found in trace amounts as a by-product in "Agent Orange" chemicals: 2,4 dichlorophenoxtacetic acid (2,4 D) and 2,4,5 trichlorophenoxyacetic acid (2,4,5 T) used as defoliant herbicides delivered by airplanes over large swaths of land during the Vietnam War, which subsequently sickened thousands of Vietnamese, as well as American troops. Much of what we know about the toxic effects of dioxins in humans has been learned from occupational exposures of workers in electrical and other industries, although accidental exposures of the public, such as those seen at Seveso, Italy, and in the Yusho incident in Japan, have provided additional data on toxicity. The reader will find details on the Seveso and Yusho disasters and more information on the toxicology of dioxins in Chapter 1 of this book.

TCDD itself is a lipophilic chemical that easily traverses cell membranes and is stored in fat. Lactation reduces dioxin levels in the breast-feeding mother, but the dioxin in breast milk increases levels in the infant. Serial measurements of TCDD in Yushchenko's blood, urine, feces, and fatty tissues were performed over the subsequent 4 years prior to *The Lancet* publication and documented a somewhat shorter elimination half-life of about 15.4 months, facilitated by liver and skin metabolism. Two metabolites 2,3,7-trichloro-8-hydroxydibenzo-*p*-dioxin and 1,3,7,8-tetrachloro-2-hydroxydibenzo-*p*-dioxin were identified in his serum, urine, and feces (Sorg et al., 2009). The feces were the major route of elimination of the TCDD in Yushchenko's case.

The toxicity of TCDD is mediated in part by its ability to induce the aromatic hydrocarbon receptor (AhR), which is a nuclear receptor and transcription factor conserved in most animal and human cells. TCDD forms a heterodimer with AhR inducing or suppressing the transcription of numerous genes (Sorg, 2014). Downstream, this toxic effect produces many cellular changes in functionality. Polychlorinated dibenzo-*p*-dioxins and polychlorinated dibenzofurans were declared Class 1 carcinogens by the International Agency for Research on Cancer (IARC) in 1997, based on animal studies, occupational data, and follow-up studies of the 1976 Seveso, Italy disaster. TCDD was unique in that it was considered by IARC as a cause of all cancers at all sites, rather than cancers associated with a few specific organ types (Steenland et al., 2004). For all of the 30 chemicals in the dioxin series of interest for their human toxicity, their "total dioxin toxic equivalency" or TEQ expresses the potency of each chemical in its ability to activate the AhR receptor, compared with TCDD (Schecter et al., 2006).

Clinical toxicology in Yushchenko's case

Yushchenko developed headaches and stomachaches within hours of the poisoned meal; he was hospitalized 5 days later, unable to walk (Sterling and Hanke, 2005). He had an elevated white cell count and elevated liver function tests, and soon thereafter suffered severe back pain and skin rashes on the face and trunk consistent with chloracne. He recovered slowly over some months with supportive care.

The skin reaction (known as "chloracne") that transformed Yushchenko's face into a confluence of cysts and lesions is not a form of acne vulgaris (Sterling and Hanke, 2005). While there are open comedones and cysts, there are few pustules or nodular lesions in chloracne. While sebaceous glands are over-active in acne vulgaris, they are atrophied in chloracne. Meibomian glands in the skin are involved in chloracne but not in acne vulgaris. The lesions in chloracne include hemartomas, multiple small growths from dermal stem cells that apparently multiply as an effect from TCDD on the AhR receptor. These prolific skin growths concentrated the TCDD and detoxified it by highly induced phase I enzymes CYP1A1 and CYP1A2 hydroxylases, probably saving his life. Chloracne lesions can persist for 2–5 years after exposure; their absence does not preclude the diagnosis of dioxin poisoning (Sorg, 2014).

Other toxic effects attributed to TCDD seen in Yushchenko's case included hepatitis, pancreatitis, neuropathy, arthritis, and gastrointestinal inflammation (Saurat et al., 2012). Other effects of occupational or environmental dioxin poisoning can include conjunctivitis, porphyria cutanea tarda, hyperpigmentation, immune deficits, endocrine disruption, diabetes, thyroid dysfunction, hirsutism, and psychiatric disturbances, including depression. See details of the clinical effects of dioxin exposure in Chapters 1.3 and 1.10.

Yushchenko underwent 26 surgical procedures—including dermabrasion, nodule and cyst excisions, and multiple punch skin biopsies (Saurat et al., 2012). While steroids and nonsteroidal antiinflammatory medications did not provide him with pain relief, infusions of the THF-alpha blockers: infliximab and adalimumab were followed by progressive improvements in his symptoms associated with inflammation (Saurat et al., 2012). There is at present no good way to reduce the body burden of dioxin.

Aftermath and lessons learned

After his remarkable recovery, Yushchenko and his "Orange Party" (the color of his campaign materials) went on to defeat the Russian-favoring candidate and he was inaugurated as president of the Ukraine in January 2005. However, he was later removed from office in a national election and his pro-western views fell out of favor with the body politic.

There were lessons to be learned for clinical toxicologists stemming from the clinical features and course of the Yushchenko case:

- Human survival after the 2nd highest recorded dose of TCDD.
- A shorter half-life (15.4 months) in this case of one-time TCDD poisoning than had been previously reported (up to 7–11 years) with small-dose chronic environmental or occupational exposures.
- The role of the skin in accumulating and metabolizing dioxin and its metabolites.

- Sebaceous gland atrophy as a biomarker specific to the rash caused by dioxin poisoning.
- The skin as a detoxifying organ for TCDD and possibly other xenobiotics.
- The role of biologic, TNF-alpha blocking antiinflammatory drugs in the treatment of dioxin poisoning.

References

McKee M. The poisoning of Victor Yushchenko. Lancet 2009;374:1132.

Piérard GE, Plomteux G, Denooz R, Charlier C. Dioxin—poisoning information or brainwashing? About the acne of Seveso and Yushchenko. Rev Med Liege 2005;60(1):18–22.

Saurat JH, Kaya G, Saxer-Sekulic N, Pardo B, Becker M, Fontao L, et al. The cutaneous lesions of dioxin exposure: lessons from the poisoning of Victor Yuashchenko. Toxicol Sci 2012;125(1):310–7.

Schecter A, Birnbaum L, Ryan JJ, Constable JD. Dioxins: an overview. Environ Res 2006;101(3):419–28.

Sorg O. AhR signaling and dioxin toxicity. Toxicol Lett 2014;230(2):225–33.

Sorg O, Zennegg M, Schmid P, Fedosyuk R, Valikhnovskyi R, Gaide O, et al. 2,3,7,8-Tetrachlorodibenzo-p-dioxin (TCDD) poisoning of Victor Yushchenko: identification and measurement of metabolites. Lancet 2009;374:1179–85.

Steenland K, Bertazzi P, Baccarelli A, Kogevinas M. Dioxin revisited: developments since the 1997 IARC classification of dioxin as a human carcinogen. Environ Health Perspect 2004;112(13):1265–8.

Sterling JB, Hanke CW. Dioxin toxicity and chloracne in the Ukraine. J Drugs Dermatol 2005;4(2):148–50.

Chapter 2.6.2

Markov incident—Ricin—London, 1978

A homicidal incident that took place in London reads like the pages of a spy novel but was all too real. This is the tragic death of 49-year-old Georgi Markov, in which ricin was likely used in the fatal poisoning. Markov was a well-known, distinguished Bulgarian author and playwright. He was also a dissident and fervent anticommunist while living in Bulgaria, where his views were not appreciated and his novels and plays suppressed. Some of his writings were banned, but he still became successful and well-known internationally for his work. After putting on a controversial play sharply critical of the Bulgarian regime, he was advised to leave the country immediately and he left for Italy the same day (Crompton and Gall, 1980). When his Bulgarian passport was not extended, he defected to Great Britain in 1971. Markov subsequently began living and working in London as a broadcaster for the BBC, Radio Free Europe, and the German Deutsche Welle Station (Fig. 2.6.3).

Markov was critical of the Bulgarian communist regime of Todor Zhivkov, who was the Bulgarian leader from 1954 to 1989. In fact, Zhivkov reportedly commented at a communist party meeting that he wanted Markov "silenced

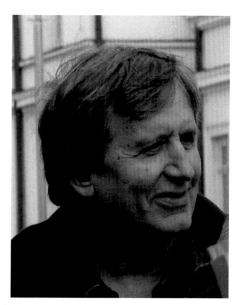

FIG. 2.6.3 Georgi Markov. *(From https://commons.wikimedia.org/wiki/File:Acad.-Georgi-Markov-20101201.jpg.)*

forever" (Papaloucas et al., 2008). Markov used his position in broadcasting as a forum for his views. He subsequently received numerous threats and two unsuccessful attempts on his life, one in Munich and the other on the island of Sardinia. Three months prior to his death, he received an anonymous threat warning him that unless he stopped working for Radio Free Europe, he would be eliminated (Papaloucas et al., 2008).

Poisoning incident

On September 7, 1978, while walking in a crowded street on the Waterloo Bridge in London, Markov was jabbed in his right thigh with an injectable umbrella by an unknown assailant who escaped in a taxi. He felt a slight pain, like an insect bite on his right thigh and discovered a small red pimple there. Within hours, he developed a high fever, tachycardia, low blood pressure, abdominal pain, vomiting, and diarrhea. He was admitted to St. James Hospital in Balham, London, where he was at first thought to be septic. He was unable to speak, had bloody vomitus, and developed a WBC count as high as 33,200. An EKG showed complete heart block and he developed anuric renal tubular necrosis. Despite supportive care, he died on September 11 (Musshoff and Madea, 2009; Crompton and Gall, 1980). The umbrella was never recovered, but a gas-propelled mechanism such as the one depicted in the Figure below was postulated to have been the weapon capable of firing the tissue-penetrating pellet-like projectile (Fig. 2.6.4).

Significantly, another Bulgarian dissident and defector to Paris, Vladamir Kostov, was attacked from behind with a blow to the back while on the Metro 2 weeks prior to Markov's umbrella attack. He developed a fever but, unlike Markov, recovered after several weeks. An identical pellet was recovered from the reddish pimple-like lesion in his back, of a similar size and borings to that embedded in Markov's thigh. Again, in this second assassination attempt, no evidence of ricin could be detected and no perpetrator could be found (Crompton and Gall, 1980).

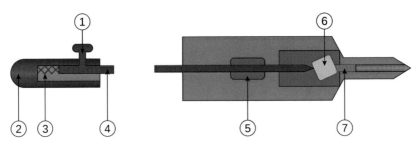

FIG. 2.6.4 Diagram of possible weaponized umbrella containing small injectable pellet. *(From https://commons.wikimedia.org/wiki/File:Markov_umbrella.PNG.)*

Markov's autopsy

At autopsy, a small round metallic pellet 1.53-mm diameter was recovered from Markov's red, indurated thigh. It had two tiny 0.34-mm holes bored into it with a total volume of about $0.28\,mm^3$. The pellet could have held a volume of about 0.5 mL, capable of carrying about 0.2–0.5 mg ricin (Papaloucas et al., 2008; Musshoff and Madea, 2009). It was covered by a sugary coating like a bubble and was designed to melt at 37°C, body temperature. Although no poison was recovered, only ricin was theorized to be toxic enough to transmit a lethal dose to the adult victim when delivered by holes of that size and volume.

Markov's autopsy showed other striking pathology. His lungs were filled with fluid indicative of heart failure, and hemorrhages were noted throughout the myocardium. His inguinal lymph nodes were swollen with hemorrhage and necrosis. His liver was fatty, intestines were necrotic, and there were interstitial hemorrhages in many tissues (Crompton and Gall, 1980).

Castor bean

The ordinary castor bean plant, *Ricinus communis* (spurge family; *Euphorbiaceae*), grows up to 12 ft in height in warm, sunny climates in the United States, although it is native to tropical Africa, China, Central and South America, India, and other locales where it is harvested for commercial purposes. It is viewed by some as a weed and by others as a cultivated red and green ornamental plant (Fig. 2.6.5).

The castor bean plant contains multiple soft, spiny seed pods. The pods grow in clusters on the shrub. Each pod contains the tick-colored, mottled brown or black and white seeds—the castor bean. The bean has a hard shell and whitish pulp which is the source of castor oil. The whole bean itself is often dyed and used to make decorative jewelry, such as necklaces and bracelets (Fig. 2.6.6).

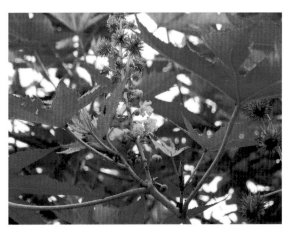

FIG. 2.6.5   Castor bean plant with spiky seed pods. *(From https://commons.wikimedia.org/wiki/ File:Castor_bean_plant_(371550056).jpg.)*

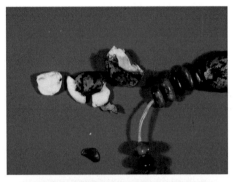

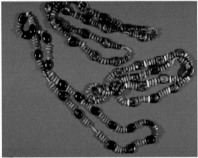

FIG. 2.6.6 Castor bean dyed in a necklace, showing whitish pulp. *(Photo by author.)*

The whitish pulp of the bean is the source of the toxic natural protein—ricin. While the entire castor plant contains small amounts of the potent cellular toxin, ricin, it is particularly concentrated in the bean (each contains 1%–5% ricin by weight, or about 0.35 mg) (Bradberry et al., 2003). Ricin is excluded in the manufacture of castor oil, a viscous, yellowish fluid that has been used as a purgative and laxative, a lubricant, and for its nutritional value. The castor bean has also been used in the manufacture of cosmetics, biofuels, and certain plastics (e.g., nylon). More than a million tons of castor beans are harvested annually for their commercial value (Vance and Mantis, 2016).

Toxicology of ricin

Ricin is a water-soluble, globular glycoprotein consisting of two polypeptide chains, A and B, connected by a single disulfide bridge. It can be inactivated by heat or anything that breaks the disulfide bond. Ricin is similar in some of its toxic actions to abrin, the active agent in the "rosary pea" plant: *Abrus precatorius* (Leguminosae) (Osnes et al., 1974). Both are phytotoxins and members of a group of natural proteins known as "type II ribosome-inactivating proteins" or RIP-II. Both are members of the "AB superfamily" of bacterial and plant toxins (including, for example, shigatoxin, anthrax, and cholera toxins) using retrograde transport to gain access to the cytosol of a cell (Yermakova et al., 2014).

Ricin is capable of entering all types of mammalian cells, attaching itself to cell membrane carbohydrates. As many as 10^6–10^8 ricin molecules can bind to a single cell (Musshoff and Madea, 2009). Ricin is transported into the cell by endocytosis; it can fully penetrate target cells within 15–30 min of presentation (Song et al., 2013). The B chain, a barbell-shaped lectin (MW 34,000), is comprised of 262 amino acids. As a haptomer, it binds to *N*-acetyl galactosamine and galactose-containing glycolipid or glycoprotein receptors on the surface of sensitive cells, allowing cellular entry by the A chain. The A chain effectomer (267 amino acids, MW 32,000) is an RNA *N*-glycosidase that is conveyed by the B-chain via retrograde transport from the plasma membrane to the Golgi Apparatus and endoplasmic reticulum. At that point, the A-chain is liberated and translocated back to the cytosol to its principal site of action: the ribosome. The A-chain enzyme binds to 28s rRNA and disrupts the 60-s subunit of ribosome. The enzymatic depurination of a single adenosine residue of the 28s rRNA within the so-called sarcin-ricin loop of the 60-s subunit interferes with protein elongation, which destroys the functional ability of the ribosome to effect protein synthesis (Morris and Wool, 1992). A single A chain molecule can thus irreversibly inactivate about 1500 ribosomes per minute, leading to impaired protein synthesis and cell death (Audi et al., 2005) (Fig. 2.6.7).

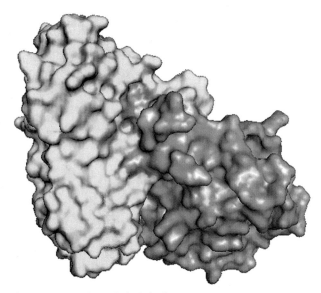

FIG. 2.6.7   Structural map of Ricin's A-chain (blue) and B-chain (yellow). *(Source: wikimedia commons https://commons.wikimedia.org/wiki/File:Ricin_structure_surface.png. Author: BSTlee using Pymol.)*

The tissue injury caused by ricin includes endothelial cell damage and death, tissue edema and reduced perfusion, the elaboration of cytokines and a resulting robust inflammatory reaction, hemorrhage, cellular apoptosis, and "vascular leak syndrome." Cells may vary in their sensitivity; for example, Kupffer cells (macrophages) in the liver are a particularly sensitive target for ricin, which accounts for its hepatotoxicity (Bradberry et al., 2003). A minimum number of about 10 ricin molecules is enough to kill a cell in culture (Osnes et al., 1974). As little as 1–20 mg/kg of body weight of ingested ricin is a lethal dose in an adult human (Audi et al., 2005). But much less, as little as 1–10 mcg/kg of body weight, may be lethal when injected intramuscularly or intravenously. The intraperitoneal LD50 for ricin in mice is 100 ng (Osnes et al., 1974). In the Markov assassination, it was estimated that about 500 mcg of ricin was injected (Crompton and Gall, 1980).

Ricin is considered an agent that can be weaponized for use in bio-chemical warfare or terrorism. It is included on the Centers for Disease Control and Prevention (CDC) Category B list of bioterrorism agents. This classifies the agent as moderately easy to manufacture and disseminate, with a moderate potential of inflicting toxic injury on people. Purified ricin is much more potent than the crude protein found in the bean. Inhaled ricin particles less than 5 μm can penetrate deep into lung tissues and be readily absorbed, with high mortality rates. The LD50 of such inhaled particles in mice is about 3–5 μg/kg (Audi et al., 2005).

Clinical toxicology

Body organs that are particularly sensitive to the toxic effects of ricin include the gastrointestinal tract, liver, kidneys, and pancreas. Ricin poisoning has usually been reported after raw castor beans are eaten, the pulp released by mastication and the raw soluble ricin swallowed. While ingestion of just a few beans is said to be toxic, the severity of the illness will of course be dependent on characteristics of the victim, the dose per body weight, and the concentration of ricin within the beans, which is variable depending on growth characteristics and size of the plant. After a period of 4–36 h, enough ricin is absorbed to produce gastrointestinal symptoms, including nausea, vomiting, hematemesis, abdominal pain, diarrhea, and melena. Other effects include cold extremities, blurred vision, dehydration, tachycardia or bradycardia, lethargy, renal dysfunction, and electrolyte imbalances (Bradberry et al., 2003). In severe poisonings, symptoms can progress to include life-threatening hypovolemic hypotension, cardiovascular collapse, hepatitis, and oliguric renal failure.

Ricin is particularly life-threatening when the exposure is by one of two routes: inhalation or injection. When tiny (a few microns in size) particles of ricin are aerosolized and inhaled, the toxin is distributed to the large surface area of the lungs where it is rapidly deposited in the terminal airways and alveoli. Its toxic effects are almost immediate, with the earliest signs being cough and dyspnea, progressing within hours. Cellular injury and death mediated by ricin provoke intense inflammatory reactions, hemorrhage, and tissue necrosis. Clinically, these toxic effects cause widespread pulmonary edema and pneumonia, with associated respiratory failure and death.

When ricin is injected, the clinical toxic effects resemble that of septic shock, including high-grade fever and hypotension. The patient can still present initially with weakness and gastrointestinal symptoms, such as abdominal cramps, nausea, vomiting, and diarrhea. Signs of toxicity quickly progress to include hemodynamic instability, hypovolemic shock, and cardiovascular collapse.

Detection of ricin

Ricin can be detected in body fluids by a variety of immunologic-based techniques such as enzyme-linked immunosorbent assays (ELISA) or radioimmunoassays (RAI), although these have only been available for research purposes. Immuno polymerase chain reaction (IPCR) is a specific ricin detection method with an LOD as low as 10 fg/mL (Musshoff and Madea, 2009).

Some methods of detecting and quantifying ricinine, another plant constituent (0.3%–0.8% of the bean) that co-locates with and can serve as a surrogate marker for ricin, have been developed (Johnson et al., 2005). Using a novel extraction method, chromatography, and tandem mass spectrometry, ricinine has been detected in urine as long as 48 h after exposure (Johnson et al., 2005). In one report of a lethal case of castor bean extract injection by a 26-year old man, ricinine was detectable in serum (16.5 ng/mL) and blood (12.9 ng/mL) within about 6 h after the injection; a urinary concentration of 81.1 ng/mL was detectable 7 h after injection (Verougstraete et al., 2019). In that report, liquid chromatography/mass spectrometry (LC-MS) was the methodology used for detection, using ricinine D3 as an internal standard.

Ricin antibodies, vaccines, cancer therapies

This unsolved assassination and other threats against prominent individuals confirmed ricin's designation by the CDC as a potential agent that could be used in biochemical warfare or terrorist attacks. Research into the phytotoxin has focused on potential technologies for treatment and prevention. Antibodies to both the A and B subunit moieties have been developed and have shown the ability to neutralize ricin's cellular toxicity in animal and in vitro models (Herrera et al., 2014; Song et al., 2013; Yermakova et al., 2014). These antibodies can have both extracellular and intracellular actions in binding ricin molecules for hours. They have been shown to aggregate toxin and interfere with its intracellular retrograde transport to target organelles (Song et al., 2013). Such specific ricin monoclonal antibodies have not yet been shown to be effective when used in humans but theoretically could be of value as postexposure therapy. There has also been an effort to develop a ricin vaccine, although this has proven to be a complex undertaking

(Doan, 2004; Herrera et al., 2014; Vance and Mantis, 2016). Additionally the use of ricin A chains as an anti-cancer therapy has been explored (Engert et al., 1997).

Aftermath

Despite an extensive investigation, there was nothing found that might connect a Bulgarian agent to Markov's murder. It was alleged that this was a state-sponsored assassination authorized and organized by the Soviet KGB and the Bulgarian secret service, since Markov was at the time considered an "enemy of the state." Years later, two former KGB agents admitted to the complicity of the Soviet spy agency in the assassination but did not name the murderer (Papaloucas et al., 2008; Musshoff and Madea, 2009). One was sentenced to 16 months in jail for destroying some 10 volumes of files on the case and the second committed suicide prior to his trial. A Bulgarian spy who was rumored to have been the commander in the plot died in a suspicious car accident.

After the fall of communism in Bulgaria, Markov was posthumously awarded the Order of Stara Planina, Bulgaria's highest honor, for his contributions to Bulgarian literature and his anticommunist activities.

References

Audi J, Belson M, Psatel M, Schier J, Osterloh J. Ricin poisoning: a comprehensive review. JAMA 2005;294(18):2342–51.

Bradberry SM, Dickers KJ, Rice P, Griffiths GD, Vale JA. Ricin poisoning. Toxicol Rev 2003;22:65–70.

Crompton R, Gall D. Georgi Markov—death in a pellet. Med Leg J 1980;48(2):51–62.

Doan LG. Ricin: mechanism of toxicity, clinical manifestations, and vaccine development: a review. J Toxicol Clin Toxicol 2004;42(2):201–8.

Engert A, Diehl V, Schnell R, et al. A phase I study of an anti-CD25 ricin A-chain immunotoxin (RFTS-SMPT-dgA) in patients with Hodgkin's lymphoma. Blood 1997;89:403–10.

Herrera C, Vance DJ, Eisele LE, Shoemaker CB, Mantis N. Differential neutralizing activities of a single domain camelid antibody (V_HH) specific for ricin toxin's binding subunit (RTB). PLoS One 2014;9(6):e99788.

Johnson RC, Lemire SW, Woolfitt AR, et al. Quantification of ricinine in rat and human urine: a biomarker for ricin exposure. J Anal Toxicol 2005;29:149–55.

Morris KN, Wool IG. Determination by systematic deletion of the amino acids essential for catalysis by ricin A chain. Proc Natl Acad Sci U S A 1992;89:4869–73.

Musshoff F, Madea B. Ricin poisoning and forensic toxicology. Drug Test Anal 2009;1(4):184–91. https://doi.org/10.1002/dta.27 [Review. Erratum in: Drug Test Anal. 2009 Jul;1(7):363-4].

Osnes S, Refsnes K, Pihl A. Mechanism of action of the toxic lectins abrin and ricin. Nature 1974;249:627–31.

Papaloucas M, Papaloucas C, Stergioulas A. Pak J Biol Sci 2008;11(19):2370–1.

Song K, Mize RR, Marrero L, Corti M, Kirk JM, Pincus SH. Antibody to ricin A chain hinders intracellular routing of toxin and protects cells even after toxin has been internalized. PLoS One 2013;8(4), e62417.

Vance DJ, Mantis NJ. Progress and challenges associated with the development of ricin toxin subunit vaccines. Expert Rev Vaccines 2016;15(9):1213–22.

Verougstraete N, Helsloot D, Deprez C, Heylen O, Casier I, Croes K. Lethal injection of a castor bean extract: ricinine quantification as a marker for ricin exposure using a validated LC-MS/MS method. J Anal Toxicol 2019;43(2):e1–5.

Yermakova A, Klokk YI, Cole R, Sandvig K, Mantis NJ. Antibody-mediated inhibition of ricin toxin retrograde transport. MBio 2014;5(2), e00995-13.

Section 3

Discovery of selected modern antidotes

Alan D. Woolf[a] and Jeffrey Brent[b]

[a]*Boston Children's Hospital & Harvard Medical School, Boston, Massachusetts, United States,*
[b]*Distinguished Clinical Professor of Medicine and Emergency Medicine, University of Colorado School of Medicine, Aurora, CO, United States*

Introduction

The term *antidote* is variously described in etymological references as from the Greek or the Latin *anti*, meaning "against" and *didonai* "to give." Antidotes can be defined as those drugs, chemicals and/or xenobiotics that, when given to a poisoned patient, improve their medical status by counteracting, at the cellular and biochemical levels, injurious effects of chemicals, poisons, drugs, stings or envenomations.

The history of antidote discovery and use dates to ancient times, although some of them worked and many of them didn't. If the poison was not lethal, often the antidote was! (See the monograph "Toxicology in Antiquity" by Philip Wexler (2019) in this Series.) The history of Greek and Roman antiquity teaches us that monarchs traditionally had a healthy respect for poisons, both for self-protection and to achieve political goals. Their fear of being poisoned led to the quest for readily available antidotes, usually in the form of a "theriac," or a "universal antidote." Generally, these were combinations of herbs, with the possibility of opium, metals, or venoms mixed in. One of the best described theriacs was developed for the Roman Emperor Nero (37–68 CE). Given the liberal use of poisonings by Nero, including an unsuccessful attempt to poison his own mother, it is little surprise that he made it a priority to have his personal physician and the botanist Andromachus develop a theriac. Nero neither appeared to be harmed nor saved by his theriac and instead died by self-ordered execution (Burks, 2020). In modern times, some traditional antidotes—such as the home remedy "universal antidote" of tea, burnt toast, and milk of magnesia—have fallen into disrepute when subjected to scientific rigor (Daly and Cooney, 1978).

Today, endeavors to formulate antidotes based on sound pharmacologic principles have resulted in lifesaving therapeutics. The development of new antidotes is evolving beyond traditional reliance on knowledge of the pathophysiology of a poisoning to the exploitation of the tremendous power and specificity of the immune system. In clinical toxicology, we utilize immunological therapies ranging from Fab fragments to treat digoxin poisoning to antivenoms to idarucizumab for the treatment of dabigatran toxicity.

This section includes compelling stories of discovery, the remarkable perseverance of brilliant scientists dedicated to finding a cure for specific poisons. We chose to focus on eight antidotes as examples of drugs with particularly remarkable, and relatively recent, histories. Some of these stories (e.g., British Anti-Lewisite, oximes) are set against a background of a military need to find answers to weaponized chemicals used in warfare. Others (e.g., methylene blue, cyanide antidotes, physostigmine) required only the inquiring, scientific minds of innovative researchers to interpret correctly what they observed of the properties of natural substances and intuitively apply them as the solution to a medical problem. Still others (e.g., N-acetyl cysteine, fomepizole, naloxone) resulted from a methodically reasoned approach to counteracting the known pathophysiology of the toxic agent. Embedded in each chapter is a story that stands as a tribute to those pioneers of clinical toxicology whose efforts gave rise to the development of these life-saving antidotes.

References

Burks R. Ancient antidotes at, https://www.chemistryworld.com/opinion/ancient-antidotes/4011771. article; 2020. [Accessed 2 October 2020].

Daly JS, Cooney DO. Interference by tannic acid with the effectiveness of activated charcoal in "universal antidote". Clin Toxicol 1978;12(5):515–22.

Wexler P, editor. Toxicology in Antiquity. 2nd ed. London, United Kingdom: Academic Press; 2019.

Chapter 3.1

N-Acetylcysteine

John Rague

Rocky Mountain Poison and Drug Safety, Denver Health and Hospital Authority, Denver, CO, United States; Department of Emergency Medicine, Denver Health and Hospital Authority, Denver, CO, United States

Introduction

N-Acetylcysteine (NAC) is a nearly ubiquitous antidote in hospitals. This is for good reason. In the United States, acetaminophen is the fifth leading cause of poisoning-related death (Gummin et al., 2019). It accounts for approximately 30,000 hospital admissions annually (Blieden et al., 2014; Manthripragada et al., 2011) and is the most common cause of acute liver failure (ALF) in North America (Stravitz and Lee, 2019). In the absence of NAC, these figures would soar. Fortunately, through a series of discoveries and clinical applications in the 1960s and 1970s, NAC proved to be an effective treatment in mitigating the harmful and sometimes fatal effects of acetaminophen poisoning.

NAC origins and mucolytic effect

The origin and synthesis of NAC are limited to the details laid forth in its patent. On August 26, 1960, biochemist Aaron Leonard Sheffner, PhD, of Mead Johnson & Company filed the patent for NAC. The invention of NAC rose from the intent to "provide a therapeutic agent which may be readily administered which has a high degree of mucolytic activity…for treating mucus whereby viscosity of the mucus is quickly and markedly reduced" (Sheffner, 1963a). Sheffner devised a simple experiment to demonstrate the mucolytic efficacy of this new agent. Globules from pulmonary secretions were placed onto a glass slide and angled at 53 degrees. The globules remained stationary at this angle and remained so when exposed to water. However, when a NAC solution was applied to the glass side, the globules immediately lost their viscosity and ran down the glass (Sheffner, 1963a). Sheffner and colleagues went on to publish additional studies on the mucolytic properties of NAC in the early 1960s. The authors concluded the mechanism of action of NAC derived from the presence of a free sulfhydryl group, which disrupted the number of disulfide bonds

History of Modern Clinical Toxicology. https://doi.org/10.1016/B978-0-12-822218-8.00002-8

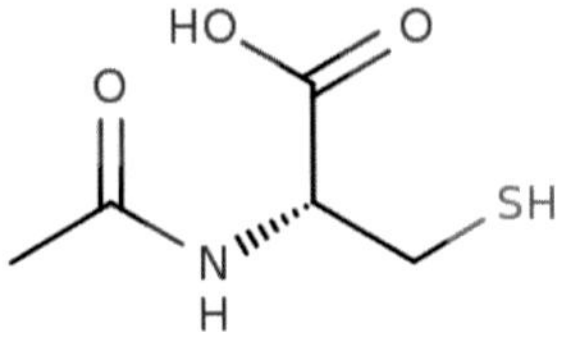

FIG. 3.1.1 Acetylcysteine.

in mucoprotein and led to a marked reduction in viscosity (Sheffner, 1963b; Sheffner et al., 1964) (Fig. 3.1.1).

The discovery of NAC's mucolytic effect came at a time when treatment modalities for cystic fibrosis (CF) were limited. Clinicians exhausted the use of existing treatments with little to no benefit in the amelioration of the respiratory complications of CF. Immediate research was conducted to evaluate the efficacy in NAC in the treatment of patients with CF given the need for an effective mucolytic agent. Research funded by Mead Johnson Medical Research Center and the National Cystic Fibrosis Research Foundation spearheaded investigations on NAC in the treatment of CF. These studies showed favorable results in reducing the viscosity of tracheobronchial secretions as well as clinical improvement in signs and symptoms (Webb, 1962; Reas, 1964; Howatt and DeMuth, 1966).

Clinicians went on to apply the mucolytic properties of NAC to other disease states where aberrations in mucus physiology resulted in physiologic disorder. From the mid-1960s to the 1970s, published cases of NAC administration in meconium ileus (Lillibridge et al., 1967; Meeker Jr., 1964; Shaw, 1969), asthma and chronic bronchitis (Anderson, 1966; Grater and Cato, 1973), postoperative atelectasis (Thomas et al., 1966; Weiner and Steinvurzel, 1966), and nasal sinusitis (Komet and Salco, 1965) appeared. NAC was effective in completely dissolving a food bezoar in a patient with pyloric stenosis (Schlang, 1970), provided symptomatic relief in a patient with keratoconjunctivitis (Messner and Leibowitz, 1971), chelated gold in rheumatoid arthritis patients receiving gold therapy (Lorber et al., 1973), prevented cyclophosphamide-induced cystitis in animals (Botta Jr et al., 1973), and treated cystinuria (Mulvaney et al., 1975). Like all antidotes, its history is intertwined with the agent it is meant to counterattack. It would not be until the widespread use of acetaminophen that NAC would come to the forefront in antidotal therapy.

Widespread use of acetaminophen

Marketed as a superior product to salicylates, acetaminophen entered the over-the-counter market in the late 1950s and early 1960s in the United States and United Kingdom (Prescott, 2000). With limited side effects at therapeutic dosing compared with salicylates, it rapidly became the preferred analgesic (Prescott, 2000). Acetaminophen's ascension into popular use for mild pain relief experienced its first setback with the publication of a sobering case report. In 1966, a publication from the United Kingdom described acute liver necrosis with fatal outcome after an overdose of paracetamol (acetaminophen) (Davidson and Eastham, 1966). Touted as the preferred choice due to its limited adverse side effect profile, the subsequent growing number of cases of hepatoxicity related to acetaminophen overdose bruised its reputation. Toxicology wards in the United Kingdom were beginning to appreciate an alarming trend. Drs. Laurie Prescott, Henry Matthew, and Alex Proudfoot of The Royal Infirmary of Edinburgh reported "the proportion of admissions involving paracetamol increased from 1.4% in 1967 to 10.4% in 1977" with "more than 1200 patients…admitted to the [Edinburgh] Regional Poisoning Treatment Centre" from 1966 to 1978 (Prescott, 1978). The Royal Infirmary group also noted that 15%–20% of their patients developed acute hepatic necrosis and death resulting from ALF (Prescott, 1978). Additionally, the Poisons Unit in Guy's Hospital in London reported "the rise in popularity of paracetamol as an analgesic [had] resulted in an increased number of admissions and deaths related to overdose of this drug" (Volans, 1976).

Acetaminophen hepatotoxicity

The identification of this troubling toxicity was delayed in the United States. The first US case report appeared in 1971 and documented hepatic necrosis after overdose (Boyer and Rouff, 1971). Dr. Barry Rumack, of the Rocky Mountain Poison Center in Denver, Colorado, postulated that the delay in recognition of this growing public health concern in the United States stemmed from the inability to screen for this toxicity. He reported "if you do not look for something, you will not diagnosis it" (Rumack and Matthew, 1975). In the spring of 1973, Rumack contacted nine US poison control centers and none had clinical experience or analytic methods to evaluate for acetaminophen toxicity (Rumack and Matthew, 1975). Rumack and Matthew reported that within Denver there were 156 acetaminophen ingestions with four fatalities (Rumack and Matthew, 1975). These findings illuminated a toxicological problem with potentially fatal sequelae that appeared to be escaping detection by many American poison control centers.

Despite supportive therapy, acetaminophen toxicity carried a mortality rate that ranged from 5% to 20% (Clark et al., 1973; Rumack, 2002; Smilkstein et al., 1988). Therapies including administration of mepyramine and corticosteroids, activated charcoal, hemodialysis, and charcoal hemoperfusion had been advocated as treatment but none appeared to have any meaningful effect on the prevention of hepatoxicity (Prescott et al., 1974). This all changed, however, after a watershed discovery was made at the National Institutes of Health (NIH) in Bethesda, Maryland.

J.R. Mitchell and colleagues from the Laboratory of Chemical Pharmacology at the NIH discovered the critical biochemical features of acetaminophen-induced hepatic necrosis. This work, published in a series of landmark papers in 1973 and 1974, illuminated essential pathways for acetaminophen-induced hepatotoxicity (Jollow et al., 1973, 1974; Mitchell et al., 1973a, b; Potter et al., 1973, 1974). In animal models, Mitchell and colleagues demonstrated toxicity from

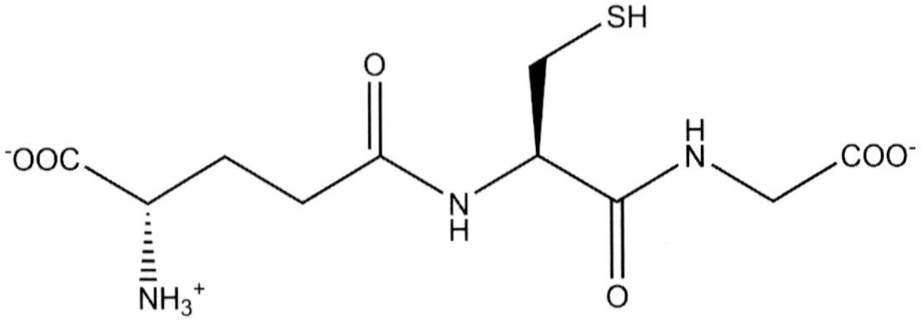

FIG. 3.1.2   Glutathione.

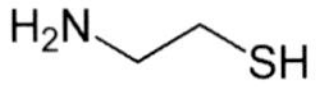

FIG. 3.1.3   Cysteamine.

acetaminophen arose from a chemically reactive metabolite formed by oxidation via cytochrome P-450 enzymes (Jollow et al., 1973; Mitchell et al., 1973a), later identified as *N*-acetyl-*p*-benzoquinoneimine (Corcoran et al., 1980). Further work showed this toxic metabolite covalently bound to hepatic macromolecules producing hepatic damage (Jollow et al., 1973). The most groundbreaking discovery came forth when the researchers added two sulfhydryl reagents, cysteine and glutathione, to the suspension of murine hepatic proteins. These reagents completely prevented covalent binding of the reactive metabolite and prevented hepatotoxicity (Jollow et al., 1974; Mitchell et al., 1973a; Potter et al., 1973, 1974). This significant observation leads to the hypothesis that physiologic stores of glutathione were critical to the detoxification of the reactive metabolite. When 70% of the glutathione store was depleted, toxicity ensued (Jollow et al., 1974; Piperno and Berssenbruegge, 1976). Their final publication included human volunteers and provided evidence that the mechanism of acetaminophen-induced hepatic injury in man is the same as in other animals (Mitchell et al., 1974). They concluded "logical treatment of patients overdosed with acetaminophen might rest on cysteamine or similar nucleophiles" (Mitchell et al., 1974). This work ignited the search for a definitive antidote (Figs. 3.1.2 and 3.1.3).

Research into antidotes for acetaminophen hepatotoxicity

The three clinical groups that characterized the growing problem of acetaminophen toxicity transitioned their efforts from describing the toxicity to treating it. Dovetailing off the findings by Mitchell and colleagues, they spearheaded the search for the most effective sulfhydryl group with the hope that one would ultimately rise to the level of an antidote. Although glutathione appeared to be the critical agent in reversing the toxicity, it lacked the ability to enter the cell readily. Therefore other sulfhydryl agents that served as a precursor needed to be considered (Mitchell et al., 1974).

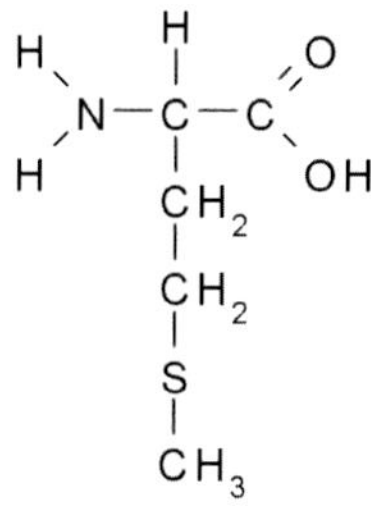

FIG. 3.1.4 Methionine.

Matthew and Prescott of the Royal Infirmary in Edinburgh published re-markable findings in April of 1974 (Prescott et al., 1974). The use of intravenous (IV) cysteamine mitigated the toxic effects of acetaminophen in five patients when compared with 11 control patients who all developed severe hepatic ne-crosis, with two of them dying from ALF (Prescott et al., 1974). Additional publications from Edinburgh went on to support their positive findings with cysteamine while suggesting other sulfhydryl-containing agents like methio-nine, penicillamine, and NAC (Prescott et al., 1974; Prescott et al., 1976a, b). However, the group expressed concern about cysteamine as a treatment. First, during treatment with this agent, clinicians stated the patients "look[ed] and felt utterly miserable" (Prescott et al., 1974). Second, IV cysteamine was not a widely available pharmaceutical formulation (Prescott et al., 1974).

Meanwhile, work out of the Poisons Unit at the Guy's Hospital in London in the early 1970s advocated for the use of oral methionine. Goulding and col-leagues demonstrated that oral methionine given within 10 h of the acetamin-ophen overdose effectively prevented death and hepatotoxicity (Crome et al., 1976) (Fig. 3.1.4).

They advocated for its use over IV cysteamine given the availability of the agent and its decreased side effect profile (Crome et al., 1976), although later findings showed delayed use increased mortality (Piperno et al., 1978). However, Prescott and his colleagues in Edinburgh strongly questioned these findings and countered this recommendation, arguing that an oral agent is "im-practical" given patients who overdose on acetaminophen invariably vomit, thereby limiting the efficacy of the antidote (Prescott et al., 1980). While con-tention between these two groups persisted in the United Kingdom over treat-ment options, momentum within the United States grew for an independent investigation of NAC. Through the efforts of Rumack, a national multicenter study was established, although first being met by a series of obstacles.

NAC as an acetaminophen antidote

Rumack obtained permission from the US Food and Drug Administration (FDA) to begin using NAC (Mucomyst, owned by Mead Johnson & Company) as an investigational new drug for acetaminophen toxicity in 1976 (Mulvaney et al., 1975; Peterson and Rumack, 1977; Rumack, 2002). The initial proposal to the FDA was for a prospective randomized controlled trial (RCT) (Rumack and Bateman, 2012). However, ethical questions were raised regarding this study design—one concern from a publication in the *New England Journal of Medicine* (Koch-Weser, 1976) and the other in an article by Dr. Prescott and colleagues (Prescott et al., 1976a, b). Both authors "expressed reservations concerning the ethics of placebo controlled trials" in acetaminophen toxicity (Prescott et al., 1976a, b). Ultimately, the FDA denied Rumack's request for a RCT because of these ethical questions. The FDA would only approve the study if it were done by utilizing historical controls. Another obstacle concerned the formulation of NAC. Already widely available as a mucolytic, NAC was not approved for IV use in the US. Mucomyst was not certified as pyrogen-free and Mead Johnson declined to undergo the expense of certification, thereby limiting the study protocol to an oral administration (Rumack and Bateman, 2012). Moreover, that same year work published by Piperno and colleagues from the Toxicology Department at McNeil laboratories showed oral NAC was an effective antidote in mice with acetaminophen toxicity (Piperno and Berssenbruegge, 1976). The FDA additionally required determination of the intensity and duration of the dose for the protocol before approval was granted. Limited pharmacokinetic data existed at this time, which necessitated Rumack and colleagues to use data from Mitchell's studies to carefully calculate a dose for the protocol based on existing data and stoichiometry (Rumack and Bateman, 2012). Given the observation that acetaminophen half-lives were well beyond 4 h and, in some patients, in excess of 12 h, the protocol submitted utilized 5 half-lives or a treatment duration of 60 h (Rumack and Bateman, 2012). The FDA added 12 h to this length as an additional safety margin, making for a total treatment duration of 72 h. After addressing the regulatory concerns, the investigation moved forward. Serving as the director of the Rocky Mountain Poison Center, Rumack in conjunction with Peterson initiated a nationwide, multicenter open-label study of oral NAC, sponsored by McNeil Consumer Products Company, enrolling patients as of September 1976 (IND, 1977; Peterson and Rumack, 1977). In 1977, they published the first case report of oral NAC in an acetaminophen overdose in the United States where hepatoxicity was successfully prevented (Peterson and Rumack, 1977). They published their pioneering findings in a series of articles in the late 1970s and 1980s. The results were clear: oral NAC effectively mitigated the hepatotoxic effects of acetaminophen when given in a timely manner and had minimal adverse effects (Rumack and Peterson, 1978; Rumack et al., 1981; Rumack, 1984). With such convincing evidence, the investigators stated oral NAC "should be considered the drug of choice as antidotal therapy" in the United States (Rumack and Peterson, 1978).

Skepticism of oral therapy remained strong in Edinburgh. Conceding the limitations of IV cysteamine, efforts transitioned to IV NAC. Building off a series of case reports demonstrating success with IV NAC (Prescott et al., 1976a,

1977), and with the support of Duncan, Flockhart and Company and McNeil Consumer Products Company, the Royal Infirmary published 3 years of experience in treating severe acetaminophen poisoning with IV NAC (trade name, Parvolex) in 1979. Unlike the United States, tight regulation did not apply in the United Kingdom at that time and it remained unclear how the IV dosing was calculated (Rumack and Bateman, 2012). Moreover, the duration of the protocol was 20.25 h, which approximated 5 four-hour half-lives of a therapeutic dose of acetaminophen, compared to the U.S. protocol of 72 h (Rumack and Bateman, 2012). The results showed IV NAC outperformed cysteamine and methionine in preventing toxicity and prompted the group to write IV NAC "is the treatment of choice for paracetamol poisoning" (Prescott et al., 1979). They went on to additionally remark that "there seems to be no place for oral treatment of severe paracetamol poisoning when effective intravenous treatment is available" (Prescott et al., 1979). However, not all groups were in agreement with this sentiment.

Efficacy of iv versus po NAC

In an exchange of published letters, the group from Guy's Hospital questioned the conclusion of superiority of IV NAC over other agents, specifically methionine. They argued oral methionine was equally as effective as IV NAC and methionine also proved to be more economic (Vale et al., 1979). In a biting response, the Edinburgh group published a letter titled "Intravenous *N*-Acetylcysteine: Still the Treatment of Choice for Paracetamol Poisoning." The authors cast doubt on the reported success and safety profile of oral methionine and asked, "how can they seriously suggest [it] is as effective as intravenous *N*-acetylcysteine?" (Prescott et al., 1980). They went on to affirm NAC "must remain the treatment of choice" and that they "make no apology for the title of [their] paper" (Prescott et al., 1980). In the same year of this publication, the Royal Infirmary published additional data from their experience with IV NAC and included oral NAC in their treatment regimen. IV NAC appeared superior with lower failure rates. The constant feature of nausea and vomiting in severe acetaminophen poisoning made oral NAC "clearly impracticable in most" patients (Prescott, 1981). Findings in the United States differed (Fig. 3.1.5).

Rumack continued his studies demonstrating oral NAC's efficacy despite the doubt emanating from the Royal Infirmary concerning this route of administration. From 1976 to 1985, Rumack and colleagues treated approximately 2000 patients with the oral formulation where acetaminophen-induced hepatotoxicity was probable based on the Rumack-Matthew nomogram showing that the oral regimen was as effective as the IV regimen when given within 10 h of ingestion (Smilkstein et al., 1988). Additionally the results showed oral NAC may be superior to IV NAC in preventing hepatotoxicity when given beyond 10 h (Smilkstein et al., 1988). These findings led to the approval of oral NAC for the treatment of acetaminophen overdose in the United States on January 31, 1985

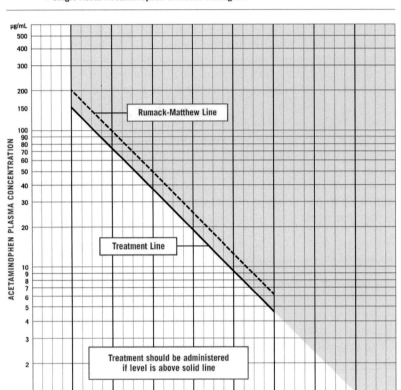

FIG. 3.1.5   Rumack-Matthew acetaminophen nomogram.

(Rumack and Bateman, 2012). It would not be until 1999, after 10-years' worth of experience of admitted patients and a meta-analysis of prior series, that the efficacy of both agents was shown to be likely equivalent (Brok et al., 2006; Buckley et al., 1999). Furthermore, a safety analysis of both formulations published in 2010 showed no serious adverse events related to NAC, with nausea and vomiting occurring more frequently with oral NAC and anaphylactoid reaction with the IV formulation (Bebarta et al., 2010). Finally the IV formulation was approved for use in the United States in 2004 and now is the most common route of administration in the country (Bronstein et al., 2010). Well-designed comparisons between the two protocols suggest superiority of the 72-h protocol in late-presenting acute acetaminophen overdose (Yarema et al., 2009). This finding is likely related to the significantly higher total dose of NAC and demonstrates both duration and intensity of NAC need to be considered in certain situations. However, no prospective randomized control trial exists between the two formulations; this limits the ability to make definitive conclusions regarding superiority and adverse effects between the two (Chiew et al., 2018).

Conclusions

The development and clinical history of NAC—from mucolytic to antidote—is storied. From the initial observation of NAC breaking the viscosity of mucus proteins positioned on an angled slide to becoming one of the most abundant and most used antidotes in the field of toxicology, the history of NAC spans many decades and fields of expertise. Ultimately, critical, groundbreaking work performed by groups from the United Kingdom and the United States catapulted NAC into the antidotal armamentarium and it became one of the most essential antidotes in the practice of modern clinical toxicology. It could be argued that no other antidote is used as frequently with equal efficacy as NAC. Although the original words were written over 40 years ago, they still remain as true as ever: NAC is the treatment of choice.

References

Anderson G. A clinical trial of a mucolytic agent—acetylcysteine—in chronic bronchitis. Br J Dis Chest 1966;60(2):101–3.

Bebarta VS, Kao L, Froberg B, Clark RF, Lavonas E, Qi M, et al. A multicenter comparison of the safety of oral versus intravenous acetylcysteine for treatment of acetaminophen overdose. Clin Toxicol (Phila) 2010;48(5):424–30.

Blieden M, Paramore LC, Shah D, Ben-Joseph R. A perspective on the epidemiology of acetaminophen exposure and toxicity in the United States. Expert Rev Clin Pharmacol 2014;7(3):341–8.

Botta Jr JA, Nelson LW, Weikel Jr JH. Acetylcysteine in the prevention of cyclophosphamide-induced cystitis in rats. J Natl Cancer Inst 1973;51(3):1051–8.

Boyer TD, Rouff SL. Acetaminophen-induced hepatic necrosis and renal failure. JAMA 1971;218(3):440–1.

Brok J, Buckley N, Gluud C. Interventions for paracetamol (acetaminophen) overdose. Cochrane Database Syst Rev 2006;2.

Bronstein AC, Spyker DA, Cantilena Jr LR, Green JL, Rumack BH, Giffin SL. 2009 annual report of the American Association of Poison Control Centers' National Poison Data System (NPDS): 27th annual report. Clin Toxicol (Phila) 2010;48(10):979–1178.

Buckley NA, Whyte IM, O'Connell DL, Dawson AH. Oral or intravenous N-acetylcysteine: which is the treatment of choice for acetaminophen (paracetamol) poisoning? J Toxicol Clin Toxicol 1999;37(6):759–67.

Chiew AL, Gluud C, Brok J, Buckley NA. Interventions for paracetamol (acetaminophen) overdose. Cochrane Database Syst Rev 2018;23:2.

Clark R, Borirakchanyavat V, Davidson AR, Thompson RP, Widdop B, Goulding R, et al. Hepatic damage and death from overdose of paracetamol. Lancet 1973;1(7794):66–70.

Corcoran GB, Mitchell JR, Vaishnav YN, Horning EC. Evidence that acetaminophen and N-hydroxyacetaminophen form a common arylating intermediate, N-acetyl-p-benzoquinoneimine. Mol Pharmacol 1980;18(3):536–42.

Crome P, Vale JA, Volans GN, Widdop B, Goulding R. Oral methionine in the treatment of severe paracetamol (acetaminophen) overdose. Lancet 1976;2(7990):829–30.

Davidson DG, Eastham WN. Acute liver necrosis following overdose of paracetamol. Br Med J 1966;2(5512):497–9.

Grater WC, Cato A. Double-blind study of acetylcysteine-isoproterenol and saline isoproterenol in non-hospitalized patients with asthma. Curr Ther Res Clin Exp 1973;15(9):660–71.

Gummin DD, Mowry JB, Spyker DA, Brooks DE, Beuhler MC, Rivers LJ, et al. 2018 annual report of the American Association of Poison Control Centers' National Poison Data System (NPDS): 36th annual report. Clin Toxicol (Phila) 2019;57(12):1220–413.

Howatt WF, DeMuth GR. A double-blind study of the use of acetylcysteine in patients with cystic fibrosis. Univ Mich Med Cent J 1966;32(2):82–5.

IND. IND status for N-acetylcysteine in acetaminophen overdosage. Bull Natl Clgh Poison Control Cent 1977;1.

Jollow DJ, Mitchell JR, Potter WZ, Davis DC, Gillette JR, Brodie BB. Acetaminophen-induced hepatic necrosis. II. Role of covalent binding in vivo. J Pharmacol Exp Ther 1973;187(1):195–202.

Jollow DJ, Thorgeirsson SS, Potter WZ, Hashimoto M, Mitchell JR. Acetaminophen-induced hepatic necrosis. VI. Metabolic disposition of toxic and nontoxic doses of acetaminophen. Pharmacology 1974;12(4–5):251–71.

Koch-Weser J. Drug therapy. Acetaminophen. N Engl J Med 1976;295(23):1297–300.

Komet H, Salco AN. A new mucolytic agent as a therapeutic adjunct in nasal sinusitis. Eye Ear Nose Throat Mon 1965;44:47–50.

Lillibridge CB, Docter JM, Eidelman S. Oral administration of n-acetyl cysteine in the prophylaxis of "meconium ileus equivalent". J Pediatr 1967;71(6):887–9.

Lorber A, Baumgartner WA, Bovy RA, Chang CC, Hollcraft R. Clinical application for heavy metal-complexing potential of N-acetylcysteine. J Clin Pharmacol 1973;13(8):332–6.

Manthripragada AD, Zhou EH, Budnitz DS, Lovegrove MC, Willy ME. Characterization of acetaminophen overdose-related emergency department visits and hospitalizations in the United States. Pharmacoepidemiol Drug Saf 2011;20(8):819–26.

Meeker Jr IA. Acetylcysteine used to liquefy Inspissated meconium causing intestinal obstruction in the newborn. Surgery 1964;56:419–25.

Messner K, Leibowitz HM. Acetylcysteine treatment of keratitis sicca. Arch Ophthalmol 1971;86(3):357–9.

Mitchell JR, Jollow DJ, Potter WZ, Davis DC, Gillette JR, Brodie BB. Acetaminophen-induced hepatic necrosis. I. Role of drug metabolism. J Pharmacol Exp Ther 1973a;187(1):185–94.

Mitchell JR, Jollow DJ, Potter WZ, Gillette JR, Brodie BB. Acetaminophen-induced hepatic necrosis. IV. Protective role of glutathione. J Pharmacol Exp Ther 1973b;187(1):211–7.

Mitchell JR, Thorgeirsson SS, Potter WZ, Jollow DJ, Keiser H. Acetaminophen-induced hepatic injury: protective role of glutathione in man and rationale for therapy. Clin Pharmacol Ther 1974;16(4):676–84.

Mulvaney WP, Quilter T, Mortera A. Experiences with acetylcysteine in cystinuric patients. J Urol 1975;114(1):107–8.

Peterson RG, Rumack BH. Treating acute acetaminophen poisoning with acetylcysteine. JAMA 1977;237(22):2406–7.

Piperno E, Berssenbruegge DA. Reversal of experimental paracetamol toxicosis with N-acetylcysteine. Lancet 1976;2(7988):738–9.

Piperno E, Mosher AH, Berssenbruegge DA, Winkler JD, Smith RB. Pathophysiology of acetaminophen overdosage toxicity: implications for management. Pediatrics 1978;62(5 Pt 2 Suppl):880–9.

Potter WZ, Davis DC, Mitchell JR, Jollow DJ, Gillette JR, Brodie BB. Acetaminophen-induced hepatic necrosis. III. Cytochrome P-450-mediated covalent binding in vitro. J Pharmacol Exp Ther 1973;187(1):203–10.

Potter WZ, Thorgeirsson SS, Jollow DJ, Mitchell JR. Acetaminophen-induced hepatic necrosis. V. Correlation of hepatic necrosis, covalent binding and glutathione depletion in hamsters. Pharmacology 1974;12(3):129–43.

Prescott LF. The chief scientist reports … prevention of hepatic necrosis following paracetamol overdosage. Health Bull (Edinb) 1978;36(4):204–12.

Prescott LF. Treatment of severe acetaminophen poisoning with intravenous acetylcysteine. Arch Intern Med 1981;141(3 Spec):386–9.

Prescott LF. Paracetamol: past, present, and future. Am J Ther 2000;7(2):143–7.

Prescott LF, Newton RW, Swainson CP, Wright N, Forrest AR, Matthew H. Successful treatment of severe paracetamol overdosage with cysteamine. Lancet 1974;1(7858):588–92.

Prescott LF, Park J, Proudfoot AT. Letter: cysteamine for paracetamol poisoning. Lancet 1976a;1(7955):357.

Prescott LF, Sutherland GR, Park J, Smith IJ, Proudfoot AT. Cysteamine, methionine, and penicillamine in the treatment of paracetamol poisoning. Lancet 1976b;2(7977):109–13.

Prescott LF, Park J, Ballantyne A, Adriaenssens P, Proudfoot AT. Treatment of paracetamol (acetaminophen) poisoning with N-acetylcysteine. Lancet 1977;2(8035):432–4.

Prescott LF, Illingworth RN, Critchley JA, Stewart MJ, Adam RD, Proudfoot AT. Intravenous N-acetylcystine: the treatment of choice for paracetamol poisoning. Br Med J 1979;2(6198):1097–100.

Prescott LF, Illingworth RN, Critchley JA, Proudfoot AT. Intravenous N-acetylcysteine: still the treatment of choice for paracetamol poisoning. Br Med J 1980;280(6206):46–7.

Reas HW. The use of N-acetylcysteine in the treatment of cystic fibrosis. J Pediatr 1964;65:542–57.

Rumack BH. Acetaminophen overdose in young children. Treatment and effects of alcohol and other additional ingestants in 417 cases. Am J Dis Child 1984;138(5):428–33.

Rumack BH. Acetaminophen hepatotoxicity: the first 35 years. J Toxicol Clin Toxicol 2002;40(1):3–20.

Rumack BH, Bateman DN. Acetaminophen and acetylcysteine dose and duration: past, present and future. Clin Toxicol (Phila) 2012;50(2):91–8.

Rumack BH, Matthew H. Acetaminophen poisoning and toxicity. Pediatrics 1975;55(6):871–6.

Rumack BH, Peterson RG. Acetaminophen overdose: incidence, diagnosis, and management in 416 patients. Pediatrics 1978;62:898–903.

Rumack BH, Peterson RC, Koch GG, Amara IA. Acetaminophen overdose. 662 cases with evaluation of oral acetylcysteine treatment. Arch Intern Med 1981;141:380–5.

Schlang HA. Acetylcysteine in removal of bezoar. JAMA 1970;214(7):1329.

Shaw A. Safety of N-acetylcysteine in treatment of meconium obstruction of the newborn. J Pediatr Surg 1969;4(1):119–25.

Sheffner AL. Mucolytic-N-acylated sulhydryl compositions and process for treating animal mucus. US 3091569A. United States Patent and Trademark Office; 1963a.

Sheffner AL. The reduction in vitro in viscosity of mucoprotein solutions by a new mucolytic agent, N-acetyl-L-cysteine. Ann N Y Acad Sci 1963b;106:298–310.

Sheffner AL, Medler EM, Jacobs LW, Sarett HP. The in vitro reduction in viscosity of human tracheobronchial secretions by acetylcysteine. Am Rev Respir Dis 1964;90:721–9.

Smilkstein MJ, Knapp GL, Kulig KW, Rumack BH. Efficacy of oral N-acetylcysteine in the treatment of acetaminophen overdose. Analysis of the national multicenter study (1976 to 1985). N Engl J Med 1988;319(24):1557–62.

Stravitz RT, Lee WM. Acute liver failure. Lancet 2019;394(10201):869–81.

Thomas PA, Lynch RE, Merrigan EH. Prevention of postoperative pulmonary atelectasis: review of 215 cases and evaluation of acetylcysteine. Am Surg 1966;32(5):301–7.

Vale JA, Meredith TJ, Crome P, Helliwell M, Volans GN, Widdop B, et al. Intravenous N-acetylcysteine: the treatment of choice in paracetamol poisoning? Br Med J 1979;2(6202):1435–6.

Volans GN. Self-poisoning and suicide due to paracetamol. J Int Med Res 1976;4:7–13.

Webb WR. Clinical evaluaton of a new mucolytic agent, acetyl-cysteine. J Thorac Cardiovasc Surg 1962;44:330–43.

Weiner AA, Steinvurzel B. Successful treatment of acute atelectasis with acetylcysteine. N Y State J Med 1966;66(11):1355–7.

Yarema MC, Johnson DW, Berlin RJ, Sivilotti ML, Nettel-Aguirre A, Brant RF, et al. Comparison of the 20-hour intravenous and 72-hour oral acetylcysteine protocols for the treatment of acute acetaminophen poisoning. Ann Emerg Med 2009;54(4):606–14.

Chapter 3.2

Fomepizole

Kenneth E. McMartin

Department of Pharmacology, Toxicology & Neuroscience, Louisiana State University Health Sciences Center, Shreveport, LA, United States

Introduction

Consumer exposure to methanol and ethylene glycol (EG) can occur because they are readily available in windshield washer fluids, camping fuels, and other automotive products such as automotive antifreeze. Although unintentional ingestions occur, human poisonings primarily happen by self-ingestion, either as an ethanol (alcohol) substitute or for reasons of self-harm. These poisonings are relatively uncommon—exposure statistics from the American Association of Poison Control Centers (Gummin et al., 2019) suggest that about 5000 cases of these poisoning require antidotal treatment in the United States per year, with about 20–30 deaths. Despite the relative rarity, these poisonings can produce significant morbidity or mortality, especially when the syndrome is not recognized or when treatment is delayed or unavailable (Jacobsen and McMartin, 1986). EG poisoning is a major problem for companion animals, particularly dogs and cats (Dial et al., 1989), while epidemics of methanol poisoning are unfortunately common world-wide due to consumption of adulterated forms of alcohol (Hassanian-Moghaddam et al., 2019).

The primary antidote for the treatment of methanol and EG poisoning prior to the development of fomepizole was ethanol, which has a higher affinity for alcohol dehydrogenase (ADH) than the other alcohols and so inhibits their oxidation to toxic metabolites. Although there has been extensive clinical experience with ethanol therapy since it was suggested (Röe, 1955), a better therapy for these poisonings has been desired for years because ethanol therapy is associated with several problems (Lepik et al., 2009). It is difficult to maintain therapeutic levels of ethanol due to interindividual variations in the metabolism of ethanol, thus requiring blood ethanol level monitoring to insure that the blood ethanol levels are neither too low nor too high. Also, ethanol is well known to exacerbate the underlying central nervous system (CNS) depression of these poisonings.

History of Modern Clinical Toxicology. https://doi.org/10.1016/B978-0-12-822218-8.00046-6

Methanol and ethylene glycol toxicity

The mechanism by which methanol and EG produce toxicity was uncovered through basic science research in the late 1970s and 1980s. Studies of methanol and EG toxicity in animals showed that neither alcohol was toxic itself but had to be metabolized to metabolites that accumulated in target organs and led to toxicity. Metabolism of methanol and EG occurs by oxidation via hepatic ADH to formaldehyde and glycolaldehyde, respectively (Jacobsen and McMartin, 1986). Formaldehyde is then rapidly metabolized to formic acid, which is the primary toxic metabolite for methanol that is responsible for metabolic acidosis as well as ocular toxicity (McMartin et al., 1977a, b; Martin-Amat et al., 1978). Glycolaldehyde is similarly further metabolized to glycolic acid, whose accumulation leads to severe metabolic acidosis in EG poisoning (Jacobsen et al., 1984). Glycolic acid is metabolized to glyoxylic acid and then to oxalic acid, which is poorly soluble in the presence of calcium and leads to the formation of calcium oxalate monohydrate (COM) crystals. Accumulation of COM crystals in the kidney is the primary mechanism for the renal toxicity of EG (Guo et al., 2007).

Discovery of 4-methylpyrazole as an alcohol dehydrogenase inhibitor

The 4-methylpyrazole (4MP) story began in the 1960s, well before the toxicities of methanol and EG were understood. 4MP was synthesized in 1960 (Table 3.2.1 for a timeline of fomepizole development) by a research group at AB Astra and the Karolinska Institute in Sweden headed by the Nobelist Hugo Theorell. This group carried out key studies of its activities in animals as well as initial studies in healthy human subjects. These studies were designed to evaluate the usefulness of pyrazoles to ameliorate the organ toxicities related to chronic ethanol use. Their hypothesis was that the pyrazoles, as inhibitors of ADH, would decrease the adverse effects of ethanol, which were thought to be related to its metabolism or its metabolites. Pyrazole itself was too toxic for such use (Torrielli et al., 1978) and numerous pyrazole derivatives, including 4MP, were synthesized to assess the structure–activity relationships as ADH inhibitors (Theorell et al., 1969). Toxicity studies in rodents showed that 4MP had much less toxicity than pyrazole (Magnusson et al., 1972). Li and Theorell (1969) subsequently showed the potency of 4MP against human liver ADH in vitro. In this paper in 1969, they made the prophetic comment "whether or not pyrazole derivatives can serve as clinically useful agents (for poisoning by both methanol and EG) remains to be determined experimentally" (Fig. 3.2.1).

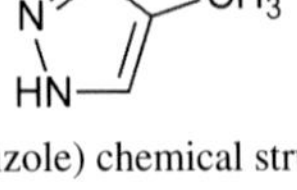

FIG. 3.2.1 4-Methyl pyrazole (fomepizole) chemical structure.

TABLE 3.2.1 Timeline for events or publications in the development of 4MP/fomepizole.

Date	Event
1960	Synthesis of 4-methylpyrazole (4MP)
1963	Inhibition of isolated horse liver alcohol dehydrogenase (ADH)
1969	Inhibition of human liver ADH in vitro—suggestion that it might be useful for treating methanol and EG poisoning
1970	Inhibition of ethanol metabolism in humans in vivo
1972	Publication of preclinical toxicology studies by AB Astra
1972–73	Metabolic studies in rodents
1970–78	Suppression of ethanol's metabolic effects in humans—Sweden and Finland
1975	Demonstration of efficacy versus methanol toxicity in animals
1978	Demonstration of efficacy versus EG toxicity in rats
1980	Dose-ranging efficacy studies establish minimally effective plasma level in animals
1983	Orphan Product Act enacted in the United States
1985	Funding of Orphan Product Research Grant from FDA for clinical studies on 4MP
1986	IND filed for Phase 1 oral dose studies (Amendment for IV doses in 1988)
1986–89	Phase 1 clinical trials with 4MP in the United States (published in 1988–1990)
1987	Superior efficacy over ethanol shown for treatment of EG poisoning in dogs
1987	Publication of first use in poisoned humans for three EG cases—France
1988	Officially designated as Orphan Product; given drug name as fomepizole
1993	Orphan Medical, Inc. sublicenses rights to 4MP from investment group
1993	Orphan Medical receives "Subpart E' designation from FDA for fomepizole
1995	Phase 2/3 clinical trials begin in the United States
1997	Antizol approved for marketing in the United States for treatment of EG poisoning

Continued

TABLE 3.2.1 Timeline for events or publications in the development of 4MP/fomepizole—cont'd

Date	Event
1999	Publication of EG clinical trial results in *New England Journal of Medicine*
2000	Antizol approved for marketing in the United States for treatment of methanol poisoning
2001	Publication of methanol clinical trial results in *New England Journal of Medicine*
2000s	Becomes standard of care for methanol and EG poisonings—used more often than ethanol in the United States
2009	Generic versions approved and start to be marketed
2013	Added to the WHO List of Essential Medicines

Initial studies in Sweden on 4MP in humans (Table 3.2.2) showed that 4MP inhibited ethanol elimination in humans (Blomstrand and Theorell, 1970) and that it suppressed ethanol's metabolic effects in animals and humans (Blomstrand and Forsell, 1971; Blomstrand and Kager, 1973). Later in the 1970s, a research group in Finland also showed that 4MP inhibited ethanol elimination and ethanol-induced redox changes in humans (Salaspuro et al., 1977, 1978; Lindros et al., 1979). This group, as well as one in Japan, subsequently demonstrated that 4MP could inhibit acetaldehyde accumulation following ethanol, thereby reducing the effects of genetic flushing and of the disulfiram-ethanol interaction (Lindros et al., 1981; Kupari et al., 1983; Inoue et al., 1984). Together in these studies, 68 human subjects were exposed to 4MP (oral or IV) in doses from 1 to 10 mg/kg with no reports of adverse effects.

Efficacy of 4MP in intoxicated animals

The prophetic comment by Theorell and the knowledge that 4MP could inhibit ethanol metabolism in humans laid the basis for animal studies in the United States that subsequently showed the potent efficacy of 4MP against both methanol and EG toxicity (Table 3.2.3). Basic mechanistic research in the early 1970s at the University of Iowa showed convincingly that accumulation of formic acid (formate) was responsible for the acidosis produced by methanol (McMartin et al., 1975), and more importantly, that formate also produced the ocular toxicity associated with methanol (Martin-Amat et al., 1978). Because the primary route of metabolism of methanol to formate in primates was ADH (Makar and Tephly, 1975), these researchers decided to test whether 4MP could block

TABLE 3.2.2 Early studies of effects of 4-methylpyrazole on ethanol in humans.

References	Number and type of subjects	Dose of 4MP	Other treatment	Results
Blomstrand and Theorell, 1970	5 healthy and 2 alcoholic	1–10 mg/kg oral	^{14}C—Ethanol (9–38 g)	Decreased E metabolism to CO_2; blocked E-induced increase L/P ratio
Blomstrand and Kager, 1973	5 healthy	180 mg IV	^{14}C—glyceryl-trioleate + Ethanol (0.55–0.9 g/kg IV)	Decreased E-induced inhibition of lipid metabolism
Salaspuro et al., 1977	10 healthy	7 mg/kg IV	Ethanol (0.6 g/kg IV)	Reduced E-induced hypoglycemia and redox changes
Salaspuro et al., 1978	9 healthy and 13 alcoholics	7 mg/kg IV	Ethanol (0.8 g/kg IV)	Decreased elimination rate of E and E-induced redox changes
Lindros et al., 1979	1 alcoholic	5 mg/kg IV	Ethanol (0.475 g/kg)	Decreased elimination rate of E
Lindros et al., 1981	4 healthy and 1 patient with Antabuse reaction	5–7 mg/kg IV	Ethanol (0.2 g/kg)+cyanamide to healthy subjects	Blocked E-induced rise in acetaldehyde and flushing effects in volunteers and patient
Kupari et al., 1983	9 healthy	7 mg/kg IV	Ethanol (0.35 g/kg PO)+cyanamide	Blocked E-induced rise in acetaldehyde and decreased cardiovascular effects
Inoue et al., 1984	9 healthy (6 flushers and 3 non-flushers)	10 mg/kg oral	Ethanol (0.5 g/kg PO)	Decreased E-induced rise in acetaldehyde and reduced flushing effects

IV, intravenous; PO, oral; E, ethanol; L/P, lactate/pyruvate.

TABLE 3.2.3 Preclinical studies of efficacy of 4-methylpyrazole in methanol or ethylene glycol toxicity.

References	Number and type of subjects	Dose of 4MP or ethanol	Other treatment	Results
McMartin et al., 1975	6 monkeys M alone, 3 monkeys with M+4MP	One dose—50 mg/kg IP	Methanol (3 g/kg) oral	Decreased M elimination from blood and metabolism to CO_2; prevented acidosis and F accumulation for 36 h, after which F accumulated and acidosis re-developed
Clay et al., 1975	Monkeys, unstated number	50 mg/kg IV every 6–48 h	Methanol (4 g/kg) IP	No acidosis observed for 48 h
McMartin et al., 1977a, 1977b	1 treated monkey	50 mg/kg IP at 10, 46, and 81 h	Methanol (3 g/kg) oral	Reversed F accumulation and acidosis post dosing—maintained protection with repeat dosing
McMartin et al., 1980	11 monkeys	2.5–50 mg/kg IM, delayed 5–22 h after M, then every 24–96 h	Methanol (2–3 g/kg) oral	Decreased M elimination from blood, reduced F accumulation and kept at zero as long as plasma 4MP >10 µmol/L; 15–20 mg/kg 4MP sufficient to prevent toxicity

TABLE 3.2.3 Preclinical studies of efficacy of 4-methylpyrazole in methanol or ethylene glycol toxicity—cont'd

References	Number and type of subjects	Dose of 4MP or ethanol	Other treatment	Results
Blomstrand and Ingemansson, 1984	7 monkeys M alone, 5 with M+4MP	20 mg/kg IM, at 5 h after M, then every 15 h	Methanol (2.5–6 g/kg) oral	Visual symptoms in M-treated monkeys, none in animals treated also with 4MP
Chou and Richardson, 1978	30 rats (6 per group)	226 mg/kg IP at −8, −4, 0, +4 and +6 h relative to EG	EG (11 g/kg) oral (and a control group)	When given prior to or with EG, 4MP blocked mortality and reduced EG metabolism; when given 4 h after EG, reduced mortality slightly; no change mortality at +6 h
Grauer et al., 1987	9 dogs, 3 per group (EG, EG+E, EG+4MP)	4MP=20 mg/kg IV at 3 h, 15 at 24 h and 5 at 36 h; E=0.9 g/kg IV at 3, 7, 14, 24 h	EG (10.7 g/kg) oral	EG only— progressively depressed, AKI EG+E— enhanced depression, given Ringers' for dehydration for 36 h EG+4MP— reversed depression— normal by 24 h Both E and 4MP reversed acidosis and AKI

Continued

TABLE 3.2.3 Preclinical studies of efficacy of 4-methylpyrazole in methanol or ethylene glycol toxicity—cont'd

References	Number and type of subjects	Dose of 4MP or ethanol	Other treatment	Results
Dial et al., 1994	11 dogs	5 given 4MP (20 mg/kg at 5 h, 15 at 17 h, 10 at 29 h and 5 at 41 h); 6 given 4MP (20 mg/kg at 8 h, then similar repeats)	EG (10.6 g/kg) oral	All treated with 5 h delay were normal by 12 h—no AKI or acidosis 2 of 6 treated with 8 h delay had acidosis and AKI, needing dialysis

M, methanol; EG, ethylene glycol; E, ethanol; 4MP, 4-methylpyrazole; IP, intraperitoneal; IV, intravenous; IM, intramuscular; F, formic acid (formate); AKI, acute kidney injury; h, hours.

methanol metabolism. Their studies showed that 4MP, when given simultaneously with methanol, prevented formate accumulation (McMartin et al., 1975) and, when given several hours after methanol, 4MP reversed the acidosis and ameliorated the toxicity produced by methanol (McMartin et al., 1977a, b). Follow-up work by Blomstrand's group in Sweden in the 1980s suggested that plasma concentrations of 4MP above $9 \mu mol/L$ prevented formate accumulation in methanol toxicity in monkeys (McMartin et al., 1980). Furthermore, 4MP doses ranging from 10 to 20 mg/kg every 12 h maintained therapeutically effective plasma 4MP concentrations (McMartin et al., 1980; Blomstrand and Ingemansson, 1984).

In 1978, 4MP was reported to reduce the mortality of EG in rats, but only when given prior to or along with EG (Chou and Richardson, 1978); efficacy of 4MP was markedly decreased when given 4 h afterwards. Two subsequent studies in dogs (Table 3.2.3) showed that 4MP, in an initial dose of 20 mg/kg at 3 to 5 h after EG (followed by smaller doses of 4MP at 12–24 h interval) was successful in treating EG toxicity. The first study showed that ethanol and 4MP were equally effective at reversing the acidosis produced by EG (Grauer et al., 1987). However, 4MP was a much superior therapy, because the adverse effects noted with ethanol in these dogs (mostly an exacerbated CNS depression for 72 h and a dehydration requiring administration of fluids) complicated the management of the intoxicated animals, while management with 4MP was relatively straight-forward (it reversed CNS depression by 24 h). The second study showed that 4MP was effective when given 5 h after EG, but was less effective when delayed until 8 h (Dial et al., 1994). The potent efficacy in these animal studies suggested that 4MP was likely to be a clinically useful agent for both methanol and EG poisonings.

Translating animal 4MP to human fomepizole

Although the preclinical studies showed that 4MP was highly effective and was relatively safe (especially compared to the adverse effects from ethanol), translational development of 4MP was slow to be pursued for a number of reasons. First, clinical toxicology research is inherently difficult because individual centers typically encounter only a small number of poisonings, such that antidotal trials require special coordination among many clinical toxicologists. Also, in the early 1980s, there was little interest to fund such studies by the National Institutes of Health and there were no independent foundations related to poisoning as a disease. Similarly, drug development was mostly conducted by the large pharmaceutical companies who were primarily interested in drugs for diseases that would bring economic returns through widespread or long-term use. Academic researchers rarely became involved in drug development until the federal government made a dramatic change.

Prior to the 1980s, development of therapeutics for rare diseases (including poisonings) was neglected. However, in 1983 due to the political action of patient groups, the federal government promulgated the Orphan Product Act, which defined "orphan drug" as one that would be annually used for < 200,000 cases. The Act provided several advantages to companies marketing orphan drugs, including Food and Drug Administration (FDA) assistance with developing approved protocols for the needed clinical trials, offering tax credits for orphan drug research, and creating a 7-year period of exclusive marketing rights after approval of the drug. This exclusive marketing period has been the main driver for orphan drug development, since it effectively provides a similar duration of exclusive marketing as that of a patented drug. The Orphan Product Act also established the Office of Orphan Product Development (OOPD) within the FDA. This office provides grant funding to academic researchers (or small companies) to conduct initial clinical studies that would then attract the attention of drug companies needed to further develop the orphan product toward marketing. 4MP would probably never have been developed as a marketed therapeutic if not for the funding of Phase 1 clinical trials by the Orphan Product Research Grant (OPRG) program.

Although 4MP's development was based on highly positive preclinical studies, serendipity was also a great contributor. The OOPD quickly identified researchers who had research experience with potential orphan drugs and might be able to further their development—hence the OOPD called in January 1984 to discuss the possibility of 4MP as an orphan drug. Our application for an FDA grant to support Phase 1 clinical studies was only successful because of the assistance by a clinical pharmacologist (Dr. Charles Defesche), who happened to be located at the local Boots Pharmaceuticals facility and also had an adjunct appointment in our department. Prior to beginning the Phase 1 studies, an Investigational Drug Application (IND) was prepared, again with help from Dr. Defesche. The complete IND included chemical information for a Good Manufacturing Practices formulation of 4-MP that we were fortunate to obtain from the manufacturer, all the available preclinical safety and efficacy information (from publications), and detailed protocols for the initial human studies. Luck also helped in developing the necessary collaboration with physicians to conduct these trials (because this PhD scientist cannot physically conduct clinical research). Precisely when the FDA approved the Phase 1 trials with 4MP, Dag Jacobsen, a physician from Ullevaal University Hospital in Oslo, Norway, had just completed his dissertation on the mechanisms and treatments of methanol and EG poisoning (Jacobsen et al., 1982a, b). Fortunately, we were able to obtain a Fogarty International Fellowship to support his postdoctoral appointment. Thus between 1986 and 1990, five Phase 1 studies of 4MP were conducted by a collaborative research group including Dag Jacobsen and several physicians at LSU Health Sciences Center—Shreveport (LSUHSC-S). The five trials were (1) a sequential, ascending, single-dose study (4 drug and 2 placebo subjects at 4 oral dose levels from 10 to 100 mg/kg) (Jacobsen et al., 1988); (2) a sequential, ascending, multiple-oral dose study (oral doses repeated over 5 days) (Jacobsen et al., 1990); (3) an ADH inhibitory study with a crossover design (four subjects given ethanol with either placebo or oral 4MP at three dose levels) (Jacobsen et al., 1996a, b); (4) an IV/oral dose kinetic study with a crossover design (five subjects given the same 4MP dose either IV or oral) (McMartin et al., 2012); (5) a 4MP IV dose study of ethanol-4MP interactions (Jacobsen et al., 1996a, 1996b). These double blind, randomized trials, involving 65 healthy subjects, showed that both oral and IV doses of 4MP in the range of 5–20 mg/kg every 12 h elicited minimal adverse effects and that such doses of 4MP inhibited ethanol metabolism in vivo as a surrogate marker of ADH activity.

Important kinetic and metabolic information was also obtained in the Phase 1 studies. In doses in the therapeutic range (5–20 mg/kg), 4MP appeared to be eliminated by nonlinear, Michaelis-Menten kinetics, with "zero order" elimination rates from 5 to 10 μmol/L/h (Jacobsen et al., 1989; McMartin et al., 2012). The nonlinear elimination kinetics for therapeutic doses of fomepizole has been confirmed in independent studies in healthy human subjects (Marraffa et al., 2007). Preclinical studies showed that 4MP was eliminated primarily by oxidation, presumably by cytochrome P450, to 4-hydroxymethylpyrazole (4OHMP) and then to 4-carboxypyrazole (4CP) (Murphy and Watkins, 1972) and that 4MP readily induced cytochrome P450 activity, particularly CYP2E1 (Winters and Cederbaum, 1992). In the Phase 1 studies, excretion of 4CP in the urine of humans was the major pathway of elimination, accounting for > 50% of the dose, while renal elimination of unchanged 4MP was minimal (< 3% of the dose) (Jacobsen et al., 1996a, b; McMartin et al., 2012). In the multiple dose study (4MP administered every 12 h for 96 h), 4MP likely induced its own elimi-nation, since 4MP plasma levels could not be maintained at a steady-state un-less the 4MP dose was increased at 48 h (Jacobsen et al., 1990). Auto-induction of elimination was further suggested by the increasing zero order elimination rates (from 3.3 μmol/L/h at 0–12 h post dosing to 13.7 μmol/L/h at 72–84 h) (McMartin et al., 2012). This increasing elimination over time was the origin for the recommended dosing schedule in use today, where the maintenance dose is recommended to be increased at 60 h. Interestingly, two studies have also demonstrated the pharmacokinetic equivalency of oral and IV doses of fomepi-zole (Marraffa et al., 2007; McMartin et al., 2012), suggesting the therapeutic usefulness of oral doses.

Technology transfer for fomepizole

Technology transfer for most antidotes is difficult because of the general lack of patent protection (the idea for the use of 4MP for treatment of methanol poi-soning had already been published in 1969 for example), meaning essentially no interest from drug companies for such development. However, the Orphan Product Act did create the Orphan Drug designation, which provides 7 years of exclusivity for the company that obtains marketing approval of the orphan drug. As such, our first step was to obtain the official Orphan Drug designation. This procedure is fairly simple (4MP required four single-spaced pages), in which one provides the indication for use (inhibition of ADH-derived toxic metabo-lites), an assessment of the number of possible uses per year (to justify it as an orphan drug) and a summary of the preclinical efficacy and safety studies. The Orphan Drug designation for the newly named "fomepizole" was obtained in late 1988, which provided us with marketing rights that could be licensed to drug companies. Despite this, our initial efforts at enticing further development by the pharmaceutical industry were widely ignored. Luckily, a group of in-vestors with pharmaceutical company experience (Mericon Investment Group) saw the great clinical usefulness and possible financial benefits of fomepizole as an orphan drug, so they licensed the rights. This group then sublicensed the rights in 1993 to Orphan Medical, Inc., which had been specifically created with the intent to develop and market orphan drugs exclusively, so was aggres-sively pursuing products like 4MP. To accelerate the development of fomepi-zole, Orphan Medical obtained "Subpart E" designation from the FDA, which is for a drug to be used for a disease with potential mortality or severely debili-tating outcome, which of course was appropriate for methanol and EG poison-ings. Subpart E designation provided for initial meetings between the FDA and Orphan Medical to agree on study protocols that provided sufficient data to allow for safety and efficacy decisions using predetermined key endpoints. Subpart E also provided for a more rapid review of the New Drug Application (NDA) submission by the FDA.

Clinical studies of efficacy lead to marketing approval

Although Phase 1 clinical studies with fomepizole were moving ahead in the United States in the 1980s, it had already been used with apparent success to treat four cases of EG poisoning in France (Baud et al., 1986–1987, 1988). Owing to the delays in obtaining various approvals from the FDA and in translating the studies to an appropriate drug company, the first clinical studies of efficacy in the United States did not begin until 1995. By necessity, the Phase 2/3 efficacy trials were conducted as a typical multicenter trial to enroll a sufficient number of patients suffering from these relatively rare poisonings. However, multicenter trials of antidotes are fairly rare within the poisoning arena, so Orphan Medical enlisted Dr. Jeffrey Brent to recruit and organize a group of about 20 clinical toxicologists associated with poison centers [the Methylpyrazole for Toxic Alcohols (META) study group]. In addition to the multiple clinical trial sites, there was a central analytical site (LSUHSC-S) that analyzed blood levels of fomepizole and of methanol, EG and their toxic metabolites. The trials were conducted in two distinct arms, one for EG and one for methanol, thus permitting separate assessment of efficacy. Both arms were conducted as open label trials with defined dosing schedules, with specific criteria for implementation of hemodialysis, and with dose adjustments in case of the use of hemodialysis [due to the known dialyzability of 4MP (Jacobsen et al., 1996a, b)]. The trials routinely evaluated acid–base status, electrolytes, renal and liver function parameters, visual function (methanol arm), and plasma levels of fomepizole, of EG/methanol and of their metabolites at predetermined intervals. Both arms of the clinical trials (Brent et al., 1999, 2001) demonstrated that fomepizole was an effective therapy against these poisonings and provided sufficient data for an NDA submission. Considering secondary endpoints, fomepizole was shown to decrease plasma formate levels in methanol patients and plasma glycolate and urine oxalate levels in EG patients. As a consequence of these trials, fomepizole was approved by the FDA for marketing as a treatment for EG poisoning in 1997 and was first sold as Antizol by Orphan Medical for this use in 1998. Because of a slower enrollment of patients in the methanol arm of the trial, it was not approved for the methanol indication until 2000.

Fomepizole today — Generics, shortages, and new uses

Once fomepizole became available, physicians had a choice for ADH inhibition, either the traditional ethanol or the new drug. Ethanol's advantages included being inexpensive plus relatively available in most settings and having a long clinical experience. However, clinicians in North America and Europe soon found that fomepizole was superior to ethanol in terms of practical use (Rietjens et al., 2014). Fomepizole was easy to dose with predictable pharmacokinetics and did not need repeated blood level monitoring (Marraffa et al., 2007; McMartin et al., 2012). Fomepizole produced few adverse effects

(Lepik et al., 2009) and could be given in general hospital settings, not needing intensive care. Fomepizole, but not ethanol, may be used without needing hemodialysis (Borron et al., 1999; Hovda and Jacobsen, 2008; Brent, 2009; Buller and Moskowitz, 2011), particularly in presymptomatic EG poisoning. Fomepizole costs more, but the overall cost of the two therapies is relatively similar due to the nursing and monitoring issues with ethanol (Rietjens et al., 2014; Sivilotti, 2009). As such, already by 2002, fomepizole was used in over 50% of the treatable cases of these poisonings in the United States and by 2012, ethanol was rarely used at all (Ghannoum et al., 2014; Sivilotti, 2009). Nevertheless, ethanol is a viable alternative where fomepizole is not available.

The rise (and temporary fall) of generics—Worldwide access issues

Because fomepizole use became widespread during the 2000s and because the cost of the trade version of fomepizole was considered by many to be excessive, it is not surprising that generic versions of fomepizole were introduced in 2009 in the United States after the exclusive marketing period for the trade product ended. Since then, at least eight different generic versions have been marketed. The initial cost of the generic versions was substantially less than that of the trade version (Antizol), mostly due to the latter being sold in four vial packs, while generics were sold as individual vials. Since 2012, the cost of some generic versions has risen nearly 50% (Mazer-Amirshahi et al., 2018). The generic fomepizole market was blunted starting March 2015, when the Sandoz product was pulled from the market due to manufacturing issues related to product sterility (Optum Rx, 2015a). By September of 2015, other fomepizole products became unavailable due to scarcity of the active ingredient (a good manufacturing practice issue) and to increased demand on the available products (Optum Rx, 2015b). This created the great national fomepizole shortage, which led to creative ways of extending its dosing, as well as a return to ethanol therapy (Boley et al., 2015). By February of 2017, the shortage was declared over by the FDA, when new or revised generic forms began to be marketed (Pharmacy Learning Network, 2017).

Worldwide, fomepizole has been widely available in North America and in Europe since the early 2000s. However, access elsewhere has been restricted by cost, availability or lack of governmental approval for use. As such, ethanol is still widely used world-wide in the treatment of methanol and EG poisonings. In epidemic methanol exposures where fomepizole access may be limited, an expert panel has recommended that, if available, fomepizole be given to more severely affected, while ethanol be provided to lesser poisoned patients. They further suggest that, where fomepizole is not available, ethanol be used since ADH inhibition is critical in these outbreaks (Hassanian-Moghaddam et al., 2019). An important step toward increased world-wide accessibility of fomepizole occurred in 2013, when fomepizole was added to the WHO Model List of Essential Medicines (WHO, 2013).

Other possible therapeutic uses of fomepizole

Fomepizole completely blocks the acidosis as well as the acute liver and kidney injury produced by diethylene glycol (DEG) and its metabolites in rats (Besenhofer et al., 2010, 2011) (See Chapter 2.1 for a review of DEG poisoning events in the United States and elsewhere.). Such data suggest that fomepizole is likely to be an effective therapy for DEG poisoning in humans, but only a few cases utilizing fomepizole have been published (Brophy et al., 2000; Borron et al., 1997; Rollins et al., 2002). It is important to note that treatment of DEG poisoning is not an FDA-approved use of fomepizole. Also, fomepizole is only going to be effective when given early after ingestion of DEG, which is not likely in most circumstances, particularly in epidemics (Sosa et al., 2014).

Fomepizole can reverse the effects of severe disulfiram-ethanol reactions (Lindros et al., 1981; Kupari et al., 1983; Inoue et al., 1984), and so could be used in these rare circumstances.

Recent studies in animals and humans have suggested an entirely new use of fomepizole, to aid in the treatment of acetaminophen overdose, based on its ability to inhibit metabolism of acetaminophen to the toxic metabolite by interacting with CYP 2E1 (Feiermann and Cederbaum, 1985, 1986, 1987). A study in 1994 confirmed that 4MP (50 or 400 mg/kg at 4 or 8 h after acetaminophen) reduced hepatotoxicity in rats (Brennan et al., 1994). These observations lay dormant until recently, when studies in mice showed that 4MP, 50 or 200 mg/kg, blocked the hepatotoxicity of acetaminophen, either when given at the same time (Akakpo et al., 2018) or when given 90 min later (Akakpo et al., 2019). Furthermore, 4MP specifically inhibited c-Jun N-terminal kinase (JNK) activation, which is critical for the liver damage induced by acetaminophen. These authors suggest that the amelioration by 4MP, when given after the metabolic phase, results from JNK inhibition rather than from CYP2E1 inhibition (Akakpo et al., 2019). Metabolic studies in healthy human subjects have confirmed that fomepizole (15 mg/kg, then 10 mg/kg at 12 h) reduces urinary excretion of oxidative metabolites, without changing that of conjugated metabolites (Kang et al., 2020). Together these studies suggest that fomepizole might be therapeutically useful to assist NAC therapy in reducing acetaminophen morbidity.

Time overcomes all obstacles in antidotal drug development

Development of antidotes for therapeutic use, even as orphan products, is not easy. What is mostly needed is time and patience (it took 30 years from the discovery of fomepizole activity until it reached the market). Advancement of fomepizole for the treatment of methanol and EG poisoning only became possible through mechanistic research showing the key role of toxic metabolites, its undeniable preclinical efficacy, a highly acknowledged therapeutic need and simple luck (such as the Orphan Product act, the serendipity of scientific collaborations, and the advance of innovative drug companies).

Acknowledgments

The author expresses his appreciation for the mentorship of Thomas Tephly and Rolf Blomstrand as well as the assistance of Stephen Fredd of the OOPD of the FDA and Charles Defesche from Boots Pharmaceuticals in Shreveport. The author also acknowledges the collaborative effort of Dag Jacobsen, Simon Sebastian, and David Dies to conduct the Phase 1 clinical trials. The author also wishes to express appreciation to a large number of students, postdoctoral fellows and research associates, as well as the META trial investigators (see lists in Brent 1999 and 2001) that have conducted the research discussed here. Grant support was provided by various Orphan Product Development Grants from the FDA, NIH (Fogarty Fellowship for Dr. Jacobsen), a Louisiana Education Quality Support Fund grant, and Orphan Medical research agreements.

Conflict of interest/disclosure

The author has received royalties from the sale of Antizol, the trade version of fomepizole for the treatment of methanol and EG poisoning, through a licensing agreement with the Mericon Investment Group.

References

Akakpo JY, Ramachandran A, Kandel SE, Ni HM, Kumer SC, Rumack BH, Jaeschke H. 4-Methylpyrazole protects against acetaminophen hepatotoxicity in mice and in primary human hepatocytes. Hum Exp Toxicol 2018;37:1310–22.

Akakpo JY, Ramachandran A, Duan L, Schaich MA, Jaeschke MW, Freudenthal BD, et al. Delayed treatment with 4-methylpyrazole protects against acetaminophen hepatotoxicity in mice by inhibition of c-Jun n-terminal kinase. Toxicol Sci 2019;170:57–68.

Baud FJ, Bismuth C, Garnier R, Galliot M, Astier A, Maistre G, Soffer M. 4-Methylpyrazole may be an alternative to ethanol therapy for ethylene glycol intoxication in man. Clin Toxicol 1986–1987;24:463–83.

Baud FJ, Galliot M, Astier A, Bien DV, Garnier R, Likforman J, Bismuth C. Treatment of ethylene glycol poisoning with intravenous 4-methylpyrazole. N Engl J Med 1988;319:97–100.

Besenhofer LM, Adegboyega PA, Bartels M, Filary MJ, Perala AW, McLaren MC, et al. Inhibition of metabolism of diethylene glycol prevents target organ toxicity in rats. Toxicol Sci 2010;117:25–35.

Besenhofer LM, McLaren MC, Latimer B, Bartels M, Filary MJ, Perala AW, McMartin KE. Role of tissue metabolite accumulation in the renal toxicity of diethylene glycol. Toxicol Sci 2011;123:374–83.

Blomstrand R, Forsell L. Prevention of the acute ethanol-induced fatty liver by 4-methylpyrazole. Life Sci 1971;10:523–30.

Blomstrand R, Ingemansson SO. Studies on the effect of 4-methylpyrazole on methanol poisoning using the monkey as an animal model: with particular reference to the ocular toxicity. Drug Alcohol Depend 1984;13:343–55.

Blomstrand R, Kager L. The combustion of triolein-1-14C and its inhibition by alcohol in man. Life Sci 1973;13:113–23.

Blomstrand R, Theorell H. Inhibitory effect on ethanol oxidation in man after administration of 4-methylpyrazole. Life Sci 1970;9:631–40.

Boley S, Schaefer S, Jones J. Treating toxic alcohols like it's 1999 (…again), https://www.acep. org/how-we-serve/sections/toxicology/news/september-2015/treating-toxic-alcohols-like-its-1999-again/; 2015. [Accessed 27 May 2020].

Borron SW, Baud FJ, Garnier R. Intravenous 4-methylpyrazole as an antidote for diethylene glycol and triethylene glycol poisoning: a case report. Vet Hum Toxicol 1997;39:26–8.

Borron SW, Mégarbane B, Baud FJ. Fomepizole in treatment of uncomplicated ethylene glycol poisoning. Lancet 1999;354:831.

Brennan RJ, Mankes RF, Lefevre R, Raccio-Robak N, Baevsky RH, DelVecchio JA, Zink BJ. 4-Methylpyrazole blocks acetaminophen hepatotoxicity in the rat. Ann Emerg Med 1994;23:487–94.

Brent J. Fomepizole for ethylene glycol and methanol poisoning. N Engl J Med 2009;360:2216–23.

Brent J, McMartin KE, Phillips S, Burkhart KK, Donovan JW, Wells M, Kulig K. Fomepizole for the treatment of ethylene glycol poisoning. N Engl J Med 1999;340:832–8.

Brent J, McMartin KE, Phillips S, Aaron C, Kulig K. Fomepizole for the treatment of methanol poisoning. N Engl J Med 2001;344:424–9.

Brophy PD, Tenenbein M, Gardner J, Bunchman TE, Smoyer WE. Childhood diethylene glycol poisoning treated with alcohol dehydrogenase inhibitor fomepizole and hemodialysis. Am J Kidney Dis 2000;35:958–62.

Buller GK, Moskowitz CB. When is it appropriate to treat ethylene glycol intoxication with fomepizole alone without hemodialysis? Semin Dial 2011;4:441–2.

Chou JY, Richardson KE. The effect of pyrazole on ethylene glycol toxicity and metabolism in the rat. Toxicol Appl Pharmacol 1978;43:33–44.

Clay KL, Murphy RC, Watkins WD. Experimental methanol toxicity in the primate: analysis of metabolic acidosis. Toxicol Appl Pharmacol 1975;34:49–61.

Dial SM, Thrall MA, Hamar DW. 4-Methylpyrazole as treatment for naturally acquired ethylene glycol intoxication in dogs. J Am Vet Med Assoc 1989;195:73–6.

Dial SM, Thrall MA, Hamar DW. Efficacy of 4-methylpyrazole for treatment of ethylene glycol intoxication in dogs. Am J Vet Res 1994;55:1762–70.

Feierman DE, Cederbaum AI. Inhibition of microsomal oxidation of ethanol by pyrazole and 4-methylpyrazole in vitro. Increased effectiveness after induction by pyrazole and 4-methylpyrazole. Biochem J 1986;239:671–7.

Feierman DE, Cederbaum AI. Increased sensitivity of the microsomal oxidation of ethanol to inhibition by pyrazole and 4-methylpyrazole after chronic ethanol treatment. Biochem Pharmacol 1987;36:3277–83.

Feiermann DE, Cederbaum AI. Increased content of cytochrome P-450 and 4-methylpyrazole binding spectra after 4-methylpyrazole treatment. Biochem Biophys Res Commun 1985;126:1076–81.

Ghannoum M, Hoffman RS, Mowry JB, Lavergne V. Trends in toxic alcohol exposures in the United States from 2000 to 2013: a focus on the use of antidotes and extracorporeal treatments. Semin Dial 2014;27:395–401.

Grauer GF, Thrall MAH, Henre BA, Hjelle JJ. Comparison of the effects of ethanol and 4-methylpyrazole on the pharmacokinetics and toxicity of ethylene glycol in the dog. Toxicol Lett 1987;35:307–14.

Gummin DD, Mowry JB, Spyker DA, Brooks DE, Beuhler MC, Rivers LJ, et al. 2018 annual report of the American Association of Poison Control Centers' National Poison Data System (NPDS): 36th annual report. Clin Toxicol 2019;57:1220–413.

Guo C, Cenac TA, Li Y, McMartin KE. Calcium oxalate, and not other metabolites, is responsible for the renal toxicity of ethylene glycol. Toxicol Lett 2007;173:8–16.

Hassanian-Moghaddam H, Zamani N, Roberts DM, Brent J, McMartin K, Aaron C, et al. Consensus statements on the approach to patients in a methanol poisoning outbreak. Clin Toxicol 2019;57:1129–36.

Hovda KE, Jacobsen D. Expert opinion: fomepizole may ameliorate the need for hemodialysis in methanol poisoning. Hum Exp Toxicol 2008;27:539–46.

Inoue K, Fukunaga M, Kiriyama T, Komura S. Accumulation of acetaldehyde in alcohol-sensitive Japanese: relation to ethanol and acetaldehyde oxidizing capacity. Alcohol Clin Exp Res 1984;8:319–22.

Jacobsen D, McMartin KE. Methanol and ethylene glycol poisoning. Mechanism of toxicity, clinical course, diagnosis and treatment. Med Toxicol 1986;1:309–34.

Jacobsen D, Jansen H, Wiik-Larsen E, Bredesen JE, Halvorsen S. Studies on methanol poisoning. Acta Med Scand 1982a;212:5–10.

Jacobsen D, Ostby N, Bredesen JE. Studies on ethylene glycol poisoning. Acta Med Scand 1982b;212:11–5.

Jacobsen D, Ovrebo S, Ostborg J, Sejersted OM. Glycolate causes the acidosis in ethylene glycol poisoning and is effectively removed by hemodialysis. Acta Med Scand 1984;216:409–16.

Jacobsen D, Sebastian CS, Blomstrand R, McMartin KE. 4-Methylpyrazole: a controlled study of safety in healthy human subjects after single, ascending doses. Alcohol Clin Exp Res 1988;12:516–22.

Jacobsen D, Barron SK, Sebastian CS, Blomstrand R, McMartin KE. Non-linear kinetics of 4-methylpyrazole in healthy human subjects. Eur J Clin Pharmacol 1989;37:599–604.

Jacobsen D, Sebastian CS, Barron SK, Carriere EW, McMartin KE. Effects of 4-methylpyrazole, methanol/ethylene glycol antidote, in healthy humans. J Emerg Med 1990;8:455–61.

Jacobsen D, Ostensen J, Bredesen L, Ullstein E, McMartin K. 4-Methylpyrazole (4-MP) is effectively removed by haemodialysis in the pig model. Hum Exp Toxicol 1996a;15:494–6.

Jacobsen D, Sebastian CS, Dies DF, Breau RL, Spann EG, Barron SK, McMartin KE. Kinetic interactions between 4-methylpyrazole and ethanol in healthy humans. Alcohol Clin Exp Res 1996b;20:804–9.

Kang AM, Padilla-Jones A, Fisher ES, Akakpo JY, Jaeschke H, Rumack BH, et al. The effect of 4-methylpyrazole on oxidative metabolism of acetaminophen in human volunteers. J Med Toxicol 2020;16:169–76.

Kupari M, Lindros K, Hillbom M, Heikkilä J, Ylikahri R. Cardiovascular effects of acetaldehyde accumulation after ethanol ingestion: their modification by beta-adrenergic blockade and alcohol dehydrogenase inhibition. Alcohol Clin Exp Res 1983;7:283–8.

Lepik KJ, Levy AR, Sobolev BG, Purssell RA, DeWitt CR, Erhardt GD, et al. Adverse drug events associated with the antidotes for methanol and ethylene glycol poisoning: a comparison of ethanol and fomepizole. Ann Emerg Med 2009;53:439–50.

Li TK, Theorell H. Human liver alcohol dehydrogenase: inhibition by pyrazole and pyrazole analogs. Acta Chem Scand 1969;23:892–902.

Lindros KO, Pikkarainen P, Salaspuro M. Effect of 4-methylpyrazole and abstinence on ethanol elimination in an alcoholic. Drug Alcohol Depend 1979;4:147.

Lindros KO, Stowell A, Pikkarainen P, Salaspuro M. The disulfiram (antabuse)-alcohol reaction in male alcoholics: its efficient management by 4-methylpyrazole. Alcohol Clin Exp Res 1981;5:528–30.

Magnusson G, Nyberg JA, Bodin NO, Hansson E. Toxicity of pyrazole and 4-methylpyrazole in mice and rats. Experientia 1972;28:8–10.

Makar AB, Tephly TR. Inhibition of monkey liver alcohol dehydrogenase by 4-methylpyrazole. Biochem Med 1975;13:334–42.

Marraffa JM, Forrest A, Grant W, Stork C, McMartin KE, Howland MA. Oral administration of fomepizole produces similar blood levels as identical intravenous dose. Clin Toxicol 2007;46:181–6.

Martin-Amat G, McMartin KE, Hayreh SS, Hayreh MS, Tephly TR. Methanol poisoning: ocular toxicity produced by formate. Toxicol Appl Pharmacol 1978;45:201–8.

Mazer-Amirshahi M, Stolbach A, Nelson LS. ACMT Position Statement: Addressing the rising cost of prescription antidotes. J Med Toxicol 2018;14:168–71.

McMartin KE, Makar AB, Martin-Amat G, Palese M, Tephly TR. Methanol poisoning I. The role of formic acid in the development of metabolic acidosis in the monkey and the reversal by 4-methylpyrazole. Biochem Med 1975;13:319–33.

McMartin KE, Martin-Amat G, Makar AB, Tephly TR. Methanol poisoning. V. Role of formate metabolism in the monkey. J Pharmacol Exp Ther 1977a;201:564–72.

McMartin KE, Martin-Amat G, Makar AB, Tephly TR. Methanol poisoning: role of formate metabolism in the monkey. In: Thurman RG, Williamson JR, Drott H, Chance B, editors. Alcohol and aldehyde metabolizing systems, vol. II. New York: Academic Press; 1977b. p. 429–40.

McMartin KE, Hedstrom KG, Tolf BR, Östling-Wintzell H, Blomstrand R. Studies on the metabolic interactions between 4-methylpyrazole and methanol using the monkey as an animal model. Arch Biochem Biophys 1980;199:606–14.

McMartin KE, Sebastian CS, Dies D, Jacobsen D. Kinetics and metabolism of fomepizole in healthy humans. Clin Toxicol 2012;50:375–83.

Murphy RC, Watkins WD. Pharmacology of pyrazoles I: structure elucidation of metabolites of 4-methylpyrazole. Biochem Biophys Res Commun 1972;49:283–91.

Optum Rx. Sandoz—recall of fomepizole injection, https://professionals.optumrx.com/content/dam/optum3/professional-optumrx/vgnlive/HCP/Assets/RxNews/Drug%20Recall_Fomepizole%20Injection_2015-0312_NAPv2.pdf; 2015a. [Accessed 27 May 2020].

Optum Rx. Antizol (fomepizole) drug shortage, https://professionals.optumrx.com/content/dam/optum3/professional-optumrx/vgnlive/HCP/Assets/RxNews/Drug%20Shortages_Antizol_2015-0925.pdf; 2015b. [Accessed 27 May 2020].

Pharmacy Learning Network. Alcohol dehydrogenase inhibitor shortage ends, https://www.managedhealthcareconnect.com/content/alcohol-dehydrogenase-inhibitor-shortage-ends; 2017. [Accessed 27 May 2020].

Rietjens SJ, de Lange DW, Meulenbelt J. Ethylene glycol or methanol intoxication: which antidote should be used, fomepizole or ethanol? Neth J Med 2014;72:73–9.

Röe O. The metabolism and toxicity of methanol. Pharmacol Rev 1955;7:399–412.

Rollins YD, Filley CM, McNutt JT, Chahal S, Kleinschmidt-DeMasters BK. Fulminant ascending paralysis as a delayed sequela of diethylene glycol (Sterno) ingestion. Neurology 2002;59:1460–3.

Salaspuro MP, Pikkarainen P, Lindros K. Ethanol-induced hypoglycaemia in man: its suppression by the alcohol dehydrogenase inhibitor 4-methylpyrazole. Eur J Clin Investig 1977;7:487–90.

Salaspuro MP, Lindros KO, Pikkarainen PH. Effect of 4-methylpyrazole on ethanol elimination rate and hepatic redox changes in alcoholics with adequate or inadequate nutrition and in nonalcoholic controls. Metabolism 1978;27:631–9.

Sivilotti ML. Ethanol: tastes great! Fomepizole: less filling! Ann Emerg Med 2009;53:451–3.

Sosa NR, Rodriguez GM, Schier JG, Sejvar JJ. Clinical, laboratory, diagnostic, and histopathologic features of diethylene glycol poisoning—Panama, 2006. Ann Emerg Med 2014;64:38–47.

Theorell H, Yonetani T, Sjöberg B. On the effects of some heterocyclic compounds on the enzymic activity of liver alcohol dehydrogenase. Acta Chem Scand 1969;23:255–60.

Torrielli MV, Gabriel L, Dianzani MU. Ethanol-induced hepatotoxicity; experimental observations on the role of lipid peroxidation. J Pathol 1978;126:11–25.

WHO. WHO model list of essential medicines. 18th list, http://www.who.int/medicines/publications/essentialmedicines/en/index.html; April 2013.

Winters DK, Cederbaum AI. Time course characterization of the induction of cytochrome P-450 2E1 by pyrazole and 4-methylpyrazole. Biochim Biophys Acta 1992;1117:15–24.

Chapter 3.3

Methylene blue

Mary Ann Howland

Clinical Professor of Pharmacy, St. John's University College of Pharmacy and Health Sciences Adjunct Professor of Emergency Medicine, New York University School of Medicine Bellevue Hospital Emergency Department Senior Consultant in Residence, New York City Poison Center New York, NY, United States

Discovery

As early as 1910, Wilson, drawing on the work of Ehrlich in 1885 and others, detailed how methylene blue, the common name for tetramethylthionine chloride, stains tissues, and in particular nerve cells in living animals (Wilson, 1910; Krafts et al., 2011). It was proposed that these nerve cells took up the methylene blue but it was not until these cells were exposed to the air that they were visibly stained blue. This was a consequence of the reduction of methylene blue to the "leucobase." Indeed, this same property—the reduction of methylene blue to its leucomethylene blue form—serves as the mechanism responsible for the ability of methylene blue to convert methemoglobin to oxyhemoglobin!

In 1932 three patients were brought to the Central Emergency Hospital in San Francisco in a coma with cyanosis after collapsing within minutes of ingesting some liquor; they died despite aggressive resuscitation. Laboratory analysis revealed the presence of cyanide (Geiger, 1932). Seeking assistance, Dr. J.C. Geiger, the director of Public Health enlisted Dr. P.J. Hanzlik, Professor of Pharmacology at the University of California Medical School to conduct a survey and then compile a list of recommended antidotes for distribution and future use (Hanzlik, 1933). Relying on work done in the 1910s by Warburg and others from the 1920s and 1930s including Brundages' Toxicology Textbook, the work of Sahlin of Lund, and of Eddy on the properties of methylene blue, they advised methylene blue as an antidote for cyanide (Eddy, 1931). Although Brooks, another researcher, had done a rat experiment using methylene blue for cyanide toxicity, her work was not cited in compiling the list, and a back and forth ensued in the press about giving due credit (Brooks, 1933, 1936; Geiger, 1933; Hanzlik, 1933). Not long thereafter a patient presented critically ill to an emergency department with evidence suggesting cyanide ingestion in a suicidal attempt (Geiger, 1932). The treating physician administered 50 mL of 1%

History of Modern Clinical Toxicology. https://doi.org/10.1016/B978-0-12-822218-8.00052-1

231

methylene blue and within minutes the patient recovered. One explanation is that this dose of methylene blue, which is seven times the dose we use today to treat methemoglobinemia, actually produced methemoglobin secondary to its ability to oxidize hemoglobin at high doses, similar to the way sodium nitrite has been used as part of the cyanide antidote kit (Alston, 2014). See Chapter 3.8 for details on the development of cyanide antidotes.

Extending the antidotal properties of methylene blue, in November 1933, Williams and Challis reported on a chemistry student who was heating para-bromoaniline and parabromorthosulfanilic acid in an experiment (Williams and Challis, 1933). An hour or so later the student noticed discolored skin. An hour and a half after that, as he drove home, he felt dizzy and developed a severe headache. By 6 h post-exposure he was in Highland Hospital in Rochester, NY comatose and cyanotic. The decision was made to treat him with glucose and 100 mL of 1% methylene blue, the experimental therapy used by Geiger. Soon thereafter, his color improved and within several hours he had recovered. Blood taken before the administration of methylene blue was chocolate brown, tested negative for carbon monoxide and tested positive for methemoglobin. An experiment with rabbits demonstrated skin absorption of the aniline dye (parabromoaniline) as the culprit (Williams and Challis, 1933). Methemoglobin was identified and the treatment of the rabbit with 1 mL of 1% methylene blue converted the methemoglobin to oxyhemoglobin. Since it was known from the experiments of Wendel (Wendel, 1933) that too much methylene blue was capable of causing methemoglobinemia, another rabbit was given 3.5 mL of 1% methylene blue and did not develop methemoglobinemia (Williams and Challis, 1933).

In June 1933 two patients were treated in Boston City Hospital with methylene blue for methemoglobinemia (Steele and Spink, 1933). One patient unintentionally mistook a red liquid for wine. Within several hours, he was hypotensive and tachycardic, with grayish-blue-brown skin and a bluish-brown tint evident in retinal vessels. His breath and gastric lavage washings smelled like aniline. Shortly thereafter, his condition deteriorated and 500 mg of oral methylene blue was administered with little improvement. Subsequently, 50 mL (undocumented concentration but 1% implied) of methylene blue solution was injected IV. Within 15 min the patient was up and awake and talking and only faintly blue. Within 30 min, his vital signs had improved. Although a methemoglobin concentration was not measured, his blood was chocolate brown before the methylene blue and normal within an hour afterwards. A second patient presented similarly after ingesting a whiskey extract. The patient was administered 100 mL of 0.5% methylene blue IV. After the first 50 mL had been injected the patient sat up and began talking and after the entire 100 mL had been infused he was nearly normal. The blood was positive for methemoglobin before the methylene blue and negative afterwards. And acetanilide, a precursor to aniline, was present in the gastric washings.

In 1934 and again in 1935, Wendel describes how methylene blue produces methemoglobin to which cyanide binds to produce cyanomethemoglobin and frees the cyanide from its reversible binding to tissue (Wendel, 1934, 1935).

This led to the study of amyl nitrite and sodium nitrite, better methemoglobin producers, and ultimately to the cyanide antidote kit which was in use for many years until hydroxocobalamin became available (Chen and Rose, 1952). It was soon recognized that methylene blue can both cause methemoglobin and also treat it, depending on the dose (Wendel, 1935, 1939).

The synthesis of methylene blue by Caro in 1876 grew out of the dye industry in England. Perkin in 1856 serendipitously discovered a beautiful purple dye called mauve, when aniline was oxidized. This led Caro to experiment with many aniline derivatives, one of which turned out to be methylene blue, a phenothiazine derivative. This then led to the synthesis of phenothiazine, the synthetic antimalarials: quinacrine and chloroquine, the potent but sedating antihistamine-promethazine, and ultimately in 1950, chlorpromazine, the first of the antipsychotic drugs (Zirkle, 1973; Shen, 1999; Krafts et al., 2012; Scheindlin, 2008).

In addition to the effects of methylene blue as a blood stain and to reverse cyanide and methemoglobinemia, it has a rich history of being recognized as a treatment for malaria since the late 1800s and is still used as part of combination therapy (Zirkle, 1973; Scheindlin, 2008; Müller et al., 2019) and as a urinary antiseptic (Scheindlin, 2008). More recently, it is being investigated for ifosfamide-induced neurotoxicity, catecholamine refractory vasoplegia, septic shock, photodynamic therapy (Ginimuge and Jyothi, 2010), hypotension associated with calcium channel blocker overdose, neuroprotection in a number of disorders including Alzheimer's disease and stroke, psychiatric disorders (Schirmer et al., 2011; Scheindlin, 2008; Wiklund et al., 2007; Tucker et al., 2018; Howland, 2016), and localization of parathyroid adenomas (van der Vorst et al., 2014).

Pharmacology

Methylene blue catalyzes the reduction of methemoglobin to oxyhemoglobin (Smith, 2019; Bodansky and Gutmann, 1947; Bodansky, 1950; Gutmann et al., 1947). The heme iron in hemoglobin is normally in the $+2$ state and carries oxygen as oxyhemoglobin. Normal processes constantly oxidize small amounts of the iron to the $+3$ state, methemoglobin, which cannot carry oxygen. By shifting the oxyhemoglobin dissociation curve to the left, methemoglobin impairs the delivery of oxygen to the tissues from oxyhemoglobin. Two pathways are responsible for converting methemoglobin back to oxyhemoglobin and in keeping the normal methemoglobin concentration around 1%. These are nicotine adenine dinucleotide (NADH) dependent methemoglobin reductase (also known as cytochrome $b5$ reductase) and nicotine adenine dinucleotide phosphate (NADPH) dependent methemoglobin reductase. NADH-dependent methemoglobin reductase is ordinarily responsible for 95% of the conversion while NADPH-dependent methemoglobin reductase accounts for the other 5%. NADPH-dependent methemoglobin reductase requires an electron carrier like flavin or a cofactor like methylene blue. Methylene blue (blue in color) is reduced to leucomethylene blue (colorless) by the NADPH-dependent reductase. The leucomethylene blue then nonenzymatically reduces methemoglobin (Smith and Thron, 1972; Sass et al., 1967). One study estimated that methylene blue decreased the time to recovery of the methemoglobin by many fold, even quoting a number of about 6.4-fold (Wuertz et al., 1964), whereas other in vitro studies suggest an even faster rate of reduction (Bradberry, 2003; Tomoda et al., 1980; Wendel, 1937; Wendel, 1939).

The usual dose of methylene blue is 1–2 mg/kg intravenously over 5–30 min, either undiluted and followed by a fluid flush or diluted in 5%D/W to avoid local pain. Sodium chloride should not be used as a diluent since this decreases the solubility of the methylene blue (Provayblue package insert 2019). The FDA approved product is now available as a 0.5% concentration while earlier preparations were available in a 1% concentration. Most patients with concentrations of methemoglobin below 50% will respond to 1 mg/kg while 2 mg/kg is usually needed for patients with higher methemoglobin concentrations (Wendel, 1937; Bodansky and Gutmann, 1947; Bradberry, 2003). Repeat dosing is often needed for drug-induced methemoglobinemia when the drug responsible is acting as a prodrug with active metabolites (such as dapsone and aniline) or when patients ingest very large doses of a methemoglobin forming xenobiotic such as sodium nitrite (Layne and Smith, 1969; Smith and Layne, 1969; Bradberry, 2003; Mudan et al., 2020; Curry, 2020). When intravenous administration is not possible, intraosseous administration has been used (Herman et al., 1999). Subcutaneous and intraspinal administration of methylene blue is contraindicated (Perry and Meinhard, 1974; Reynolds et al., 2014; Raimer et al., 1999; Provay blue package insert).

Adverse effects

Adverse effects of methylene blue are best described by an experiment performed by Nadler et al. in 1934. They administered 50 mL of a 1% methylene blue solution IV over 5–30 min to 18 normal adult volunteers (Nadler et al., 1934). Assuming an average weight of 70 kg this dose is approximately 7 mg/kg. Several patients received multiple doses 3–5 days after the urine was no longer blue-green. The EKG demonstrated only a reduction in the height of both the T and R waves which reversed within 2 h. Some patients reported chest pressure/pain with an increased heart rate. The skin and mucous membranes, saliva, and gastric contents became blue not long after the start of the infusion. Other complaints included "burning" in the mouth and a feeling of warmth in the stomach as well as occasional nausea and vomiting, restlessness, anxiety, facial and extremity tremors, and paresthesias. Some patients complained of an altered mental status, headache, and minimal GI effects that lasted for about 12 h. In one patient, the dose was stopped at 25 mL (250 mg; 3.5 mg/kg) due to extreme anxiety and the feeling of impending doom. Methylene blue urinary excretion often produces burning and dysuria and in two patients caused severe scrotal and groin pain. Methemoglobin concentrations ranged from 0.6% to 8.3% of total hemoglobin.

In 1961, a 2.3-kg infant without methemoglobinemia was administered approximately 16 mg/kg of methylene blue over several minutes (Goluboff and Wheaton, 1961). As expected the infant's skin looked bluish but without the presence of methemoglobinemia. By 2½ h the skin color was described as slightly grayish blue and a second dose was administered. Again, the infant became blue all over with the exception of the ears and his body and urine remained blue in color for the next 4 days. Other than his cyanotic appearance and occasional twitching and poor feeding for several days the infant remained well with no evidence of methemoglobinemia. However, 4 days later, the infant became jaundiced; by 8 days his hemoglobin had dropped by half secondary to acute hemolysis. Another child was administered 5 mg/kg of methylene blue and remained intensely blue for 6 days; his stool was dark blue for 4 days (Blass and Fung, 1976).

Adverse effects of methylene blue include local toxicity, allergy (rare), inaccurate interpretation of pulse oximetry, blue discoloration of the skin and urine, the risk of producing methemoglobin and/or hemolysis, and the risk of serotonin toxicity (Bradberry, 2003; Coleman and Coleman, 1996). It can cause skin necrosis if extravasation occurs (Lee et al., 2014; Wendel, 1939). Because methylene blue is a dye it transiently interferes with the pulse oximeter reading and the Bispectral Index used in anesthesiology after IV administration (Coleman and Coleman, 1996; Matisoff and Panni, 2006). In addition, it has been known for decades that methylene blue turns the urine blue-green; this attribute was even once suggested as a way to assess compliance (Kraus et al., 1987; Prischl et al., 1999).

Methylene blue can act as an oxidant when given in a large enough dose or when there is not enough reducing power to form leucomethylene blue (Goluboff and Wheaton, 1961). The reduction to leucomethylene blue depends on NADPH-dependent methemoglobin reductase (Beutler, 1991, 1994; Frank, 2005; Nkhoma et al., 2009; Luzzatto and Seneca, 2014). Without NADPH, this pathway is compromised. The red blood cell (RBC) also depends on NADPH to replenish glutathione and catalase, two important antioxidants. The formation of NADPH is dependent on the action of glucose-6-phosphate dehydrogenase (G6PD) which catalyzes the production NADPH in the pentose monophosphate shunt. Without G6PD the RBC is susceptible to oxidant stresses. Worldwide the prevalence of G6PD deficiency is estimated at almost 5%. It is an X-linked hereditary deficiency with many variants ranging in quantity and quality (Luzzatto and Seneca, 2014). The variants are classified on the basis of enzyme activity from Class 1 (most severe, but uncommon) to Class V (none). Class II (G6PD Mediterranean, severe, < 10% of normal activity, mostly in Asian and Mediterranean populations) and Class III (G6PD A-, moderate, 10%–60% of normal activity, in 10% of US black males) are the two most common (Frank, 2005). Now that methylene blue is being used in conjunction with other antimalarials to reduce the gametocyte production of *Plasmodium falciparum*, a renewed interest in its potential for causing hemolysis in G6PD A-deficiency has arisen. A recent analysis suggested methylene blue at an oral dose of 15 mg/kg/day was responsible for a drop in hemoglobin which reached a minimum of 8.5 g/dL with limited clinical relevance (Müller et al., 2019). The decision to administer methylene blue to a patient with methemoglobinemia is almost always made without knowing their G6PD status. However once 1–2 mg/kg of intravenous methylene blue has been administered without any effect on the methemoglobin then an alternate diagnosis (sulfhemoglobin, hemoglobin M, NADPH methemoglobin reductase deficiency) or the possibility of G6PD deficiency should be entertained and other treatment measures undertaken (Noor and Beutler, 1998; Rosen et al., 1971; Gharahbaghian et al., 2009).

When faced with patients who exhibit methemoglobinemia from xenobiotics that produce prolonged or recurring methemoglobin it is often difficult to determine whether the inciting xenobiotic is the culprit or if methylene blue is making the situation worse (Kearney et al., 1984; Bradberry, 2003). Stossel and Jennings in 1966 were unable to induce methemoglobinemia in dogs administered 20 mg/kg IV methylene blue or in rats administered an LD50 of methylene blue intraperitoneally (Stossel and Jennings, 1966). As mentioned above Nadler administered approximately 7 mg/kg of methylene blue intravenously to volunteers in 1934 and the maximum methemoglobin concentration achieved was 8.3% of total hemoglobin. A similar case reported the maximal production of 7% methemoglobin after 5 mg/kg (Whitwam et al., 1979). When 4 mg/kg of methylene blue was administered to cats a small but significant increase in methemoglobin occurred (Harvey and Keitt, 1983). In vitro and presumably in vivo, the balance favoring the production of methemoglobin by methylene blue is dependent on dose and the presence of hemolysis (Smith and Thron, 1972).

Methylene blue is a potent MAOI inhibitor in vitro and many case reports now support its role in producing serotonin toxicity when combined with serotonin reuptake inhibitors (SRIs). https://psychotropical.com/methylene-blue-serotonin-toxicity-syndrome/ accessed August 22, 2020 (Gillman, 2006). The first report of an association between methylene blue and central nervous system toxicity occurred in 2003 in the form of a letter describing a patient who had received 7.5 mg/kg of methylene blue to stain abnormal parathyroid glands before surgery. Dr. Gillman took up the cause and with colleagues established that methylene blue is a potent and preferential MAO-A inhibitor (Gillman, 2006; Ramsay et al., 2007; Stanford et al., 2010; Gillman, 2011). Most cases of severe serotonin toxicity have been associated with large doses of methylene blue administered preoperatively to patients undergoing parathyroidectomy surgery (7.5–9 mg/kg doses) (Bach et al., 2004; Top et al., 2014; Shopes et al., 2013) but recently even a 1 mg/kg dose was associated with serotonin toxicity (Schwiebert et al., 2009). Other factors may be at play since not all patients on SRIs receiving methylene blue develop serotonin toxicity (Sweet and Standiford, 2007). The Provayblue package insert contains a warning about the potential for serotonin toxicity when methylene blue is used in patients on SRIs. In patients with consequential methemoglobinemia who are also on SRIs it is reasonable to use small doses of methylene blue and monitor for and quickly treat any ensuing serotonin toxicity (Curry, 2020).

Comparative safety and effectiveness

Dogs were used to compare the effects of methylene blue, ascorbic acid, and dimercaprol (BAL) on the time required to reduce methemoglobin induced by the IV injection of *p*-aminopropiophenone in propylene glycol to one half the maximal concentration (Bodansky and Gutmann, 1947). Most dogs that achieved a maximal methemoglobin concentration of 89% without therapy died between 1 and 3 h. Control dogs brought to about 60% methemoglobin took 4 h to drop to 30%. Those that received 1 mg/kg methylene blue took about 35 min to drop by 50% from maximal concentrations of 50% methemoglobin. Higher doses (5–10 mg/kg) dropped the concentrations even faster. Ascorbic acid at very large doses in those dogs reduced the maximal concentration in about 1½ to 2 h. Although BAL had some affect, the doses necessary were too close to toxic doses. Case reports have used various doses of ascorbic acid to reduce methemoglobin concentrations when methylene blue is unavailable or suspected contraindications exist (Carnrick et al., 1946; Rehman et al., 2018). The reduction in methemoglobin concentrations is slower with ascorbic acid compared with methylene blue.

Special populations (pregnancy, children, elderly)

The current FDA approved package insert of Provayblue states that the use of methylene blue may cause fetal harm when administered to pregnant women (Provayblue, 2019). A 2017 textbook on drugs in pregnancy states that methylene blue may cause fetal harm in the second and third trimesters (Briggs et al., 2017). The intra-amniotic injection of methylene blue to detect ruptured membranes should be avoided. This use has led to fetal abnormalities including hemolytic anemia, hyperbilirubinemia, methemoglobinemia, deep blue staining of the fetal skin, multiple ileal occlusions, and jejunal and ileal atresia. There are no data regarding breastfeeding; the current manufacturer of Provayblue suggests discontinuing breastfeeding for 8 days after administration (Briggs et al., 2017; Provayblue, 2019).

Development

Provepharm SAS, a French company, received orphan drug designation for Provayblue (methylene blue 0.5%, 2 mL, 10 mL) in 2013 and received new drug approval status on April 8, 2016, under an accelerated drug approval process. It retains manufacturing exclusivity rights until 2023. Provayblue is now the only FDA-approved methylene blue product. Previously methylene blue 1%, USP was available for many decades as an unapproved FDA drug. The evidence for efficacy of Provayblue was based on demonstrating bioequivalence to the 1% product, case reports, retrospective case reports and a literature review. Efficacy is determined by a 50% reduction in methemoglobinemia within 1 h of administration and a normalization of vital signs within 2 h. Complete information on this process and a summary review are available at: https://www.accessdata.fda.gov/drugsatfda_docs/nda/2016/204630Orig1_toc.cfm https://www.accessdata.fda.gov/drugsatfda_docs/nda/2016/204630Orig1s000SumR.pdf.

Recent history

An expert consensus panel recommends that all emergency departments have methylene blue stocked for immediate availability (Dart et al., 2018). The WHO List of Essential Medicines 2019 lists methylene blue 1% 10 mg/mL (10 mL) (WHO, 2020). The US national stockpile does not contain methylene blue. A comparison of the last 10 years of available US poison control center data reveals a similar pattern of use (Bronstein et al., 2009; Gummin et al., 2019). Data for 2018 shows a total of 239 uses for methylene blue, most often in those over the age of 20 years (Gummin et al., 2019).

Methylene blue is an excellent drug with a very long history. Its efficacy as an antidote in the treatment of methemoglobinemia is undeniable. Starting with a low dose and titrating upward when an effect is clearly demonstrable and stopping when no effect is appreciable should maximize the benefit while minimizing the adverse effects. Contraindications should be respected. Close monitoring for adverse effects like serotonin toxicity should be observed with early and aggressive treatment undertaken as needed.

References

Alston TA. Why does methylene blue reduce methemoglobin in benzocaine poisoning but beneficially oxidize hemoglobin in cyanide poisoning? J Clin Anesth 2014;26:702–3.

Bach KK, Lindsay FW, Berg LS, Howard RS. Prolonged postoperative disorientation after methylene blue infusion during parathyroidectomy. Anesth Analg 2004;99:1573–4.

Beutler E. Glucose-6-phosphate dehydrogenase deficiency. N Engl J Med 1991;324:169–74.

Beutler E. G6PD deficiency. Blood 1994;84:3613–36.

Blass N, Fung D. Dyed but not dead—methylene blue overdose. Anesthesiology 1976;45:458–9.

Bodansky O. Mechanism of action of methylene blue in treatment of methemoglobinemia. JAMA 1950;142:923.

Bodansky O, Gutmann H. Treatment of methemoglobinemia. J Pharmacol Exp Ther 1947;90:46–56.

Bradberry SM. Occupational methaemoglobinaemia. Mechanisms of production, features, diagnosis and management including the use of methylene blue. Toxicol Rev 2003;22:13–27.

Briggs GG, Freeman RK, Towers CV, Forinash AB, editors. Drugs in pregnancy and lactation: a reference guide to fetal and neonatal risk—methylene blue. In: Methylene blue monograph. 11th ed. New York: Wolters Kluwer; 2017. p. 935–6.

Bronstein A, Spyker D, Cantilena L, et al. 2008 annual report of the American Association of Poison Control Centers' National Poison Data System (NPDS): 26th annual report. Clin Toxicol 2009;47:911–1084.

Brooks MM. Methylene blue as antidote for cyanide and carbon monoxide (letter). JAMA 1933;100:59.

Brooks MM. Mechanism of Methylene blue in CO-Poisoning. Am J Phys 1936;34:659–61.

Carnrick M, Polis BD, Klein T. Methemoglobinemia; treatment with ascorbic acid. Arch Intern Med 1946;78:296–302.

Chen KK, Rose CL. Nitrite and thiosulfate therapy in cyanide poisoning. JAMA 1952;149:113–9.

Coleman MD, Coleman NA. Drug-induced methaemoglobinaemia. Treatment issues. Drug Saf 1996;14:394–405.

Curry S. The tox and the hound. Methylene blue, https://emcrit.org/toxhound/refractory-methemo-globinemia/; 2020. [Accessed 15 August 2020].

Dart RC, Goldfrank LR, Erstad BL, et al. Expert consensus guidelines for stocking of antidotes in hospitals that provide emergency care. Ann Emerg Med 2018;71:314–25.

Eddy NB. Regulation of respiration. The antagonism between methylene blue and sodium cyanide. J Pharmacol Exp Ther 1931;41:449–64.

Frank JE. Diagnosis and management of G6PD deficiency. Am Fam Physician 2005;72:1277–82.

Geiger JC. Cyanide poisoning in San Francisco (letter). JAMA 1932;99:1944–5.

Geiger JC. Methylene blue as antidote for cyanide and carbon monoxide poisoning (letter). JAMA 1933;100:59.

Gharahbaghian L, Massoudian B, Dimassa G. Methemoglobinemia and sulfhemoglobinemia in two pediatric patients after ingestion of hydroxylamine sulfate. West J Emerg Med 2009;10:197–201.

Gillman PK. Methylene blue implicated in potentially fatal serotonin toxicity. Anaesthesia 2006;61:1013–4.

Gillman PK. CNS toxicity involving methylene blue: the exemplar for understanding and predict-ing drug interactions that precipitate serotonin toxicity. J Psychopharmacol 2011;25:429–36.

Ginimuge PR, Jyothi SD. Methylene blue: revisited. J Anaesthesiol Clin Pharmacol 2010;26:517–20.

Goluboff N, Wheaton R. Methylene blue induced cyanosis and acute hemolytic anemia complicat-ing the treatment of methemoglobinemia. J Pediatr 1961;58:86–9.

Gummin D, Mowry J, Spyker D, et al. 2018 annual report of the American Association of Poison Control Centers' National Poison Data System (NPDS): 36th annual report. Clin Toxicol 2019;57:1220–413.

Gutmann HR, Jandorf BJ, Bodansky O. The role of methylene blue and pyridine nucleotides in the reduction of methemoglobin in hemolyzates. Fed Proc 1947;6(1 Pt 2):257.

Hanzlik PJ. Methylene blue as antidote for cyanide poisoning (letter). JAMA 1933;100:357.

Harvey JW, Keitt AS. Studies of the efficacy and potential hazards of methylene blue therapy in aniline-induced methaemoglobinaemia. Br J Haematol 1983;54:29–41.

Herman MI, Chyka PA, Butler AY, Rieger SE. Methylene blue by intraosseous infusion for methe-moglobinemia. Ann Emerg Med 1999;33:111–3.

Howland RH. Methylene blue: the long and winding road from stain to brain: part 1. J Psychosoc Nurs Ment Health Serv 2016;54:21–4.

Kearney TE, Manoguerra AS, Dunford Jr JV. Chemically induced methemoglobinemia from aniline poisoning. West J Med 1984;140:282–6.

Krafts K, Hempelmann E, Skórska-Stania A. From methylene blue to chloroquine: a brief review of the development of an antimalarial therapy. Parasitol Res 2012;111:7.

Krafts KP, Hempelmann E, Oleksyn BJ. The color purple: from royalty to laboratory, with apologies to Malachowski. Biotech Histochem 2011;86:7–35.

Kraus RP, Grof P, Arana GW, Workman RJ, Harvey KJ, Hux M. Methylene blue: a reliable and practical marker for validating compliance on the DST. J Clin Psychiatry 1987;48:224–9.

Layne WR, Smith RP. Methylene blue uptake and the reversal of chemically induced methemoglo-binemias in human erythrocytes. J Pharmacol Exp Ther 1969;165:36–44.

Lee JH, Chang CH, Park CH, Kim JK. Methylene blue dye-induced skin necrosis in immediate breast reconstruction: evaluation and management. Arch Plast Surg 2014;41:258–63.

Luzzatto L, Seneca E. G6PD deficiency: a classic example of pharmacogenetics with on-going clinical implications. Br J Haematol 2014;164:469–80.

Matisoff AJ, Panni MK. Methylene blue treatment for methemoglobinemia and subsequent dramatic bispectral index reduction. Anesthesiology 2006;105:228.

Mudan A, Repplinger D, Lebin J, et al. Severe methemoglobinemia and death from intentional sodium nitrite ingestions. J Emerg Med 2020. [online ahead of print]. S0736-4679(20)30580-1.

Müller O, Lu G, Jahn A, Mockenhaupt FP. How worthwhile is methylene blue as a treatment of malaria? Expert Rev Anti-Infect Ther 2019;17:471–3.

Nadler JE, Green H, Rosenbaum A. Intravenous injection of methylene blue in man with reference to its toxic symptoms and effect on the electrocardiogram. Am J Med Sci 1934;188:15–21.

Nkhoma ET, Poole C, Vannappagari V, Hall SA, Beutler E. The global prevalence of glucose-6-phosphate dehydrogenase deficiency: a systematic review and meta-analysis. Blood Cells Mol Dis 2009;42:267–78.

Noor M, Beutler E. Acquired sulfhemoglobinemia. An underreported diagnosis? West J Med 1998;169:386–9.

Perry PM, Meinhard E. Necrotic subcutaneous abscesses following injections of methylene blue. Br J Clin Pract 1974;28:289–91.

Prischl FC, Hofinger I, Kramar R. Fever, shivering…and blue urine. Nephrol Dial Transplant 1999;14:2245–6.

Provayblue. Methylene blue package insert. Shriley, NY: American Regent; 2019.

Raimer, Sharon S, Quevedo EM, Johnston RV. Dye rashes. Cutis 1999;63(2):103–7.

Ramsay RR, Dunford C, Gillman PK. Methylene blue and serotonin toxicity: inhibition of monoamine oxidase a (MAO A) confirms a theoretical prediction. Br J Pharmacol 2007;152:946–51.

Rehman A, Shehadeh M, Khirfan D, Jones A. Severe acute haemolytic anaemia associated with severe methaemoglobinaemia in a G6PD-deficient man. BMJ Case Rep 2018. bcr2017223369.

Reynolds PM, MacLaren R, Mueller SW, Fish DN, Kiser TH. Management of extravasation injuries: a focused evaluation of noncytotoxic medications. Pharmacotherapy 2014;34:617–32.

Rosen PJ, Johnson C, McGehee WG, Beutler E. Failure of methylene blue treatment in toxic methemoglobinemia. Association with glucose-6-phosphate dehydrogenase deficiency. Ann Intern Med 1971;75:83–6.

Sass MD, Caruso CJ, Axelrod DR. Accumulation of methylene blue by metabolizing erythrocytes. J Lab Clin Med 1967;69:447–55.

Scheindlin S. Something old…something blue. Mol Interv 2008;8:268–73.

Schirmer RH, Adler H, Pickhardt M, Mandelkow E. Lest we forget you—methylene blue…. Neurobiol Aging 2011;32:2325.e7.

Schwiebert C, Irving C, Gillman PK. Small doses of methylene blue, previously considered safe, can precipitate serotonin toxicity. Anaesthesia 2009;64:924.

Shen WW. A history of antipsychotic drug development. Compr Psychiatry 1999;40:407–14.

Shopes E, Gerard W, Baughman J. Methylene blue encephalopathy: a case report and review of published cases. AANA J 2013;81:215–21.

Smith RP, Layne WR. A comparison of the lethal effects of nitrite and hydroxylamine in the mouse. J Pharmacol Exp Ther 1969;165:30–5.

Smith RP, Thron CD. Hemoglobin, methylene blue and oxygen interactions in human red cells. J Pharmacol Exp Ther 1972;183:549–58.

Smith MT, McHale CM. Toxic responses of the blood. In: Klaassen CD, editor. Casarett and Doull's toxicology: the basic science of poisons. 9th ed. NY: McGraw-Hill Education; 2019 [Chapter 11].

Stanford SC, Stanford BJ, Gillman PK. Risk of severe serotonin toxicity following co-administration of methylene blue and serotonin reuptake inhibitors: an update on a case report of post-operative delirium. J Psychopharmacol 2010;24:1433–8.

Steele CW, Spink WW. Methylene blue in the treatment of poisonings associated with methemoglobinemia. N Engl J Med 1933;208:1152–3.

Stossel TP, Jennings RB. Failure of methylene blue to produce methemoglobinemia in vivo. Am J Clin Pathol 1966;45:600–4.

Sweet G, Standiford SB. Methylene-blue-associated encephalopathy. J Am Coll Surg 2007;204:454–8.

Tomoda A, Ida M, Tsuji A, Yoneyama Y. Mechanism of methaemoglobin reduction by human erythrocytes. Biochem J 1980;188:535–40.

Top WM, Gillman PK, de Langen CJ, Kooy A. Fatal methylene blue associated serotonin toxicity. Neth J Med 2014;72:179–81.

Tucker D, Lu Y, Zhang Q. From mitochondrial function to neuroprotection—an emerging role for methylene blue. Mol Neurobiol 2018;55:5137–53.

van der Vorst JR, Schaafsma BE, Verbeek FP, et al. Intraoperative near-infrared fluorescence imaging of parathyroid adenomas with use of low-dose methylene blue. Head Neck 2014;36(6):853–8.

Wendel WB. Oxidations by erythrocytes and the catalytic influence of methylene blue part 1—the oxidation of lactate to pyruvate and part 2—methemoglobin and the effect of cyanide. J Biol Chem 1933;102:373–83. 373-401.

Wendel WB. The mechanism of the antidotal action of methylene blue in cyanide poisoning. Science 1934;80:381–2.

Wendel WB. Methylene blue, methemoglobin and cyanide poisoning. J Pharmacol Exp Ther 1935;54:283–98.

Wendel WB. Use of methylene blue in methemoglobinemia from sulfanilamide poisoning. JAMA 1937;109:1216.

Wendel WB. The control of methemoglobinemia with methylene blue. J Clin Invest 1939;18:179–85.

Whitwam JG, Taylor AR, White JM. Potential hazard of methylene blue. Anaesthesia 1979;34:181–2.

Wiklund L, Basu S, Miclescu A, Wiklund P, Ronquist G, Sharma HS. Neuro- and cardioprotective effects of blockade of nitric oxide action by administration of methylene blue. Ann N Y Acad Sci 2007;1122:231–44.

Williams JR, Challis FE. Methylene blue as an antidote for aniline dye. J Lab Clin Med 1933;19:166–71.

Wilson JG. Intra vitam staining with methylene blue. Anat Rec 1910;4:267–77.

World Health Organization (WHO), https://apps.who.int/iris/bitstream/handle/10665/325771/WHO-MVP-EMP-IAU-2019.06-eng.pdf?ua=1; 2020. [Accessed 15 August 2020].

Wuertz RL, Frazee Jr WH, Hume WG, et al. Chemical cyanosis-anemia syndrome. Diagnosis, treatment, and recovery. Arch Environ Health 1964;9:478–91.

Zirkle CL. To tranquilizers and antidepressants from antimalarials and antihistamines chapter 5 in how modern medicines are discovered. Mt Kisco, NY: Futura; 1973. p. 55–77.

Chapter 3.4

British anti-lewisite (dimercaprol)

Marissa Hauptman and Alan D. Woolf
Boston Children's Hospital & Harvard Medical School, Boston, Massachusetts, United States

Discovery

British anti-lewisite (BAL, dimercaprol, 2,3-dimercaptopropanol, 2,3-dithiolpropanol, 2,3-dimercaptopropan-1-ol) is a metal-chelating agent with a rich history of discovery dating back 100 years. BAL was the first chelating agent to be used in clinical medicine. The fact that it is still in use today as a therapeutic agent is a testament to its enduring scientific legacy in the annals of the history of clinical toxicology research and discovery.

Lewisite

World War I (WWI) saw the introduction of chemical weapons, such as mustard gas, phosgene, and chlorine, to the battlefields of Europe by the German military (Fig. 3.4.1). Thousands of troops were disabled or killed by toxic effects of these gases by inhalation and/or dermal, conjunctival, or mucous membrane exposures. The chlorination of arsenoxides led to a dangerous new agent, lewisite. The discovery of lewisite can be traced to a dissertation thesis by a chemistry doctoral student, Father Julius Arthur Nieuwland, working in the chemistry laboratories at Catholic University of America in Washington, DC, in 1904 (Vilensky and Redman, 2003). He was reacting different substances with acetylene gas in 1903 and happened upon its mixture with arsenic trichloride in the presence of aluminum chloride, leading to the synthesis of 2-chlorovinyldichloroarsine ($ClCH=CHAsCl_2$), now known as lewisite. When mixed with water, it delivered a noxious odor and turned the flask black. Inhaled vapors from this new synthetic compound were so toxic as to hospitalize Father Nieuwland for a few days; he subsequently abandoned the compound because of this intense toxicity (Vilensky and Sinish, 2005).

History of Modern Clinical Toxicology. https://doi.org/10.1016/B978-0-12-822218-8.00050-8

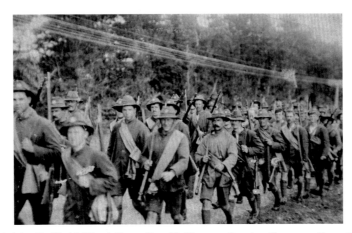

FIG. 3.4.1 "A World War 1 Story, Part 5" *(Source: Creative Commons (https://search. creativecommons.org/photos/bec59ec5-2150-4fa0-8eca-259e0cbdf77e).) Credit: InMemoriam:Phillip Capper licensed under CC by 4.0*

As a trivalent arsenic-derived compound, lewisite exerted its toxicity by binding sulfhydryl groups and disrupting sulfhydryl-dependent enzymatic systems (Oehme, 1972); lewisite also acted through its toxic breakdown products: arsine oxide and hydrochloric acid. As a potent vesicating and inflammatory agent, its vapors were capable of causing extensive, painful blistering of the skin and mucous membranes (Li et al., 2016) and destroying sensitive eye tissues, causing blindness (Tewari-Singh et al., 2016). It is lipophilic and rapidly absorbed through skin, leading to systemic hypovolemia from vascular leaks and death from "lewisite shock." Lewisite inhalation results in extensive damage to lungs, with impaired oxygenation and disrupted pulmonary function.

Although Nieuwland's dissertation was published, the new chemical was forgotten until rediscovered by Captain Winford Lee Lewis, a chemist who directed a chemical warfare research laboratory at the same university in the latter days of WWI. Father Nieuwland's former thesis advisor, Rev. John Griffin, mentioned the publication to Captain Lewis. He read the dissertation and proposed the manufacture of the chemical, now renamed "lewisite" (Vilensky and Sinish, 2005). It was produced in large quantities in a secret Ohio laboratory. In fact, it was said that 150 tons of lewisite, also known as the "dew of death," were on-board a ship headed for Europe when the war ended (the vessel was sunk after the war) (Vilensky and Redman, 2003). Fortunately, the WWI armistice in 1918 prevented the intended deployment of lewisite as a weapon. However, after the war, many of the major nations began to manufacture weapons-grade lewisite.

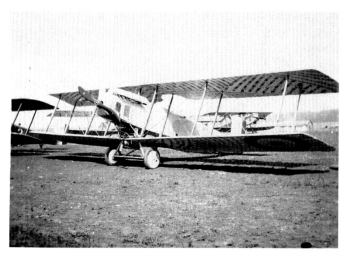

FIG. 3.4.2 Dorand AR1 French World War 1 reconnaissance biplane. *Source: Wikimedia Commons: https://commons.wikimedia.org/w/index.php?search=World+War+1+biplane&title= Special:MediaSearch&go=Go&type=image Author: San Diego Air & Space Museum archives*

Discovery of British anti-lewisite

Lewisite could be dropped by planes over enemy soldiers as explosive bombs containing the chemical which would subsequently be dispersed in an explosion as a vapor, aerosol, or liquid (Fig. 3.4.2). The possible stockpiling of lewisite as a chemical weapon more lethal than mustard gas was worrisome to the British. In anticipation of the use of weaponized lewisite in World War II, the British government, specifically the Ministry of Supply, commissioned scientists in the Department of Biochemistry at Oxford University to develop an effective antidote to the arsenic-based gas. As noted previously, the toxicity of arsenical compounds correlated with their binding to sulfhydryl groups of cellular enzymes, inactivating them. Monothiol compounds had previously been well-studied but found to be ineffective in the treatment of arsenic toxicity. Some sulfhydryl donors, such as glutathione or cysteine, could delay or partially protect, but not entirely reverse arsenic's effects. For example, even when present in excess amounts, monothiols could not prevent the toxic effects of arsenic on the brain's pyruvate dehydrogenase enzyme system (Oehme, 1972). A breakthrough moment came while those researchers were investigating the binding of arsenic to keratein—a reduced, dithiol-containing form of the compound, keratin, found in hair that they had obtained from nearby barber shops (Eagle et al., 1946; Vilensky and Redman, 2003). Arsenic formed stable bonds with keratein at two thiol sites—which the metal could not do with monothiol-containing compounds. Thus these researchers tested various dithiol-containing chemicals to see which might have the properties necessary for a therapeutic agent to be used in humans. Such chemicals should be of small molecular size, able to penetrate skin quickly, and form a stable and permanent 5-member or 6-member ring with arsenic (Oehme, 1972).

Development

On July 21, 1940, L.A. Thompson and R.A. Stocken under the direction of Sir Rudolph Peters, produced results, with the discovery of 2,3-dithiolpropanol (or 2,3-dimercaptopropanol) or dimercaprol (Peters et al., 1945; Vilensky and Redman, 2003). Heralded as an answer to lewisite, hence informally named by the Americans as "British anti-lewisite" or BAL, it was intended solely for military purposes. Original work was carried out to demonstrate its effectiveness in reversing lewisite toxicity. BAL was shown by Peters and his colleagues, Stocken and Thompson, to protect cellular pyruvate dehydrogenase (known in the 1940s as pyruvate oxidase) enzyme systems from arsenite and lewisite (Stocken and Thompson, 1946a, b). Although the experiments initially involved dermal exposure studies in rats and guinea pigs, human volunteer experiments were subsequently also carried out. The forearm skin was burned with lewisite and then BAL was used in an attempt to reverse the damage (Stocken and Thompson, 1946a, b). While the original discovery came from British scientists, including Stocken and Thompson, working in Peters' laboratory, the results were confirmed by scientists in America (Waters and Stock, 1945).

BAL was not water-soluble and was incompatible with vehicles like propylene glycol. However, studies found that it could be easily dissolved in peanut oil with benzyl benzoate as a stabilizer. This mixture could be sterilized in glass ampoules and given parenterally by deep muscular injection in patient care; an acceptable dose range of about 2.5–3.0 mg/kg given every 4 h was established (Eagle and Magnuson, 1946). BAL was successful in preventing skin vesiculation in humans when given as late as an hour after lewisite contamination. Hughes (1946) demonstrated BAL's ability to reverse injury to the eye in a rabbit model when applied shortly after lewisite exposure. Others confirmed that BAL was stable in peanut oil and, when given parenterally, was successful in reversing systemic toxicity and lowering mortality rates in arsenic-dosed animals (Stocken and Thompson, 1946a, b; Eagle et al., 1946). The research group at Johns Hopkins Hospital in Baltimore extended their studies of BAL as an antidote for arsenic exposure to humans (Eagle and Magnuson, 1946; Wexler et al., 1946). BAL's local and systemic toxicity in humans, and its ability to inhibit certain enzyme systems in experimental studies, were also recognized early on as unwanted contributors to its adverse effects profile (Eagle and Magnuson, 1946; Stocken and Thompson, 1946a, b; Peters et al., 1947; Webb and Van Heyningen, 1947). The human studies of BAL also took note of its associated adverse reactions. By 1947, there were more than 30 published articles by these and other investigators reporting the results of studies of the effects of BAL on heavy metals poisoning. All these studies confirmed BAL's clinical utility at achievable doses in human arsenic poisoning. The use of BAL was now incorporated into instructions on how to treat victims of lewisite poisoning in the event of a military attack (Chiesman, 1944).

Originally, stocks of BAL were manufactured by, and only available in Britain through the Ministry of Supply. Distribution was strictly controlled by application to the British Medical Research Council. Plans for the military use of BAL as an antidote included its bulk manufacture, up to 200,000 pounds per year, by the DuPont Chemical Company in the United States (Vilensky and Redman, 2003). However, it was fortunately never needed since the war was already drawing to a close.

BAL: Other uses

However, soon its therapeutic value for other medical conditions outside of its original military use became apparent to scientists and clinicians. Thompson and Whittaker (1947) described its value as an antidote for the toxic effects of gold, antimony, and mercury in an experimental pyruvate oxidase system in pigeon brain tissue. Stocken demonstrated its effectiveness in reducing mortality in rats poisoned with mercuric chloride given either orally or via parenteral routes (Stocken, 1947). In other animal studies, Graham and Hood (1948) showed that BAL had protective effects in animals (rats, mice, guinea pigs, and rabbits) poisoned with arsenic, mercury, antimony, and chromium, but a toxic effect on those poisoned with lead, gold, or bismuth. Rabbits poisoned with arsenic had rapid reversal of its toxic effects when given BAL (Eagle et al., 1946).

Arseno-therapy had been used for decades to treat a number of bacterial and parasitic infections, including syphilis. However, a range of toxic side-effects complicated arsenical antisyphilitic therapy, including a severe exfoliative dermatitis. Peters et al. (1947) documented the effectiveness of BAL in treating 44 patients suffering from arsenic therapy-related dermatitis, although they noted local abscess formation as an infective complication in some cases. Luetscher et al. (1946) demonstrated BAL's ability to produce an arsenic diuresis in 18 patients treated with arsenicals, 16 of whom were suffering from arsenical dermatitis. Clinicians in the United States also reported success in treating patients suffering from arsenic-related encephalopathy. A 1949 report described a man suffering from side-effects from the use of bismuth and arsenic to treat his syphilis (Reeke, 1949). A 5% BAL solution seemed to improve his bismuth toxicity-related stomatitis almost immediately on application.

Wilson's Disease (also known as hepatolenticular degeneration) was named after Samuel Alexander Kinnier Wilson who, in 1912, described it as a uniformly fatal, familial disease involving neurological dysfunction (a progressive movement disorder and lenticular degeneration) and cirrhosis (Wilson, 1912). Its pathogenesis was later determined to be excessive copper deposition in the brain, eyes, and liver associated with genetic defects in copper metabolism (Cumings, 1948). In 1949, the neurologist, Huntington Porter, observed an improvement of neurological functioning of two patients with Wilson's Disease after administration of BAL. In 1951, Drs. Denny-Brown and Porter in the United States and Cumings in Britain reported that BAL successfully and dramatically improved the movement disorder in patients suffering from Wilson's Disease, with increased copper excretion in the urine (Denny-Brown and Porter, 1951a, b; Cumings, 1951). This was held to be a significant advance in the field, moving neurology from a mostly palliative, descriptive subspecialty, to one with curative possibilities. Five years later, John M. Walshe demonstrated the efficacy of a much less toxic compound, D-penicillamine (dimethylcysteine), in the treatment of Wilson's Disease (Walshe, 1956). Subsequently, D-penicillamine and other newer, effective copper-chelating oral agents have largely supplanted the use of BAL (Aggarwal and Bhatt, 2018).

Inorganic mercury compounds were used as antiseptic agents in the 1900s. One such mercuric chloride product, sold as "corrosive sublimate" in pill form, was commonly used to commit suicide in the 1920–40s (Kosnett, 2013). Investigators Longcope and Luetscher (1949) reported a case series of no deaths among 42 mercuric chloride (≥ 1 g) poisoned patients treated with BAL within 4 h of ingestion, as opposed to a case fatality rate of 31.4% in comparable, historical controls.

BAL was also reported to be a successful treatment for children suffering from acute arsenic ingestion. Woody and Kometani (1948) reported its use in a case series of 42 children aged 6 months to 10 years. Childhood arsenic poisoning was common, since it was often used in an insecticide syrup (particularly as an ant poison) in the home. The authors also described frequent, dose-related adverse effects of BAL, including hypertension, convulsions, and coma in children receiving the highest doses of 25 mg/kg or more.

Later on, BAL was found to be effective in reducing blood lead levels while promoting a urinary lead diuresis in both children and adults with acute lead poisoning. With the introduction of BAL chelation alone or combined with calcium disodium ethylenediamine tetra-acetic acid (CaNa2EDTA) therapy in children suffering with severe lead encephalopathy, their case-fatality rate was cut in half (Chisholm, 1970).

Recent history

BAL was made available for use in everyday medical practice in the late 1940s and early 1950s. Dimercaprol is still used, although uncommonly, as an antidote for severe childhood lead poisoning and poisonings from other metals, such as acute or chronic elemental mercury, acute inorganic mercury or arsenic (Kosnett, 2013). It has been FDA-approved since 1946 for the treatment of acute arsenic, gold, and mercury poisoning, and it is indicated in life-threatening lead poisoning when used concomitantly with CaNa2EDTA (FDA, 2006). It is of questionable value in poisoning from other heavy metals such as bismuth or antimony. It is still recognized as an important antidote to be stockpiled in case of chemical warfare. Dimercaprol is ineffective in poisoning from other metals, including thallium, tellurium or vanadium, and organic lead (e.g., tetraethyl lead). It should not be used in iron, cadmium, or selenium poisoning because the resulting dimercaprol-metal complexes are more toxic than the metal alone, especially to the kidneys. Dimercaprol is included on the 2019 World Health Organization's List of Essential Medicines (WHO, 2019). Currently the antidote is marketed by Akorn Pharmaceuticals as sterile BAL in Oil Injection USP in 3 mL (100 mg/mL) single-use ampoules. Each 1 mL contains 100 mg dimercaprol in 700 mg peanut oil and 200 mg benzyl benzoate (Akorn Pharmaceuticals, 2016).

Mechanism of action

This antidote works as a chelating chemical, with its sulfhydryl groups forming a heterocyclic ring with a heavy metal, which is then excreted through the kidneys (Fig. 3.4.3). When two molecules of BAL bind with a metal ion, a 5-member heterocyclic ring is formed, which is a very stable configuration. By tightly binding with a metal ion that has higher affinity for BAL than for the enzyme's sulfhydryl group, BAL removes it from tissue ligands where it can exert its interference with enzyme systems and other subcellular functions to cause its toxic effects. The BAL-metal complex is then excreted in urine, lowering the body burden of the toxic metal. Lipoic acid, a dithiol, is an essential cofactor for functional subcellular enzyme systems: succinoxidase and pyruvate dehydrogenase systems. Substitution of a metal, such as lead, renders the enzyme system nonfunctional. BAL, by attracting the lead to form a stable mercaptide ring, pulls it off the enzyme and returns lipoic acid to its role as cofactor.

Toxicology

BAL is readily absorbed from intramuscular injection and reaches peak blood levels in about 30–60 min. It is lipophilic and is distributed into intracellular spaces in many body systems, including the brain, with highest concentrations in the liver and kidneys. The dithiol-metal complex is then excreted into urine within a few hours in patients with normal renal function. However, BAL in therapeutic concentrations also can redistribute some metals to the brain (Kosnett, 2013). Because of this, dimercaprol is considered contraindicated in chronic inorganic and organic mercury exposure (Bjorklund et al., 2019; Dawn and Whited, 2020). Berlin and Rylander (1964) reported chronic exposure to organic (aryl- or alkyl-) mercury with dimercaprol therapy doubles the amount

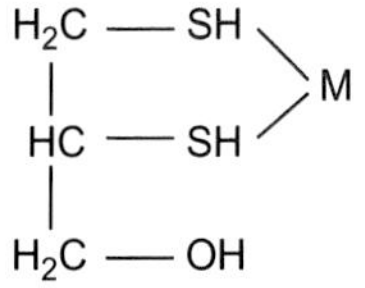

FIG. 3.4.3 Chemical structure of dimercaprol, where "M" is a metal being chelated.

of mercury deposited in the brain compared with animals only receiving mercury. Therefore, an alternative oral chelator, such as dimercaptosuccinic acid (succimer), which does not redistribute arsenic or mercury to the brain, may be a better agent in these cases (Kosnett, 2013).

Contraindications

The commercial preparation of BAL uses peanut oil as a miscible vehicle. Thus patients who are allergic to peanuts should not be given the drug. Dimercaprol should be used cautiously in patients who are dehydrated or oliguric or those who have underlying hypertension. It may be contraindicated in patients who are in renal failure or who manifest hepatotoxicity. It is also contraindicated for use in patients known to have continuing exposure to the metal of concern. The adverse effects of BAL in pregnancy are not well understood; it is not recommended for use in pregnancy unless absolutely necessary. It is unknown if BAL is excreted in breast milk. BAL is ineffective in patients suffering from selenium, iron, or cadmium poisoning, as the complexes formed are themselves nephrotoxic (Akorn Pharmaceuticals, 2016). It is also ineffective in patients suffering from argyria or thallium, uranium, tellurium, or vanadium poisoning.

Adverse side-effects

Dimercaprol is a parenteral antidote; it must be delivered by deep intramuscular injection. There are both local and systemic side-effects that occur in up to half of treated patients (as many as two-thirds of patients at higher doses). Common local reactions include warmth, redness, and pain at the site of injection (see Table 3.4.1). Occasionally, hematomas and painful sterile abscesses may form. Patients may report sweating or burning of the face, throat, lips, or other parts of the body (Akorn Pharmaceuticals, 2016). BAL also is associated with a rapid increase in blood pressure and both tachycardia and tachypnea, which are dose-related. Lacrimation, blepharospasm, and headache are other reported adverse effects. Since the chelant dissociates in an acidic environment, the urine must be kept alkaline during metals diuresis to prevent its nephrotoxicity (Akorn Pharmaceuticals, 2016). Nausea and vomiting are relatively common side-effects of BAL administration. BAL use in children can cause fever or leukopenia. Patients who are given an overdose of BAL may experience seizures and stupor or lapse into coma. Iron therapy needs to be discontinued because dimercaprol and iron form a complex that causes vomiting. Adequate patient hydration and good urine flow during chelation therapy with dimercaprol are of paramount importance, given its risk of renal toxicity.

Place in modern therapeutics

BAL has been used in the recent past in the treatment of acute poisoning by the inorganic salts of arsenic, gold, and mercury (Table 3.4.1). It is ineffective in the

TABLE 3.4.1 Summary of clinical uses and known toxicity of dimercaprol (BAL).

Agent	Approved use	Toxicity
British anti-lewisite (BAL [2,3-dimercatopropanol])	• Only given parenterally (deep intramuscular) • Arsenic, gold, mercury, acute lead poisoning (when used concomitantly with calcium disodium edetate)	•Toxicities are dose dependent and doses require small fractional dosages in pediatric population • Contraindicated in children allergic to nuts (as medication dissolved in peanut oil) • Contraindicated in children with glucose-6-phosphatae deficiency as can lead to hemolysis in this patient population • Can cause nausea, emesis, fever, rashes, significant hypertension/tachycardia; headache; burning sensation in lips, mouth, throat; feeling of throat, chest, or hand constriction; transient decline in percent polymorphonuclear leukocyte count •Can cause liver and kidney dysfunction or zinc deficiency •Can cause pain or sterile abscesses at the injection site •Children often develop fever, which abates with cessation of treatment

treatment of poisoning by arsine gas and has largely been replaced by less toxic agents now used as primary therapy in patients with Wilson's Disease. Other challenges with the use of BAL, in addition to its requirement for parenteral administration, its contraindications, and its toxic side-effects, include its own liver and kidney toxicity, its limited availability, and its rising cost (Heindel et al., 2017).

While BAL still is uncommonly used in children with life-threatening, severe lead poisoning who have developed seizures or encephalopathy, other chelating agents are preferable in most patients. US poison control centers only recorded

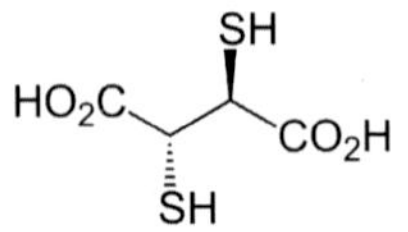

FIG. 3.4.4 Chemical structure of meso-dimercaptosuccinic acid.

18 cases in which BAL had been used in the treatment of acute poisonings in 2017 (Gummin et al., 2018), although that is likely an underestimate since physicians treating hospitalized patients may not notify a poison control center.

A congener of dimercaprol, dimercaptosuccinic acid (succimer) was approved in 1991 by the FDA under the trade name, Chemet as an oral chelating agent. It is hydrophilic and is used as a first-line therapeutic agent in the treatment of lead, mercury, and certain other poisonings with heavy metals. Succimer has a higher therapeutic index than BAL, is associated with fewer adverse effects, and so has largely replaced BAL in the management of metals-poisoned patients (Kosnett, 2013) (Fig. 3.4.4).

References

Aggarwal A, Bhatt M. Advances in treatment of Wilson disease. Tremor Other Hyperkinetic Mov 2018. https://doi.org/10.7916/D841881D.

Akorn Pharmaceuticals. BAL package insert, https://www.akorn.com/prod_detail. php?ndc=17478-526-03; 2016. [Accessed 9 October 2020].

Berlin M, Rylander R. Increased brain uptake of mercury induced by 2,3-dimercaptopropanol (BAL) in mice exposed to phenylmercuric acetate. J Pharmacol Exp Ther 1964;146:236–40.

Bjorklund G, Crispani G, Murchi VM, Cappai R, Djordjevic AB, Aaseth J. A review of coordination properties of thiol-containing chelating agents towards mercury, cadmium, and leas. Molecules 2019;24:3247. https://doi.org/10.3390/molecules24183247.

Chiesman WE. Diagnosis and treatment of lesions due to vesicants. Br Med J 1944;2(4359):109–12.

Chisholm JJ. Treatment of acute lead intoxication—choice of chelating agents and supportive measures. Clin Toxicol 1970;3(4):527–40.

Cumings JN. The copper and iron content of brain and liver in the normal and in hepato-lenticular degeneration. Brain 1948;71:410–5.

Cumings JN. The effects of B.A.L. in hepatolenticular degeneration. Brain 1951;74:10–22.

Dawn L, Whited L. Dimercaprol. Treasure Island, FL: StatPearls Publishing; 2020. Available from: https://www.ncbi.nlm.nih.gov/books/NBK549804/. [Accessed 11 November 2020].

Denny-Brown D, Porter H. The effect of BAL (2,3-dimercaptopropanol) on hepatolenticular disease (Wilson's disease). N Engl J Med 1951a;245:917–25.

Denny-Brown D, Porter H. The effect of BAL (2,3-dimercaptopropanol) on hepatolenticular degeneration (Wilson's disease). Trans Am Neurol Assoc 1951b;56:79–84.

Eagle H, Magnuson HJ. The systemic treatment of 227 cases of arsenic poisoning (encephalitis, dermatitis, blood dyscrasias, jaundice, fever) with 2,3-dimercaprol (BAL). Am J Syph Gonorrhea Vener Dis 1946;30:420–41.

Eagle H, Magnuson HJ, Fleischman R. Clinical uses of 2,3-dimercaptopropanol (BAL). I. the systemic treatment of experimental arsenic poisoning (mapharsen, lewisite, phernyl arsenoxide) with BAL. J Clin Invest 1946;25(4):451–66.

Food and Drug Administration. BAL in oil ampules: dimercaprol injection, USP. Food and Drug Administration; 2006. Available from: https://www.accessdata.fda.gov/drugsatfda_docs/label/2007/005939s007lbl.pdf. [Accessed 11 November 2020].

Graham JDP, Hood J. Actions of British anti-lewisite (2,3-dimercaptopropanol). Br J Pharmacol 1948;3:84–90.

Gummin DG, Mowry JB, Spyker DA, Brooks DE, Osterhaler KM, Banner W. 2017 annual report of the American Association of Poison Control Centers' National Poison Data System (NPDS): 35th annual report. Clin Toxicol 2018;56(12):1213–415.

Heindel GA, Trella JD, Osterhoudt KC. Rising cost of antidotes in the U.S.: cost comparison from 2010 to 2015. Clin Toxicol 2017;55(5):360–3.

Hughes WF. Clinical uses of 2,3-dimercaptopropanol (BAL). IX. The treatment of lewisite burns of the eye with BAL. J Clin Invest 1946;25(4):541–8.

Kosnett MJ. The role of chelation in the treatment of arsenic and mercury poisoning. J Med Toxicol 2013;9:347–54.

Li C, Srivastava RK, Weng Z, Croutch CR, Agarwal A, Elmets CA, et al. Molecular mechanism underlying pathogenesis of Lewisite-induced cutaneous blistering and inflammation. Am J Pathol 2016;186(10):2637–49.

Longcope WT, Luetscher J. The use of BAL (British anti-lewisite) in the treatment of the injurious effects of arsenic, mercury, and other metallic poisons. Ann Intern Med 1949;31:545–53.

Luetscher JA, Eagle H, Longcope WT, Watson EB. Clinical uses of 2,3 dimercaptopropanol (BAL). VIII. The effect of BAL on the excretion of arsenic in arsenical intoxication. J Clin Invest 1946;25(4):534–40.

Oehme FW. British anti-lewisite (BAL), the classic heavy metal antidote. Clin Toxicol 1972;51(5):215–22.

Peters RA, Stocken LA, Thompson RHS. British anti-lewisite (BAL). Nature 1945;156:616–9.

Peters RA, Bennet J, King AJ, Carleton AB, Dixon M, Cameron GR, et al. British anti-lewisite—a report on its use and therapeutic value in arsenical intoxications from the BAL research conference, Medical Research Council. Br Med J 1947;520–1.

Reeke AAM. Treatment of bismuth stomatitis with BAL (British anti-lewisite). Br Med J 1949;1213.

Stocken LA. British anti-lewisite as an antidote for acute mercury poisoning. Br Med J 1947;358–60.

Stocken LA, Thompson RHS. British anti-lewisite. Br Med J 1946a;40:535–48.

Stocken LA, Thompson RHS. British anti-lewisite. Dithiol compounds as antidotes for arsenic. Biochem J 1946b;40:535–48.

Tewari-Singh N, Croutch CR, Tuttle R, Goswami DG, Kent R, Peters E, et al. Clinical progression of ocular injury following arsenical vesicant lewisite exposure. Cutan Ocul Toxicol 2016;35(4):319–28.

Thompson RHS, Whittaker VP. Antidotal activity of British anti-lewisite against compounds of antimony, gold, and mercury. Br Med J 1947;342–6.

Vilensky JA, Redman K. British anti-lewisite (Dimercaprol): an amazing history. Ann Emerg Med 2003;41:378–83.

Vilensky JA, Sinish PR. Weaponry: lewisite—America's World War 1 chemical weapon. MHQ Spring. https://www.historynet.com/weaponry-lewisite-americas-world-war-i-chemical-weapon.htm; 2005.

Walshe JM. Penicillamine, a new oral therapy for Wilson's disease. Am J Med 1956;21(4):487–95.

Waters LL, Stock C. BAL (British anti-lewisite). Science 1945;102:601.

Webb EC, Van Heyningen R. The action of British anti-lewisite (BAL) on enzyme systems. Br Med J 1947;74–8.

Wexler J, Eagle H, Tatum HJ, Magnuson HJ, Watson EB. Clinical uses of 2,3-dimercaptopropanol (BAL). II. The effect of BAL on the excretion of arsenic in normal subjects and after minimal exposure to arsenical smoke. J Clin Invest 1946;25(4):467–73.

Wilson RAK. Progressive lenticular degeneration—a familial nervous disease associated with cirrhosis of the liver. Brain 1912;34:295–509. https://doi.org/10.1093/brain/34.4.295.

Woody NC, Kometani JT. BAL in the treatment of arsenic ingestion of children. Pediatrics 1948;1(3):372–8.

World Health Organization (WHO). Model list of essential medicines. 21st list 2019. WHO-MVP-EMP-IAU-2019.06-eng   https://www.google.com/search?source=hp&ei=JFStX9HPCejm_QaVzomgC Q&q=who+list+of+essential+medicines&gs_ssp=eJzj4tLP1TeoKs8qTrE0YPSSL8_IV8jJLC5 RyE9TSC0uTs0ryUzMUchNTclMzsxLLQYAWw8P7Q&oq=WHO+List+of+&gs_lcp=CgZw-c3ktYWIQARgAMggILhDJAxCTAjICCAAyAggAMgIIADICCAAyAggAMgIIADICCAAyAgg AMgIIADoICAAQsQMQgwE6DgguELEDEIMBEMcBEKMCOgUIABCxAzoLCC4QsQMQx-wEQowI6AgguOg4ILhCxAxDHARCjAhCTAjoECAAQAzoICC4QxwEQrwE6EAgAELEDE-IMBEMkDEEYQ-wE6BQgAEMkDUNQLWN49YPBbaABwAHgAgAFRiAG6BpIBAjEymAE AoAEBqgEHZ3dzLXdpeg&sclient=psy-ab; 2019. [Accessed 12 November 2020].

Chapter 3.5

Pralidoxime and oximes

Alexander F. Barbuto[a] and Michele M. Burns[b]

[a]*Department of Emergency Medicine, Carl R. Darnall Army Medical Center, Ft. Hood, TX, United States,* [b]*Harvard Medical Toxicology Fellowship/Division of Emergency Medicine, Boston Children's Hospital, Boston, MA, United States*

Background

Introduction

Oximes are a class of medications that are used to treat organophosphate nerve agent poisonings. They work by rescuing acetylcholinesterase (AChE), the critical enzyme inhibited by organophosphates. First developed in 1955, they are now stockpiled by public health agencies and militaries around the globe, ready for use in the event of a nerve agent incident.

Origins: Nerve agents

In 1936, tabun, the first of the deadly chemical weapons known as organophosphate nerve agents, was produced in Germany. Shortly thereafter, German chemists developed soman, sarin, and cyclosarin (often referred to as the G-series of nerve agents). British chemists developed the V-series: VG, VE, VM, and VX in the 1950s, and a Russian program developed the novichok agents between the 1970s and 1990s (Chai et al., 2018). Although nerve agents were not used in warfare until the Iran-Iraq war in 1988, the observed lethality of these nerve agents in accidents and in animal studies prompted the need for rapid development of antidotal treatments in the 1950s. In 1955, scientists would publish their findings on the first of these antidotes, pralidoxime.

Mechanism of action: Nerve agents

Nerve agents work by interfering with a key enzyme of the nervous system, AChE. AChE, which is found at junctions between neurons and at the neuromuscular junction (NMJ), degrades the neurotransmitter acetylcholine.

History of Modern Clinical Toxicology. https://doi.org/10.1016/B978-0-12-822218-8.00030-2

After acetylcholine binds to receptors on the postsynaptic cell and initiates an action potential, this synapse must "reset," and AChE serves to degrade acetylcholine and thereby prevent repetitive signal generation.

When nerve agents inhibit AChE, acetylcholine builds up at these nerve junctions, and causes an array of symptoms due to uncontrolled activity at two types of receptors: muscarinic and nicotinic. Activity at the muscarinic receptors causes increased secretions from the eyes, mouth, lungs, and gastrointestinal tract, and slows heart rates. Nicotinic receptors are located at the NMJ and the central nervous system. Uncontrolled activity at the NMJ affects the muscles, ranging from twitching to weakness to frank paralysis by depolarization blockade. The combination of muscle weakness and secretions in the lungs ultimately leads to ineffective respiration, hypoxia, and, potentially, death. This entire process can happen within minutes. While atropine, a muscarinic antagonist, is an effective treatment for excess acetylcholine at muscarinic receptors, it has no ability to treat overstimulation of nicotinic receptors. Another antidote would be needed to treat organophosphate poisoning at this second group of receptors.

Nerve agent aging

Interestingly, in medical practice we use medications that inhibit AChE in treating conditions like myasthenia gravis. These medications, such as the carbamate pyridostigmine, are reversible AChE inhibitors, meaning they intermittently block its activity. (see Chapter 3.7 Physostigmine for additional information about AChE inhibitors). However, nerve agents become irreversible inhibitors if given sufficient time.

When a nerve agent reaches AChE's active site, a bond forms between the enzyme and the phosphoryl moiety of the nerve agent. The nerve agent then deposits a substituted-phosphoryl group on this site, rendering the enzyme inactive. This early agent-enzyme complex is reversible. However, over time, an alkyl side-chain of the substituted-phosphoryl moiety can be nonenzymatically lost. When this happens, the bond between the enzyme and the phosphoryl moiety strengthens; for all practical purposes the enzyme is now permanently inhibited. This process is called "aging," and each nerve agent takes a different amount of time to age. While VX has an aging half-time of 22 days, tabun's is 14 h, sarin's 3–4 h, and soman ages in 2 min (Barbuto and Chai, 2020).

Hydrolysis is able to remove this substituted-phosphoryl group prior to aging, though by a very slow process. This process is so slow that it is faster for the body to synthesize new AChE than to wait for phosphorylated enzymes to be regenerated. Trials began looking for new chemicals which could remove the phosphoryl group from AChE.

Development of oximes

Nachmansohn lab and operation eel

Governments around the world, but notably in the United States and the United Kingdom were eager to study nerve agent toxicity and antidotal therapy. In the United States, research at New York's Columbia University led the way in developing antidotes. David Nachmansohn, a Russian-born German-Jewish scientist, devoted much of his academic career to studying electrical impulses in nervous tissue and describing the role of acetylcholine in nerve impulse transmission. He looked to natural sources of highly electric creatures, like the marbled electric ray (*Torpedo marmorata*) or the electric eel (*Electrophorus electricus*), as sources rich in AChE on which to experiment (Nachmansohn et al., 1941). Nachmansohn's work on AChE in the 1940s made his laboratory a perfect incubator for scientists who would later go on to develop the oxime organophosphate reactivator, pralidoxime.

Wilson and Ginsburg

Both Irwin B. Wilson and Sara Ginsburg were pivotal leaders in the field of oxime development. Wilson received a B.S. degree in chemistry from the City College of New York in 1941, graduating *cum laude*, and then obtained his PhD in physical chemistry from Columbia University, where Nachmansohn had his laboratory, in 1949. Sara Ginsburg attended the Taganzew School in St. Petersburg, Russia, before fleeing the communists to Germany where she graduated from the Hohenzollern Lyceum in Berlin in 1929. Her PhD in chemistry was obtained at the Friedrich-Wilhems University in Berlin in 1934 where she worked in the laboratory of Professor Peter Rona, who had also taught Nachmansohn (Petroianu, 2012). She then fled Germany through France and Spain, taking a ship to New York where she found employment at Columbia. It was at Columbia's College of Physicians & Surgeons that Wilson and Ginsburg developed and first synthesized 2-pyridine aldoxime methyl chloride, otherwise known as pralidoxime (2-PAM), realizing the importance of this medication to treat warfare gases and insecticide poisonings (Wilson and Ginsburg, 1955).

Operation eel

The Nachmansohn laboratory's in-depth work on nervous system biochemistry made it a natural pick when the Army Chemical Corps required a site for developing top-secret antidotes to nerve agents. A procurement officer asked Dr. Nachmansohn if he needed any special materials for his project. He replied "Yes, please. One hundred electric eels" (Kobler, 1957). Electric eels were, perhaps not surprisingly, hard to come by in the 1950s.

An exposé, "The Terrible Threat of Nerve Gas," published in the Saturday Evening Post in 1957, describes the US government's going to great lengths of hiring, equipping, and funding freelance animal collectors. Contacts through the New York Aquarium and their main supplier of exotic fish led to an expedition through the Brazilian Amazon by a French fisherman, J. Auguste Rabaut. He required passports, re-entry permits, and special flights out of the Amazon, capable of carrying fish tanks full of over 100 electric eels (Kobler, 1957).

From hydroxylamine to pralidoxime

When the eels arrived at the lab at Columbia University, a large supply of AChE became available for ongoing work. Nachmansohn used tetraethylpyrophosphate (TEPP), an organophosphate insecticide, to inhibit the enzyme. Similar to the organophosphate nerve agents, it phosphorylates the serine residue at the enzyme's active site. Wilson's team had already identified that water was capable of hydrolyzing this bond, though too slowly to be clinically useful. Wilson explored other, more strongly nucleophilic reagents, and discovered hydroxylamine could regenerate enzymatic activity of TEPP-inhibited AChE (Wilson, 1951). They noted, importantly, that hydroxylamine could regenerate the enzyme and restore its function, but when doing so, it did not regenerate TEPP itself.

The AChE esteric site has a nearby anionic (electronegatively charged) pocket, and this region would become a helpful tool in designing a faster reactivator. Wilson, Ginsburg, and another partner, Estelle Meislich, created additional molecules combining hydroxylamine with a positively charged quaternary amine, approximately three carbons apart (O'Brien, 1960). Presumably, this anionic site helps to guide the oxime into a proper configuration for nucleophilic attack at the inhibited enzyme. They created nicotinhydroxamic acid (Wilson et al., 1955), nicotinhydroxamic acid methiodide (Wilson and Meislich, 1953), and picolinhydroxamic acid (Wilson and Ginsburg, 1955), before determining what would become the oxime that countries would continue to use 60 years later.

Simultaneous discovery

In 1955, Wilson and Ginsburg announced their discovery of 2-pyridine aldoxime methyl chloride, or pralidoxime, and found it was a potent reactivator, regenerating alkyl phosphate inhibited AChE within minutes (Wilson and Ginsburg, 1955). Independently and nearly simultaneously, Albert Lawrence Green synthesized the same compound in Britain. Green worked with Anthony F. Childs, a senior member of the Chemical Defense Experimental Establishment, and their laboratory included Daniel R. Davies and John P. Rutland, who would do the preliminary reactivation experiments (Petroianu, 2012) (Fig. 3.5.1).

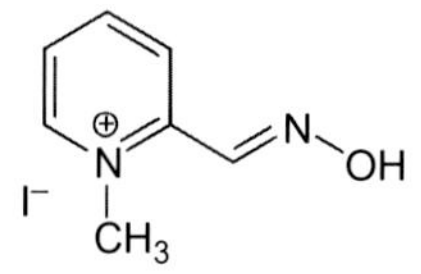

FIG. 3.5.1 Pralidoxime (2-pyridine aldoxime methyl iodide). *(Source: Wikimedia Commons.)*

Development of other oximes

Several other oximes were developed in the late 1950s and beyond. Trimedoxime, or TMB-4, was a *bis*-pyridinium oxime developed in 1957 by Poziomek and colleagues in the United States (Poziomek et al., 1958) and Hobbiger and Sadler in the United Kingdom (Hobbiger et al., 1958). It is a broad reactivator and is used in autoinjectors distributed to the public in Israel (Kozer et al., 2005).

The so-called "Hagedorn series" were developed in Germany in the 1960–80s. Arthur Lüttringhaus and Ilse Hagedorn first developed obidoxime, or LüH-6, in 1964 (Luettringhaus and Hagedorn, 1964). It was effective at treating tabun, sarin, and VX, though not soman (Antonijevic and Stojiljkovic, 2007). As with most other oximes, its adverse effects include paresthesias and increases in both heart rate and blood pressure.

Asoxime, or HI-6 was the first oxime which showed ability to reactivate soman-poisoned AChE, also developed by Hagedorn. However, evidence of its ability at reversing tabun-induced AChE inhibition was mixed. Of the oximes, it has the least toxic effects, with minimal cardiovascular or hepatic toxicity.

HLö-7, named after Hagedorn and Marianne Löffler, was synthesized in Germany in 1986 (Löffler, 1986). It is a broad reactivator of sarin, soman, tabun, VX, and cyclosarin poisoning, though when compared head-to-head with other oximes, it had slight differences in efficacies for each agent (Stojiljković and Jokanović, 2006).

MMB4, or methoxime, is a broadly active oxime undergoing investigation. In animal models, it has been shown to be more effective in reactivating AChE exposed to sarin and VX when compared with 2-PAM (Wilhelm et al., 2018) and may also be superior to obidoxime (Lundy et al., 2011).

The K-series of oximes are the newest, developed by Kamil Kuca and Kamil Musilek in the Czech Republic in the 2000s (Nurulain, 2012). Over 200 K-oximes have been developed since 2003 (Kassa et al., 2008), with several candidates demonstrating broad reactivating potential.

Place in modern therapeutics

Military auto-injectors

Oximes are an important component of military treatment algorithms for nerve agent exposure. Since early administration of antidotal therapy increases their efficacy in reversing nerve agent toxicity, it is important for soldiers to be able to rapidly self-treat, and so auto-injectors were developed. These are either single-medication or combination ampoules, and are spring-loaded with a needle capable of penetrating military uniforms. In the United States, the Mark I NAAK (Nerve Agent Antidote Kit) contained separate auto-injectors containing 2 mg of atropine and 600 mg of 2-PAM. The Mark I kit was gradually phased out starting in 2002, replaced with the ATNAA (Antidote Treatment Nerve Agent Auto-injector) which was a single syringe that included both medications. Combined syringe kits can be administered more rapidly and with fewer errors than kits which contain separate syringes (Rebmann et al., 2009).

Other countries have selected different oximes to be their first-line oxime reactivator for military use. Several factors impact a country's choice of oxime, including cost, commercial availability, and safety profile. For instance, Canada, Sweden, and the Czech Republic use HI-6 (Lundy et al., 2011), while Germany, Finland, and Norway use LüH-6 (Stojiljković and Jokanović, 2006). While 2-PAM, TMB-4, and LüH-6 are stable in aqueous solutions, HI-6 and HLö-7 are not (Marrs et al., 1996). Since it is not shelf-stable in an aqueous solution, HI-6 must be stored in a more complex, two-compartment wet-dry injector, perhaps keeping it from being more widely adopted (EMEA/CPMP Guidance Document, 2003). Additionally, pralidoxime is formulated in four different salts, used in different countries: chloride, mesylate, iodide, and methylsulfate (Sharma et al., 2015).

Strategic National Stockpiles

The US Strategic National Stockpile (SNS), formerly called the National Pharmaceutical Stockpile, is the national repository for chemical antidotes, vaccines, antibiotics, antitoxins, and other critical medical supplies for the United States. Previously managed by the Centers for Disease Control and Prevention, it is now operated under the guidance of the Office of the Assistant Secretary for Preparedness and Response within the Department of Health and Human Services as of October 1, 2018. There are 12 secret locations across the nation which warehouse these materials, with both 12-h push packs and CHEMPACKs available (www.cdc.gov) (Center for Disease Control, n.d.).

The 12-h push packs, which weigh 50 t each, contain pharmaceuticals, respiratory equipment, and general medical supplies; they are delivered within 12 h of the federal decision to utilize them to augment a hospital's supply in the event of a disaster. Because of the concern that a nerve agent incident may rapidly deplete a hospital's supply of antidotes (Barbuto and Chai, 2020), 1960 CHEMPACKs, containing 2-PAM and other antidotes, are distributed across the country. Large metropolitan areas may have multiple CHEMPACKs, and 90% of the US population lives within 1 h of a CHEMPACK site (PHE, 2020). All of the medical products are regulated by the US Food and Drug Administration. An investigational new drug application must be submitted for those agents not yet approved or for expanded access (i.e., compassionate use) (Bhavsar et al., 2018). Some notable deployments of the SNS include after the terrorist attacks on September 11, 2001, anthrax terrorist attacks of 2001, Hurricanes Katrina and Rita along the Gulf coast in 2005, the H1N1 pandemic of 2009, and most recently, during the coronavirus (COVID-19) pandemic of 2020 (https://www.phe.gov/about/pages/default.aspx).

Treatment of nonweaponized organophosphate poisoning

Organophosphate compounds are also used as insecticides, which remain in common use in many parts of the world. In addition to unintentional exposures, suicidal ingestions are tragically common. Parathion, malathion, chlorpyrifos, and dichlorvos are some examples of organophosphate pesticides in wide use. Pralidoxime is the most frequently studied oxime for treating agricultural organophosphate poisoning, though evidence for its efficacy is mixed.

Conclusions

The development of oximes is particularly interesting because oximes are not an obvious antidote. They do not directly antagonize effects at a receptor or enhance the elimination of a poison. Rather, oximes were the product of a deep knowledge of chemistry, combining a reactive nucleophile capable of removing a nerve agent from AChE with a backbone molecule which would help to make the nucleophile acquire its target more rapidly and reliably. Since there is no "universal" reactivator for all of the nerve agents, research on this family of antidotes will continue, hunting for the ideal combination of broad-spectrum efficacy, safety, and shelf stability for stockpiling and military use.

Acknowledgment

We thank Lydia Bunker, MD, for her edifying comments and insightful proofreading of this chapter.

Disclaimer

The views presented are those of the author (AFB) and do not necessarily represent the views of the Department of Defense or its components.

References

Antonijevic B, Stojiljkovic MP. Unequal efficacy of pyridinium oximes in acute organophosphate poisoning. Clin Med Res 2007;5(1):71–82. https://doi.org/10.3121/cmr.2007.701.

Barbuto AF, Chai PR. Recent developments in the clinical management of weaponized nerve agent toxicity. In: Martellini M, Trapp R, editors. 21st century prometheus. Cham: Springer; 2020. p. 287. https://doi.org/10.1007/978-3-030-28285-1_13.

Bhavsar TR, Esbitt DL, Yu PA, Yu Y, Gorman S. Planning considerations for state, local, tribal, and territorial partners to receive medical countermeasures from CDC's strategic national stockpile during a Public Health Emergency. Am J Public Health 2018;108(S3):S183–7.

Center for Disease Control. Strategic National Stockpile 12-hour push package product catalog. n.d. [Accessed 1 June 2020]. https://ftp.cdc.gov/pub/MCMTraining/Miscellaneous%20Resources%20and%20Documents/SNS_Push%20Package%20Catalogl_2-1-12.pdf.

Chai PR, Hayes BD, Erickson TB, Boyer EW. Novichok agents: a historical, current, and toxicological perspective. Toxicol Commun 2018;2(1):45–8.

EMEA/CPMP Guidance Document. EMEA/CPMP Guidance Document on the Use of Medicinal products for the treatment of patients exposed to terrorist attacks with chemical agents; 2003. p. 12–3. London 25 April, 1255(03) https://www.ema.europa.eu/en/documents/other/european-medicines-agency/committee-proprietary-medicinal-products-guidance-document-use-medicinal-products-treatment-patients_en.pdf. [Accessed 1 June 2020].

Hobbiger F, O'Sullivan DG, Sadler PW. New potent reactivators of acetocholinesterase inhibited by tetraethyl pyrophosphate. Nature 1958;182(4648):1498–9.

Kassa J, Kuca K, Karasova J, Musilek K. The development of new oximes and the evaluation of their reactivating, therapeutic and neuroprotective efficacy against tabun. Mini-Rev Med Chem 2008;8(11):1134–43.

Kobler J. The terrible threat of nerve gas. Saturday Evening Post 1957;(27 July):28–9. 75–77.

Kozer E, Mordel A, Haim SB, Bulkowstein M, Berkovitch M, Bentur Y. Pediatric poisoning from trimedoxime (TMB4) and atropine automatic injectors. J Pediatr 2005;146(1):41–4.

Löffler M. Quaternary salts of pyridinium-4-aldoxime as antidotes for organophosphate poisonings [QuartäreSalze von Pyridin-2,4-dialdoxim als Gegenmittel für Organophosphat-Vergiftungen] [Dissertation in German]. Freiburg, Germany: University of Freiburg; 1986.

Luettringhaus A, Hagedorn I. Quaternary hydroxyiminomethylpyridinium salts. The dischloride of bis-(4-hydroxyiminomethyl-1-pyridinium-methyl)-ether (LueH6), a new reactivator of acetyl-cholinesterase inhibited by organic phosphoric acid esters. Arzneimittelforschung 1964;14:1–5.

Lundy PM, Hamilton MG, Sawyer TW, Mikler J. Comparative protective effects of HI-6 and MMB-4 against organophosphorous nerve agent poisoning. Toxicology 2011;285(3):90–6.

Marrs T, Maynard R, Sidell F. Chemical warfare agents: toxicology and treatment. Chicester, England: John Wiley & Sons Ltd; 1996. p. 104–5.

Nachmansohn D, Coates CW, Cox RT. Electric potential and activity of choline esterase in the electric organ of *Electrophorus electricus* (Linnaeus). J Gen Physiol 1941;25(1):75–88.

Nurulain SM. Different approaches to acute organophosphorus poison treatment. J Pak Med Assoc 2012;62(7):712–7.

O'Brien RD. Toxic phosphorous esters: chemistry, metabolism, and biological effects. Academic Press; 1960. p. 101–3.

Petroianu GA. The history of cholinesterase reactivation: hydroxylamine and pyridinium aldoximes. Pharmazie 2012;67:874–9.

Poziomek EJ, Hackley BE, Steinberg GM. Pyridinium aldoximes. J Org Chem 1958;23(5):714–7. https://doi.org/10.1021/jo01099a019.

Public Health Emergency (PHE). U.S. Department of Health and Human Services. Stockpile products, https://www.phe.gov/about/sns/Pages/products.aspx; 2020. [Accessed 1 June 2020].

Rebmann T, Clements BW, Bailey JA, Evans RG. Organophosphate antidote auto-injectors vs. traditional administration: a time motion study. J Emerg Med 2009;37(2):139–43.

Sharma R, Gupta B, Singh N, et al. Development and structural modifications of cholinesterase reactivators against chemical warfare agents in last decade: a review. Mini-Rev Med Chem 2015;15(1):58–72.

Stojiljković MP, Jokanović M. Pyridinium oximes: rationale for their selection as causal antidotes against organophosphate poisonings and current solutions for auto-injectors. Arh Hig Rada Toksikol 2006;57(4):435–43.

Wilhelm CM, Snider TH, Babin MC, Platoff Jr GE, Jett DA, Yeung DT. Evaluating the broad-spectrum efficacy of the acetylcholinesterase oximes reactivators MMB4 DMS, HLö-7 DMS, and 2-PAM Cl against phorate oxon, sarin, and VX in the Hartley Guinea pig. Neurotoxicology 2018;68:142–8.

Wilson IB. Acetylcholinesterase. XI. Reversibility of tetraethyl pyrophosphate inhibition. J Biol Chem 1951;190(1):111–7.

Wilson IB, Ginsburg S. A powerful reactivator of alkylphosphate-inhibited acetylcholinesterase. Biochim Biophys Acta 1955;18(1):168–70. https://doi.org/10.1016/0006-3002(55)90040-8. 13260275.

Wilson IB, Meislich EK. Reactivation of acetylcholinesterase inhibited by alkylphosphates. J Am Chem Soc 1953;75(18):4628–9.

Wilson IB, Ginsburg S, Meislich EK. The reactivation of acetylcholinesterase inhibited by tetraethyl pyrophosphate and diisopropyl fluorophosphate. J Am Chem Soc 1955;77:4286.

Chapter 3.6

Naloxone

David Toomey and Edward W. Boyer
Department of Emergency Medicine, Brigham and Women's Hospital, Harvard Medical School, Boston, MA, United States

Morphine and other opioids

Morphine is the prototypical alkaloid isolated from the opium poppy; morphine and its congeners comprise the opioid class of medications. Opioids have a long-standing role in human history both as medications for the treatment of pain and as substances of abuse. Since their earliest therapeutic use as early as 3400 BCE, opioids have been recognized for their euphoric and analgesic effects, as well as their lethality when consumed in overdose (Bushak, 2016). In the Hippocratic work "Fistulas," compounds of "white meconium" (white poppy) are suggested as a method of treating severe pain caused by inflammation (Potter, 1995), but are also noted for their hypnotic ability to produce sleep. The historical use of opioids, therefore, involves a duality of two co-occurring but often overlapping conditions, comprising medically guided treatment of acute pain and illicit use.

Addiction

Dependence and poisoning from both acute and protracted opioid use are well-described phenomena in historical and contemporary medical literature. Regarding acute effects, agonism of central and peripheral endogenous opioid receptors produces analgesia, euphoria, pupillary constriction, and derangement of respiratory activity, resulting in respiratory depression. At higher doses, opioids can induce frank apnea culminating in death from hypoxic respiratory failure (Boom et al., 2012). In contrast, chronic exposure to opioids can cause a wide number of adverse effects including constipation, nausea, hyperalgesia, as well as physical dependence and compulsive use consistent with addiction (Benyamin et al., 2008). In their search for an optimal treatment for pain, chemists sought to preserve analgesia while eliminating respiratory depression and constipation. Historically the efforts to modulate the adverse effects of the opiates in the early 20th century, particularly addiction, led to the development of opioid antagonists.

History of Modern Clinical Toxicology. https://doi.org/10.1016/B978-0-12-822218-8.00042-9

Morphine, heroin, opium, and cocaine use, already growing in the early 1900s in the United States, had become endemic by the start of World War I. The association of opium with Chinese immigrants, cocaine with African Americans, and morphine addiction with careless physicians triggered increasingly restrictive access to these drugs that culminated in the Harrison Anti-Narcotics Act of 1914. The availability of psychoactive drugs was thought to be an important contributor to substance abuse. Regulations derived from the Harrison Act dictated that maintaining addicts on narcotics to avoid withdrawal was no longer a legitimate medical practice. In the wake of the Harrison Act and bolstered by American Medical Association recommendations, clinics that sold opioids to addicts were closed (Musto, 1996). Addicts were left without a legitimate source of opioids. At the same time, the Social Hygiene Movement emerged in the United States in the late 19th and early 20th centuries. Adherents, who emphasized controlling social ills through scientific research, proposed identifying new analgesics that lacked the respiratory depressant and dependence-inducing qualities of opioids, an additional approach focused on modulating adverse effects through the development of opioid antagonists.

Nalodeine and nalorphine

The first opioid antagonist, a codeine derivative N-allylnorcodeine, later renamed Nalodeine, was discovered by Julius Pohl in 1915. Early chemists correctly ascertained that allyl substitution for the methyl group on the nitrogen bridging the phenanthrene rings conferred respiratory stimulatory properties on the target molecule. In studies of the interactions between codeine derivatives and morphine, Pohl observed that N-allylnorcodeine partially reversed morphine-induced respiratory depression. These findings were largely ignored until a reexamination of the literature in 1942 by Weijlard and Erickson and their associates led to the synthesis of N-allylnormorphine, which became known as nalorphine (Weijlard and Erickson, 1942). In the following year, N-allylnormorphine was demonstrated as having significant antagonism to the effects of morphine by Unna (1943), effects that were further investigated in 1944 by Hart and McCawley (1944). Despite these findings, the use of nalorphine as an antidote for opiate poisoning was not recognized until 1951, when Eckenhoff and colleagues described a case study in which opioid-induced respiratory depression was reversed by nalorphine in a series of patients who received boluses of 90 mg morphine as an adjunct to nitrous oxide anesthesia for minor surgery (Eckenhoff et al., 1951). Based on this finding, clinicians readily adopted nalorphine (Nalline) as the opioid reversal agent of choice in hospital settings. Sadly, nalorphine also gained notoriety in the 1950s and 1960s through its implementation in controversial police drug surveillance programs in California, where the compound was injected as a provocative test to identify opioid abusers by intentionally inducing opioid withdrawal (Campbell, 2019). Interestingly, law enforcement nalorphine programs may have had the unintended consequence of paradoxically increasing methamphetamine use, a drug that could not be "detected" by nalorphine challenge.

Ultimately the dysphoric withdrawal precipitated by nalorphine was determined to be a cruel and unusual punishment by the U.S. Supreme Court in Robinson vs. California (1962); causing the compound to be removed from clinical practice (U.S. Supreme Court, 1962).

Discovery of naloxone

Despite the relative efficacy of nalorphine, research continued throughout the 1950s to develop agents that would be effective in relieving constipation from long-term opioid use. By the end of the 1950s, research conducted by Harold Blumberg (Endo Laboratories) concluded that novel opioid reversal agents derived from synthetic opioids were feasible. This work was continued by Mozes Lowenstein and Jack Fishman, colleagues of Dr. Blumberg working at a private pharmaceutical laboratory (Yardley, 2013). This work culminated in the production of N-allyl-14-hydroxydihydro-nor-morphinone in 1961, which was ultimately generically named "naloxone." Despite having been intended as a therapy for opioid-induced constipation, the original patent for naloxone notes that the compound and its related components were "more potent antagonists to the respiratory depressive effects of potent analgesics than the antagonists hitherto known" (Lewenstein and Fishman, 1966). Despite proven efficacy and potency of the compound for reversing opioid overdose, developers saw little market for naloxone; not until 1971 did FDA approve naloxone (under the trade name Narcan) for use in the reversal of opioid-induced respiratory depression. At that time, Narcan had been developed in intravenous, intramuscular, and subcutaneous formulations for use in hospital settings (Jiang, 2018).

Naloxone was briefly used as a vasopressor. Endorphins, a class of naturally occurring opioid agonists thought to be released from the pituitary during shock states, decrease cardiac contractility (Holaday and Faden, 1978). In early clinical studies, administration of naloxone caused transient increases in blood pressure. Because of perceived similarities between opioid overdose and shock as well as the belief that endorphin release was important in shock states, naloxone was briefly used in the 1970s to treat shock at doses of up to 2 mg/kg. Well-controlled studies, however, identified that naloxone offered little clinical benefit and this indication was dropped from clinical practice.

Naloxone enjoyed widespread use in emergency medicine and anesthesia, due to its considerable efficacy in reversing acute opioid intoxication. Based on the early successes in multiple clinical settings, the WHO listed naloxone as an essential medicine in 1983.

Inranasal naloxone

The dramatic rise in the use of heroin and prescription opioids in the 1980s heralded a rise in overdose deaths in Europe; this, in turn, was followed by a nearly sixfold increase in opioid poisoning deaths in the United States (Warner et al., 2011; Davoli et al., 1993). The pandemic of opioid overdose deaths forced a reorientation of treatment priorities. For example, inadvertent needlestick injury leading to increased risk of HIV transmission led to changes in preferred routes of delivery. Intravenous administration, which required the insertion of an intravenous catheter followed by injection of drug, maximized the use of sharps and, hence, the opportunity for needle-stick incidents. In contrast, the use of subcutaneous and intramuscular naloxone increased, particularly in the prehospital setting (Sporer, et al. 1996). This switch in route of delivery decreased exposure to needles but did not eliminate the threat of needlestick. By 1994, Loimer and associates developed an intranasal delivery device (Loimer et al., 1994), based on highly concentrated naloxone solutions that eliminated entirely the use of sharps.

Bystander naloxone kits

The observation that most overdoses occurred in group settings, coupled with the safety of intranasal naloxone, created the potential for "bystander naloxone" as a harm reduction intervention. The unabated growth in the number of overdose fatalities accelerated discussions about the utility of bystander naloxone programs. These discussions, however, remained largely theoretical until a 1996 *British Medical Journal* editorial by John Strang confronted common misconceptions regarding the use of naloxone by the general population. More importantly, Strang laid the foundation for naloxone distribution as a nonprescription medication (Strang et al., 1996). This approach resonated with overdose intervention activists in the United States. In May of 1996, the Chicago Recovery Alliance began traininsg injection heroin users to reverse overdose with preloaded syringes of the antidote as part of take-home overdose treatment kits. Similar programs emerged in Germany and Italy shortly thereafter that trained heroin users to recognize opioid overdose and reverse it with naloxone (Strang and McDonald, 2016). These early bystander naloxone programs focused solely on heroin use and ignored reversal of poisoning from therapeutic use of prescribed opioid analgesics.

In a tragic and ironic twist of fate, Johnathan Stampler, the stepson of naloxone's inventor, Jack Fishman, died of an opioid overdose in Miami in 2003. The event was witnessed by bystanders; unfortunately, take-home naloxone programs had not been developed by that time, so bystanders could not resuscitate him (Andrey Smith, 2016).

Proliferation of bystander naloxone programs in widespread locations such as New Mexico, California, Spain, and the United Kingdom raised questions about the legal status of naloxone, liability of bystanders administering a prescription medication, and whether physicians could even prescribe a medication to someone other than its intended recipient (Burris et al., 2001). In the United States, the legal status of naloxone and laws regulating its use have been established on a state-by-state basis; a majority have adopted practices to increase legal access to naloxone, such as third party prescribing and standing orders. In addition, many states have enacted Good Samaritan laws which confer legal protection to nonmedical personnel who have used naloxone to prevent or treat opioid overdose (Gabay, 2016). These legal and regulatory solutions have been adapted for use in Europe, spurring a general expansion in government sponsored take-home naloxone programs from 2005 to 2015 (Strang and McDonald, 2016). Moreover, in the United Kingdom, naloxone has been incorporated into Schedule 7 of the Medicines Act in 2005, formally qualifying it as a rescue medication and providing full legal protection to members of the general public administering naloxone for the aim of saving a life. The successes of naloxone distribution programs prompted further research into advanced naloxone delivery devices (U.S. FDA, 2018). Unfortunately, dramatic increases in the price of naloxone or naloxone-containing devices—in some cases over 500% from an already exorbitant initial cost—may be due to questionable business practices intended to inflate drug prices (Gupta et al., 2016).

Naloxone is increasingly viewed as an effective clinical tool as well as an instrument for population-wide harm reduction. Unfortunately the adulteration of heroin with fentanyl or its congeners in the late 2010s led to striking increases in the rate of opioid overdose deaths through the inability of even large doses of the antidote to reverse opioid poisoning. This has triggered a search for antidotes with greater potency and longer durations of action. Approaches such as naloxone-laden nanoparticles may have the ability to better reverse overdose. Because the antidote is still naloxone, however, this and related approaches lack the potency to reverse molecules with high affinity for the mu-opioid receptor such as fentanyl and its congeners. The introduction of new opioid antagonists of ultrahigh affinity and long duration awaits further research.

References

Andrey Smith P. Why the inventor of the antidote naloxone lost his stepson to heroin. Retrieved 7 August 2020, from: https://www.newsweek.com/jack-fishman-naloxone-opioids-overdose-heroin-466355; 2016.

Benyamin R, Trescot AM, Datta S, Buenaventura R, Adlaka R, Sehgal N, Glaser SE, Vallejo R. Opioid complications and side effects. Pain Physician 2008;11(2 Suppl):S105–20.

Boom M, Niesters M, Sarton E, Aarts L, Smith TW, Dahan A. Non-analgesic effects of opioids: opioid-induced respiratory depression. Curr Pharm Des 2012;18(37):5994–6004. https://doi.org/10.2174/138161212803582469. PMID: 22747535.

Burris S, Norland J, Edlin BR. Legal aspects of providing naloxone to heroin users in the United States. Int J Drug Policy 2001;12:237–48.

Bushak L. How did opioid drugs get to be so deadly? A brief history. Retrieved 15 June 2020, from: https://www.medicaldaily.com/opioid-drugs-heroin-epidemic-prescription-painkillers-abuse-history-392747?rel=most_shared5; 2016. [Accessed 9 June 2020].

Campbell ND. Naloxone as a technology of solidarity: history of opioid overdose prevention. Can Med Assoc J 2019;191(34):E945–6.

Davoli M, Perucci CA, Forastiere F, Doyle P, Rapiti E, Zaccarelli M, Abeni DD. Risk factors for overdose mortality: a case-control study within a cohort of intravenous drug users. Int J Epidemiol 1993;22:273–7.

Eckenhoff JE, Elder JD, King BD. Effect of N-allylnormorphine in the treatment of opiate overdose. Am J Med Sci 1951;222:115–7.

Gabay M. Increasing access to naloxone and legal issues. Hosp Pharm 2016;51(8):633–4.

Gupta R, Shah ND, Ross JS. The rising price of naloxone—risks to efforts to stem overdose deaths. N Engl J Med 2016;375(23):2213–5.

Hart ER, McCawley EL. The pharmacology of N-allyl-normorphine as compared with morphine. J Pharmacol Exp Ther 1944;82:339–48.

Holaday J, Faden A. Naloxone reversal of endotoxin hypotension suggests role of endorphins in shock. Nature 1978;275:450–1.

Jiang T. Clinical and regulatory overview of naloxone products intended for use in the community [powerpoint slides]. Retrieved from: https://www.fda.gov/media/121189/download; 2018. [Accessed 9 June 2020].

Lewenstein M, Fishman J. Morphine Derivative. US 3254088A. United States Patent and Trademark Office; 1966. https://patents.google.com/patent/US3254088A/en. [Accessed 9 June 2020].

Loimer N, Hofmann P, Chaudhry HR. Nasal administration of naloxone is as effective as the intravenous route in opiate addicts. Int J Addict 1994;29:819–27.

Musto DF. Pathways of addiction: opportunities in drug abuse research. Institute of Medicine Committee on Opportunities in Drug Abuse Research, Washington, DC: National Academies Press (US); 1996.

Potter P, editor. Hippocrates. Fistulas. In: Hippocrates vol VIII: places in man. Glands. Fleshes. Prorrhetic 1–2. Physician. Use of liquids. Ulcers. Haemorrhoids. Fistulas. Cambridge, MA: Harvard University Press; 1995 [section 7].

Sporer KA, Firestone J, Isaacs SM. Out-of-hospital treatment of opioid overdoses in an urban setting. Acad Emerg Med 1996;3:660–7.

Strang J, McDonald R. Preventing opioid overdose deaths with take-home naloxone. Luxembourg: Publications Office of the European Union; 2016. p. 49–66 [European Union, European monitoring Centre for Drugs and Drug Addiction, EMCDDA Project Group].

Strang J, Darke S, Hall W, Farrell M, Ali R. Heroin overdose: the case for take-home naloxone. Br Med J 1996;312:1435.

U.S. Supreme Court. Justia: Robinson v. California 370, U.S. 660, https://supreme.justia.com/cases/federal/us/370/660/; 1962. [Accessed 9 April 2020].

United States (U.S.) Food & Drug Administration. Press Announcements—FDA moves quickly to approve easy-to-use nasal spray to treat opioid overdose. Retrieved 27 June 2020, from: https://www.fda.gov/news-events/press-announcements/fda-approves-first-generic-naloxone-nasal-spray-treat-opioid-overdose; 2018.

Unna K. Antagonistic effect of N-allyl-normorphine upon morphine. J Pharmacol Exp Ther 1943;79:27–31.

Warner M, Chen L, Makuc DM, Anderson RN, Miniño AM. Drug Poisoning Deaths in the United States, 1980–2008. NCHS Data Brief 2011;81(81):1–8.

Weijlard J, Erickson AE. N-allylnormorphine. J Am Chem Soc 1942;64:869–70.

Yardley W. Jack Fishman dies at 83; saved many from overdose. Retrieved 23 June 2020, from: https://www.nytimes.com/; https://www.nytimes.com/2013/12/15/business/jack-fishman-who-helped-develop-a-drug-to-treat-overdoses-dies-at-83.html?_r=0 [Accessed 9 June 2020]; 2013.

Chapter 3.7

Physostigmine

Nathan Kunzler[a] and Timothy B. Erickson[b]

[a]*Department of Emergency Medicine, Medical Toxicology Fellowship Program, Regions Hospital, St. Paul, MN, United States,* [b]*Chief, Division of Medical Toxicology, Department of Emergency Medicine, Mass General Brigham, Harvard Medical School, Harvard Humanitarian Initiative, Boston, MA, United States*

Introduction

Many modern pharmaceuticals have roots in ethnobotanical practices. Physostigmine represents a case of a modern medical drug that was developed as a result of these traditional practices. Furthermore, it represents an important milestone in our understanding of agonist-antagonist relationships in pharmacology and physiology and therefore demonstrates the value that ethnobotanical research can provide in the development of pharmaceuticals and natural remedies for use in modern medicine.

Discovery

The human quest for an objective means to ascertain the veracity of statements is as ancient as humanity itself. "Trial by ordeal" involves subjecting a person to painful or unpleasant experiences to determine guilt. Varied means have been used in trial by ordeal including fire, water, combat, and notably ingestion of a poison. It is because of the tradition of trial by ordeal that physostigmine came to be known throughout the western world. Specifically the practice of the Efik Uburutu people, in what is now south-east Nigeria, of administering the extract of the Calabar bean lead to the discovery of physostigmine (Proudfoot, 2006). Ingestion of this extract was used to determine guilt whereby those who lived were considered innocent and those who died, guilty.

This trial by ordeal first came to the attention of western medicine around 1846 when missionaries traveling in what was then known as Old Calabar began to take note of the trial being used as a test for witchcraft. These missionaries, who were mostly of Scottish descent, noted that as many as 120 people a year died in Old Calabar as a result of the trial (Proudfoot, 2006). The first formal investigation of the mechanism underlying the bean's clinical effects came from

History of Modern Clinical Toxicology. https://doi.org/10.1016/B978-0-12-822218-8.00059-4
271

Robert Christison, a toxicologist in the 1800s (Proudfoot, 2006). His methods of study included ingesting the bean himself to study and describe its various effects on a human. In 1861, John Hutton Balfour formally described and named the plant that gave rise to the Calabar bean, choosing *Physostigma venenosum*, which remains its currently accepted binomial botanical name (Balfour, 1861) (Fig. 3.7.1).

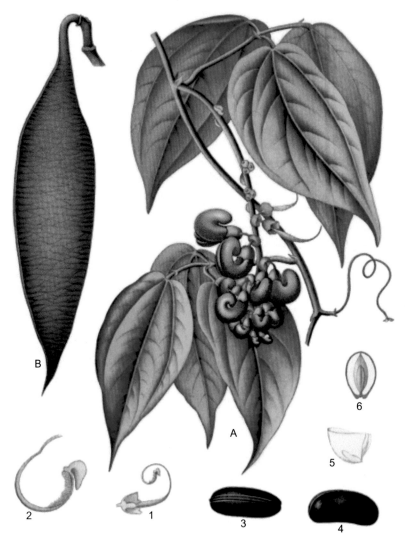

FIG. 3.7.1 Calabar Bean *Physostigma venenosum. Source: Wikimedia Commons https:// commons.wikimedia.org/w/index.php?search=calabar+bean&title=Special:MediaSearch&go= Go&type=image. Author: Franz Eugen Köhler, Köhler's Medizinal-Pflanzen.*

Development

Shortly after the formal taxonomy of the plant was described, uses beyond trial by ordeal began to appear. Dr. Argyll Robertson, a Scottish surgeon and ophthalmologist, noted in 1863 that an extract of the Calabar bean caused constriction of the pupil of the eye (Proudfoot, 2006). His discovery was contemporaneous with those in several other publications at the time discussing the ophthalmological effects of the bean. During this period of study, the extract of the Calabar bean itself came to be known as "physostigma" (or, alternatively, physostigmine). In the time period after the discovery of the use of physostigmine for ophthalmological purposes, its effects on other organ systems and its systemic toxicity were also investigated. In particular, a physician named Dr. Thomas Fraser began an extensive study of the effects of the Calabar extract and ultimately laid the groundwork for our modern understanding of neuromuscular physiology (Proudfoot, 2006).

Fraser, along with other contemporaries such as George Harley, began to publish extensively on the effect of physostigmine (Proudfoot, 2006). He notably advanced the idea that physostigmine and atropine were antagonistic in their actions. The effect was most likely first noticed by an ophthalmologist, Bernd Kleinwachter, who published as early as 1864 that he had treated a patient with atropine poisoning with physostigmine, the first antidotal use of the extract (Kleinwachter, 1864). Fraser, however, took this work further by experimenting with animals and showing convincingly that atropine and physostigmine were in-fact antagonistic in their effects (Proudfoot, 2006). This basic principle, while not completely novel, ultimately underlies our modern understanding of the basic physiology that describes most neurotransmitter communications in the human body.

Other than its use as an occasional antidote for atropine poisoning, the next significant use of physostigmine as a therapeutic agent was published in 1876 when a German ophthalmologist, Ludwig Laqueur (Fig. 3.7.2), began to use physostigmine to treat glaucoma (Proudfoot, 2006). Then in the 1920s physostigmine would again revolutionize our understanding of human physiology. Otto Loewi was studying the effect of the parasympathetic nervous system and found that its actions were controlled by chemicals, specifically acetylcholine (Mccoy and Tan, 2014). His work demonstrated that physostigmine acted by preventing the metabolism of acetylcholine. Loewi and his colleague, Sir Henry Hallett Dale, would go on to win the Nobel Prize in Physiology and Medicine in 1936 for their efforts in advancing our understanding of the transmission of neural impulses.

In 1934, Dr. Mary Walker (Fig. 3.7.3) discovered that by injecting physostigmine subcutaneously, she could temporarily reverse the weakness associated with myasthenia gravis. She was working at St. Alfege's hospital in London at the time and published her finding in *The Lancet* (Walker, 1934). She was also the first to recognize that the weakness associated with myasthenia gravis was

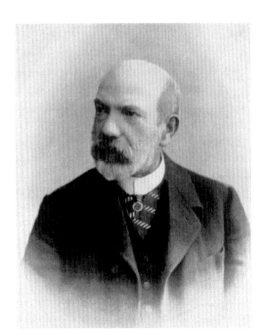

FIG. 3.7.2 Dr. Ludwig Laqueur. *Source: Wikimedia Commons https://commons.wikimedia. org/w/index.php?search=Ludwig+LaQueur&title=Special:MediaSearch&go=Go&type=image. Unknown author.*

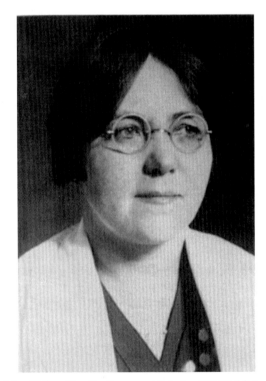

FIG. 3.7.3 Dr. Mary Walker. *(Creative Commons Attribution (CC BY 4.0) terms and conditions https://creativecommons.org/licenses/by/4.0 Credit: Portrait; Mary Broadfoot Walker (1888–1974). Credit: Wellcome Collection. Attribution 4.0 International (CC BY 4.0).)*

similar to that seen in those suffering from curare poisoning and she advocated for the use of physostigmine as an antidote. This was the second use of physostigmine as an antidote to poisoning. Our current understanding of the physiology of both atropine and curare make the reason for reversal of the clinical effects of these poisons by physostigmine more evident, placing physostigmine in rare company as an antidote for two distinct poisonings.

With an increased knowledge of human physiology, and the role that physostigmine might play, the focus of the scientific community shifted to the synthesis of this important tertiary amine carbamate (Fig. 3.7.4). Dr. Percy Lavon Julian was the first to synthesize physostigmine. Julian (Fig. 3.7.5) received his PhD in 1931 while working at DePauw University as a research fellow. In 1935,

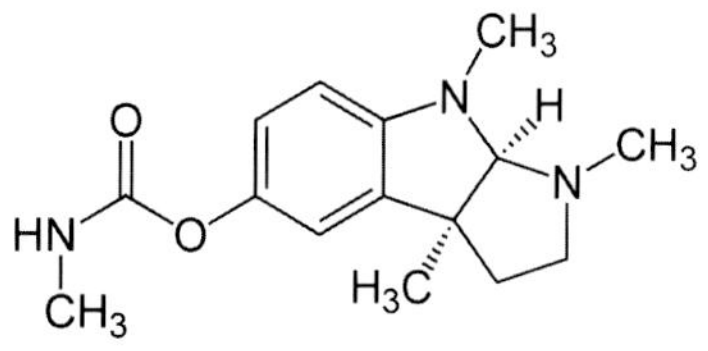

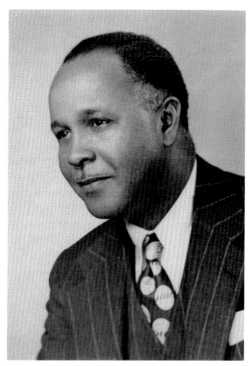

FIG. 3.7.4 Physostigmine molecular structure. *(Wikimedia Commons.)*

FIG. 3.7.5 Dr. Percy Lavon Julian. *(The Science History Institute, Philadelphia, Pennsylvania, USA. used with permission.)*

he synthesized physostigmine and published his work in a landmark article titled *Studies in the Indole Series. V. The Complete Synthesis of Phsyostigmine (Eserine)* (Julian et al., 1934; Julian and Pikl, 1935). Unfortunately, likely due to the racial politics in the United States at the time, after his grant funding expired Julian was denied a teaching position at DePauw, this despite the fact that his synthesis paper was widely recognized at the time as a landmark study (Julian and Pikl, 1935). Julian persevered and went on to pioneer the industrial chemical synthesis of the human hormones: progesterone and testosterone from plant sterols. In 1950, Julian moved his family to the Chicago suburb of Oak Park, becoming the first African-American family to reside there. Owing to racial tensions, his house was firebombed and later attacked with dynamite. These malicious attacks galvanized the community, and a social network was formed in response to support the Julian family (Grossman, 2020). Ultimately Julian overcame incredible barriers and received more than 130 chemical patents (Wiktop, 1980). He was one of the first African-Americans to receive a doctorate in chemistry and was the first African-American chemist inducted into the National Academy of Sciences (Wiktop, 1980).

Recent history

Physostigmine began to see increasing use in the 1970s because it was able to produce an arousal effect on the central nervous system (CNS). While traditional use of the drug for the treatment of antimuscarinic delirium was well-established by this time (Trade name "Antilirium"), its use as a therapy in cases of nonantimuscarinic altered mental status began to grow (Arens and Kearney, 2019).

It began to see use in the emergency department as a general arousal agent in patients presenting with signs of overdose of benzodiazepines, opioids, gamma-hydroxy-butyrate, and baclofen. The effect seen in these cases does not stem from its antagonism of antimuscarinic effects, but rather more likely from increased acetylcholine concentrations in areas such as the reticular activating system, although this effect has not been conclusively proven (Nilsson, 1982).

Physostigmine use and controversy shifted when asystole and death followed the administration of physostigmine in two published tricyclic antidepressant (TCA) overdoses (Pentel and Peterson, 1980). After these reports the use of physostigmine declined precipitously, especially in nonantimuscarinic cases of altered mental status (Arens and Kearney, 2019). Analysis of physostigmine as a potential cause, and its subsequent exoneration, in these deaths helped to elucidate the complex physiological mechanisms underlying cyclic antidepressant toxicity.

Place in modern therapeutics

Since its discovery and development, physostigmine has had a preeminent place in the parthenon of toxicological controversy in the modern era. The use of physostigmine as an antidote for anticholinergic poisoning is still discussed and hotly debated. Its use in purely antimuscarinic poisoning, however, is logical, backed by abundant evidence of safety and clinical efficacy (Arens et al., 2018; Boley et al., 2019).

What complicates the clinical picture is that few patients present with such pure toxic syndromes, and physostigmine interacts with numerous drugs in an antagonistic fashion. While its use may be common among medical toxicologists, others relegate the use of physostigmine as an antidote to that of a simple historical footnote. Physostigmine may be used for treatment of antimuscarinic-induced delirium. Multiple observational studies have found that patients with pure antimuscarinic poisoning have their delirium well-controlled with physostigmine with superior efficacy compared to traditional doses of benzodiazepines and other potent neuroleptic agents (Boley et al., 2019). Physostigmine remains the antidote of choice for delirium-induced poisonings from natural toxins such as *Datura stramonium* (Jimson weed) and isolated antimuscarinic toxicity from pharmaceutical agents (e.g., diphenhydramine).

As previously described, rare cases of asystole have been reported after physostigmine use in TCA toxicity, particularly in patients with bradycardia and AV block. While these patients likely died from their TCA toxicity, some toxicologists have advised clinicians not to administer this antidote to patients with QRS or QTc prolongation following TCA overdose. However, it should be considered in patients with delirium of unclear etiology who are therapeutically taking anticholinergic agents and in whom toxicity from these agents is suspected. When used diagnostically in an antimuscarinic poisoned patient, a rapid clinical response can be expected within 10–15 min. A positive response to physostigmine administration, with near complete reversal of delirium, may confirm diagnostic suspicions of the clinician and decrease the need for more invasive testing and costly intensive care monitoring. Overall, physostigmine should be considered as a safe diagnostic and therapeutic intervention in patients with antimuscarinic toxicity, especially when the drug-induced delirium places the patient or healthcare providers at risk.

Conclusion

The history of physostigmine forces us to consider so much about our place in medicine. Its use as an essential part of a "trial by ordeal" ritual allows us to consider our relationship to truth and the sordid past of baseless accusation and death of countless innocent victims. Its relationship with the Efik people allows us to consider our obligations to the indigenous people whose ethnobotanical knowledge has so often improved the lives of those of us in the rest of the world while offering little recompense for those from whom we gained the knowledge. Its laboratory synthesis and the subsequent refusal of recognition for the enormity of the contribution of its first synthesizer, Dr. Julian, also reminds us of the ugly history of racism in the United States.

The first use of physostigmine to treat myasthenia and as an antidote for curare poisoning also invites us to consider the contributions of women to the world of medicine and the science, technology, engineering, and mathematics disciplines, especially in a time when those contributions were less often recognized. The fact that the incredible, rich, and important scientific history of physostigmine yielded only a single Nobel Prize, one awarded to a White man (despite its initial synthesis by a Black man), is worth noting.

Finally the controversy around its use in altered mental status and the resultant decrease in its use remind us that ultimately science must be reconciled with the contemporary practice environment in which it takes place. While it is impossible to know what the future of physostigmine holds, it seems certain that this important historical compound will continue to find new ways to teach us about our own physiology, find new uses for our patients, and create new controversy.

References

Arens AM, Kearney T. Adverse effects of physostigmine. J Med Toxicol 2019;15(3):184–91.

Arens AM, Shah K, Al-Abri S, Olson KR, Kearney T. Safety and effectiveness of physostigmine: a 10-year retrospective review. Clin Toxicol 2018;56:101–7.

Balfour J. IX. Description of the plant which produces the ordeal bean of Calabar. Trans R Soc Edinb Earth Environ Sci 1861;22(2):305–12. https://doi.org/10.1017/S0080456800030623.

Boley SP, Olives TD, Bangh SA, Fahrner S, Cole JB. Physostigmine is superior to non-antidote therapy in the management of antimuscarinic delirium: a prospective study from a regional poison center. Clin Toxicol 2019;57:50–5.

Grossman R. Chemist Percy Julian pushed past racial barriers—Amid attacks on his oak park home. Available from: https://www.chicagotribune.com/opinion/commentary/ct-perspec-flashback-percy-julian-chemist-oak-park-20190206-story.html; 2020. [Accessed 30 October 2020].

Julian PL, Pikl J. Studies in the indole series. III. On the synthesis of physostigmine. J Am Chem Soc 1935;57(3):539–44. https://doi.org/10.1021/ja01306a046.

Julian PL, Pikl J, Boggess D. Studies in the indole series. II. Alkylation of 1-methyl-3-formyloxindole and a synthesis of the basic ring structure of physostigmine. J Am Chem Soc 1934;56(8):1797–801. https://doi.org/10.1021/ja01323a046.

Kleinwachter. Beobachtung uber die Wirkung des Calabar-Extracts gegen Atropin-vergiftung. Berl Klin Wochenschr 1864;1:369–71.

Mccoy AN, Tan SY. Otto Loewi (1873–1961): dreamer and Nobel laureate. Singap Med J 2014;55(1):3–4.

Nilsson E. Physostigmine treatment in various drug-induced intoxications. Ann Clin Res 1982;14(4):165–72.

Pentel P, Peterson CD. Asystole complicating physostigmine treatment of tricyclic antidepressant overdose. Ann Emerg Med 1980;9(11):588–90.

Proudfoot A. The early toxicology of physostigmine: a tale of beans, great men and egos. Toxicol Rev 2006;25(2):99–138. https://doi.org/10.2165/00139709-200625020-00004. 16958557.

Walker MB. Treatment of myasthenia gravis with physostigmine. Lancet 1934;1(5779):1200–1. https://doi.org/10.1016/S0140-6736(00)94294-6.

Wiktop B. Percy Lavon Julian: a biographical memoir. 52. National Academy of Sciences; 1980. http://www.nasonline.org/publications/biographical-memoirs/memoir-pdfs/julian-percy.pdf.

Chapter 3.8

Cyanide antidotes

Patrick C. Ng[a,b,c,d], Joseph K. Maddry[a,b,e], and Vikhyat S. Bebarta[f,g,h,i,j]

[a]*Department of Emergency Medicine, Brooke Army Medical Center, San Antonio, TX, United States,* [b]*Emergency Medicine, Uniformed Services University of the Health Sciences, Bethesda, MD, United States,* [c]*Emergency Medicine, University of Colorado Anschutz Medical Campus, Aurora, CO, United States,* [d]*En Route Care Research Center, 59th Medical Wing/Science and Technology, Joint Base San Antonio, San Antonio, TX, United States,* [e]*United States Army Institute of Surgical Research, San Antonio, TX, United States,* [f]*Center for Combat Medicine and Battlefield (COMBAT) Research, Aurora, CO, United States,* [g]*Translational Research, Innovation, and Antidote Development (TRIAD) Research, Aurora, CO, United States,* [h]*Department of Emergency Medicine, Anschutz Medical Campus, University of Colorado, Aurora, CO, United States,* [i]*Rocky Mountain Poison and Drug Safety, Denver Health and Hospital Authority, Denver, CO, United States,* [j]*Office of the Chief Scientist, 59th Medical Wing/Science and Technology, Joint Base San Antonio, San Antonio, TX, United States*

Introduction

Cyanide is a potentially deadly chemical and exposure to the toxin has been reported in several different scenarios (Borron et al., 2007a, b; Brenner et al., 2017; Lee et al., 2016). Cyanide is used in suicide and its use as an agent in homicide has been reported (Petrikovics et al., 2019). Industrial exposures to cyanide as well as occupational exposures in the metal, mining, petrochemical, and electroplating industries have also been reported. Cyanogenic glycosides are naturally found in various plants and are a major source of exposure to cyanide world-wide. Exposure to cyanide can occur when various medications including nitroprusside and succinonitrile are administered and with the combustion of organic material in residential and industrial fires.

Cyanide toxicity is characterized by respiratory and cardiovascular collapse, metabolic acidemia, and hyperlactatemia secondary to cytochrome *a*3 inhibition. In lower exposures, nonspecific symptoms such as headache, nausea, vomiting, chest pain, and shortness of breath can occur. In more chronic exposures such as in patients with tobacco amblyopia, tropical ataxic neuropathy and Leber's hereditary optic atrophy, visual and neurological symptoms are the mainstay (Petrikovics et al., 2015). Given the potential for the debilitating and potentially deadly effects of cyanide both chronically and acutely, an interest

History of Modern Clinical Toxicology. https://doi.org/10.1016/B978-0-12-822218-8.00034-X

in antidote development was born. Strategies of treatment, in addition to supportive care, focus around two major therapeutic targets: promoting enzymatic detoxification of cyanide and the direct binding of cyanide in vivo with compounds such as ferrihemoglobin (methemoglobin) and hydroxocobalamin.

Methemoglobin inducers

Early chemical binders of cyanide stemmed from studies involving methylene blue (Geiger, 1933) (See Chapter 3.3 for additional details on the use of methylene blue as an antidote for cyanide.). Experimentally, animals with higher methemoglobin concentrations needed higher doses of cyanide to cause severe toxicity (Chen et al., 1933) and it was postulated that the formation of methemoglobin by methylene blue was the reason why it was protective against cyanide poisoning. Other studies demonstrated that methemoglobin had a high affinity for cyanide and that this was the potential mechanism of action of possible antidotes such as methylene blue. Further studies performed in dogs and mice showed that the degree of protection against cyanide was proportional to the degree of methemoglobinemia (Jandorf and Bodansky, 1946). With more data supporting the protective effect of methemoglobinemia in cyanide poisoning, other compounds that promoted the formation of methemoglobin were explored.

Amyl nitrite, which is a methemoglobin inducer, is an early compound that was explored as an antidote for cyanide toxicity. In the late 1800s, it was found that dogs that were exposed to amyl nitrite were protected against cyanide poisoning. Further studies were done in the 1930s. Chen and Rose (1952) looked at other nitrite compounds including inhaled amyl nitrite and intravenous (IV) sodium nitrite. Intravenous nitrites were effective in inducing methemoglobinemia; however, some limitations included the need for an IV for administration and the extra steps involved with reconstitution of the substance before infusion. Furthermore, it was noted that nitrites were limited in their use for cyanide poisoning because the rate of methemoglobin formation by some nitrites was out-paced by the rapid inhibition of cytochrome oxidase by cyanide. Authors noted that nitrites formed methemoglobin too slowly to be truly effective in rapid, severe cyanide toxicity (Kiese, 1969; Christel et al., 1977). As a result, after initial studies involving nitrites, other agents that could more rapidly generate methemoglobin were explored (Kiese, 1969; Eyer et al., 1974). Various aminophenols including 2-aminophenol hydrochloride, 2-amino-4-chlorophenol hydrochloride, 2-amino-4,6-dichlorophenol hydrochloride, 2-dimethylaminophenol hydrochloride, 4-aminophenol hydrochloride, *bis*-(4-methylaminophenol)sulfate, and dimethylaminophenol hydrochloride were investigated. The rates of formation of ferrihemoglobin by aminophenol were compared with the rate of ferrihemoglobin formed by sodium nitrite; 4-dimethylaminophenol more rapidly formed methemoglobin compared with sodium nitrite. In a canine model, it was found that animals poisoned with cyanide and then treated with 4-dimethylaminophenol had a rapid induction of ferrimethemoglobinemia and a subsequent decrease in serum cyanide concentrations and return to spontaneous ventilation (Christel et al., 1977). This line of investigation was expanded to other compounds that produced methemoglobin, such as hydroxylamine (Kruszyna et al., 1982).

Despite the rapid formation of ferrimethemoglobin with compounds such as 4-dimethylaminophenol and hydroxylamine, other studies continued to support the use of sodium nitrite. Sodium nitrite was thought to have other mechanisms that were protective against cyanide intoxication including the inhibition of methemoglobin reductase which in turn allowed for a more sustained methemoglobinemia. Sodium nitrite also promoted the formation of nitric oxide which competes with cyanide for binding to cytochrome C oxidase (Johnson et al., 1989; Pearce et al., 2003). Compared with other agents such as the aminophenols and hydroxylamine, sodium nitrite was found to cause a more sustained methemoglobinemia, which was thought to be more effective when treating cyanide poisoning compared with agents that formed methemoglobin more rapidly (Kruszyna et al., 1982).

In the 1980s, further studies were conducted to improve the treatment of cyanide poisoning. Stroma-free methemoglobin (SFM) was explored as a potential solution. SFM is described to be a solution that is made by oxidizing ferrous iron in stroma free hemoglobin. An advantage of using SFM over agents that induce methemoglobinemia in vivo is that, unlike sodium nitrite or aminophenols, SFM would not affect the patient's overall oxygen-carrying capacity as it would not affect a patient's endogenous hemoglobin. Ten Eyck et al. (1985–1986) demonstrated that the administration of SFM was efficacious in improving survival in rats poisoned with cyanide. The authors proposed SFM as a potential treatment alternative to nitrites. Data from a rat study in 1985 supported this (Ten Eyck et al., 1985). In this study, authors compared nitrite/sodium thiosulfate versus SFM for cyanide poisoning. They found that nitrite was only effective when given prior to cyanide exposure which they highlighted as a major limitation compared with SFM, which was effective in when administered after the cyanide exposure (Ten Eyck et al., 1985). Similar effects of SFM on cyanide poisoning were demonstrated in a large animal model (Breen, 1996).

Thiosulfate

Rhodanese and mercaptopyruvate-cyanide-*trans*-sulfurase are enzymes found in the kidney and liver of humans that had been identified to detoxify cyanide by converting it to thiocyanate when in the presence of a sulfur donor (Himwich and Saunders, 1948). In several experiments, it was noted that combining thiosulfate and rhodanese was effective in treating cyanide poisoning (Clemedson et al., 1955).

The combination of sodium thiosulfate and sodium nitrite for cyanide poisoning was studied in dogs (Chen and Rose, 1952). The combination of the two was found to be more effective than either of the agents alone. Chen proposed a treatment combination of inhaled amyl nitrite, which could be administered early, followed by sodium nitrite and then followed by sodium thiosulfate once intravenous access was obtained. The combination treatment of amyl nitrite, sodium nitrite, and sodium thiosulfate was eventually commercially produced as the Cyanide Antidote Kit, the Taylor kit, the Lily kit, and the Pasadena Kit (Uhl et al., 2006). In 2010, Hope Pharmaceuticals (London, UK) filed a New Drug Application with the FDA for the use of Nithiodote for sequential use for the treatment of acute cyanide poisoning that is judged to be life threatening. Nithiodote contains one 10-mL vial of 30 mg/mL sodium nitrite and one 50-mL vial of 250 mg/mL sodium thiosulfate solutions for injection. As of the writing of this text, the Nithiodote kit had FDA approval for the treatment of cyanide toxicity in the United States.

Cobalt compounds

The earlier reports of cobalt salts' ability to form stable complexes with cyanide date back to the late 1800s (Antal, 1984). Various cobalt containing compounds including dicobalt acetate, hydroxocobalamin, dicobalt edetate, and cobinamide have been explored (Evans, 1964).

Dicobalt acetate in combination with thiosulfate was found to be effective in reducing mortality in mice and rabbits. Cobalt EDTA and cobalt histidine were noted to be of limited benefit in cyanide toxicity secondary to the potential antidotes' inherent toxicity. Out of the cobalt containing compounds studied, it was noted that the naturally occurring, relatively nontoxic compound, vitamin B12, contained a tightly bound cyanide moiety (Brink, 1950) and that its hydroxy-derivative, vitamin B12a or hydroxocobalamin, did not. This led to a series of experiments to investigate the reaction between hydroxocobalamin and cyanide (Kaczka et al., 1950). In vitro studies performed by Kaczka and colleagues of Merck and Co. demonstrated that the combination of hydroxocobalamin and cyanide formed cyanocobalamin. Further studies highlighted the antidotal potential of hydroxocobalamin for cyanide poisoning (Paulet and Oliver, 1962; Silvestroni and Fimiani, 1964). Additionally, hydroxocobalamin was shown to be nontoxic in animal models and it was already being used in humans to treat conditions such as pernicious anemia (Winter and Mushett, 1950).

Further investigation of hydroxocobalamin for cyanide poisoning was performed in canines. Hydroxocobalamin was found to delay onset of toxicity, prolong survival and prevented one death in dogs poisoned with cyanide (Rose et al., 1965). Given the studies demonstrating the efficacy of hydroxocobalamin and previous studies showing the efficacy of sodium thiosulfate, Friedberg et al. investigated the efficacy of a combination of hydroxocobalamin and sodium thiosulfate in cats (Friedberg and Shukla, 1975), noting that sodium thiosulfate had a delayed onset of action because the enzymatic detoxification of cyanide via rhodanese was slow. Given the rapid onset of cyanide toxicity, monotherapy with sodium thiosulfate was limited. A combination of hydroxocobalamin and sodium thiosulfate was more effective in cats poisoned with cyanide compared with hydroxocobalamin alone. The authors proposed that a combination of the two would be a feasible method to treat cyanide poisoning. Similarly,

Burrows et al. found that the combination of a cobalt compound and sodium thiosulfate was more efficacious than a single agent for the treatment of cyanide intoxication in sheep (Burrows, 1979). Although several cobalt containing compounds were found to be effective for treating cyanide poisoning, some had inherent toxicities that limited their use as antidotes. Hydroxocobalamin, a vitamin derivative already administered for other diseases such as pernicious anemia, became the forerunner for further investigation into the treatment of cyanide poisoning. In vitro studies using rat cardiac papillary muscles demonstrated the antidotal efficacy of hydroxocobalamin for cyanide poisoning (Riou et al., 1990). Its safety profile was of utmost importance given the potentially rapid and deadly nature of cyanide which often necessitated empiric treatment in the prehospital setting. Furthermore, reports of the potential toxic effects of sodium nitrite continued to be published (Hall et al., 1989). Animal studies comparing the toxicity of hydroxocobalamin to that of other cobalt containing compounds showed that hydroxocobalamin was potentially safer than the other compounds (Riou et al., 1993). Using a canine model, Riou and colleagues described the lack of unfavorable hemodynamic effects induced by hydroxocobalamin at therapeutic doses (Riou et al., 1991). Compared with cobalt edetate, hydroxocobalamin had a more favorable side-effect profile (Riou et al., 1993).

Since it was licensed in 1996, hydroxocobalamin has been used in France for cyanide poisoning. In 2006, Uhl et al. reported data generated from a randomized, double-blind, placebo-controlled, ascending-dose study in healthy volunteers to assess the safety of hydroxocobalamin. They found that the side-effect profile of the compound (rash, headache, erythema, and a rise in blood pressure) was minor compared with other antidotes (Uhl et al., 2006). In 2006, EMD Pharmaceuticals submitted an application to the FDA for approval of the Cyanokit, which contains 5.0 g of hydroxocobalamin as a lyophilized powder to be reconstituted and administered intravenously for the treatment of adult cyanide poisoning victims. Several studies published after FDA approval demonstrated its efficacy in patients with cyanide intoxication (Borron et al., 2007a, b). Hydroxocobalamin has FDA approval for the treatment of suspected cyanide poisoning in the United States and is marketed by Meridian Medical Technologies, a Pfizer company, as the Cyanokit. Hydroxocobalamin is listed on the World Health Organization (WHO) list of essential drugs, but is listed under treatments for anemia, not cyanide poisoning (WHO Model List of Essential Medicines, 2013).

Recent investigations

There is continued investigation into alternative antidotes for cyanide poisoning. Given its potentially deadly nature and its potential for use in a large-scale chemical attack, cyanide has been a chemical of interest of various governmental agencies including but not limited to the U.S. Departments of Defense and Homeland Security (Bebarta et al., 2014a, b). Concerns about inadequate stocking of cyanide antidotes, and the limitations of current antidotes for mass casualty application in the event of a large-scale exposure have been highlighted (Gasco et al., 2013). Some limitations of IV hydroxocobalamin include the need for intravenous access, high volume administration, and the need for reconstitution of the lyophilized compound prior to administration. Given these limitations, other routes of administration of antidotes have been explored (Bebarta et al., 2014a, b, 2017). In addition to studying the intraosseous and intramuscular routes of administration of established cyanide antidotes, further studies have been directed at understanding the effect of these antidotes with other routes of exposure to cyanide, particularly oral exposure (Brenner et al., 2017; Ng et al., 2018, 2019).

With the current need to prepare for a potential mass exposure event, efforts have been directed toward finding an effective antidote that can be administered in a small volume intramuscularly. The intramuscular administration of sodium tetrathionate and dimethyl trisulfide in animal models of acute cyanide toxicity has been reported (Hendry-Hofer et al., 2019, 2020). There are studies of hydroxocobalamin derivatives, such as cobinamide, a precursor to hydroxocobalamin. Structurally, cobinamide has two potential binding sites for cyanide compared with hydroxocobalamin's single site. Cobinamine is more water-soluble compared with hydroxocobalamin, allowing a smaller volume of administration making it a better candidate for intramuscular injection which would be more practical in the prehospital, mass casualty scenario. Both small and large animal studies have demonstrated the efficacy of cobinamide in the treatment of acute cyanide poisoning (Lee et al., 2016; Bebarta et al., 2014a, b; Petrikovics et al., 2019).

Summary

Cyanide is a potentially deadly chemical that can be found in various settings. The development of treatments for cyanide toxicity is ongoing. Methemoglobin inducers such as aminophenol and nitrites, substrates for biotransformation such as sodium thiosulfate and dimethyl trisulfide, and compounds that directly bind cyanide such as hydroxocobalamin and cobinamide have been explored. The larger areas of investigation include antidotes that can be ideally used in the prehospital, mass casualty setting and that can be administered without advanced procedures (e.g., IV access) and in a small volume.

References

Antal M. The application of cobalt labelling to electron microscopic investigations of serial sections. J Neurosci Methods 1984;12(1):69–77.

Bebarta VS, Pitotti RL, Boudreau S, Tanen DA. Intraosseous versus intravenous infusion of hydroxocobalamin for the treatment of acute severe cyanide toxicity in a swine model. Acad Emerg Med 2014a;21(11):1203–11.

Bebarta VS, Tanen DA, Boudreau S, Castaneda M, Zarzabal LA, Vargas T, Boss GR. Intravenous cobinamide versus hydroxocobalamin for acute treatment of severe cyanide poisoning in a swine (*Sus scrofa*) model. Ann Emerg Med 2014b;64(6):612–9.

Bebarta VS, Brittain M, Chan A, Garrett N, Yoon D, Burney T, Mukai D, Babin M, Pilz RB, Mahon SB, Brenner M, Boss GR. Sodium nitrite and sodium thiosulfate are effective against acute cyanide poisoning when administered by intramuscular injection. Ann Emerg Med 2017;69(6):718–25.

Borron SW, Baud FJ, Barriot P, Imbert M, Bismuth C. [b] Prospective study of hydroxocobalamin for acute cyanide poisoning in smoke inhalation. Ann Emerg Med 2007a;49(6):794–801.

Borron SW, Baud FJ, Megarbane B, Bismuth C. Hydroxocobalamin for severe acute cyanide poisoning by ingestion or inhalation. Am J Emerg Med 2007b;25(5):551–8.

Breen PH. Protective effect of stroma-free methemoglobin during cyanide poisoning in dogs. Anesthesiology 1996;85(3):558–64.

Brenner M, Azer SM, Oh KJ, Han CH, Lee J, Mahon SB, Du X, Mukai D, Burney T, Saidian M, Chan A, Straker DI, Bebarta VS, Boss GR. Oral glycine and sodium thiosulfate for lethal cyanide ingestion. J Clin Toxicol 2017;7(3):355.

Brink NG. Vitamin B12: the identification if vitamin B12 as a cyano-cobalt coordination complex. Science 1950;112(2909):354.

Burrows GE. Cyanide intoxication in sheep: enhancement of efficacy of sodium nitrite, sodium thiosulfate and cobaltous chloride. Am J Vet Res 1979;40(5):613–7.

Chen KK, Rose CL. Nitrite and thiosulfate therapy in cyanide poisoning. JAMA 1952;149(2):113–9.

Chen KK, Rose CL, Clowes HA. Methylene blue, nitrites and sodium thiosulphate against cyanide poisoning. Exp Biol Med 1933;31(2):250–1.

Christel D, Eyer P, Hegemann M, Kiese M, Lorcher W, Weger N. Pharmacokinetics of cyanide in poisoning of dogs, and the effect of 4-dimethylaminophenol or thiosulfate. Arch Toxicol 1977;38(3):177–89.

Clemedson C, Hultman HI, Sorbo B. A combination of Rhodanese and Ethanethiosulfonate as an antidote in experimental cyanide poisoning, research Institute of National Defense, Medical Development, Sundbyberg, Sweden and the Biochemical Department of the Medical Nobel Institute. Acta Physiol Scad 1955;35(1):31–5.

Evans JC. Cobalt compounds as antidotes for hydrocyanic acid. Br J Pharmacol Chemother 1964;23(3):455–75.

Eyer P, Kiese M, Lipowsky G, Weger N. Reactions of 4-dimethylaminophenol with hemoglobin, and autoxidation of 4-dimethylaminophenol. Chem Biol Interact 1974;8(1):41–59.

Friedberg KD, Shukla UR. The efficiency of aquocobalamine as an antidote in cyanide poisoning when given alone or combined with sodium thiosulfate. Arch Toxicol 1975;33(2):103–13.

Gasco L, Rosbolt MB, Bebarta VS. Insufficient stocking of cyanide antidotes in US hospitals that provide emergency care. J Pharmacol Pharmacother 2013;4(2):95–102.

Geiger JC. Methylene blue solutions in potassium cyanide poisoning. JAMA 1933;101(4):269.

Hall AH, Kulig KW, Rumack BH. Suspected cyanide poisoning in smoke inhalation complications of sodium nitrite therapy. J Toxicol Clin Exp 1989;9(1):3–9.

Hendry-Hofer TB, Witeof AE, Lippner DS, Ng PC, Mahon SB, Brenner M, Rockwood GA, Bebarta VS. Intramuscular dimethyl trisulfide: efficacy in a large swine model of acute severe cyanide toxicity. Clin Toxicol 2019;57(4):265–70.

Hendry-Hofer TB, Witeof AE, Ng PC, Mahon SB, Brenner M, Boss GR, Bebarta VS. Intramuscular sodium tetrathionate as an antidote in a clinically relevant swine model of acute cyanide toxicit. Clin Toxicol 2020;58(1):29–35.

Himwich WA, Saunders JP. Enzymatic conversion of cyanide to thiocyanate. Am J Phys 1948;153(2):348–54.

Jandorf BJ, Bodansky O. Therapeutic and prophylactic effect of methemoglobinemia in inhalation poisoning by hydrogen cyanide and cyanogen chloride. J Ind Hyg Toxicol 1946;28:125–32.

Johnson WS, Hall AH, Rumack BH. Cyanide poisoning successfully treated without 'therapeutic methemoglobin levels. Am J Emerg Med 1989;7(4):437–40.

Kaczka EA, Wolf DE, Kuehl FA, Folkers K. Vitamin B12: reactions of cyano-cobalamin and related compounds. Science 1950;112(2909):354–5.

Kiese M. Formation of ferrihaemoglobin with aminophenols in the human for the treatment of cyanide poisoning. Eur J Pharmacol 1969;7(1):97–105.

Kruszyna R, Kruszyna H, Smith RP. Comparison of hydroxylamine, 4-dimethylaminophenol and nitrite protection against cyanide poisoning in mice. Arch Toxicol 1982;49(3–4):191–202.

Lee J, Mahon SB, Mukai D, Burney T, Katebian BS, Chan A, Bebarta VS, Yoon D, Boss GR, Brenner M. The vitamin B12 analog cobinamide is an effective antidote for oral cyanide poisoning. J Med Toxicol 2016;12(4):370–9.

Ng PC, Hendry-Hofer TB, Witeof AE, Brenner M, Mahon SB, Boss GR, Bebarta VS. Characterization of a swine (Sus scrofa) model of oral potassium cyanide intoxication. Comp Med 2018;68(5):375–9.

Ng PC, Hendry-hofer TB, Witeof AE, Mahon SB, Brenner M, Boss GS, Bebarta VS. Efficacy of oral administration of sodium thiosulfate and glycine in a large, swine model of oral cyanide toxicity. Ann Emerg Med 2019;74(3):423–9.

Paulet G, Oliver M. On the subject of the therapeutic value of hydroxocobalamin in hydrocyanic acid poisoning. Ann Pharm Fr 1962;21:133–7.

Pearce LL. Reversal of cyanide inhibition of cytochrome c oxidase by the auxiliary substrate nitric oxide: an endogenous antidote to cyanide poisoning. J Biol Chem 2003;278(52):52139–45.

Petrikovics I, Budai M, Kovacs K, Thompson DE. Past, present and future of cyanide antagonism research: from the early remedies to the current therapies. World J Methodol 2015;5(2):88–100.

Petrikovics I, Kiss L, Chou CE, Ebrahimpour A, Kovacs K, Kiss M, Logue B, Chan A, Manage ABW, Budai M, Boss GR, Rockwood GA. Antidotal efficacies of the cyanide antidote candidate dimethyl trisulfide alone and in combination with cobinamide derivatives. Toxicol Mech Methods 2019;29(6):438–44.

Riou B, Baud FJ, Astier A, Barriot P, Lecarpentier Y. In vitro demonstration of the antidotal efficacy of hydroxocobalamin in cyanide poisoning. J Neurosurg Anesthesiol 1990;2(4):296–304.

Riou B, Gerard JL, La Rochelle CD, Bourdon R, Berdeaux A, Giudicelli JF. Hemodynamic effects of hydroxocobalamin in conscious dogs. Anesthesiology 1991;74(3):552–8.

Riou B, Berdeaux A, Pussard E, Giudicelli JF. Comparison of the hemodynamic effects of hydroxocobalamin and cobalt edetate at equipotent cyanide antidotal doses in conscious dogs. Intensive Care Med 1993;19(1):26–32.

Rose CL, Worth RM, Chen KK. Hydroxo-cobalamin and acute cyanide poisoning in dogs. Life Sci 1965;4(18):1785–9.

Silvestroni A, Fimiani R. Use of hydroxocobalamin in experimental cyanide poisoning. Folia Med 1964;47:667–80.

Ten Eyck R, Schaerdel AD, Ottinger WE. Stroma-free methemoglobin solution: an effective antidote for acute cyanide poisoning. Am J Emerg Med 1985;3(6):519–23.

Ten Eyck R, Schaerdel AD, Ottinger WE. Comparison of nitrite treatment and stroma-free methemogobin solution as antidotes for cyanide poisoning in a rat model. J Toxicol Clin Toxicol 1985–1986;23(7–8):477–87.

Uhl W, Notling A, Golor G, Rost KL, Kovar A. Safety of Hydroxocobalamin in healthy volunteers in a randomized, placebo-controlled study. Clin Toxicol 2006;44(1):17–28.

WHO Model List of Essential Medicines. WHO model list of essential medicines; April 2013.

Winter CA, Mushett CW. Absence of toxic effects from single injections of crystalline vitamin B12. J Am Pharm Assoc Am Pharm Assoc 1950;39(6):360–1.

Section 4

Clinical toxicology and poison control in the United States

Alan D. Woolf

Boston Children's Hospital & Harvard Medical School, Boston, Massachusetts, United States

Introduction

The origins and growth of poison control in the United States, along with the growth of clinical toxicology as a specialty in medicine, are reviewed in this section. Although the origins of both predate the 1950s, we chose this decade to start our review because it marks the post-World War II beginnings of the formal organization of U.S. poison control centers (PCCs). Initially, pediatricians and pharmacists sparked the professionalization of clinical toxicology. Since then, clinical toxicology as a specialty has grown and flourished, with contributions from leaders in basic and clinical research, as well as those intent on improving the provision of poisoning-related personal and public health care services.

The U.S. poison control movement started with rudimentary resources: notes on products and poisons kept on index cards in a file, with some poison handbooks and pharmacology texts as references. It has matured over the subsequent 70 years into an integrated, organized system, with expert consultation and advice accessible to both health professionals and the general public 24 h daily.

The PCCs, at first, were staffed by a few volunteer health professionals armed only with a specific interest in poisoning. Later, a cadre of health professionals was trained using a more organized and comprehensive toxicology curriculum. They came from diverse backgrounds and disciplines: in pharmacy, pharmacology, nursing, military medicine, occupational and preventive medicine, forensic medicine, pediatrics, emergency medicine, internal medicine, nephrology, surgery, other medical specialties, veterinary science, and others. These specialists acquired their credentials in clinical and medical toxicology as a newly recognized field in medicine. They now comprise the workforce staffing the PCCs, toxicology treatment centers, and other clinical services.

This section is divided into five chapters, each covering a different era in the development of poison control: the origins and growth (1950s and 1960s), an era of consolidation and standardization (1970s and 1980s), an era of computerization, continued regionalization, and improvements in surveillance and clinical services (1990s), and finally, the advent of stable Federal funding and the continuing revolution in information technology (2000s to today). We devote a separate fifth chapter to describe the growth of professional expertise, research, and societies devoted to clinical toxicology. We have also included here Tables 1 and 2 which include the timelines of legislation and professional societies, as well as some important milestones in the development of PCCs and clinical toxicology in the U.S.

TABLE 1 TimeLine: U.S. poison control and clinical toxicology.

Year	Event
1952	American Academy of Pediatrics establishes Accident Prevention Committee
1953	First U.S. Poison Control Center—Chicago, Illinois
1957	National Clearinghouse for Poison Control Centers (NCHPCC) established
1957	*The Clinical Toxicology of Commercial Products* book, 1st edition sponsored by FDA
1958	American Association of Poison Control Centers (AAPCC) founded
1962	First "National Poison Prevention Week"—3rd week in March annually (PL 87–319 [75 Stat. 681])
1966	Baby aspirin packaging limited to 36 tablets and 81 mg each
1968	American Academy of Clinical Toxicology (AACT) founded
1970	FDA requires first patient package insert (oral contraceptives)
1974	Poisindex product database on microfiche

TABLE 1 TimeLine: U.S. poison control and clinical toxicology—cont'd

Year	Event
1974	American Board of Medical Toxicology (ABMT) established
1975	First ABMT Certification Exam in Medical Toxicology offered to physicians
1978	AAPCC introduces quality standards to certify PCC
1982	CPSC requires tamper-resistant packaging
1983	First AAPCC Certification Exam for Specialist in Poison Information
1983	First TESS annual report published
1985	Poisindex available on CD-ROM for computers
1987	NCHPCC terminated by FDA
1987	American Board of Applied Toxicology (ABAT) founded by AACT
1992	Computerized retrieval of poison information introduced
1992	American Board of Medical Specialties (ABMS) recognizes Medical Toxicology
1993	ABMT is dissolved
1993	American College of Medical Toxicology (ACMT) founded and replaces ABMT
1994	First ABMS Certification Exam in Medical Toxicology offered for physicians
1995	FDA improves imprint coding of medications to allow easier identification
1997	Iron supplement medication packaging requires changes to protect children
2000	Accreditation Council in Graduate Medical Education (ACGME) approves Medical Toxicology as a specialty training program
2001	Federal funding of U.S. Poison Control Centers
2001	First U.S. nation-wide toll-free telephone number activated 1-800-222-1222
2003	Real time analyses of national data on poisoned cases introduced
2014 and 2015	WebPoisonControl and poisonhelp.org both launched

Modified Box 4-1: Institute of Medicine. Forging a Poison Prevention and Control System. Chapter 4: Historical Context of Poison Control. The National Academies Press, Washington DC, 2004.

TABLE 2 U.S. clinical toxicology-related agencies, legislation.

1906—Pure Food & Drug Act ('Wiley' Act)

1927—The Federal Caustic Poison Act

1930—Food & Drug Administration (FDA) created (previously Food, Drug & insecticide Administration, Bureau of Chemistry) (https://www.fda.gov)

1938—U.S. Food, Drug & Cosmetic Act

1947—Federal Insecticide, Fungicide, & Rodenticide Act (FIFRA)

1951—Humphrey-Dunham Drug Prescription Act

1960—Federal Hazardous Substances Act (FHSA)

1961—National Poison Prevention Week (3rd week in March) (PL 87–319 (745 Stat. 681))

1963—Clean Air Act

1966—Child Protection Act

1970—Poison Prevention Packaging Act (creates Consumer Product Safety Commission [CPSC])

1970—EPA and NIOSH (https://www.epa.gov, https://www.osha.gov, https://www.cdc.gov/niosh/index.htm)

1971—Lead-Based Paint Poisoning Prevention Act (LBPPPA)

1971—U.S. OSHA created (https://www.osha.gov)

1972—Clean Water Act

1973—Emergency Medical Services Act of 1973 (PL 93–154)

1976—Toxic Substances Control Act (TSCA)

1978—National Toxicology Program (NTP)

1980—Comprehensive Environmental Response, Compensation & Liability Act (CERCLA)

1994—DSHEA—Dietary Supplement Health & Education Act

1997—FDA Modernization Act

2000—Poison Control Center Enhancement & Awareness Act (Pl 106–174) (Feb 25th)

2002—Homeland Security Act of 2002 (Sec 505)

2003—Poison Control Center Enhancement and Awareness Act Amendments of 2003 (PL 108–194) 117 Stat. 2888 (December 19th)

2008—Poison Center Support, Enhancement and Awareness Act of 2008 (PL 110–377)

2014—Poison Center Network Act (PL 113–77)

2018—Poison Center Network Enhancement Act of 2018 (never enacted)

2019—The Poison Center Network Enhancement Act of 2019, H.R. 501 & S. 1199

Author created table.

1906—Pure Food and Drug Act (Wiley Act)

Created the Food, Drug, and Insecticide Administration (which, in 1930, became the FDA). Required governmental oversight and approval of foods and drugs, leading to a ban on most 'patent medicines'. Protected the public from adulterated foods and misbranded patent medicines. The Wiley Act was later strengthened by the 1938 Food, Drug & Cosmetic Act. (source: https://catalog.archives.gov/id/5716297 accessed on June 17, 2020.).

1927—The Federal Caustic Poison Act

Stipulated that lye, acids, and other caustic-containing commercial products available to the public had to prominently display a "poison" warning on the label. The legislation was intended to protect children from unintentional poisoning with household caustic cleaning agents.

1938—Federal Food, Drug, and Cosmetic Act

Passed as a direct result of the 1937 sulfanilamide tragedy (see Chapter 2.1). Required pharmaceutical companies to submit a 'new drug application' with scientific data confirming the drug's safety prior to interstate shipment for marketing to the general public. It banned drugs that were dangerous to the public and prohibited false or misleading advertising and package labeling. Labeling required listing of active ingredients and directions for use for any over-the-counter products available without prescription. However, the legislation did not require proof of efficacy of the drug for the health condition or disease; it did not extend to pre-marketing clinical trials in humans; animal testing was not standardized. While penalties for infractions of the law were increased, if the FDA did not act on a new drug application within 60 days, it was automatically approved for sale to the public. United States Pharmacopeia (USP), an independent organization, was recognized in the 1938 Act as the public, good manufacturing standard-setting agency for all prescription medications, non-prescription drugs, and other healthcare products sold in the U.S. (source: https://research.archives.gov/description/299847 accessed on June 17, 2020).

1951—Humphrey-Dunham Drug Prescription Act

Categorized drugs into those requiring a prescription by a physician and those that could be purchased 'over-the-counter' without a prescription. This act codified trends in the commercial availability of drugs; previously most drugs (except narcotics) could be purchased by consumers without any restrictions. As a barrier to obtaining potent medications such as antibiotics without authorization, it altered the patient-doctor relationship (source: http://www.gpo.gov/fdsys/pkg/STATUTE-65/pdf/STATUTE-65-Pg648.pdf accessed on June 17, 2020).

1960—Federal Hazardous Substances Act (Title 15 U.S. Code, Section 1261)

This Act required proper precautionary labeling of a broad array of commercial products intended for use by consumers in the home or farm. Included were those substances that were toxic, corrosive, flammable, combustible, a strong irritant or sensitizer, or one that would generate pressure through heating or other means. It required listing of their contents and relative toxicity. The intent was to warn consumers about hazardous chemicals that might pose a danger to young children and what they needed to do to protect themselves and their children. Implementation of the Act was later assigned to the Consumer Product Safety Commission. At first the Act did not prevent the sale of products containing chemicals too hazardous for home use regardless of the labeling warnings. Amendments later allowed the CPSC to ban products so dangerous that labeling warnings would be insufficient to protect the public (source: https://www.govinfo.gov/app/details/USCODE-2013-title15/USCODE-2013-title15-chap30-sec1261 accessed on June 17, 2020).

1961—National Poison Prevention Week (PL 87-319)

Established on September 26, 1961 and endorsed by Present Kennedy. It set the 3rd week in March as the annual National Poison Prevention week to focus public education campaigns on protecting young children from household hazards (source: https://www.govtrack.us/congress/bills/87/hjres358/text accessed on June 17, 2020).

1962—Kefauver new drug amendments

Required comprehensive animal studies of drugs by pharmaceutical companies for safety and efficacy prior to any human testing. It required FDA monitoring of all stages of pre-marketing research into new drugs, including Phase 3 clinical trials. Any time constraints for FDA actions regarding new drug applications were removed (source: http://www.gpo.gov/fdsys/pkg/STATUTE-76/pdf/STATUTE-76-Pg780.pdf accessed on June 17, 2020).

1966—Child Protection Act

This piece of legislation gave the Secretary of Health Education & Welfare the power to interdict interstate commerce of some chemicals and products deemed too hazardous for use in households regardless of labeling and to put a hold on the distribution of a suspect substance during a legal appeals process (source: https://legislation.lawi.us/child-protection-act-of-1966/ accessed on June 17, 2020).

1970—Poison Prevention Packaging Act (PPA)

This landmark legislation was directed towards the prevention of childhood poisoning by setting forth standards of safe packaging that were mandated for pharmaceuticals and consumer products before they were marketed to the public. It included the technology of "child resistant containers" (CRCs), which was intended to prevent the unintentional poisoning of a young child. A young child would developmentally not have attained the fine and gross motor skills required to open the container. Yet opening the container would not be so difficult as to prevent its use by the adult and elderly population. CRCs were intended to remind adults of the need to prevent poisoning in the home by restricting the access of young children to drugs and household products (source: https://www.cpsc.gov/Regulations-Laws--Standards/Statutes/Poison-Prevention-Packaging-Act accessed on June 17, 2020).

1971—Lead-Based Paint Poisoning Prevention Act (LBPPPA; PL 91-695)

This Act specified lead-based paint chips as a health hazard, defined "lead-based paint" as that containing $> 1\%$ lead (later amended to 0.06% or 600 ppm), set the level of lead in blood of concern at $60\,\mu g/dL$ (later lowered several times and set in 2012 at $5\,\mu g/dL$), and set standards for abatement (later amended to be much more rigorous). It required the Secretary of Health Education & Welfare (later Department of Health & Human Services) to prohibit the use of lead-containing paint in any residential structures either newly constructed or rehabilitated by the Federal government or with Federal assistance (source: https://uscode.house.gov/view.xhtml?path=/prelim@title42/chapter63&edition=prelim accessed on June 17, 2020).

1972—Consumer Product Safety Act (PL 92-573)

The enactment of this piece of legislation led to the formation of the U.S. Consumer Product Safety Commission (CPSC). The CPSC was charged with protecting the public against unreasonable risks of injury associated with consumer products, to assist them in assessing comparative safety of products, to develop uniform safety standards, and to encourage research into the causes and prevention of product-related mishaps. The CPSA also provided for a national Advisory Committee which made recommendations concerning product labeling and safety. Members included Drs. Arena, Haggerty and Rumack (see Chapters 4.1 and 4.2) (source: https://www.cpsc.gov/Regulations-Laws--Standards/Statutes/Summary-List/Consumer-Product-Safet-Act accessed on June 17, 2020).

1973—National Emergency Services System Act (PL 93-154-93 Stat 2410)

This legislation mandated a systems approach to emergency care. It included critical care systems for such emergencies as burns, spinal cord injuries, life-threatening cardiac events, and poisonings. The Act promoted regionalized trauma and burn centers and indirectly funded some poison control activities, promoting the integration of PCCs into emergency medical services (EMS) (source: https://www.govinfo.gov/app/details/STATUTE-87/STATUTE-87-Pg594 accessed on June 17, 2020).

1994—DSHEA—Dietary Supplement Health and Education Act

This legislation defined the term "dietary supplement" and exempted manufacturers of such products from the need for pre-marketing testing to demonstrate their safety or effectiveness. Manufacturers were not required to collect or report adverse effects involving their dietary supplement products. DSHEA largely prohibited the Food & Drug Administration from any regulatory oversight of these products unless they presented a clear and immediate danger to the public's health (source: https://ods.od.nih.gov/About/DSHEA_Wording.aspx accessed on June 23, 2020).

2000—Poison Control Center Enhancement and Awareness Act (PL 106-174; EO 12372)

This legislation addressed the crisis in funding of U.S. PCCs by allocating funds to support universal toll-free telephone access to regional poison control services, support PCC operations, and encourage the upgrade of non-certified PCCs to certified status (source: https://www.govinfo.gov/app/details/PLAW-106publ174 accessed on May 28, 2020).

2003—Poison Control Center Enhancement and Awareness Act Amendments (PL 108–194)

This law was intended to stabilize the funding of PCCs and maintain access to a nationwide toll-free emergency phone number. It was occasioned by the tragic events of September 11, 2001 and the subsequent terrorism-inspired cases of anthrax identified in October of the same year.

A 2001 Presidential Task Force on Citizen Preparedness in the War on Terrorism recommended that PCCs be used as the source of public information and education regarding potential biological, chemical and nuclear domestic terrorism. Subsequently, PL 108–194 was enacted. It also enhanced the roles of the CDC and ATSDR Federal Agencies in the maintenance of a national system of toxic exposure surveillance. It allocated $2,000,000 annually from 2000 to 2009 for maintenance of a nationwide toll-free number, $600,000 annually for a media campaign to promote PCCs, and $25,000,000 for years 2000–2004 and $27,500,000 for 2005–2009 for sustaining PCCs and promoting their progress towards AAPCC certification (source: https://www.govinfo.gov/app/details/PLAW-108publ194 accessed on May 28, 2020).

2008—Poison Center Support, Enhancement and Awareness Act (PL 110–377)

This legislation reauthorized the national toll-free telephone number and public education campaign and extended the previous direct funding of PCCs at about 15%–20% of their operating budget (source: https://www. govinfo.gov/app/details/PLAW-110publ377 accessed on May 28, 2020).

2014—Poison Center Network Act (PL 113-77—113th congress)

This legislation reauthorized the national toll-free telephone number and public education campaign and extended the previous direct funding of PCCs at about 15%–20% of their operating budget. https://www.govinfo. gov/app/details/PLAW-113publ77

2018—Poison Center Network Enhancement Act of 2018 (HR 5329—115th congress)

This law would have enhanced poison control center capacity to address the opioid crisis by coordinating its efforts with other health care agencies. It was passed by the House but was not advanced by the Senate and so was never enacted. https://www.govtrack.us/congress/bills/115/hr5329

2019—Poison Center Network Enhancement Act of 2019 (HR 501; S 1199—116th congress) would reauthorize federal funds used to support poison control. Its provisions are similar to such legislation in the past. https://www.congress.gov/bill/116th-congress/senate-bill/1199/all-info

Further reading

Institute of Medicine. Historical context of poison control. In: Forging a poison prevention and control system. Washington, DC: The National Academies Press; 2004. https://doi.org/10.17226/10971 [chapter 4].

U.S. Federal Register. Poison control stabilization and enhancement grant program. Vol. 66, number 44; 2001. p. 13548–50. Tuesday March 6. https://www.federalregister.gov/ documents/2001/03/06/01-5500/poison-control-stabilization-and-enhancement-grant-program.

Chapter 4.1

U.S. Poison Control Centers get organized: 1950s–1960s

Alan D. Woolf

Boston Children's Hospital & Harvard Medical School, Boston, Massachusetts, United States

Pediatric origins

Young children have always been an age group with a very high incidence of unintentional poisonings and toxic exposures. They rely on adults for their supervision to protect them from harm and help them escape from hazardous situations. Their curiosity, energy, oral exploratory behaviors, and inability to discriminate between edibles and nonedibles all make them vulnerable to a poisoning exposure event. Their immature body systems, including a growing, developing nervous system, are sensitive to injury. Their lungs, liver, and kidneys are not fully functional in their roles in detoxifying and eliminating substances; these organs continue to develop throughout the early childhood years.

Hazardous products, such as leaded paint, kerosene used in space heating, and arsenicals in indoor pesticides had been commonly stored in households for decades (Haggerty, 1970). Mishaps in the home accounted for numerous childhood poisonings and deaths every year. A pediatrician in the 1930s, Dr. Jay Arena, developed an interest in the prevention of childhood poisoning during his residency under the mentorship of a prominent pediatrician at Duke University, Dr. Wilbur C. Davison (Fig. 4.1.1). Together these early pioneers in the poison control movement described new treatments for children suffering from caustic injuries secondary to lye ingestion. Liquid lye was a common cause of childhood poisoning in the 1920s and 1930s, because it was easily mistaken for milk and was often stored in open containers. Poisonings remained a prominent cause of childhood injury and death throughout the 1930s and 1940s.

History of Modern Clinical Toxicology. https://doi.org/10.1016/B978-0-12-822218-8.00018-1

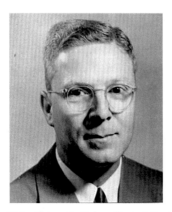

FIG. 4.1.1   Dr. Jay Arena, Duke University Poison Control Center. *(Photo: Duke University Medical Center Archives, with permission.)*

By the 1950s, Americans were experiencing a post-World War II boom in housing and consumerism, with an unprecedented demand for household conveniences. This expansion spawned a rise in the manufacturing of new chemicals and commercial products, some of which (e.g., caustics, petroleum distillates used in cleaners, and kerosene used in heating) were potentially quite toxic. There were over 250,000 different trade-name substances on the market (Scherz and Robertson, 1978). With so many products coming into homes, it was an impossible task for any one practitioner to be informed about all of them and give expert advice to the public. A centralized storehouse of scientific knowledge about drugs, chemicals, household products, plants, and other substances could fill in that knowledge gap. At the same time, a "baby boom" of increased numbers of children being born in the post-World War II era produced a spike in the age group most vulnerable to unintentional poisoning: that is, young children. Consequently, there were more than 800 childhood poisoning deaths recorded each year in the 1950s (Haggerty, 1957).

Thus it is no surprise that pharmacists and pediatricians were in the vanguard of the poison control movement in the United States. They led the way in seeking new strategies to prevent some of these poisoning incidents. Mr. Louis Gdalman, a pharmacist in Chicago, was another such pioneer in poison control. He had already established a poison information service in the pharmacy at St. Luke's Hospital in Chicago in the 1930s, providing information to nurses and physicians working in the emergency department (Botticelli and Pierpaoli, 1992). By the 1950s, he had accumulated a library of resources covering over 9,000 commercial and consumer products and a standard form to be used in recording information about a poisoning incident (IOM, 2004). Later, when the American Academy of Pediatrics (AAP) established the first poison control center (PCC) in Chicago in 1953, he was the only pharmacist involved (Fig. 4.1.2).

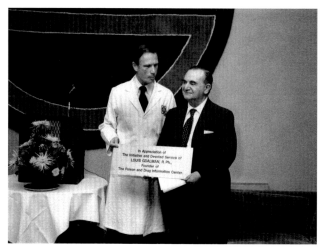

FIG. 4.1.2   Louis Gdalman, RPh. *(Courtesy Rush Medical School Archives.)*

First US Poison Control Center—Chicago, IL

Another prominent pediatrician, Dr. George Wheatley, was a vice president for health at the Metropolitan Life Insurance Company for 33 years, where he pursued his interest in childhood injury prevention. A leader in the AAP, he advocated for lowering the amount of harmful lead in house paint, for child-resistant enclosures for medicines, and for nonflammable children's clothing. He was also an early proponent of childhood poisoning prevention (Fig. 4.1.3).

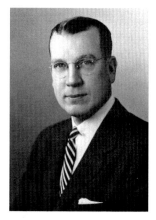

FIG. 4.1.3   Dr. George Wheatley. *(Courtesy AAP Publications.)*

In 1950, the Illinois Branch of the AAP commissioned a work group, the Accident Prevention Advisory Committee, led by Dr. Wheatley as committee chairman and including Drs. Edward Press and Jay Arena and Louis Gdalman. The work group's charge was to study the occurrence and epidemiology of accidents involving children (Mofenson, 1975; IOM 2004). Collaborating with other representatives from national organizations such as the National Safety Council, the US Children's Bureau, and Metropolitan Life Insurance Company, the group used available sources of data to study the rate of childhood injury and explore ways to prevent such accidents. Findings confirmed the prominence of poisoning; it comprised 51% of childhood accidents. The group's report noted the particular problem of baby aspirin, which was implicated in far too many inadvertent and sometimes lethal, childhood poisonings (Arena, 1963).

Subsequently, the nation's first PCC was established 3 years later in 1953 in Chicago, IL, and called the Chicago Area Poisoning Control Program. This was a pilot program sponsored by the Illinois Chapter of the AAP, in collaboration with the Illinois Health Department, and treatment and referral centers at seven local hospitals (Mofenson, 1975; Botticelli and Pierpaoli, 1992). The new PCC was led by Dr. Edward Press. Besides the hospitals and health department, the new center also forged ties with the State Toxicology Laboratory, also located in Chicago, and the City Board of Health Laboratory (Press and Mellins, 1954). Dr. Press developed a poisoning case report form which included questions about the toxic substance involved, the victim and circumstances of the poisoning. A separate follow-up report form was created. Completed reports were sent to the health department to be archived, summarized and analyzed (Press and Mellins, 1954). Dr. Press and the AAP also began to publish a monograph listing ingredients and toxic properties of common household products. It became a popular reference for clinical toxicologists and PCC staff. By 1961, 11 hospital-based drug and poison information centers in Chicago had been consolidated into one PCC based at Presbyterian-St. Luke's Hospital with Dr. Joseph Christian as the medical director and pharmacist Gdalman as operations director (IOM, 2004). Its scope of services had been broadened by its advisory committee to include telephoned consultations from the general public.

While the Chicago PCC was at first set up only as a pilot project, soon the idea caught fire, with the opening of many hospital-based PCC manned by a variety of professionals around the country. Dr. Arena founded the Duke University Poison Control Center, the second PCC in the country, in 1954 and directed it for the next 25 years. The third US PCC, a consortium involving seven different Massachusetts hospitals, was founded in 1955 and coordinated by Dr. Robert Haggerty, its Director from 1955–1964 (Fig. 4.1.4). The Cleveland Information Center, founded by Dr. Irving Sunshine, was opened shortly thereafter. By the end of 1956, there were 17 such centers in operation in the United States.

From the beginning, PCCs in the United States were seen as a resource that should be accessible for consultation 24 h each day. Centers were usually

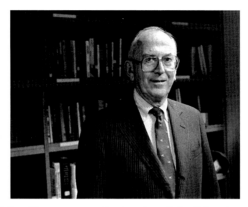

FIG. 4.1.4 Dr. Robert Haggerty, an early champion of the U.S. poison control movement. *(Courtesy: Archives of the University of Rochester Miner Library History of Medicine Section, with permission.)*

based in academic hospitals or affiliated with schools of pharmacy or medicine. They relied on physicians, health care (pharmacy, nursing, or medical) students, nurses, and/or pharmacists to staff the requests for telephone consultations coming in. Although originally intended to provide only consultations to health professionals, soon the users of PCC services expanded. The clientele was seen not only as health professionals but also the lay public, unlike in Europe where similar centers were intended to provide consultation to physicians, who remained in charge of their patient (Govaerts, 1970). In contrast, as many as 80%–90% of the calls to US PCCs were from the general public (Lovejoy Jr and Alpert, 1970).

Proliferation of U.S. Poison Control Centers—1960s

PCCs as a resource for health professionals and the public were an idea whose time had come. Their value was immediately recognized and PCCs proliferated throughout the country. In the beginning, their development was erratic and uncoordinated. Although state health departments in theory had to approve such initiatives, every hospital wanted to offer this benefit to their clientele, and public health officials acquiesced to these demands. By 1960 there were over 347 such centers situated in hospitals around the United States; by 1961 there were 450 centers; by 1962 there were 490 centers; and by the end of the decade there were 661 PCC in the United States (Anonymous, 1962; Robb et al., 1963; Scherz and Robertson, 1978). Such spectacular growth was encouraged by health care professionals and the hospitals in which they worked. Lacking were any local, state, or national standards as to how such a PCC should operate. There was no one model for how they should be staffed, what qualifications should be expected of those giving advice, what facilities should be available to PCCs, or how they should be financed beyond what the sponsoring hospital could provide, which was quite variable.

There was no directive as to which clientele the PCC should serve and how such encounters should be documented and archived. Some centers served a catchment area of only a few 1000 people, whereas others served millions. They duplicated each other's work and there was little coordination or sharing of information or resources. There was little assurance that the centers would be adequately publicized to make sure that the community was aware of their existence and could be encouraged to use them. While the creation of a new PCC would occasion feature stories in newspapers or on the radio, there was no systematic approach to marketing their services to the public or health professionals (Robb et al., 1963). While some PCCs saw a steady growth in their utilization and handled up to 80 calls/day, others received only one or two, if any, calls in any given day (Crotty and Vehulst, 1970; Scherz and Robertson, 1978).

Some centers only employed pediatric resident trainees, supported by clerical staff, in answering calls. Many PCCs did not have a full-time medical director. Since the service was an "add-on" to the resident's other hospital responsibilities, they were sometimes unable to respond to questions immediately. One 1960 survey of families noted delays as a frequent complaint about the service (Robb et al., 1963). In a 1970 national survey, poison information was given out by nurses (43%), doctors (32%), house-staff (9%), pharmacists (14%), and secretaries (2%) (Lovejoy Jr and Alpert, 1970). Many PCCs did not have access to a toxicology laboratory that could reliably assay body fluid specimens for the quantification of chemicals, drugs, or poisons; such expertise did not exist in many areas of the country.

There was marked variation in the quality of the information received by the public from the PCC. There was little accountability or oversight regarding whether the advice they gave over the telephone was accurate, let alone whether following that advice would lead to safer decision-making in an emergency situation. This shortcoming was recognized nationally and the Secretary of the Department of Health, Education and Welfare established an infrastructure for the sharing of such information. This entity became known as the National Clearinghouse for Poison Control Centers (NCHPCC).

National Clearinghouse for Poison Control Centers 1957–1987

NCHPCC was established by the Surgeon General within the Bureau of Product Safety, a division of the Food & Drug Administration under the direction of Henry L. Verhulst, PharmD, in 1957 to distribute information on commercial products to PCCs and collect and analyze reports of poisoning from them (Anonymous, 1962; Arena, 1963). NCHPCC became the first national agency to collect data systematically from the 17 existing PCCs, using a templated paper carbon-copy data form. The NCHPCC also compiled toxicity information on consumer products on 5″ × 8″ index cards for use by PCCs and published a monthly newsletter summarizing new scientific advances in clinical toxicology. It published the textbook *The Clinical Toxicology of Commercial Products,* edited by Drs. Harold Hodge, Marion Gleason, and Robert Gosselin (Gleason, Gosselin, & Hodge, 1957). This was a compendium with ingredient information on more than 25,000 household products, both as generic ingredients and by trade name, as a reference guide for PCCs (Scherz and Robertson, 1978). NCHPCC also published the AAP's *Handbook of Common Poisonings in Children* (Crotty and Armstrong, 1978). Even in the 1960s, NCHPCC and others were exploring rudimentary ways to encode, store, and retrieve poison information and poison case data in computer systems, using state-of-the-art machines (at the time) such as the IBM360 (Thoman, 1998) (Figs. 4.1.5 and 4.1.6).

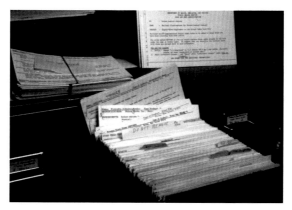

FIG. 4.1.5 NCHPCC card file system. *(Courtesy Dr. Barry Rumack.)*

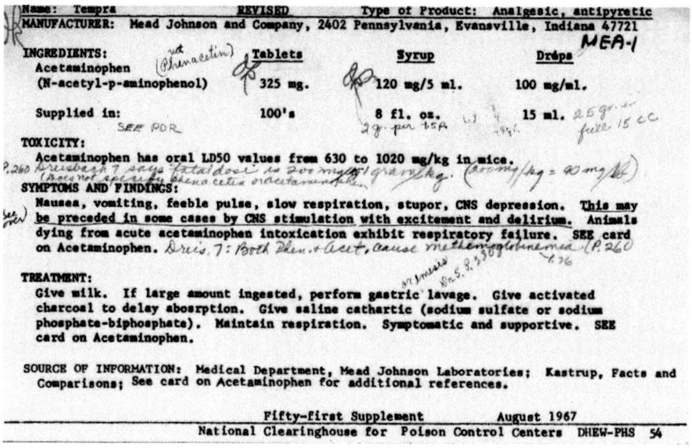

Name: Tempra REVISED Type of Product: Analgesic, antipyretic
MANUFACTURER: Mead Johnson and Company, 2402 Pennsylvania, Evansville, Indiana 47721
MEA-1

INGREDIENTS:	Tablets	Syrup	Drops
Acetaminophen (N-acetyl-p-aminophenol)	325 mg.	120 mg/5 ml.	100 mg/ml.
Supplied in:	100's	8 fl. oz.	15 ml.

SEE PDR

TOXICITY:
Acetaminophen has oral LD50 values from 630 to 1020 mg/kg in mice.

SYMPTOMS AND FINDINGS:
Nausea, vomiting, feeble pulse, slow respiration, stupor, CNS depression. This may be preceded in some cases by CNS stimulation with excitement and delirium. Animals dying from acute acetaminophen intoxication exhibit respiratory failure. SEE card on Acetaminophen.

TREATMENT:
Give milk. If large amount ingested, perform gastric lavage. Give activated charcoal to delay abosrption. Give saline cathartic (sodium sulfate or sodium phosphate-biphosphate). Maintain respiration. Symptomatic and supportive. SEE card on Acetaminophen.

SOURCE OF INFORMATION: Medical Department, Mead Johnson Laboratories; Kastrup, Facts and Comparisons; See card on Acetaminophen for additional references.

Fifty-first Supplement August 1967
National Clearinghouse for Poison Control Centers DHEW-PHS 54

FIG. 4.1.6 Typical NCHPCC card. *(Courtesy Dr. Barry Rumack.)*

By the 1970s, over 150,000 poisoning exposure cases were being submitted annually to NCHPCC from 480 of 580 PCCs in 47 states (Waldman et al., 1976; Crotty and Armstrong, 1978). The NCHPCC collected the limited data from participating centers and published an aggregated report every 2 years in an attempt to portray the scope of poisoning exposures in the United States (IOM, 2004). However, the process was fragmented, with erratic voluntary reporting, incomplete standardization of data, and ambiguous definitions. NCHPCC reporting forms were complicated, cumbersome to complete and submit, and often ignored by PCC staff. NCHPCC was neither charged with oversight of the quality of poison control services delivered by the centers, nor did it have authority over how PCCs were run, whether they had adequate staffing, or what should be the qualifications of the people running them. As time went on, the constraints of limited NCHPCC authority, an inadequate number of staff, and reduced funding undermined its effectiveness. Its mandate within the FDA was gradually scaled back even more, to just providing periodic poisoning information, until the program itself ended in 1987. By then the Toxic Exposure Surveillance System, a much more standardized and efficient data collection system sponsored by the American Association of Poison Control Centers, was up and running (see Chapter 4.2).

Other information sources

Besides NCHPCC resources, clinical toxicologists and PCCs had a variety of other sources of information about chemicals and poisons. Robert Dreisbach had first published his widely used "little black book," *Handbook of Poisoning: Diagnosis and Treatment* in 1955 (Dreisbach et al., 1955). Edward Press, with the AAP's Committee on Accident Prevention, published *Accidental Poisoning in Children* in 1956 (Press et al., 1956). Jay Arena's *Poisoning*, Clinton H. Thienes and Thomas J. Haley's *Clinical Toxicology,* and the *Textbook of Toxicology* by Dubois and Geiling were three others in use by the late 1960s or early 1970s. PCCs themselves had also been collecting and archiving index cards documenting their own cases and experience, but these were incomplete and disorganized at many centers or not kept at all in others. A national survey of PCCs in 1962 found that adequate information on ingested products was not available in 8.2% of 17,873 telephone consultations (Lovejoy Jr and Alpert, 1970).

The National Library of Medicine (NLM) improved its information services during the 1960s with initiatives such as creation of the "Medical Literature Analysis and Retrieval System" (MEDLARS), the Toxicology Bibliography, and the Toxicology Information Program (TIP) databases. NLM offered its resources to PCCs as a central repository of scientific toxicological information collected from a variety of sources (Rice, 1969).

In 1968, a new international journal, *Clinical Toxicology*, was founded by leaders in clinical toxicology and was published quarterly by Marcel Dekker Publisher. Dr. Richard T. Rappolt Sr was its founding executive editor and the journal was informally affiliated with the American Academy of Clinical Toxicology. Its principal aim was "to present authoritative and critical articles, notes, case histories, and reviews dealing with all medical and scientific aspects of toxicology" (Rappolt, 1968). From the start, it enjoyed a wide readership across many professional disciplines.

By 1969, 16 poisoning handbooks, 9 drug reference manuals, and 31 other references covering chemicals, pesticides, plants, animals, and pharmacology and metabolism were recommended to PCCs to be curated for consultation as needed (Dacre, 1969).

Poisoning prevention in the United States

- Poisoning prevention education

    The poison control movement in America has always included the goal of poisoning prevention. The pioneering clinical toxicologists of the 1950s who founded PCCs recognized the importance of preventing as many childhood poisonings as possible. Of first importance was increasing access of the public and health professionals to the telephone number of the PCC. Even by 1970, 72% of surveyed PCCs did not have a listing in their local telephone directories (Lovejoy Jr and Alpert, 1970). There was a great need to "market" the services of poison control both to health professionals and the general public. This would not be accomplished until later, when the organizational infrastructure of PCCs improved in the 1970s and 1980s.

    However, PCCs had already begun to get involved in poison prevention education outreach at the community level even in the 1950s (Press and Mellins, 1954). Families were warned about potential hazardous chemicals and products in the home. Medical practitioners were urged to limit the amount of drug dispensed, counsel parents about their safe storage up and out of reach in cupboards, and provide them with first aid charts and pamphlets outlining what to do in case of an emergency at home (Anonymous, 1962). Interestingly, in 1964 the Poison Control Branch of the Public Health Service's Division of Accident Prevention published "*A Guide for Teaching Poison Prevention in Kindergartens*" which was adopted by several states (U. S. DHEW, PHS, 1965).

- Child-resistant containers

    Poisoning prevention uses three overarching strategies: technology, regulation, and education. Mitigating the hazard that baby aspirin posed to young children is an example of the application of all three. During the 1940s, when "flavored" baby aspirin was first marketed to parents, children were poisoned when they ate the drug thinking it was candy. Several hundred children died from aspirin poisoning each year. The invention of child-resistant containers (CRCs) and tamper-proof packaging are examples of technology aimed at preventing mishaps involving household medicines and products. The idea of CRCs was fostered by pediatricians and clinical toxicologists, with support from the AAP, other national organizations, and industry itself. Dr. Jay Arena worked with drug companies to develop this approach to childhood poisoning prevention (Arena, 1959; Arena, 1963). In 1958, the FDA held a meeting with manufacturers who voluntarily agreed to lower the baby aspirin dosage and reduce the number of tablets to 36 in each bottle.

Later, Dr. Henri Breault from Tecumseh, Ontario Canada invented the "Palm 'n Turn" locking child-resistant enclosure (Breault, 1974). This CRC and two others required that the caps be effective in preventing toddlers from opening medicines while at the same time not being overly difficult for the elderly population to use. These devices were studied by a committee formed by the FDA in 1966. The Industry-FDA Safety Closure Committee, chaired by Dr. Press and including Drs. Arena and Verhulst, as well as representatives from the pharmaceutical industry, container manufacturers, and liaisons from the U.S. Children's Bureau, FDA, AAP, and U.S. Public Health Service (Industry—FDA Safety Closure Committee, 1969) culminated in the passage of the "Poison Prevention Packaging Act" by Congress in 1970. This piece of legislation codified the responsibility of manufacturers to insure the safety features of their products prior to marketing. CRCs have become the standard enclosure for prescribed medications. The public was educated about the dangers of medications like aspirin and were instructed on the need for and proper use of CRCs. All of these measures were successful in lowering the childhood aspirin fatality rate from 25% in the 1950s to less than 1% by the late 1970s. Since their widespread introduction in 1974, CRCs were shown to reduce substantially the rate of inadvertent childhood medicine poisonings and aspirin-related deaths (Breault, 1974; Palmisano, 1981; Walton, 1982) (Fig. 4.1.7).

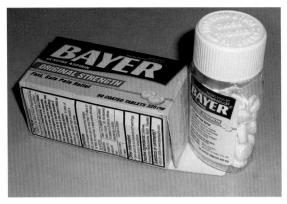

FIG. 4.1.7 Example of "twist and turn" child-resistant cap on a bottle of aspirin. *(Source: Wikimedia Commons.)*

- Poison prevention week

  Other nationwide efforts to inform the public about the dangers drugs and chemicals posed for young children and how to contact the local PCC in an emergency, led to extensive public education campaigns. Even in the early 1960s, there were still more than 500 childhood poisoning deaths and 500,000 childhood poisonings occurring in the United States each year (Haggerty, 1963). The passage of federal legislation (PL 87-319) on September 26, 1961, marked the beginning of an annual national public education campaign by declaring the 3rd week in March of each year to be "Poison Prevention week." President Kennedy endorsed the legislation and the first Poison Prevention Week was held in March of 1962, with oversight from the National Poison Prevention Week Council, a group of nonprofit organizations addressing safety issues.

- Pill and tablet imprinting

  The identification of unlabeled medicine or free tablets or pills found in the home that were suspected to be involved in a poisoning posed a serious challenge to clinical toxicologists. The director of the Washington PCC in Seattle, Dr. Bill Robertson, devoted much of his free time to advocating for better pill identification throughout the 1960s and 1970s. He worked directly with the pharmaceutical industry on perfecting a system of unique codes to be imprinted on tablets and, later on, capsules to facilitate their identification. This would require an expensive re-engineering of the manufacturing process that was resisted by the industry for many years.

- Home storage of ipecac

  Health care providers also had traditionally recommended as a first aid measure the evacuation of an ingested poison by vomiting to prevent its absorption and reduce the possibility of serious injury. Clinical toxicologists recognized in the 1950s that this first aid measure could begin in the home. Although several emetics: salt water, apomorphine, copper sulfate, and ipecac had been used in the past to evacuate the stomach, ipecac was the safest, least expensive, and could be stored at home for poisoning emergencies. The FDA recognized this by removing the prescription requirement for syrup of ipecac, thus making it easily obtained by the public. A very concentrated and much more toxic product, ipecac extract, could easily be mistaken for the syrup. It was removed from most pharmacies and hospital formularies. The dose of syrup of ipecac was adjusted to insure over 90% efficacy in inducing emesis. PCCs soon began to advocate for the storage of syrup of ipecac in the homes of families with young children so that, in case of a poisoning emergency and only upon the recommendation of a PCC, it could be given at home.

Progress of poison control in the 1960s

Despite the many shortcomings of individual PCCs, the 1960s still saw promising signs of positive outcomes from these national efforts. The rate of child poisoning deaths in the United States fell from 2.3/100,000 in 1961 to 1.7/100,000 population by 1967—a 25% drop (Haggerty, 1970). And this decline occurred before child-resistant packaging legislation had been enacted. While some of the decline could be attributed to trends away from using some particularly dangerous products in the home, such as liquid lye, it was apparent that PCCs were making a difference.

But by the end of the 1960s, the need to make poison control advice more consistent and based on scientific evidence, to professionalize the clinical toxicology workforce, and to set standards for the operations of PCCs was recognized. These widely recognized weaknesses of the poison control movement needed to be addressed (Teitelbaum, 1968). Improvements in PCC operations became the focus of the 1970s and 1980s, the subject of Chapter 4.2.

References

Anonymous. N Engl J Med 1962;267(26):1371–2.

Arena JM. Safety closure caps. JAMA 1959;169:1187–8.

Arena JM. Poisoning: chemistry, symptoms, treatments. Springfield, IL: Charles C. Thomas; 1963.

Botticelli JT, Pierpaoli PG. Louis Gdalman, a pioneer in hospital pharmacy poison information services. Am J Hosp Pharm 1992;49(6):1445–50.

Breault HJ. Five years with 5 million child resistant containers. Clin Toxicol 1974;7(1):91–5.

Crotty JJ, Armstrong G. National clearinghouse for poison control centers. Clin Toxicol 1978;12(3):303–7.

Crotty JJ, Vehulst HL. Organization and delivery of poison information in the United States. Pediatr Clin North Am 1970;17:741.

Dacre JC. Recommended reference books for poison control/information centers. Clin Toxicol 1969;2(2):165–9.

Dreisbach RH. Handbook of poisoning: diagnosis and treatment. Los Altos, CA: Lange Publishers; 1955.

Gleason MN, Gosselin RE, Hodge HC. Clinical toxicology of commercial products: acute poisoning (home and farm). Baltimore, MD: Williams & Wilkins Publishers; 1957.

Govaerts M. Poison control in Europe. Pediatr Clin North Am 1970;17:729–39.

Haggerty RJ. The Boston poison information center. N Engl J Med 1957;257:1050–1.

Haggerty RJ. National Poison Prevention Week: 1963. N Engl J Med 1963;268(10):559–60.

Haggerty RJ. Childhood poisoning: an overview. Pediatr Clin North Am 1970;17(3):472–5.

Industry—FDA Safety Closure Committee. Progress report on the industry-FDA safety closure committee. Clin Toxicol 1969;2(3):345–6.

IOM (Institute of Medicine); Forging A Poison Control And Prevention System. Chapter 4: Historical context of poison control (pp. 81-105). National Academies Press, Washington DC, 2004.

Lovejoy Jr FH, Alpert JJ. A future direction of poison centers: a critique. Pediatr Clin North Am 1970;17(3):747–53.

Mofenson HC. The American Association of Poison Control Centers (founded 1958). Clin Toxicol 1975;8(1):77–9.

Palmisano PA. Targeted intervention in the control of accidental drug overdoses by children. Pub Heal Rep 1981;96(2):150–6.

Press E. Accidental poisoning in children. Springfield, IL: Charles C. Thomas; 1956.

Press E, Mellins RB. A poison control program. Am J Public Heal 1954;44:1515–25.

Rappolt RT. Clinical Toxicology: aims and scope. Clin Toxicol 1968;1:1.

Rice CN. The role of specialized information centers in toxicological information systems. Clin Toxicol 1969;2(1):105–9.

Robb GL, Elwood HS, Haggerty RJ. Evaluation of a poison center. Am J Pub Heal 1963;53(11):1751–60.

Scherz RG, Robertson WO. The history of poison control centers in the United States. Clin Toxicol 1978;12(3):291–6.

Teitelbaum DT. New directions in poison control. Clin Toxicol 1968;1:3–13.

Thoman M. The American Academy of Clinical Toxicology: a historic pediatric perspective. J Toxicol Clin Toxicol 1998;36(5):399–400.

U. S. DHEW, PHS. United States Department of Health, Education, and Welfare, Public Health Service, Division of Accident Prevention, A Guide for Teaching Poison Prevention in Kindergartens and Primary Grades. Publ. 1381; September 1965.

Waldman JM, Mofenson HC, Greensher J. Evaluating the functioning of a poison control center. Clin Toxicol 1976;15(1):75–9.

Walton W. An evaluation of the Poison Prevention Packaging Act. Pediatrics 1982;69(3):363–70.

Chapter 4.2

Era of regionalization and standardization: 1970s–1980s

Alan D. Woolf

Boston Children's Hospital & Harvard Medical School, Boston, Massachusetts, United States

Redefining the mission of PCCs

The control of morbidity and mortality from poisonings, and their prevention, would include educational outreach to both the public and health professionals practicing primary care. The concept of the *control* of such events was incorporated into the scope of a center's services, so that instead of "poison information centers," a more apt description of these centers of expertise would be "poison control centers." However, some toxicologists felt the word "control" limited their scope of operations, and they marketed their services simply as those of a "poison center."

It was recognized by the 1970s that PCCs could and should play an important role in the education of health professionals at all levels—from developing curricula for students and clinical trainees to offering continuing education for health care practitioners (Temple, 1977). Training of their own staff and the next generation of health professionals in clinical toxicology was central to the goals adopted by many PCCs. The faculty, acquiring toxicology expertise that would set them apart from other practitioners, participated in the education of health care students and more advanced trainees (see Chapter 4.5). Faculty could provide students with opportunities for contact with a diverse group of health care professionals, with specialized knowledge in such areas as environmental and industrial toxicology, mycology, herpetology, marine biology, acute and intensive care medicine, extracorporeal methods for poison removal, and toxicokinetics. The PCC gave the student a unique educational experience, showcasing a model of daily inter-professional interactions between nurses, pharmacists, physicians, first responders, and others. The range of learners included students coming from schools of pharmacy, nursing, public health, and medicine, as well as public health staff, health care practitioners, trainees (interns, residents, and clinical fellows) from teaching hospitals, and other community-based health professionals.

History of Modern Clinical Toxicology. https://doi.org/10.1016/B978-0-12-822218-8.00005-3

Early on, pharmacists were enlisted in the management of patients with acute poisoning, and clinical toxicology was included in their pharmacy school curriculum (Kinnard, 1971). In some hospitals, pharmacists and pharmacology departments had created separate "drug information" services, focusing on drug identification, drug-drug interactions, dosing and kinetics, and the concerns of special populations, such as pregnant and lactating women. As pharmacists became increasingly involved with the development of PCCs, many such drug information centers eventually merged staff, forming one unified source of information and training (Czajka et al., 1979; Wilson, 1980; Troutman and Wanke, 1983). And yet some hospital-based pharmacy programs, often affiliated with schools of pharmacy or medicine, continued to offer telephone-based drug information centers to assist callers with the rational use of medicines. One report identified 194 such centers still operating in the United States in the early 1990s (Beaird et al., 1992). Some of these centers answered poison information calls as well, but most would triage such callers directly to PCCs.

The Motherisk program, originally established in 1985 at the Hospital for Sick Children in Toronto, Canada, also operated a telephone-based consultative service to women of reproductive age and pregnant and lactating women concerned about potential toxic exposures. PCCs often would triage such callers to the Motherisk program, which could provide more detailed and specialized information about teratogenicity and other concerns. While some PCCs answered callers with questions about poisoning exposures involving animals, most referred such callers to dedicated animal hotlines maintained by veterinarians.

Research and PCCs

New professional societies and innovative infrastructures to support the science of clinical toxicology and poison control emerged nationally in the 1970s and accelerated in the 1980s (see Chapter 4.5). The mission of PCCs, operating within professional schools and academic medical centers, also often included research aims, to extend the science of clinical toxicology and thereby improve medical treatments, saving lives and affording poisoning victims a better chance for recovery.

Clinical toxicologists quickly realized the value of PCC-generated data in advancing research in the epidemiology, triage, and treatment of poisoning. The PCC adopted the additional mission of serving as a source of information about trends in poisoning, the frequency products were implicated, profiles of the victims of specific exposures, and signals offered by the data. In this way, PCCs could identify new, unappreciated toxicity, new hazardous agents, adverse and toxic effects of newly introduced drugs, and newly described vulnerable subpopulations of patients. Postmarketing product surveillance was soon demonstrated to be an additional PCC function.

Data collected by PCCs could be used by Federal agencies (e.g., EPA, FDA, CPSC, and CDC) or private industry (e.g., pharmaceutical companies) seeking additional surveillance methods for agent categories such as pesticides or newly marketed drugs. For example, while the FDA had operated a system of reporting adverse drug reactions (ADRs), Medwatch, the reporting mechanism was detailed and cumbersome; under-reporting was an enormous problem. With the wider participation of emergency departments, outpatient clinics, and other venues reporting their ADRs directly to a PCC, those reported ADRs could supplement the FDA's data and provide a second "early warning system" for drug-related safety concerns (Holland and Marcus, 1987).

New methodologies were required to measure the impact of centers on the communities they served. Clinical research in the 1970s and 1980s documented the need for and effectiveness of PCCs (Sagotsky et al., 1977; Geller and Looser, 1985). One such study of 1744 pediatric poisoning episodes found that less than 1% of PCC callers versus 28% of noncallers made unnecessary visits to an emergency department (Chafee-Bahamon and Lovejoy Jr., 1983). Studies found that PCCs meeting the AAPCC's provisional criteria for certification provided better and more consistent poison information than did noncertified centers, and were more often utilized by people in their catchment areas than those served only by small local centers (Thompson et al., 1983; Marcus et al., 1984).

Who will pay?

Challenges inherent in sustaining 24-h availability of services were insurmountable for some PCCs. Operating in small hospitals without much in the way of staff or funding, they might only get 1 call per day. Many PCCs were dependent for financing solely on the budgets of the institutions (hospitals or academic schools of medicine or pharmacy) in which they were housed. That funding was often inadequate to cover the expenses they incurred and many relied on staffing by students and volunteer health care professionals.

It was recognized by the 1970s that the constraints of cost inefficiencies, unpredictable staff availability, limited physical space, and insufficient marketing would close some centers. If hospitals were threatened with financial losses themselves because of changes in the economic climate, administrators often viewed poison control as an elective line item that could be deleted to maximize cost containment. Thus some PCCs began to explore a variety of financing mechanisms to support their services and diversify their funding streams. For example, a model of annual member hospital dues was adopted in Massachusetts in 1979 to supplement state funding and private donations (Chafee-Bahamon and Lovejoy Jr., 1984). This model was sustained throughout the 1980s, although it later proved to be unstable. As affiliated hospitals faced their own crisis-level fiscal challenges throughout the 1980s and into the 1990s, some closed and others merged, reducing both the number of hospital members and the amount of funding they could commit to this purpose. Other financing models were adopted by other centers. In Utah, a telephone surcharge was levied on the public to pay for the 24-h accessibility of telephone emergency services, including poison control.

Some state governments were willing to provide funds for emergency services to PCCs through their departments of public health. The passage of the Federal Emergency Health Services Act in 1973 provided an infusion of federal funds to emergency medical services and PCCs, administered through state health departments. Still the availability of those funds to PCCs varied by state. Other funding sources included county or city funding, charitable grants, and contracts with pharmaceutical firms, pesticide and household product manufacturers, or other companies interested in tracking adverse events involving their products. Some PCCs operated industry-sponsored "hotlines" for managing safety inquiries from consumers. Some PCCs contracted with state-level departments of public health to create dedicated lines for specific consultations—for example, inquiries about possible exposures to animals with rabies or, later in the 1980s, operating an HIV/AIDS hotline.

Regionalization

Toward the end of the 1960s, prominent clinical toxicologists such as Dan Teitelbaum, Fred Lovejoy, Joel Alpert, and Bob Haggerty, had called for the regionalization of PCCs to address redundancies and inefficiencies of their operations, while improving the quality and consistency of the medical advice being given to both the public and health professionals alike (Teitelbaum, 1968; Haggerty, 1970; Lovejoy Jr and Alpert, 1970). However, the impetus to create additional centers continued unabated into the 1970s. Hospitals saw their entrance into the provision of poison control services as a sign of distinction and marketed their PCC as evidence of their commitment to the community. Some of these "centers" consisted only of a telephone line, part-time clerical staff, and a few volunteer students and health care professionals with little toxicology expertise and limited resources. Most centers were not well-publicized and were under-utilized; fewer than 6% of PCCs received more than 9–10 calls/day (Manoguerra and Temple, 1984). By 1978 there were still 661 PCCs throughout the United States (Scherz and Robertson, 1978). Early studies evaluated the effectiveness of PCCs and gave mixed reviews as to their ability to triage poisonings appropriately to stay home or seek emergency medical services. There were delays in the PCC's response to an inquiry. There was a lack of public awareness of simple poisoning prevention strategies. Clerks could nort always identify the product, plant or mushroom involved in the exposure (Waldman et al., 1976; Sagotsky et al., 1977). It was soon appreciated that the needs of both health professionals and the public transcended the provision of simple (and sometimes delayed or inaccurate) telephone advice.

Cost constraints, staffing limits, overlapping population service catchment areas, and variability in the quality of information provided ushered in a new emphasis on efficiencies in operations (Lerner and Warner, 1988). Many hospitals could no longer support the costs of providing the service, and PCCs were closed or combined to become a more regionalized, statewide center of excellence (or one covering multiple states) (Schleich and McIntire, 1984). For example, 11 hospitals formed a single Rocky Mountain Poison Center in Colorado (Rumack et al., 1978); one regional center covered all of Utah (Temple and Veltri, 1978); the Pittsburgh Poison Center established and coordinated seven "satellite" facilities (Moriarty, 1978); and Massachusetts consolidated seven hospital-based PCCs into one system serving the entire state (Lovejoy Jr et al., 1979). Consolidation along the political and funding units of state-wide resources occurred, such that there were only 384 PCCs operating in 1983.

AAPCC certification criteria

The American Association of Poison Control Center (AAPCC), founded in 1958 and centered in Washington, DC, became the primary professional organization representing the specialty (Mofenson, 1975). One of its goals was to develop an infrastructure that promoted a more consistent level of expert advice and poisoning response by member centers. It should not matter where you live; if you suffered a poisoning, you should receive the same quality of medical advice. To achieve this goal nationally, the AAPCC formulated standards for regional PCCs starting in 1978, and the Executive Committee of the AAPCC's Board of Directors had approved a set of minimal national standards of operations. Only those member centers meeting these metrics of outstanding service were eligible to be certified:

- A regional poison information service available at all times, with toll-free telephone accessibility.
- A regional system for providing comprehensive poisoning care, including at least one comprehensive poison treatment center having a direct relationship with the poison information service for regionalized referral and transport.
- Availability of comprehensive analytical toxicology services and an appropriate transport system for severely poisoned patients.
- Management protocols for the initial management of public calls and standardized recommendations for health professional calls.
- Documentation of calls through a regional poisoning data collection and reporting system.
- An outreach health professional education program.
- An outreach public education program.

Beyond these mandatory general requirements, details were included regarding the determination of the optimal size of a catchment region by geography and population served (usually not less than 1 million people or more than 10 million), qualifications of the PCC staff, what regional poisoning treatment capabilities should be available, and how such services should be coordinated with those of the PCC. Sixteen PCCs met these newly promulgated criteria (Table 4.2.1).

TABLE 4.2.1 Original 16 certified US Poison Control Centers.

Cardinal Glennon Poison Center, St. Louis, MO

Children's Hospital of Michigan Poison Control center, Detroit, MI

Children's Mercy Hospital Poison Center, Kansas City, MO

Children's Orthopedic Hospital Poison Center, Seattle, WA

Georgia Poison Center (Grady Memorial Hospital), Atlanta, GA

Hennepin Poison Center, Minneapolis, MN

Inter-mountain Poison Control Center, Salt Lake City, UT

Life Line, University of Rochester Medical Center, Rochester, NY

Massachusetts Poison Control System, Boston, MA

Nassau County Medical Center Poison Center, East Meadow, NY

Nebraska Poison Center, Children's Hospital, Omaha, NE

Texas State Poison Center, Galveston, TX

University of California at Davis, Sacramento, CA

University of California at San Diego, San Diego, CA

University of New Mexico Poison Center, Albuquerque, NM

West Michigan Poison Center, Grand Rapids, MI

Source: Notes of Dr. William Robertson.

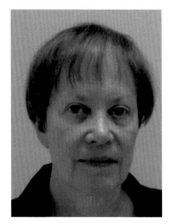

FIG. 4.2.1   Dr. Toby Litovitz.

The certification of PCCs accelerated in the 1980s under the influence of AAPCC and its leader, Toby Litovitz. Dr. Litovitz, an emergency medicine physician at Georgetown University and a clinical toxicologist, had founded the National Capital Poison Center in Washington, DC, in 1980 and thereafter served in various leadership capacities in the AAPCC from 1984 to 2005, including the position of its president from 1990 to 1992 and executive director from 1994 to 2004 (Fig. 4.2.1). Her efforts were spurred on by pressure to elevate the quality of clinical services PCCs provided. The creation of AAPCC certification criteria for regional PCCs provided leverage for individual centers to recruit state public health officials and legislators to support meeting the criteria by granting the facility adequate annual funding. Another influential clinical toxicologist, Dr. Anthony Temple, a pediatrician, became the medical director of the Intermountain (later, Utah) Regional PCC. He later joined the medical department of McNeil Consumer Products Company in 1979 and secured funding from McNeil to help some centers reach the high standards required to become certified.

Poison information retrieval

The original impetus for the development of poison control was the need for detailed information about a toxin or the ingredients of a commercial product and what adverse health effects might result from a human exposure. No one health care professional could be expected to have ready access to such specialized information that was crucial to making good medical decisions, and so centralized resources of such guidance were established starting in the 1950s. Those health professionals interested in clinical toxicology relied on textbooks and handbooks describing poisons and poisoning. Many clinical toxicologists kept $3'' \times 5''$ or $5'' \times 7''$ index card file systems with product or chemical information and, separately, index cards describing decontamination methods, enhanced elimination, use of antidotes, and other medical management measures. Some kept informal records of their cases which they archived and referred to when they were confronted with new patients who had similar clinical presentations. As early as the 1960s, researchers were investigating the use of computers to archive and retrieve toxicology information for use by PCCs or drug information services (Kwok and Ledley, 1968; Anderson and Tester, 1969). By the 1970s, the National Library of Medicine had organized journal articles into an online format called MEDLINE. Clinicians worked with librarians to adapt such resources for use in responding to the poisoning information needs in a busy emergency department (Schaap and Sunshine, 1975).

Poisindex

As PCCs got more organized, new tools were developed to assist these specialists in their work. Immediate access to sources of detailed, accurate information about specific drugs, commercial products, or other potential toxins and

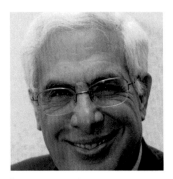

FIG. 4.2.2 Dr. Barry Rumack.

xenobiotics was tremendously important to everyday PCC operations (Temple, 1977). Various systems of written information were developed to assist clinicians, including the NCHPCC Card System. Dr. Barry Rumack, director of the Rocky Mountain Poison Center, introduced a change in the information retrieval paradigm in 1974 with the proprietary system, Poisindex (Fig. 4.2.2). Poisindex contained ingredient information on 50,000 products, linked to a microfiche reader system for easy retrieval (Rumack, 1975). Each microfiche card might carry over 2000 entries. Many companies, but not all, voluntarily provided lists of ingredients contained in their products and their toxicities. There was no government mandate to provide proprietary information and some manufacturers did not reveal their products' contents.

Medical advisors with toxicology expertise devised algorithms that paired product ingredients, poisons, venoms, and others with appropriate medical treatment recommendations. These experts ensured that the treatment guidance, whether in the home or in the emergency department, was based on the best scientific evidence at the time. This microfiche poison information system was originally designed for use only in Colorado. Dr. Rumack then reached out to his colleague, Dr. Frederick H. Lovejoy Jr., the medical director of the Boston Poison Control Center. Together they installed the microfiche system there as a second test site. It proved so successful that, by 1977, Poisindex was disseminated widely to well over 550 hospitals throughout the United States, Canada, and more than 10 foreign countries. Poisindex was publishing ingredient information on 160,000 products and updating managements coded directly to those products, assisted by an editorial board of 43 toxicologists and consultants.

A parallel microfiche-based database of product ingredients, botanicals, chemicals, and other potential poisons, Toxfile, was developed in Chicago and the NCHPCC continued to distribute poisoning information to PCCs, but neither of these tools was as comprehensive or widely accepted as Poisindex (Fig. 4.2.3).

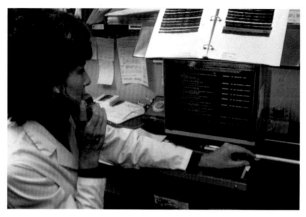

FIG. 4.2.3   Specialist in Poison Information using microfiche system. *(Courtesy: Dr. Barry Rumack.)*

Responding to a potential poisoning exposure call using the microfiche reader involved two steps: detailed ingredient or chemical class information, including symptoms and signs of typical poisoning, was located on one microfiche film, and then medical management guidance organized by chemical category was detailed on a separate microfiche film. Information retrieval from microfiche was tedious and time consuming, and especially awkward with a parent waiting for advice on the telephone. By 1985, Poisindex had abandoned the two-step microfiche process and the database was published for the first time on CD-ROM for use with personal computers. Again, it was piloted first at the two PCCs: by Rumack at Rocky Mountain Poison Center in Denver and Lovejoy at the Massachusetts Poison Control system. This new format featured rapid access to extended, referenced information that was updated quarterly. It now served as the primary reference tool utilized by most PCCs in the United States and those in many other countries.

The activities of PCCs had expanded in the 1980s to include drug identification information to callers even when an exposure had not occurred. The Micromedex Corporation, makers of Poisindex, responded by introducing complementary databases: Identidex in 1974 and Drugdex in 1979, to assist in such activities.

Other sources of poisoning information

In addition, dissemination of the progress in scientific research in clinical toxicology was facilitated by the development of new resources. There was an explosion of new, authoritative textbooks on the science of toxicology and the diagnosis and management of poisonings. The NLM expanded its toxicology offerings, including the *Toxicity Bibliography*, extracting articles from 2500 journals, starting in 1970 and a few years later introduced Toxline, a compendium of abstracts from technical reports (Rice, 1969; Scherz and Robertson, 1978). The *Toxic Effects of Chemical Substances* was published annually by the National Institute for Occupational Safety and Heath (NIOSH), with information on over 26,700 generic chemical compounds. Also, the National Toxicology Program, initiated in 1978, provided a central repository of the results of toxicology research into chemicals and other substances coming from the NIH, NIEHS, FDA, CDC, and other Federal agencies (Huff, 1980).

In 1981, under the leadership of its second editor, Dr. Helmut M. Redetski, the specialty journal *Clinical Toxicology* changed its name to *The Journal of Toxicology: Clinical Toxicology* and promised to broaden its scope by accepting analytical and animal-based toxicology research that included dose-response relationships or kinetic data that directly related to human toxicology (Redetski, 1981). The journal also sought to increase its international readership by accepting contributions from toxicologists worldwide and including clinical toxicologists from other countries on its editorial board. Under its third editor-in-chief Dr. Carol Angle, the journal was formally named the official journal of the American Academy of Clinical Toxicology (AACT) (Angle, 1991). Two years later the European Association of Poisons Centres and Clinical Toxicologists was welcomed as a sponsor. Equal numbers of representatives from each society sat on the editorial board and a portion of the annual member dues of each was dedicated to the support of the journal's publication. Dr. Angle, as the editor-in-chief from 1989 to 2002, provided enormous leadership in shaping the journal's mission, scientific quality, style, and content to become what it still is today.

Another widely read, more informal clinical toxicology journal, *Veterinary & Human Toxicology,* was published by Dr. Frederick Oehme in Manhattan Kansas from 1977 to 2004 and sponsored by the American College of Veterinary Toxicology. It included research on animal as well as human poisonings and, for a time, published the abstracts of the annual clinical toxicology meeting, NACCT. It also served as a repository for information from the two societies: AACT and AAPCC.

Collecting and reporting poison exposures

Throughout the 1970s case histories were documented by individual PCCs but there was no governmental involvement or directives; there did not exist any consistency or uniformity in such PCC activities. Caller-related information might exist only on 3″ × 5″ or 5″ × 7″ paper index cards. The information collected varied from center to center. In 1982, the Poison Surveillance & Epidemiology Section of the FDA awarded funds to the AAPCC Data Collection Committee to develop a functional, uniform data collection system. Joseph Veltri, PharmD, director of the Intermountain Regional PCC (Salt Lake City) worked closely with Dr. Litovitz, to harmonize the data collection records used by PCCs. The resulting template contained details defining the main elements of any poison exposure: date, time, and identification of the toxic agents involved, amount, route(s) and duration of exposure, age and gender of the victim(s), circumstances and environment in which the incident occurred, clinical effects, triage and medical interventions, and the clinical outcome. There were also blank areas where narrative notes could be hand-written. Information characterizing the product, chemical, botanical, or other substance involved in the incident was integrated into the new format, using the seven-digit Poisindex product codes. The template was created in a side-by-side format: information could be collected in the left side during the poisoning call; during or after the call, "bubble" codes were filled in on the detachable right side of the form with an optically readable Sharpie marker. A long-arm hole punch was used to correct coding errors, a tedious process at best. These forms were archived in the PCC. The machine-readable bubble form was optically scanned into an aggregated file and sent to the AAPCC in Washington DC quarterly for conversion to 9-track tapes which were then compiled by Micromedex into the larger national data base for analysis. The standardized data collection tool was launched by AAPCC in 1983 and named the Toxic Exposure Surveillance System (TESS). Successive AAPCC presidents through the 1980s—Anthony Temple, MD, Barry Rumack MD, Regine Aronow, MD, Anthony Manoguerra, PharmD, and William O. Robertson, MD—each worked with Dr. Litovitz to enable the initial development, then later the widespread adoption of uniform data collection by US poison centers (Fig. 4.2.4).

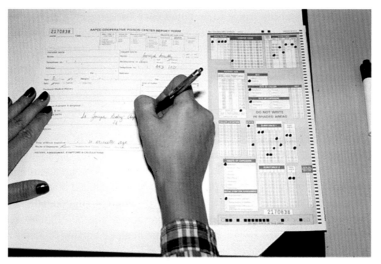

FIG. 4.2.4 Typical AAPCC data collection paper "bubble" form used in the 1980s and 1990s. *(Figure Courtesy Dr. Barry Rumack.)*

Toxic Exposure Surveillance System

TESS data reported by the PCCs were summarized by Dr. Litovitz and her colleagues starting in 1983 (Veltri and Litovitz, 1984), and subsequently published annually by the AAPCC in the *American Journal of Emergency Medicine*. Elements within the dataset were also made available to both private industry and government agencies. By 1984, 47 PCCs (15 certified) were participating in the data collection system; these PCCs still represented less than 50% of the US population. Submission of data on all human poison exposure cases to the TESS database was subsequently required by AAPCC as a mandatory certification criterion. It soon became apparent that there was a market for selected information extracted and compiled from TESS. The AAPCC was able to recoup its costs and return some monies to individual reporting PCCs by charging for data reports. Clients included Federal agencies such as the EPA, CDC, FDA, pharmaceutical companies, and consumer product manufacturers wanting to track postmarketing experience with their commercial products.

Two-tiered approach to PCC staffing

Poison control centers expanded their staffing using mainly three interprofessional sources of expertise: nurses, pharmacists, and physicians. Starting in the 1960s, no longer were telephone calls managed by clerical staff with little toxicology training. Most PCCs adopted a two-tiered approach—the calls were first answered and triaged by a group of intermediary providers—usually nurses, pharmacists, or students in the health professions working under direct supervision. For those poisoning exposure calls deemed by staff to be more serious, especially those requiring triage to an emergency department, a second tier of response was invoked: timely consultation to PCC staff by physicians with expertise in clinical toxicology was sought.

A cadre of specialists in poison information

The explosive growth of PCCs in the 1960s and 1970s created a workforce issue: the need for nonphysician professionals with expertise in clinical toxicology who would answer the phones and serve as the frontline consultants in the PCC. A curriculum centered on the tenets of clinical toxicology and unique to the needs of the public and health professionals was developed by the AAPCC, which sponsored and promoted this specialized training with educational materials and developed criteria to be met before one would be eligible to take the exam (Litovitz et al., 1984). Pharmacy, medical, or nursing students who assisted in answering telephone calls but were still learning the fundamentals of clinical toxicology were known as *poison information providers (PIPs)*. In 1983, the AAPCC's personnel proficiency committee, chaired by Dr. Litovitz, created and administrated the first annual certifying written examination specific to the needs of those nurses, pharmacists, and other health care professionals who were answering the phone calls—the *specialists in poison information (SPIs)*. If you passed your certifying exam, you were then elevated to the rank of *CSPI*. SPI certification was time-limited, so that study and updating by the individual was necessary for his/her recertification every 5 years (more recently extended to every 7 years). CSPIs gave knowledgeable, consistent, and medically correct advice to callers and carried out triage and follow-up of cases, relying on physician-level medical toxicologists who were on-call 24 h daily when the need arose. From 1984 to 1999, AAPCC's annual CSPI exam was prepared by an all-volunteer team of clinical toxicologists, led by Wendy Klein-Schwartz, PharmD, who chaired the personnel proficiency committee for 15 years.

Subsequent studies of the proficiency of SPIs who passed the certification exam were favorable: scores on the certifying exam were higher among SPIs (77%) than the scores of emergency physicians (57%) serving as a control group (Litovitz et al., 1984). Those taking the exams who were nurses or pharmacists fared better with higher pass rates than those who were less well-prepared, such as college graduates, emergency medical technicians, or licensed practical nurses. SPIs staffing regional PCCs and those from PCCs handling more than 15,000 calls per year had higher certification pass rates, arguing for the continued regionalization of poison control (Litovitz et al., 1984).

Poisoning prevention

- Poison prevention education and educators

Poisoning prevention efforts intensified during the 1970s, as PCCs incorporated this goal as an integral part of their mission. Community-based surveys were conducted to determine whether the public knew about their local PCC and how to contact them in an emergency, as well as knowledge about how to prevent such poisoning incidents from involving their children (Waldman et al., 1976; Lacouture et al., 1978). It was recognized that PCCs needed to market themselves to both the public and health care providers as a resource with expertise for consultation for *all* toxic exposures, not just those involving children. PCCs saw increased utilization by physicians in hospitals caring for adults with occupational exposures, patients suffering from adverse effects of medications, distressed individuals attempting suicide by poisoning, and those exhibiting clinical toxicity related to substance abuse. As PCCs matured and gained more professional staff, many hired professional health educators experienced in providing outreach to community members.

- Child-resistant and tamper-proof packaging

The Federal "Poison Prevention Packaging Act" of 1970 combined technology and regulation through legislation to address the public health issue of accidental childhood poisoning. Child-resistant containers (CRCs), unit-dose dispensing (strip packaging), and limiting the number of tablets in a bottle of medicines such as aspirin all made a measurable difference in the incidence of life-threatening poisonings among children, as documented by subsequent studies of their effectiveness (McIntire et al., 1976; Temple, 1978; Walton, 1982). Further packaging changes on many over-the-counter pharmaceuticals and other consumer products were mandated to make them tamper-proof following the Tylenol cyanide murders in Chicago in 1982 (see Chapter 2.3).

- Home storage of ipecac syrup

PCCs continued to recommend home storage of ipecac, with the intent of managing medically low-risk poisonings of young children at home. PCCs would advise caregivers simply to administer the emetic at home. Vomiting would remove enough unabsorbed poison from the stomach so that transfer to a hospital emergency department would be unnecessary. In this way, unnecessary health care visits and costs could be averted. Studies confirmed that home ipecac was effective in inducing vomiting > 98% of the time and children could be kept home without adverse consequences (Veltri and Temple, 1976). There were risks; vomiting is contraindicated in caustic ingestions (Dershewitz and Niederman, 1981) or those involving hydrocarbons or volatile substances.

- Poison warning logos

From ancient times the skull and crossbones have served as the symbol of warning on product containers, chemical-containing bags or drums, and other receptacles containing a potential poison or hazardous substance (Fig. 4.2.5).

The need for another symbol to convey the hazards of household products led to the creation of "Mr. Yuk" stickers and symbols by the Pittsburgh Poison Center in 1971. Mr. Yuk or other logos, such as "Officer Ugg," were adopted by PCCs and incorporated into their public education campaigns. No single national logo had yet emerged (Fig. 4.2.6).

- Uniform, unique medication imprinting

Another poisoning prevention idea was advanced by clinical toxicologists in this era. PCCs were getting increasing numbers of calls asking specialists

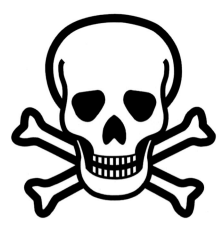

FIG. 4.2.5 Skulls and crossbones poison warning symbols. *(Source: Wikimedia Commons)*

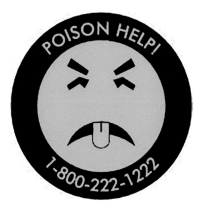

FIG. 4.2.6 The Mr. Yuk logo is a registered trademark of Children's Hospital of Pittsburgh of UPMC. *(Used with permission.)*

to identify a pill or a tablet for them, without any poisoning exposure event. In response, clinical toxicologists, led by Dr. Bill Robertson of the Washington PCC in Seattle, continued to advocate with industry for the uniform imprinting of unique codes on medication capsules, pills, and tablets to make easier their identification (Robertson, 1974).

Advances in research and clinical applications

Throughout the 1970s and 1980s, research in clinical toxicology was yielding new advancements in the science of toxicology and the diagnosis and management of human poisoning. Clinical toxicology was becoming much more evidence-based. Traditional approaches to treatment were being challenged and, when patient benefit could not be substantiated, abandoned. Analytical toxicology employed more precise methodologies in the laboratory to make dramatic progress in the detection and quantification of toxic agents, enabling the use of such information in clinical diagnosis and management. Such progress in clinical toxicology and PCC functioning would continue in the 1990s, spurred on by the rapidly evolving computer age, as described in Chapter 4.3.

References

Anderson HC, Tester WW. A computerized poison information retrieval system. Clin Toxicol 1969;2(1):b81–97.

Angle C. Toxicologists of the world unite. J Toxicol Clin Toxicol 1991;29(1):vii–ix.

Beaird SL, Coley MR, Crea KA. Current status of drug information centers. Am J Hosp Pharm 1992;49:103–6.

Chafee-Bahamon C, Lovejoy Jr FH. Effectiveness of a regional poison control center in reducing excess emergency room visits for children's poisonings. Pediatrics 1983;72:164–9.

Chafee-Bahamon C, Lovejoy Jr FH. Member hospital network for poison control. Vet Human Toxicol 1984;26(Suppl 2):20–3.

Czajka PA, Skoutakis VA, Wood CC, Autian J. Clinical toxicology consultation by pharmacists. Am J Hosp Pharm 1979;36(8):1087–9.

Dershewitz RA, Niederman LG. Ipecac at home-a health hazard? Clin Toxicol 1981;18(8):969–72.

Geller RJ, Looser RW. Cost savings from poison center use by medical consumers. Vet Hum Toxicol 1985;27:521.

Haggerty RJ. Childhood poisoning: an overview. Pediatr Clin North Am 1970;17(3):472–5.

Holland B, Marcus S. Monitoring adverse drug reactions using a state poison control center data base. Drug Information J 1987;21(3):331–4.

Huff JE. National Toxicology Program, Public Health Service, Department of Health Education and Welfare. Clin Toxicol 1980;16(3):405. 406.

Kinnard WJ. The role of the pharmacist in the control of acute poisoning. Clin Toxicol 1971;4(4):659–63.

Kwok RHM, Ledley RS. A computer communication system in the poison control center. Clin Toxicol 1968;1(1):31–7.

Lacouture P, Minisci M, Gouveia WA, Lovejoy FH. Evaluation of a community-based poison education program. Clin Toxicol 1978;13(5):623–9.

Lerner WM, Warner KE. The challenge of privately financed community health programs in an era of cost containment: a case study of poison control centers. J Pub Heal Policy 1988;9:411–28.

Litovitz TL, Klein-Schwartz W, Oderda GM, Easom JM. Poison information providers. An assessment of proficiency. Am J Emerg Med 1984;2(2):129–37.

Lovejoy Jr FH, Alpert JJ. A future direction of poison centers: a critique. Pediatr Clin North Am 1970;17(3):747–53.

Lovejoy Jr FH, Caplan DL, Rowland T, Fazen L. A statewide plan for the care of the poisoned patient: The Massachusetts Poison Control System. N Engl J Med 1979;300:363–5.

Manoguerra AS, Temple AR. Observations on the current status of poison control centers in the United States. Emerg Med North Am 1984;2:185.

Marcus SM, Chafee-Bahamon C, Arnold VW, Lovejoy Jr FH. Effect of a regional poison control system in response to poisoning incidents. Am J Dis Child 1984;138:1010–3.

McIntire MS, Angle CR, Grush ML. How effective is safety packaging? Clin Toxicol 1976;9(3):419–25.

Mofenson HC. The American Association of Poison Control Centers (founded 1958). Clin Toxicol 1975;8(1):77–9.

Moriarty RW. Regionalization: the Pittsburgh experience. Clin Toxicol 1978;12(3):271–6.

Redetski HM. Clinical Toxicology—reflections on the past and future. Clin Toxicol 1981;18(10):iii–v.

Rice CN. The role of specialized information centers in toxicological information systems. Clin Toxicol 1969;2:105–9.

Robertson WO. Drug imprinting. Clin Toxicol 1974;7(4):407–8.

Rumack B. POISINDEX: an emergency poison management system. Drug Inf J 1975;9(2–3):171–80.

Rumack BH, Ford P, Sbarbaro J, Bryson, Winokur M. Regionalization of poison centers—a rational role model. Clin Toxicol 1978;12(3):367–75.

Sagotsky R, Gouveia WA, Lovejoy Jr FH. Evaluation of the effectiveness of a poison information center. Clin Toxicol 1977;11:581–6.

Schaap AL, Sunshine I. Computer retrieval of articles on the therapy of poisonings. Clin Toxicol 1975;8(3):301–10.

Scherz RG, Robertson WO. The history of poison control centers in the United States. Clin Toxicol 1978;12(3):291–6.

Schleich C, McIntire M. Poison control and definitive cost containment. Vet Human Toxicol 1984;26:101–4.

Teitelbaum DT. New directions in poison control. Clin Toxicol 1968;1:3–13.

Temple AR. Testing of child-resistant containers. Clin Toxicol 1978;12(3):357–65.

Temple AR. Poison control centers: prospects and capabilities. Ann Rev Pharmacol Toxicol. 1977;17:215–22.

Temple AR, Veltri JC. One year's experience in a regional poison control center: The Regional Inter-Mountain Regional Poison Center. Clin Toxicol 1978;12(3):277–89.

Thompson DF, Trammel HL, Robertson NJ, Reigart JR. Evaluation of regional and non-regional poison centers. N Engl J Med 1983;308:191–4.

Troutman WG, Wanke LA. Advantages and disadvantages of combining poison control and drug information centers. Am J Hosp Pharm 1983;40(7):1219–22.

Veltri JC, Litovitz TL. 1983 annual report of the American Association of Poison Control Centers National Data Collection System. Am J Emerg Med 1984;2:420.

Veltri JC, Temple AR. Telephone management of poisonings using syrup of ipecac. Clin Toxicol 1976;9(3):407–17.

Waldman JM, Mofenson HC, Greensher J. Evaluating the functioning of a poison control center. Clin Toxicol 1976;15(1):75–9.

Walton W. An evaluation of the Poison Prevention Packaging Act. Pediatrics 1982;69(3):363–70.

Wilson JT. Concepts to promote a combined program of clinical pharmacology and clinical toxicology. Clin Toxicol 1980;16(3):371–6.

Chapter 4.3

The information technology revolution: 1990s

Alan D. Woolf

Boston Children's Hospital & Harvard Medical School, Boston, Massachusetts, United States

By the 1990s the work of PCCs had expanded and many were providing complex consultations spanning diverse areas of clinical toxicology. In total, they were taking almost 2 million calls each year regarding potential poisoning incidents and another one million drug identification and other nonexposure inquiries. They were widely recognized as the lead entities advocating for the best practices in the diagnosis and management of acute or chronic poisonings, as well as in organizing and promoting community-wide efforts at poisoning prevention. They were also engaged in research in clinical toxicology, surveillance of trends in poisoning, and the education of health professionals at every stage of training, from students to practitioners.

Advent of the computer age

By the 1990s, PCCs had ready access to the Internet for use in their daily operations. Instantaneous availability of information resources via free search engines (e.g., Yahoo was an online start-up in 1994, AltaVista in 1995) quickly became limitless. Websites allowed users to search for scientific descriptions of toxicities related to drugs, chemicals, botanicals, or any other substances. Many proprietary resources, such as Poisindex, ToxED, and others used every day by PCC staff issued computer-compatible versions of their materials. The NLM, through its Toxicology and Environmental Health Program (TEHP) now provided online repositories [e.g., Hazardous Substances Data Bank (HSDB), TOXNET and TOXLINE] of freely accessible toxicology information, chemical nomenclature, and other references (Hung and Nelson, 1997; Wexler and Phillips, 2002). US government agencies such as the EPA, ATSDR, CDC, CPSC, OSHA, NIOSH, the NIEHS National Toxicology Program (NTP), Integrated Risk Information System (IRIS), Registry of Toxic Effects of Chemical Substances (RTECS), the EPA's Toxic Chemical Release Inventory (TRI) and the FDA all developed online searchable databases of toxicological

History of Modern Clinical Toxicology. https://doi.org/10.1016/B978-0-12-822218-8.00006-5

information, regulations and policies, updated regulatory actions, and toxic releases. Academic centers, schools of medicine, nursing, and pharmacy, and other institutions developed websites that contained toxicology-related information resources available to both the public and health professionals. Scientific journals were digitalized and, for a subscription price, allowed access to their latest table of contents, as well as archived past issues. All of these new resources transformed not only the daily operations of PCCs but also how clinical toxicologists and, frankly, all health professionals went about their daily lives.

Computerizing onsite case data collection and improving the toxic exposure surveillance system

As early as the 1970s, halting attempts were made at entering data from poisoning cases using an IBM360 mainframe computer (Gregory and Boss, 1974). PCCs quickly computerized their operations in the 1990s as more compact and sophisticated table-top computers became commercially available. By the year 2000, only a few PCCs were still collecting case histories on paper forms. PCCs migrated to several new commercially available electronic templates for case information in databases. The most commonly used of these new proprietary data collection systems was Toxicall. Aggregated data were still sent quarterly to be included in the national *Toxic Exposure Surveillance System* (TESS) database. Toxicall was integrated with the Poisindex 7-digit coding of brand-named and generic products, biologicals, household products, and other substances. TESS also harmonized the clinical variables related to the date and time of the call and the exposure, whether it was an acute, acute-on-chronic or chronic event, the age and sex of the person involved, the possible toxic agent(s) and amount implicated and exposure route, the venue (e.g., work, school, home, and daycare), geographical location, and the reason for the poisoning. Workgroups within AAPCC also regularly updated TESS training manuals and held workshops to promote consistent and accurate coding of poison exposure case data.

While the AAPCC collaborated with public health agencies in reporting out data of interest, TESS was not a government database. Improvements to TESS were made throughout the 1990s by the AAPCC itself, sometimes with contributions of funding from the CDC or ATSDR. AAPCC also conducted training workshops on TESS for PCCs at the NACCT annual meetings. The AAPCC made TESS reporting of aggregated data from regional PCCs a required element for eligibility for certification in the early 1980s. The number of certified PCCs and those reporting data annually to TESS grew considerably over the next two decades. By 1999, the 64 regional poison control centers shown in Fig. 4.3.1 were reporting well in excess of 2 million poisoning exposure calls annually, as shown in Fig. 4.3.2.

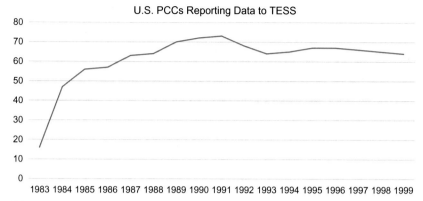

FIG. 4.3.1 Changes in the number of US Poison Control Centers reporting data to TESS, 1983–99. *(Source: data from Gummin DG et al. Clin Toxicol 2020)*

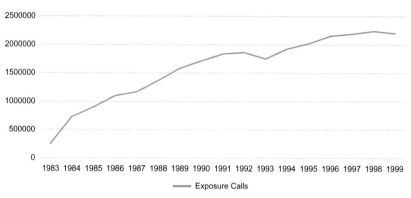

FIG. 4.3.2 Growth in exposure calls reported from US Poison Control Centers 1983–99. *(Source: data from Gummin DG et al. Clin Toxicol 2020)*

TESS critiques

There were limitations inherent to TESS that were the source of critiques by researchers and epidemiologists in the 1990s and 2000s (Soslow and Woolf, 1992; Hamilton and Goldfrank, 1997; Woolf, 2001; Hoffman, 2007; Bronstein, 2007).

- TESS case data were collected by passive reporting. Reporting poisoning exposure events to a PCC was never mandatory. Instead, both the public and health professionals called PCCs for triage, diagnostic, or treatment guidance. Generally that meant that when guidance was no longer needed (common poisonings, for example), under-reporting would increase. Thus TESS from its inception could only capture a fraction of actual poisoning exposure incidents, including serious poisonings. Incidents would always be under-counted locally, regionally, and nationally due to its voluntary nature.

- Many telephoned poison exposures could not be confirmed, and so were *potential* exposures, but may in fact have been "near misses" rather than actual poisonings. Further, many calls involved substances that were inherently nontoxic or implicated in an amount so small that toxicity was unlikely. Retrospective studies using such data have inherent limitations.

- Undercounting by TESS was especially true with respect to poisoning fatalities. Out of hospital deaths or those occurring immediately in emergency departments or in the hospital were often not reported to a PCC, even though a drug or poison might have been the immediate or contributing cause of death. Deaths not recognized as poisoning incidents by health care providers would also be missed. Medical examiners or coroners might not process toxicological samples before attributing death to other causes.

- The reliability of data collection required constant attention to training and updating the staffs of contributing PCCs on data elements, so that data coding was consistent. Variations between regional PCCs in details of data collecting and patient triage were a continuing concern.

Most recently, such inherent limitations have been acknowledged by the AAPCC itself in disclaimers accompanying its annual reports. Independent "quality assurance (QA)" activities by individual PCCs have also been designated by AAPCC as a required element for continued PCC accreditation. Such QA programs have included routine self-audits of PCC data accuracy before uploading to the national database, along with automated logic-based rejections of cases with inconsistent coding. Advanced training models intended to improve the accuracy and consistency of PIP and SPI reporting have continued well into the 2000s (Krenzelok et al., 2014).

Disaster planning

Events such as the Chernobyl nuclear disaster in the Ukraine in 1986 (Savelkoul et al., 1989), the Loma Prieta earthquake in California in 1989 (Nathan et al., 1992), and the Gulf War in 1990 prompted PCCs to examine their readiness for and role in disaster preparedness. The maturing of PCCs as a national network covering most of the population gave rise to concerns about disruptions of service in the event of local or regional disasters. One 1995 survey of 72 certified and noncertified PCCs reported that less than half had a disaster plan in place (Vilke et al., 1996). Larger PCCs and those that were certified were more likely to have written disaster plans, redundant phone systems and back-up arrangements with other poison centers.

In disaster emergencies, PCCs were capable of providing the public with accurate and timely information with 24-h accessibility. This capacity was newly identified as a core function. There was recognition that PCCs were not yet integrated into the regional hazardous materials (HAZMAT) teams and the emergency medical services (EMS) system. They needed to be included in the disaster planning activities of the communities they served (Woolf, 1996). PCCs were encouraged to harden their physical plants against failure and formalize ties with other PCCs so that, in the event of a surge or a service disruption, they could transfer calls to the partner PCC. PCCs were also urged to forge closer ties with EMS, HAZMAT, and other local and state-level public health resources. It was suggested that meeting minimal requirements for such participation in disaster planning be included among the AAPCC's mandatory certification requirements for PCCs. Partnering with the Arizona Emergency Medicine Research Center in the University of Arizona College of Medicine and led by Dr. Frank Walter, the American Academy of Clinical Toxicology initiated the Advanced Hazmat Life Support (AHLS) training program in 1999. It has since trained over 15,000 health care providers and military personnel in 64 countries in the principles of emergency management of toxic disaster situations [https://www.ahls.org/ahls/ecs/subpage/about.html].

The recognition of the key role of PCCs in national surveillance and emergency preparedness was yet another compelling argument for Federal participation in assuring the financial sustainability of the US poison control system.

Poisoning prevention

- Effectiveness of poison prevention education

Public education outreach continued to emphasize safe storage of drugs and household products and awareness of PCC 24-h availability. PCC utilization was higher in those communities in which PCC educational materials had been widely disseminated (Youniss et al., 2000). However, the profile of PCC consultations had changed over time as their services became more widely known and they became more integrated into the relatively new specialty of emergency medicine (Caravati and McElwee, 1991). While there were still plenty of calls regarding inadvertent poison exposures among preschool children, a growing number of calls concerned victims of the adverse effects of substance abuse, more calls from health professionals regarding suicide attempts, and more calls concerning serious, even life-threatening poisonings among adults, especially involving potent psycho-pharmaceuticals and opioids. These calls were more complex, required more follow-up, and took up more time of PCC staff. These poisonings were much more difficult to prevent through educational outreach, and their frequency would only escalate in the 2000s.

- CRCs and prenatal iron poisoning

Progress was made in other technologies aimed at poisoning prevention. By the 1990s, research comparing mortality rates before and after the introduction of child-resistant and tamper-proof packaging showed reductions in the incidence of childhood poisoning deaths by 45% (Rodgers, 1996, 2002).

PCCs advocated for other changes in pharmaceutical dispensing. For example, prenatal iron tablets were highly concentrated and the pills resembled hard candies. PCCs received calls of serious iron poisonings and deaths among toddlers who had found their mother's iron pills. One study of TESS data found that iron poisonings represented greater than 30% of children's pharmaceutical poisoning fatalities (Litovitz and Manoguerra, 1992). Clinical toxicologists advocated for changes to blister-style, unit dose packaging, reformulation of prenatal iron products to make them less attractive to toddlers, education of both obstetricians and pregnant women, and other safeguards to avoid inadvertent childhood exposures. Some of these provisions were later reversed in legal action.

- Drug identification and unique imprinting

PCCs continued to be challenged by the many requests from both the public and health professionals simply looking for drug identification (i.e., no exposure incident had occurred). Dr. Bill Robertson, introduced in Chapter 4.1, had effectively advocated for improved pill imprinting measures after years of effort. Pill identification with unique codes had become more uniform through industry-wide voluntary manufacturing changes. The advent of dedicated websites on the Internet now allowed the public to confirm a medicine's identification by simply entering its description. However, even by 2000, PCCs annually received more than 700,000 information calls (Litovitz et al., 2001). The majority of such inquiries sought to identify a pill or tablet, or to gather information about a drug's dosing, medical indications, or side-effects.

- Bittering agents

Strategies that were passive (i.e., they required no active, repetitive behaviors by adults, such as safe storage of hazardous products in the home or securing child-resistant caps on pill bottles after each use) were attempted in poison prevention. For example, the addition of aversive bittering agents to household products was investigated in an attempt to make them unpalatable and discourage their ingestion by toddlers (Lawless et al., 1982). One study showed that 95% of preschool children had aversive reactions to liquids spiked with small amounts of one of the bitterest agent known to man: denatonium benzoate (Sibert and Frude, 1991). In 1991, Oregon passed the first legislation requiring the addition of the bittering agent, denatonium benzoate (trade name Bitrex or Aversion) at 30–50 ppm to antifreeze and other automotive products containing ethylene glycol or methanol. Sixteen other states followed suit. But while addition of bittering agents might discourage ingestions by preschoolers in such controlled palatability studies, it did not seem to impact actual poisoning frequency or outcome (White et al., 2009) or deter adults who were intent on drinking antifreeze in a suicide attempt (White et al., 2008).

Ethylene glycol is slightly sweet, posing a risk also to pets and small animals, which were killed in great numbers each year by accidental ingestion of antifreeze. In 2012, the Humane Society and Consumer Products Specialty Association reached a voluntary nationwide agreement with manufacturers to add denatonium to ethylene glycol-containing antifreeze and automotive coolant solutions despite unproven efficacy in the prevention of either unintentional or intentional poisonings (Consumer Specialty Products Association, 2012).

Unstable PCC finances

The 1990s ushered in a time of more consolidation as PCCs continued to struggle with issues of staffing and capital expenses. Some lost institutional sponsorship and closed. As academic hospitals housing PCCs and states pulled back in their support, leadership scrambled to find other sources of support (Lerner and Warner, 1988). A mixed revenue stream included donations from member hospitals, surcharges on telephone services, funding from state departments of health, and private grants from nonprofit organizations (e.g., the United Way). Some states stepped in to provide funding from Federal block grants or other short-term fixes; others were reluctant to commit to adequate funding to maintain the PCC's standard of clinical service. States in total provided only about 47.9% of PCC funding (Youniss et al., 2000). Some novel state-level strategies worked, such as, in Utah, linking poison control services to a modest surcharge added to every monthly residential telephone bill, much like that attached for the availability of other EMS. This state-level approach to PCC funding via telephone surcharges or 911 or license fees was adopted by 13 states by 1998 (Youniss et al., 2000).

Cost containment could only go so far in reconciling a budget without sacrificing core functions and lowering the PCC's ability provide a high standard of clinical care. A 1995 survey of 83 PCCs reported that, whereas adequate poison control funding to cover the entire US population was calculated at $120 million annually, PCCs only had $74.6 million available to them (Felberg et al., 1996). Nationally only 63.1% of the population had access to certified poison control services in 1995; 4 PCCs had closed and the only center serving Hawaii was threatened with closure. By 1998 there were 73 PCCs in total, but only 52 were AAPCC-certified, covering only 35 states and the District of Columbia and serving only 78.5% of the US population (Youniss et al., 2000). Of the 73 centers, 41% anticipated a decline in funding levels from state governments and other sources; 33% had experienced a budget reduction within the previous five years; and 47.9% had faced threats of closure (Youniss et al., 2000).

PCC certification and effectiveness

Paradoxically, at the same time PCCs were struggling financially to keep their doors (and phone lines) open, health services-related research studies concluded that they were reliable sources of accurate information and were extremely cost-effective in their operations (Filandrinos et al., 1993; Mvros et al., 1994; Krenzelok et al., 1998). Louisiana's loss of a PCC in 1988 resulted in $1.4 million in higher medical costs for the state (estimated at more than threefold higher costs than the PCC's annual $400,000 budget) due to the unnecessary self-referral of patients to more expensive out-patient and emergency care services (King and Palmisano, 1991). Almost 75% of poison exposure calls received by PCCs were assessed to be either nontoxic or have minimal risk and could be kept home.

One study evaluating the accuracy of PCCs versus advice given out by emergency department personnel in a simulated telephone consultation found that emergency departments responded accurately 64% of the time, whereas PCCs were accurate 94% of the time (Wigder et al., 1995). Certification of PCCs by the AAPCC had achieved goals of upgrading their standards: 65.8% of certified PCCs were staffed by certified specialists in poison information versus 34.9% of uncertified PCCs; 48% of certified PCC managers were ABAT board-certified versus 15% of directors of noncertified centers; 84% of certified PCCs employed educators on staff versus 56% of noncertified centers (Felberg et al., 1996).

Reframing poison control—Drive for National Funding and National Toll-Free Access

The drive to secure Federal funding for a more integrated, national system of PCCs in the United States accelerated throughout the 1990s. The continuing erosion of financial support for a system clearly benefitting everyone was the impetus to develop an approach to sustainability for PCCs at a national level. The patchwork strategy of more than 28 different sources of public and private revenue streams was insufficient to guarantee a sustainable national poison control network. There were calls for a national solution (Tong and Soloway, 1994). A parallel and equally compelling issue, besides the threatened imminent closure, was the inability of some PCCs to mobilize enough resources to attain the certification status required by the AAPCC to assure the public of a PCC's high quality and reliable services. Another challenge was that access to poison control was complicated by multiple local and/or state-wide toll-free telephone numbers, none of which could be easily remembered in an emergency. Invaluable time could be lost simply looking up the right phone number. Catchment areas sometimes overlapped, creating confusion as to which center would assume responsibility for case management.

A stakeholders' group of poison control leadership was formed by AAPCC in the early 1990s and met regularly throughout the decade, developing strategies to pursue to reach a goal of Federal support of poison control. The services of consultants familiar with the legislative process on Capitol Hill were enlisted by the AAPCC. The ex-senator from Nebraska, David Karnes, and his colleagues played a key role in bringing poison control advocates together with legislators from both sides of the aisle in a series of meetings. PCC stakeholders and advocates were instrumental in winning new Congressional interest during hearings held in 1994 (Kearney, 1994; Litovitz et al., 1994; Landis, 1994; Miller, 1994). They met frequently with Congressional staffers,

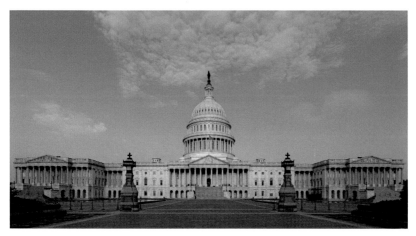

FIG. 4.3.3 Congress and White House mandate funding of US poison control centers. *(Source: Wikimedia Commons)*

representatives, and senators, prepared with talking points and authoritative research studies confirming the cost-effectiveness of the PCCs (Chafee-Bahamon, 1983; King and Palmisano, 1991; Lovejoy Jr et al., 1994; Harrison et al., 1995; Harrison et al., 1996; Kelly et al., 1997). One 1997 study concluded that PCC activity in the United States averted more than 350,000 unnecessary emergency department visits annually (Miller, 1997). It was widely recognized that PCCs provided services that benefitted greatly local and state public health agencies, as well as the Federal government (e.g. Medicaid, Medicare, and the State Children's Health Insurance Program (SCHIP))., insurance companies, hospitals and medical schools, and the general public. And yet some of these beneficiaries provided little or no financial support for their operations. In an era focused primarily on cost containment, it was estimated that each $1 dollar spent on poison control saved $7.75 dollars in averted health care costs (Miller, 1994). These compelling arguments convinced lawmakers of the plight of the poison control movement and the lack of sustainable funding to insure its viability as an indispensable health care asset to the nation. A line-item appropriation was authorized by Congress in 1999 and administered by the Health Resources Services Administration (HRSA) with an initial funding of about $21.5 million in 2000 (Fig. 4.3.3).

New millennium

Building on the progress made in the five previous decades, changes have come rapidly to the poison control movement in the United States since 1999. The first two decades of the new millennium have brought startling new advancements and serious challenges. These are described in Chapter 4.4.

References

Bronstein AC, Spyker DA, Cantilena LR, Green JL, Rumack BH, Heard SE. 2006 annual report of the American Association of Poison Control Centers' National Poison Data System (NPDS): 25th annual report. Clin Toxicol 2007;45(8):815–917.

Caravati EM, McElwee NE. Use of clinical toxicology resources by emergency physicians and its impact on poison control centers. Ann Emerg Med 1991;20(2):147–50.

Chafee-Bahamon C, Caplan D, Lovejoy FH Jr. Pattern in hospitals' use of a poison information center. Am J Pub Heal 1983;73(4):396–400.

Consumer Specialty Products Association. Antifreeze and engine coolant being bittered nationwide, https://web.archive.org/web/20121228225407/http://www.cspa.org/news-media-center/news-releases/2012/12/antifreeze-and-engine-coolant-being-bittered-nationwide; 2012. [Accessed 3 May 2020].

Felberg L, Litovitz TL, Soloway RA, Morgan J. State of the nation's poison centers: 1994 American Association of Poison Control Centers survey of U.S. poison centers. Vet Human Toxicol 1996;38(3):214–9.

Filandrinos DT, Zunker RJ, Sioris LJ. Costs incurred from unnecessary emergency department visits for treatment of poisonings. Vet Human Toxicol 1993;35:323.

Gregory AR, Boss IDJ. Direct input of toxicological data to the computer. Clin Toxicol 1974;7(4):395–400.

Gummin DD, Mowry JB, Beuhler MC, Spyker DA, Brooks DE, Dibert KW, Rivers LJ, Pham NPT, Ryan ML. 2019 annual report of the American Association of Poison Control Centers' National Poison Data System (NPDS): 37th annual report. Clin Toxicol 2020;58(12):1360–541.

Hamilton RJ, Goldfrank LR. Poison center data and the Pollyanna phenomenon. J Toxicol Clin Toxicol 1997;35(1):21–3.

Harrison DL, Draugalis JR, Slack MK, Tong TG. The production model as a basis for conducting economic evaluations of regional poison control centers. Clin Toxicol 1995;33(3):233–7.

Harrison DL, Draugalis JR, Slack MK, Langley PC. Cost-effectiveness of regional poison control centers. Arch Intern Med 1996;156:2601–8.

Hoffman RS. Understanding the limitations of retrospective analyses of poison center data. Clin Toxicol 2007;45(8):943–5.

Hung O, Nelson LS. Toxnet—A guide to clinical toxicology resources available on the Internet. J Toxicol Clin Toxicol 1997;35(6):677–9.

Kearney TE. Testimony on behalf of the American Association of Poison Control Centers, to the Subcommittee on Human Resources and Inter-Government Relations, Committee on Government Operations, U.S. House of Representatives; March 1994.

Kelly NR, Ellis MD, Kirkland RT, Holmes SE, Kozinetz CA. Effectiveness of a poison center: impact on medical facility visits. Vet Human Toxicol 1997;39(1):44–8.

King WD, Palmisano PA. Poison control centers: can their value be measured? South Med J 1991;84(6):722–6.

Krenzelok EP, Schexnayder S, James LP, Kearns GL, Farrar HC. Do poison centers save money? What are the data? J Toxicol Clin Toxicol 1998;36(6):545–7.

Krenzelok EP, Reynolds KM, Dart RC, Green JL. A model to improve the accuracy of U.D. poison center data collection. Clin Toxicol 2014;52(8):889–96.

Landis NT. Poison center's plight gets national attention. Am J Hosp Pharm 1994;51:1755–61.

Lawless HT, Hammer LD, Corina MD. Aversions to bitterness and accidental poisonings among preschool children. J Toxicol Clin Toxicol 1982;19(9):951–64.

Lerner WM, Warner KE. The challenge of privately financed community health programs in an era of cost containment: a case study of poison control centers. J Pub Heal Policy 1988;9:411–28.

Litovitz T, Manoguerra A. Comparison of pediatric poisoning hazards: an analysis of 3.8 million exposure incidents. A report from the American Association of Poison Control Centers. Pediatrics 1992;89:999–1006.

Litovitz T, Kearney TE, Holm K, Soloway RA, Weisman R, Oderda G. Poison control centers: is there an antidote for budget cuts? Am J Emerg Med 1994;12(5):585–99.

Litovitz TL, Klein-Schwartz W, White S, Cobaugh DJ, Youniss J, Omslaer J, et al. 2000 annual report of the American Association of Poison Control Centers Toxic Exposure Surveillance System. Am J Emerg Med 2001;19(5):337–95.

Lovejoy Jr FH, Robertson W, Woolf AD. Poison centers, poison prevention and the pediatrician. Pediatrics 1994;94:220–4.

Miller TR. Children's Safety Network. The costs of poisoning and the savings from poison control centers: a cost-benefit analysis. Testimony presented at the Human Resources and Inter-Governmental Relations Subcommittee, House Committee on Government Relations hearing on "Poison Control Centers: Is There An Antidote for Budget Cuts?"; March 1994.

Miller TR. Costs of poisoning in the United States and savings from poison control centers: a benefit-cost analysis. Ann Emerg Med 1997;29:239–45.

Mvros R, Dean BS, Krenzelok EP. Poison center funding—Who should pay? J Toxicol Clin Toxicol 1994;32:503–8.

Nathan AR, Olson KR, Everson GW, Kearney TE, Blanc PB. Effects of a major earthquake on calls to regional poison control centers. West J Med 1992;156:278–80.

Rodgers GB. The safety effects of child-resistant packaging for oral prescription drugs. Two decades of experience. JAMA 1996;275(21):1661–5.

Rodgers GB. The effectiveness of child-resistant packaging for aspirin. Arch Pediatr Adolesc Med 2002;156(9):929–33.

Savelkoul TJF, Leenhouts HP, Sangster B. The role of poison control centers in radiation accidents. J Toxicol Clin Toxicol 1989;27(4–5):305–10.

Sibert JR, Frude N. Bittering agents in the prevention of accidental poisoning: children's reactions to Bitrex (denatonium benzoate). Arch Emerg Med 1991;8:1–7.

Soslow A, Woolf AD. Reliability of data sources for poisoning deaths in Massachusetts. Am J Emerg Med 1992;10:124–7.

Tong TG, Soloway RA. Fiscal antidotes needed. J Toxicol Clin Toxicol 1994;32:509–11.

Vilke GM, Jacoby I, Manoguerra AS, Clark R. Disaster preparedness of poison centers in the United States. J Toxicol Clin Toxicol 1996;34(1):53–8.

Wexler P, Phillips S. Tools for clinical toxicology on the World Wide Web: review and scenario. J Toxicol Clin Toxicol 2002;40(7):893–902.

White NC, Litovitz T, White MK, Watson WA, Benson BE, Horowitz Z, Marr-Lyon L. The impact of bittering agents on suicidal ingestions of antifreeze. Clin Toxicol 2008;46(6):507–14.

White NC, Litovitz T, Benson BE, Horowitz BZ, Marr-Lyon L, White MK. The impact of bittering agents on pediatric ingestions of antifreezer. Clin Pediatr 2009;48(9):913–21.

Wigder HN, Erickson T, Morse T, Saporta V. Emergency department poison advice telephone calls. Ann Emerg Med 1995;25(3):349–52.

Woolf A. The specter of variation in poison control center triage practices: Where do we go from here? Clin Toxicol 2001;39(5):439–40.

Woolf AD. Disaster planning—our finest hour? J Toxicol Clin Toxicol 1996;34(1):59–60.

Youniss J, Litovitz T, Villanueva P. Characterization of U.S. poison centers: a 1998 survey conducted by the American Association of Poison Control Centers. Vet Human Toxicol 2000;42(1):43–53.

Chapter 4.4

New millennium, new directions: 2000–2020

Alan D. Woolf

Boston Children's Hospital & Harvard Medical School, Boston, Massachusetts, United States

By 2000, the poison control movement had fully matured and was widely acknowledged as the preeminent source of authoritative information on poisonings in America. Collectively, 63 Poison Control Centers (PCCs) were reporting over 2.1 million human exposures annually (Litovitz et al., 2001). By then, the American Association of Poison Control Centers had archived more than 29 million cases, a rich central repository of poisoning-related information routinely shared with public health partners, researchers, and clinical toxicologists everywhere. PCCs had expanded their activities to those listed in Table 4.4.1.

Federal funding

In the 1990s, the national PCC task force took their case to lawmakers for a more integrated national system, one with stability and sustainability. Their advocacy finally came to fruition; lawmakers were convinced by the argument that PCCs were unfairly excluded from receiving Federal funding, even though they served government-insured patients (i.e., Medicare, Medicaid, and the State Children's Health Insurance Program) and saved the government millions of dollars by diverting patients from using unnecessary, expensive health care services.

The "Poison Control Center Enhancement and Awareness Act" (PL 106-174), administered by the Health Resources Services Administration (HRSA), was enacted in 2000 and reauthorized in 2003 and 2008 (see Table 2 in the Section 4—Introduction).

The 2003 amendment to Title XII of the Public Health Services Act provided a specific authorization to support PCCs and authorized $2 million annually through FY09 to support a nationwide toll-free telephone number. It also provided $600,000 annually through 2005 for a media campaign to educate the public and health care providers on poison prevention and how to access the new toll-free number. $25 million was appropriated through HRSA annually

History of Modern Clinical Toxicology. https://doi.org/10.1016/B978-0-12-822218-8.00028-4

TABLE 4.4.1 Activities of poison control centers.

Administration, leadership, finance, and human resources
Nonhealth care facility patient management
Health care facility patient management
Information and referral services
Data collection and management
Health professional training in clinical toxicology
Government and public agency resource
Professional educational outreach
Public education and outreach for poisoning prevention
Research into topics in clinical toxicology
Disaster, surge, and HAZMAT preparedness
Real-time toxico-surveillance and risk assessment

Table adapted from Woolf AD. Challenge and promise: the future of poison control services. Toxicology 2004;198:285–9.

through fiscal year 2004 and $27.5 million annually in fiscal years 2005–09 for grants to certified regional PCCs to help them achieve financial stability, develop standard patient management guidelines and poisoning prevention promotion programs, improve national surveillance, expand toxicological expertise, and improve PCC capacity to answer high volumes of calls (surges) during times of national crisis. Funding was also available to enable some PCCs to reach the AAPCC standards required for certification.

Federal funding was reauthorized in 2008 by PL 110-377 and again in 2014 by PL 113-77, but at reduced spending levels. The advent of Federal funding, while it certainly helped, did not in itself solve funding issues of PCCs and did not stabilize funding through implementation of a single payer system per se (IOM, 2004). Federal funds only accounted for about 15% of total PCC funding. They were earmarked to improve services and support a national toll-free telephone number but were, in fact, never meant to supplant state-level funding or other funding streams available to PCCs to deliver existing services. Maintenance of Federal involvement has continued to require vigilance and advocacy on behalf of poison control (Giffin and Heard, 2009; Woolf et al., 2011; Dart, 2012).

Case mix and cost effectiveness

Recent studies have analyzed the types of exposure calls received by PCCs annually and have discovered changes in case-mix over time. While two-thirds of PCC calls involved pediatric cases in 1983, by year 2000 just over 52% of PCC cases and by 2018 only 44% involved young children. Conversely, the number of intentional poisoning cases involving adolescents or adults increased from 11.3% to 17.6% from 2000 to 2015 (Anderson and Seung, 2018). The numbers of calls involving toxic exposures from the intentional use or abuse of multiple drugs and other substances by adolescents and adults increased, as did the mortality associated with such serious cases (Greenwald et al., 2016). These poisoning exposures were more medically complex and required more time and expertise in consultation and follow-up both by medical toxicologists and SPIs. While the overall number of poison exposure calls to PCCs nationwide had been dropping since 2008, the complexity of those cases and consequent workload demands on PCC staff had both been increasing (Anderson and Seung, 2018).

Justification of PCCs by demonstrating their cost effectiveness has continued to be a focus of health services research. A host of studies confirmed their return-on-investment (Blizzard et al., 2008), their benefit in lowering costs by reducing unnecessary hospital visits (LoVecchio et al., 2008; Litovitz et al., 2010a, b) and their effectiveness in reducing length of stay of hospitalized poisoned patients (Vassilev and Marcus, 2007; Kostic et al., 2010; Friedman et al., 2014). A revised savings calculation in 2012 estimated that for every dollar spent on PCC funding, there was a return on investment of $13.39 in unnecessary medical costs averted (The Lewin Group, 2012). That study detailed a number of savings:

- $752.9 million per year due to avoided medical utilization
- $441.1 million per year due to reduced hospital length of stay
- $23.9 million per year due to in-person outreach
- $603 million per year due to reduced work-loss days

In total, the US poison center system saved over $1.8 billion per year in medical costs and productivity (The Lewin Group, 2012).

With stabilized funding, some PCCs were able to gain regional certification status with the AAPCC and/or expand their operations to serve more effectively people in their catchment areas. However, consolidation continued. As Fig. 4.4.1 shows, there were 60 PCCs reporting to NPDS by 2010; by 2015, this number had fallen to the current 55 centers.

Post-2001 emergency preparedness and poison control

An Institute of Medicine (IOM) monograph: *Forging a New Poison Control System,* published by the National Academy of Sciences in 2004, was instrumental in the push for the integration of poison control services into a national plan of emergency preparedness. The IOM report specified "core" functions that mandated Federal support, including:

- manage telephone calls about poison exposure and information,
- prepare and respond to "all-hazards" emergency needs, especially those arising from biological or chemical terrorism,

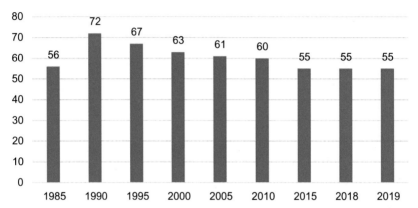

Number of U.S. Poison Control Centers 1985-2019

FIG. 4.4.1   Number of Poison Control Centers contributing data to NPDS. *(Table created from data in Gummin et al., Clin Toxicol 2020.)*

- capture, analyze, and report data on poison exposures,
- train personnel, including specialists in and providers of poison information,
- perform continuous quality improvement, and integrate the centers' services into the public health system.

As the IOM report pointed out, "public health agencies, for the most part, had little involvement with poison control centers until 2001, when bioterrorism and related activities created interest…" (IOM, 2004). Resources were made available to PCCs and the AAPCC after the September 11, 2001, terrorist attack on the World Trade Center in New York City. That event, and the new toll-free nationwide telephone number (1-800-222-1222), ushered in a new era of greater integration of poison control-derived data into emergency disaster planning and real-time national surveillance related to homeland security. The national poison control system was recognized as an equal partner in disaster planning; PCCs were now included in newly organized state and local disaster preparedness planning efforts.

NPDS and surveillance

Real-time monitoring of cases submitted to TESS was initiated in March 2003, with most centers submitting data every 4–10 min (Watson et al., 2005). Data from individual PCCs could now be uploaded into one central repository of the National Poison Data System (NPDS) every few minutes and the aggregated data were available for analysis of national trends and events of public health significance. This allowed for real-time analysis of trends in exposures to specific products/product categories, syndromic patterns, and other all-hazard assessments. In 2006, the AAPCC database changed its name from the Toxic Exposure Surveillance System (TESS) to the National Poison Data System (NPDS) (Bronstein et al., 2007).

One of the services provided by the national PCC network through the AAPCC and by individual PCCs since the 1990s has been one of surveillance: the PCC's ability to provide data on toxic exposures to public health agencies, nonprofits, industry, and other organizations. For example, PCCs have collaborated with public health agencies like the Occupational Safety & Health Administration (OSHA) in uncovering hazardous workplace situations in violation of OSHA standards (Tustin et al., 2018). With regard to potentially hazardous products, examples detailed how NPDS data were used to inform the decisions of governmental regulators and manufacturers of laundry detergent pods, button batteries, and e-cigarettes about changes needed to improve product safety (Litovitz et al., 2010b; Wang et al., 2018).

PCCs and national disasters

The terrorist attack on the United States on September 11, 2001, was a turning point that expanded the mission of the poison control movement to include a "sentinel" function. Its real-time data collection system was recognized by public health officials as an asset both in early detection of warnings of newly emerging illnesses, newly recognized product hazards, or a coming disaster. PCCs could be a key partner to public health agencies in monitoring the aftermath of regional or national catastrophic events, providing 24-h support services to both the public and health care providers.

PCCs needed to address such issues as manpower needs, communication redundancy, and other capacity-related issues to deal with the anticipated "surge" in anxious callers during a local, state-wide or national emergency (Klein et al., 2007). Building alliances with public health and other nonprofits and community-based helping agencies proactively was also recommended preparation (Geller and Lopez, 1999). The NPDS has also served as a national biosurveillance tool described in the Pandemic All-Hazards Preparedness Act (PAHPA) and Homeland Security Presidential Directive 21 (HSPD-21). One study cited 11 instances of call volume spikes between 2003 and 2011 detected by NPDS, some involving microbial outbreaks such as food poisoning with *Escherichia coli* or *Salmonella* or H1N1 influenza (Dart, 2012).

Surveillance algorithms assist the AAPCC in monitoring trends in reported poisoning exposures in real-time. Unusual, statistically significant peaks in the frequency of certain types of exposures or involvement of certain chemicals or products can alert public health authorities early on to an unusually suspicious activity or a potential mass poisoning event.

The AAPCC has collaborated with the CDC in such monitoring activities and could detect deviations from expected numbers of poison exposure calls. For example, PCCs served as a source of information for the public in the Deepwater Horizon oil drilling platform accident in April of 2010 in the Gulf of Mexico. Hazardous petroleum-based chemicals were generated, spilling from the destroyed platform and washing ashore along the coast (Wang et al., 2018). Notification of CDC officials of real-time data in that evolving public event promoted situational awareness, which could then be shared with local and state health departments and other agencies. One study of 5 years of NPDS data highlighted 138 such reportable regional incidents, including 58 that involved gases and fumes (most often carbon monoxide) (Law et al., 2014).

When explosions at the Fukushima Daiichi nuclear power plant followed the March 11, 2011, Tohoku earthquake and tsunami, there was widespread nuclear contamination. The AAPCC staff partnered with clinical toxicologists working at the CDC in offering guidance to Japanese colleagues on the medical management of radiation toxicity and the proper use of countermeasures, potassium iodide, and antidotes (Law et al., 2013; Kazzi and Miller, 2013).

At no time was the new PCC role in public health more evident than in the 2020 pandemic of illnesses, many of them life-threatening, involving a novel virus: severe acute respiratory syndrome corona virus 2 (SARS-CoV-2). The disease caused by the virus (known as COVID-19) became a national concern in the United States at the beginning of March 2020. Since PCCs were accessible to both the general public and health care providers 24 h daily, they partnered with public health agencies as another source of reliable COVID-19 related information. By April 1 2020, PCCs had already received over 45,550 exposure calls related to cleaners and disinfectants, representing an overall increase of 20.4% from the year before (Chang A et al., 2020). Many calls related to the misuse of disinfectants, including their ingestion, and the use of methanol, mistakenly substituted for ethanol, as a viral disinfectant ingredient in hand sanitizers. The AAPCC reported in 2021 that PCCs handled 23% more telephone inquiries regarding bleach, hand sanitizers, and disinfectants in the first 5 months of 2021 as compared to the first 5 months of 2019 (source: www.aapcc.org). Many PCC's, in collaboration with state-level public health agencies, set up dedicated hotlines to answer the public's questions and concerns about COVID-19. One PCC in New Jersey alone recorded 57,579 calls to a dedicated COVID-19 line between January and October 2020 (Meaden et al., 2021).

Environmental toxicology

Environmental toxicology has long been within the purview of clinical toxicologists and has been included in the most recent iterations of core curricular content for the training of medical toxicologists. Poison control centers have been urged to adopt a "sentinel" role in the identification of environmental contaminants affecting the health of children (Pronczuk de Garbino, 2002). Since the 1950s, the importance of preservation of the natural ecology of the earth's environments, and more recently in the face of man's contributions to climate change, has become more compelling. Disasters outlined in Chapter 1, such as that at Minamata Bay in Japan in the 1950s, and the writings and testimony of environmental champions like Rachel Carson in the 1960s brought the issue of environmental contamination by manmade pollutants into public consciousness and lent an urgency to the need to address environmental toxicants. These concerns culminated in the creation of the Environmental Protection Agency in 1970, charged with protecting the natural environment by issuing and enforcing regulations governing commercial and industrial enterprises. The passage of such legislation as The Clean Air Act in 1970, The Clean Water Act in 1977, The Comprehensive Environmental Response, Compensation & Liability Act (CERCLA) Superfund Act in 1980 and many others ushered in a paradigm shift in regulatory oversight to preserve the environment.

Pediatric environmental health specialty units

Pediatric Environmental Health Specialty Units (PEHSUs; *www.pehsu.net*) were established by the Agency for Toxic Substances & Disease Registry (ATSDR) in 1998 by then Assistant Surgeon General Barry Johnson. Dr. Johnson viewed PEHSUs as an efficient and cost-effective mechanism for providing expert advice and consultation on pediatric and reproductive environmental health matters. The mission of each PEHSU is to provide education and consultation for families, health care professionals, communities, and policy makers on environmental threats to children's health. The 10 regional U.S. PEHSUs (mapped to the EPA's regional offices) are clinically oriented centers of excellence. Each is based in an academic center and staffed by board-certified pediatricians, occupational physicians, maternal fetal medicine experts, and/or medical toxicologists with expertise in environmental exposures. PEHSUs also may include educators, nurses, and other experts; many have formed partnerships with nearby PCCs. PEHSUs provide education in children's environmental health for students and health care trainees. By 2006, 17 physicians had completed pediatric environmental health fellowships at PEHSU sites (Landrigan et al., 2007); by 2018, 56 physicians and scientists were trained (Landrigan et al., 2019). Through outreach activities between 1999 and 2014, PEHSUs reached an estimated 298,936 health professionals, 61,947 health professional trainees, 323,817 members of the public, and 17,806 government officials and others (Woolf et al., 2016). The most frequent environmental topics addressed in these clinical consultations included lead, mold and fungus, phthalates, pesticides, and mercury. The PEHSU model has been replicated in other countries, including Canada, Mexico, Spain, and Argentina.

Poisoning prevention

- Updated logos, PCC reach, and poisoning prevention

    Under the direction of AAPCC staffer Rose Ann Soloway, an intense national public education campaign followed the introduction of the nationwide toll-free telephone number for poison control in 2000. A new logo (Fig. 4.4.2) was rolled out by the AAPCC in brochures, phone stickers, and other educational materials. Public education outreach marketing

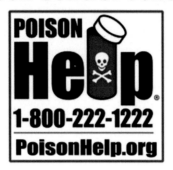

FIG. 4.4.2 National poison control logo disseminated starting in 2002.

by individual regional PCCs continued to emphasize safe storage of drugs and household products and awareness of PCC 24-h availability (Krenzelok et al., 2008). On-line toolkits, such as *Be Poison Smart* were shown to be effective in raising parental awareness on strategies for poisoning prevention (Polivka et al., 2006).

- Disparities in PCC use

  During the 1990s and 2000s, new concerns were raised as to how PCC could respond to racial, ethnic, and socioeconomic and cultural determinants of PCC utilization. Studies have raised issues in disparities as reflected in under-utilization of PCC consultation services by racial and ethnic minorities, as well as those living in poverty (Clark et al., 2002; Litovitz et al., 2010a; Kelly et al., 2014). Preexisting health beliefs, mistrust of organized medical care, and ethnic cultural practices may preclude the use of a PCC when those families confront an illness or a medical emergency. Barriers to the use of a PCC may include the lack of awareness of the PCC's free services, lack of access to a telephone, and perceived lack of non-English interpreter services.

- Abandoning Ipecac

  The messaging has changed in some aspects of poisoning prevention over the past 20 years. Home storage of ipecac was recommended for decades. However, numerous scientific studies did not support its benefit versus its risks and disadvantages. It was abandoned by US PCCs as a first-aid measure, in favor of early triage to the emergency department for poison exposures serious enough to require monitoring and more effective treatments. A revised position statement issued jointly by the AACT and EAPCCT in 2013 affirmed their 2004 recommendation to avoid ipecac as first aid for most poisonings, either at the site of ingestion or in the emergency department (Höjer et al., 2013).

- Poison prevention packaging

    The year 2020 marked the 50th anniversary of passage of the Poison Prevention Packaging Act in the US. New safe packaging measures, such as the use of blister style unit dose packaging, labeling measurements using metric units, promotion of "Up and Away" storage education campaigns, and use of "flow restrictors" for liquid medications, are all recommended (Budnitz et al., 2020).

- Medication identification

    The role of PCCs in medication identification for callers has always been controversial (Jaramillo et al., 2004). Some PCCs refused to provide such services; they felt that such information, often involving drugs of abuse, facilitated diversion of controlled substances or violated patient confidentiality. Others took hundreds of such calls as a courtesy to the public and health professionals, expending considerable time and effort by their staffs. One study of 2002–07 information calls to all US PCCs reported that nonexposure calls had increased by 44%, with 90% of the increase related to pill identification (64% of which involved drugs with abuse potential) (Spiller and Griffith, 2009).

    However, the advent of Internet websites now offering picture-aided identification of tablets, pills, and capsules has allowed users to identify drugs themselves without calling a PCC. And some PCCs have employed automated, self-service "interactive voice response" (IVR) systems to answer such inquiries without taking staff time to do it (Benson, 2011). One study demonstrated that the availability of an IVR system reduced such calls by 84.1% and reduced the staff time of manual documentation of such requests by 97.9% (Krenzelok and Mrvos, 2011). PCCs responded to only 47,170 drug ID requests and 70,179 drug information requests in 2019 (Gummin et al., 2020), compared with the more than 1 million such calls registered in 2007 (Spiller and Griffith, 2009).

The Internet Age — Immediate information retrieval

By the early 2000s, updates to Internet-based resources were being transmitted electronically, so that PCC staff could retrieve new information instantaneously. These electronic resources have now largely replaced physical books, journals, and references as sources consulted by PCC staff in their everyday work. *Poisindex* continues to expand its entries as new products and chemicals come onto the market and into households and other settings. The database now includes more than a million commercial products, chemicals, drugs, toxic plants, and animals and has been adapted for use on a mobile smartphone. It has over 850 detailed management/treatment protocol entries and 2000 searchable slang drug terms (Watson IBM, 2018). Other proprietary online databases offer immediate access to updated toxicological information from reliable sources. For example, *Hazard Navigator* provides rapidly searchable hazmat information culled from authoritative books and other sources in the United States and the United Kingdom on over 7000 hazardous chemicals (Walter, 2012). *ToxED* (Elsevier Publishers) is another electronic database with drug-related information used as a reference in many PCCs. The *Natural Medicines Database* is another used for descriptions of herbal preparations and dietary supplements.

All of the clinical toxicology societies: AAPCC, ACMT, AACT, AOEC, EAPCCT, APAMT, and IUTOX have public and professional information on various poisoning and toxicological topics at their websites. Reference books and journals have adapted to the digital age. Toxicology textbooks are available in hard-cover but also as *electronic* books. The AACT journal *Clinical Toxicology* and the newer ACMT *Journal of Medical Toxicology* are published and delivered to subscribers on-line; back-issues are digitally archived and accessible electronically. In 2017, the APAMT joined the three other societies: AACT, AAPCC, and EAPCCT as official sponsors of the journal which in 2005 reverted back to its former title: *Clinical Toxicology*.

Internet-based clinical toxicology education

The Internet has ushered in an era of innovation in education in clinical toxicology targeting every level of health care professional, from the student to the house-staff trainee to the practitioner. Electronic newsletters, and *e*-learning modules, podcasts, synchronous and asynchronous webinars, and forums offer up-to-date information. The websites of toxicology societies such as AACT and ACMT, using a variety of learning management system platforms, have contributed to the democratization of online access to toxicology information around the world. The Global Educational Toxicology Uniting Project (GETUP) developed in 2016 is one example of a free online curricular resource in toxicology that can reach professional audiences in less-developed countries who are without such expertise locally (Wong et al., 2017).

Era of social media

By the early 2000s, the electronic media had integrated itself into the lives of Americans. New social media networks, such as Facebook, Snapchat, Twitter, and LinkedIn, were becoming popular as vehicles for crowdsourcing materials and widely disseminating ideas and information with real-time accessibility. Patterns of the public's searches within Internet search engines have shown intriguing results. There was a notable spike in internet searches for "dioxin" at the time of Ukrainian Viktor Yushchenko's poisoning in 2004 (see Chapter 2.6) and another spike in queries for the novel substance of abuse, "bath salts" (i.e., cathinone-containing compounds), in 2010 (Yin and Ho, 2012). Often these spikes correlated in time and geographical location to regional spikes in calls to PCCs. Some remained skeptical that social media sites can provide forewarning signs of an impending toxicological disaster, because they are most often reactive and dependent on the public's curiosity over what's new and different, only to fade over time as people move on to the next novelty (Juurlink, 2012).

The advent of mobile smart-phones with Internet connectivity in 2010 heralded a new era of information services and "just-in-time" capabilities. So far, conventional PCCs have been cautiously adapting to these new interactive applications. By 2013, more than half of PCCs had developed Facebook and Twitter accounts and were distributing poisoning information, often measures for poison prevention, via regular postings (Vo and Smollin, 2015; Gussow, 2015). One 2017 survey of US PCCs queried their utilization of short-messaging service (SMS or text-messaging) and online chatting. Of 51 PCC (93% response), only 6 (12%) had experience in using these modalities to field public inquiries (Su et al., 2019). Responders indicated that the benefit was to offer an alternative means of accessibility, but they cited disadvantages as staff reluctance, technology start-up costs, legal liability issues, and a lack of public awareness of its availability. Toxicology societies themselves have moved into the era of social media since 2008: ACMT—@acmtmedtox April 2008; AAPCC—@AAPCC September 2009; AACT—@AACTinfo February 2013; APAMT—@asiatox August 2013; and EAPCCT—@eapcct November 2018.

Recent trends in poison control

The poison control movement in America continues to evolve over time. The advent of new Internet sources of information about drugs, chemicals, plants, botanicals, dietary supplements, herbal and other ethnic remedies, commercial products, and other potentially hazardous substances has increased the "just-in-time" accessibility of information to the general public.

As Fig. 4.4.3 demonstrates, poisoning calls to PCCs peaked in 2008 at just under 2.5 million human exposure cases but have since then shown a decline nationally to 2.1 million calls in 2019. Coincidentally, Internet resources have shown explosive growth in the past 20 years, along with the proliferation of mobile devices connected to the Internet enabling instantaneous access to poisoning-related information. The electronic environment in America has changed from a largely static Internet in the 1990s to a mobile one in recent years, as shown in Fig. 4.4.4. By 2019, more than 96% of US adults possessed a cell phone and 81% had a smart phone, capable of Internet access to a multitude of other electronic software applications. As one can see from comparing Figs. 4.4.3 and 4.4.4, the rise in cell phone and smart phone access has mirrored the fall in PCC calls.

While there may be many reasons for the decline, the change in Americans' behavior regarding how they use the Internet to obtain information, how they use social media to interact with others when seeking information, and how they use telephone calling versus "texting" or "e-mailing" in crisis situations may account for at least some of that change in PCC utilization.

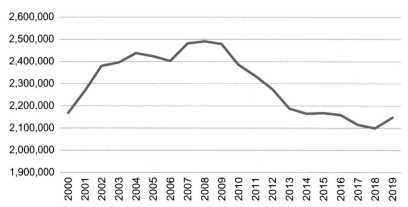

FIG. 4.4.3 Trends in exposure cases reported to NPDS by US Poison Control Centers: 2000–19. *(Data source: Gummin et al., Clin Toxicol 2020.)*

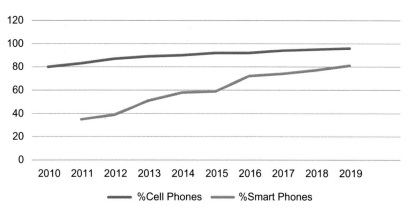

FIG. 4.4.4 Trends in acquisition of cell phones and "smart" phones by Americans: 2010–19. *(Data source: Pew Research Center survey data.)*

Smart algorithms, artificial intelligence (AI) & clinical decision-making: Internet-based automated poison control

One of the recent responses of poison control to the new and evolving landscape of the mobile electronic environment has been the creation of on-line resources of emergency poison control information. In 2015, clinicians at the AAPCC developed an online tool for consumers to obtain simple, individualized poisoning information (including phone access to a poison specialist) while also guiding consumers in avoiding errors of self-diagnosis and treatment from possibly unreliable, web-based resources. The tool, **poisonhelp.org**, was launched to the public during National Poison Week with the express goals of providing access to trustworthy, fast, easy-to-use information from a variety of devices (Gummin et al., 2020). In 2015, another Internet-based tool: web**POISONCONTROL®** was also created by Dr. Toby Litovitz and her colleagues, Jess Benson, PharmD and Susan Smolinske, PharmD. (Litovitz et al., 2016).

These innovative triage tools guide users faced with a poison emergency through a series of simple questions to determine the toxicity, using ingredient-based, automated algorithms and decision trees to help the public decide what to do when substances are swallowed, splashed in the eye or on the skin, inhaled, or injected or in cases of bites or stings. Such tools are designed only to handle uncomplicated cases. Complicated cases (e.g., high dose, multiple substances involved, pregnancy, patients with underlying medical conditions) are referred to SPIs at poison control centers.

Future of clinical toxicology and poison control

Clinical toxicology in the United States continues to evolve, employing transformative technological advances such as artificial intelligence, smart algorithms, 'big data' analysis, increasingly sophisticated Internet-based platforms, and progress in genomics and precision medicine. The future holds the inevitable introduction of new drugs and xenobiotics and their toxicities, as well as increasing threats posed by environmental pollution and climate change. Clinical toxicologists will need to develop new and better poisoning management strategies and continue to respond to new and unforeseen regional and national disasters.

But if there is one thing to be learned from the last 70 years, it is that people in our specialty are innovative, resolute, and resilient; they will continue to make progress and figure things out.

References

Anderson BD, Seung H. Klein-Schwartz W. Trends in types of calls managed by U.S. poison centers 2000–2015. Clin Toxicol 2018;56(7):640–5.

Benson BE. Interactive voice response systems for medication identification requests: poison or cure? Clin Toxicol 2011;49(9):799–800.

Blizzard JC, Michels JE, Richardson WH, Reeder CE, Schulz RM, Holstege CP. Cost-benefit analysis of a regional poison center. Clin Toxicol 2008;46(5):450–6.

Bronstein AC, Spyker DA, Cantilena LR, Green J, Rumack BH, Heard SE. 2006 annual report of the American Association of Poison Control Centers' National Poison Data System (NPDS). Clin Toxicol 2007;45(8):815–917.

Budnitz DS, Lovegrove M, Geller RJ. Prevention of unintentional medication overdose among children: time for the promise of the Poison Prevention Packaging Act to come to fruition. JAMA Netw 2020. https://doi.org/10.1001/jama.2020.2152. e1, e2 [Accessed 25 July 2020].

Chang A, Schnall AH, Law R, Bronstein AC, Marraffa JM, Spiller HA, et al. Cleaning and disinfectant chemical exposures and temporal associations with Covid-19 - National Poison Data System, United States, January 1, 2020-March 31,2020. Morbidity and Mortality Weekly Report (MMWR), CDC. 2020;69(16):496–98.

Clark RF, Phillips M, Manoguerra AS, Chan TC. Evaluating the utilization of a regional poison center by Latino communities. J Toxicol Clin Toxicol 2002;40(7):855–60.

Dart RC. The secret life of America's poison centers. Ann Emerg Med 2012;59(1):62–6.

Friedman LS, Krajewski A, Vannoy E, Allegretti WM. The association between U.S. poison center assistance and length of stay and hospital charges. Clin Toxicol 2014;52(3):198–206.

Geller RJ, Lopez GP. Poison center planning for mass gatherings: the Georgia poison center experience with the 1996 Centennial Olympic Games. J Toxicol: Clin Toxicol 1999;37(3):315–9.

Giffin S, Heard SE. Budget cuts and U.S. poison centers—regional challenges create a nationwide problem. Clin Toxicol 2009;47:790–1.

Greenwald PW, Farmer BM, O'Neill M, et al. Increasing frequency and fatality of poison control center reported exposures involving medication and multiple substances: data from reports of the American Association of Poison Control Centers 1984–2013. Clin Toxicol 2016;54:590–6.

Gummin DD, Mowry JB, Beuhler MC, Spyker DA, Brooks DE, Dibert KW, Rivers LJ, Pham NPT, Ryan ML. 2019 annual report of the American Association of Poison Control Centers' National Poison Data System (NPDS): 37th annual report. Clin Toxicol 2020;58(12):1360–541.

Gussow L. "My child ate poop!"—How one poison center established its social media presence. Clin Toxicol 2015;53(5):419–20.

Höjer J, Troutman WG, Hoppu K, Erdman A, Benson BE, Mégarbane B, et al. Position paper update: ipecac syrup for decontamination. Clin Toxicol 2013;51:134–9.

Institute of Medicine. Forging a poison prevention and control system. Washington, DC: The National Academies Press; 2004.

Jaramillo JE, Anderson HG, Jaramillo P, Nester ML, Shum S. Drug identification: a survey of Poison Control Centers. J Toxicol: Clin Toxicol 2004;42(4):371–81.

Juurlink DN. What the Internet can and cannot tell us about emerging toxicologic outbreaks. Clin Toxicol 2012;50:805–6.

Kazzi ZN, Miller CW. The role of toxicologists and poison centers during and after a nuclear power plant emergency. Clin Toxicol 2013;51:1–2.

Kelly NR, Harding JT, Fulton JE, Kozinetz CA. A randomized controlled trial of a video module to increase U.S. poison center use by low-income parents. Clin Toxicol 2014;52(1):54–62.

Klein KR, Herzog P, Smolinske S, White SR. Demand for poison control center services "surged" during the 2003 blackout. Clinical Toxicology 2007;45(3):248–54.

Kostic MA, Oswald J, Gummin DD, et al. Poison center consultation decreases hospital length of stay and inpatient charges. Clin Toxicol 2010;48:605.

Krenzelok E, Mrvos R, Mazo E. Combining primary and secondary poison prevention in one initiative. Clin Toxicol 2008;46(2):101–4.

Krenzelok EP, Mrvos R. A regional poison information center IVR medication identification system: Does it accomplish its goal? Clin Toxicol 2011;49(9):858–61.

Landrigan PJ, Woolf ADS, Gitterman B, Landrigan B, Forman J, Karr K, Moshier EL, et al. The Ambulatory Pediatric Association Fellowship in pediatric environmental health. Environ Heal Persp 2007;115:1383–7.

Landrigan PJ, Braun J, Forman J, Galvez M, Karr C, Paulson J, Woolf AD, Lanphear B, Wright RO. The APA training programs in pediatric environmental health: a 15-year assessment. Acad Pediatr 2019;19(4):421–7.

Law RK, Schier JG, Martin CA, Olivares DE, Thomas RG, Bronstein AC, Chang AS. National surveillance for radiological exposures and intentional potassium iodide and iodine product ingestions in the United States associated with the 2011 Japan radiological incident. Clin Toxicol 2013;51:41–6.

Law RK, Sheikh S, Bronstein TAR, Spiller HA, Schier JG. Incidents of potential public health significance identified using national surveillance of US poison center data (2008–2012). Clin Toxicol 2014;52(9):958–63.

Litovitz T, Benson BE, Youniss J, Edward ME. Determinants of U.S. poison center utilization. Clin Toxicol 2010a;48(5):449–57.

Litovitz T, Whitaker N, Clark L, White NC, Marsolek M. Emerging battery-ingestion hazard: clinical implications. Pediatrics 2010b;125(6):1168–77.

Litovitz T, Benson BE, Smolinske S. webPOISONCONTROL: can poison control be automated? Am J Emerg Med 2016;34:1614–9.

Litovitz TL, Klein-Schwartz W, White S, Cobaugh DJ, Youniss J, Omslaer J, et al. 2000 annual report of the American Association of Poison Control Centers Toxic Exposure Surveillance System. Am J Emerg Med 2001;19(5):337–95.

LoVecchio F, Curry SC, Waszolek K, Klemens K, Hovseth K, Glogan D. Poison control centers decrease emergency healthcare utilization costs. J Med Toxicol 2008;4(4):221–4.

Meaden CW, Ramdin C, Ruck B, Nelson LS, Soukas C, Hirsch M, et al. The poison center as a pandemic response establishment and characteristics of a COVID-19 hotline through the New Jersey poison center. Clin Toxicol 2021. https://doi.org/10.1080/15563650.2021.1905163.

Polivka BJ, Casavant MJ, Erika Malis E, Baker D. Evaluation of the Be.Poison.Smart.® poison prevention intervention. Clin Toxicol 2006;44(2):109–14.

Pronczuk de Garbino J. The sentinel role of poisons centers in the protection of children's environmental health. J Toxicol Clin Toxicol 2002;40(4):493–7.

Spiller HA, Griffith JRK. Increasing burden of pill identification requests to U.S. poison centers. Clin Toxicol 2009;47(3):253–5.

Su MK, Howland MA, Alam M, Ha C, Guerrero K, Schwartz L, Hoffman RS. Poison control centers and alternative forms of communicating with the public: what's all the chatter about? Clin Toxicol 2019;57(7):657–62.

The Lewin Group. Final report on the value of the Poison Control System. Alexandria, VA: American Association of Poison Control Centers; 2012. [cited 2017 June 20]. Available at: https://www.illinoispoisoncenter.org/value_of_poison_center_systems. [Accessed 21 May 2020].

Tustin AW, Jones A, Lopez GP, Ketcham GR, Hodgson MJ. Occupational chemical exposures: a collaboration between the Georgia Poison Center and the Occupational Safety and Health Administration. Clin Toxicol 2018;56(1):55–62.

Vassilev ZP, Marcus SM. The impact of a poison control center on the length of hospital stay for patients with poisoning. J Toxicol Environ Health A 2007;70:107–10.

Vo K, Smollin C. Online social networking and US poison control centers: Facebook as a means of information distribution. Clin Toxicol 2015;53(5):466–9.

Walter FG. Website review. Clin Toxicol 2012;50(1):81–5.

Wang A, Law R, Lyons R, Choudhary E, Wolkin A, Schier J. Assessing the public health impact of using poison center data for public health surveillance. Clin Toxicol 2018;56(7):646–52.

Watson IBM. Poisindex, https://www.micromedexsolutions.com/micromedex2/4.85.0/WebHelp/Document_help/Toxicology_Management_document.htm; 2018. [Accessed 23 May 2020].

Watson WA, Litovitz TL, Belson MG, Funk Wolkin AB, Patel M, Schier JG, et al. Toxic Exposure Surveillance System (TESS): risk assessment and real-time toxicovigilance across United States poison centers. Toxicol Appl Pharmacol 2005;207:S604–10.

Wong A, Vohra R, Dawson AH, Stolbach A. Impact of online toxicology training on health professionals: the Global Educational Toxicology Uniting Project (GETUP). Clin Toxicol 2017;55(9):981–5.

Woolf AD, Karnes DK, Kirrane BM. Preserving the United States's poison control system. Clin Toxicol 2011;49:284–6.

Woolf AD, Sibrizzi C, Kirkland K. Pediatric environmental health specialty units: an analysis of operations. Acad Pediatr 2016;16(1):25–33.

Yin S, Ho M. Monitoring a toxicological outbreak using Internet search query data. Clin Toxicol 2012;50(9):818–22.

webPoisonControl, https://www.webpoisoncontrol.org/about-us. [Accessed 2 May 2020].

Chapter 4.5

Professionalism in US Clinical Toxicology—Training, practice, consultation, and societies

Alan D. Woolf

Boston Children's Hospital & Harvard Medical School, Boston, Massachusetts, United States

Professional societies

The creation of professional societies accompanied and encouraged the growth of the field of clinical toxicology and the poison control network. The Society of Toxicology was founded in 1961 and the Society of Forensic Toxicologists was founded 9 years later, in 1970. Both attracted a variety of researchers and scientists interested in the field of toxicology broadly defined. But there was a recognized need in America for the convening of groups of health professionals with expertise in clinical toxicology. Table 4.5.1 shows the timeline of the creation of different professional organizations in the fields of toxicology and medical and clinical toxicology.

American Association of Poison Control Centers

The need for an organization convening regularly those health care professionals with a special interest in clinical toxicology and poisoning prevention was first proposed by members of the American Academy of Pediatrics (AAP) and the American Public Health Association at a joint meeting in the mid-1950s. The American Association of Poison Control Centers (AAPCC) was established at the 1958 meeting of the AAP. It also held its first meeting in October of 1958; 75% of its founding members were pediatricians (Arena, 1983). It was chartered as a nonprofit, nongovernmental voluntary organization, and it began to hold annual meetings to present scientific reports and discuss administrative challenges and issues. The first three presidents during its founding and first years from 1958 to 1960 were Edward Press, George Wheatley, and Robert Grayson.

The AAPCC gained prominence over time. Its membership evolved to include representatives from poison control centers (PCCs) across the United States, and

History of Modern Clinical Toxicology. https://doi.org/10.1016/B978-0-12-822218-8.00025-9

TABLE 4.5.1 Growth of professional societies in clinical toxicology— United States.

AAP "Accident Prevention Committee"—1952

American Association of Poison Control Centers—1958

Society of Toxicology—1961

American Academy of Clinical Toxicology—1968

Society of Forensic Toxicology—1970

American Board of Applied Toxicology—1987

American Board of Medical Toxicology—1975–1992

First Medical Toxicology Examination—1975

American College of Medical Toxicology—1993

American Board of Medical Subspecialties Medical Toxicology 1st Subboard Exam—1994

its mission also evolved to one based in the concerns and needs of a PCC. The AAPCC was charged by its leadership with advancing goals in the appropriate diagnosis and treatment of poisoning, the setting of standards for the operation of a PCC, and the promotion of education, lay and professional, to promote poison prevention (Anonymous, 1962; Mofenson, 1974). It developed minimum standards of PCCs to be eligible for certification by the AAPCC and it also developed a number of educational materials for both the public and health professionals. Such initiatives were critically important to inform the public and health care professionals regarding how to access poison control in an emergency. AAPCC initiated a modest grants program for sponsoring toxicology research, and it pursued a dialogue with the U.S. Congress in support of constructive legislative action. By 1969, the AAPCC had almost 280 individual and institutional members (Anonymous, 1970). In 1975, the AAPCC joined the AACT in joint sponsorship of the annual clinical toxicology meeting, the North American Congress of Clinical Toxicology (NACCT); that meeting heralded the subsequent close collaboration of the two societies.

Beginning in the 1970s, AAPCC addressed the immediate challenges confronting the poison control movement: regionalization, standards for operating centers, and certifying center personnel (see Chapters 4.1 and 4.2). The need for a standardized data set used to document poison center calls and a centralized system of aggregating PCC experience was also recognized early in the history of the AAPCC, which led first, to the development of the Toxic Exposure Surveillance System (TESS), and later, the National Poison Data System (NPDS) (see Chapters 4.2–4.4). AAPCC became the primary organization advocating for Federal involvement in the financing of poison control in the 1990s. It also recognized the need to enhance and expand PCC operations to include disaster preparedness and response (see Chapters 4.3 and 4.4).

American Academy of Clinical Toxicology

The present day American Academy of Clinical Toxicology (AACT) was formed by a small group of four physicians (R.T. Rappolt, D. Teitelbaum, E. Comstock, and R. Okun) and an industry representative (J. Pepper) who had an abiding passion for clinical toxicology and were seeking a vehicle to promote its growth as a new specialty and the advance of its science. They organized themselves into a chartered nonprofit organization at the October 22, 1968, meeting of the AAPCC/AAP with Dr. Eric Comstock as the first president (Thoman, 1998). There were many controversies: the length of the annual meetings, their scientific content, whether to focus more on poisonings in adults versus children, and others. They held their first national meeting that year, and then annually thereafter. In 1968, AACT members also started to publish the widely read international journal *Clinical Toxicology,* with Dr. Richard T. Rappolt, Sr., as its first editor. By 1972, the AACT had 254 dues-paying members (Anonymous, 1972). At its meeting in Aspen Colorado that year, the AACT voted to allow nonphysician members into the organization, making it officially interdisciplinary and interprofessional (Aldrich, 1998).

By 1975, the AACT and AAPCC were holding one annual, joint clinical toxicology meeting known as the North American Congress of Clinical Toxicology (NACCT). In 1976, the Canadian Academy of Clinical Toxicology became a participant in NACCT. Since then, a number of other societies, including ACMT, EAPCCT, and APAMT, have joined the NACCT, offering symposia, speakers, and organizational support. Today, NACCT is the premier international conference in clinical toxicology, offering the presentation of scientific research abstracts, lectures by noted toxicologists, and a variety of committee meetings and workshops.

By 1993, the AACT included 417 active members, 79 of whom had been accorded the honor of being named "fellows" of the Academy (Lovejoy et al., 1994). In the recent past, the AACT has begun offering its members regular distance-learning events and a variety of educational resources and has also sponsored research grants to toxicology trainees and faculty-level researchers. The AACT has since grown into a diverse interprofessional group of more than 700 individuals, representing such disciplines as nursing, physicians, first-responders (emergency medical technicians, paramedics), veterinarians, pharmacists, pharmacologists, students and clinical trainees, and scientists interested in toxicology.

American Board of Applied Toxicology

The American Board of Applied Toxicology (ABAT) was organized as a standing committee of AACT in 1987 with the goal of establishing and maintaining credentialing standards of excellence in clinical toxicology. ABAT ensures the competency for nonphysician clinical toxicologists, such as pharmacists, nurses, and PhD scientists working in the field. Eligibility requires either a doctorate degree or 5 years of full-time work in clinical toxicology. Many candidates will have completed a 12-month fellowship training program in clinical pharmacology and toxicology offered by some regional PCCs affiliated with schools of pharmacy in academic medical centers. ABAT conducts a rigorous credentialing and examination process to certify its diplomates. It provides guidance on how to prepare and a list of potential exam topics designed to prepare and support prospective candidates for its board examination.

Candidates who pass the board examination are conferred the title: Diplomate of the American Board of Applied Toxicology (DABAT), and are thereafter members of ABAT. ABAT members possess the requisite knowledge, experience, and competence to provide their expertise to PCCs, emergency departments, critical care services, government agencies, and others in need of clinical toxicology expertise. They are recognized as clinical toxicologists demonstrating exceptional knowledge, experience, and expertise. ABAT is committed to continuing professional development and serves as a resource for the education of health care professionals. It administers board re-certification exams periodically to its diplomates to ensure that their knowledge of clinical toxicology is current.

American College of Medical Toxicologists

The American College of Medical Toxicologists (ACMT) was formed as a new, physician-only nonprofit society immediately after the American Board of Medical Toxicology (ABMT) was dissolved in 1993. The president of the ABMT from 1990 to 1992, Dr. Lewis Goldfrank, and the president of the new ACMT from 1992 to 1994, Dr. William Banner, both presided over this transition. ACMT's mission statement on its website has the twin goals: "advancing the toxicologic care of patients and populations; and advocating for the specialty of medical toxicology." ACMT was chartered to further the interests of research and education in toxicology and to be a resource for physicians in training to become medical toxicologists and those in the clinical practice of medical toxicology. It began to hold annual meetings separate from the NACCT at which scientific abstracts of research were reviewed, didactic lectures presented, and the organization's committees could meet. ACMT also sponsors national webinars, workshops and seminars. Originally the ACMT created the *Internet Journal of Medical Toxicology* in 1998 but it recognized the need for a print version and, in 2005, founded the *Journal of Medical Toxicology (JMT)* to publish scientific studies of interest to its members. ACMT also publishes its position statements and abstracts from its annual scientific meeting in *JMT*. It co-sponsors international toxicology seminars with other societies and has organized special research groups such as the ToxICs group (described later). It offers travel and research grants within its Medical Toxicology Foundation. The ACMT now has more than 800 members.

Collaborations, consortia, partnerships

EXTRIP (**EX**tracorporeal **TR**eatments **I**n **P**oisoning)—an international group of recognized experts (medical toxicology, pharmacology, emergency medicine, nephrology, pediatrics, critical care) representing a number of different international professional societies first convened in October 2010. Their purpose was to use a rigorous evidence-based methodology to provide guidance statements regarding the clinical indications for the use of advanced, invasive extracorporeal treatments—such as hemodialysis, hemoperfusion, sustained low efficiency dialysis, plasma exchange, and exchange blood transfusion—in the management of the patient suffering from an acute, severe, life-threatening poisoning (Lavergne et al., 2017). Opinions from over 30 national and international professional societies have been solicited; many have endorsed and sponsored the initiative. Funding was acquired from industry with careful restrictions to avoid a conflict of interests. Members of the workgroup are not paid honoraria; they donate their time and effort. The group uses a formal methodology with a systematic approach to the review and grading of the extant scientific literature for its scientific rigor. It carefully considers the risks, costs, and benefits of the intervention in the context of each particular poisoning. It then uses a modified Delphi system of two rounds of voting among its experts before reaching consensus decisions on the clinical utility of the intervention (Lavergne et al., 2017). So far, the workgroup has published its recommendations for a series of toxic agents, such as salicylates, phenytoin, acetaminophen, lithium, metformin, and others.

ToxIC (Toxicology Investigators Consortium)—In 2010, leaders of the ACMT (led by Dr. Jeffrey Brent, a prominent medical toxicologist in Denver) created the Toxicology Investigators Consortium (ToxIC) case registry and multicenter research database, attracting over 50 participating sites within its first 2 years (ACMT ToxIC, 2020). Medical toxicologists enter poisoning cases admitted to in-patient medical toxicology services in hospitals or treated in outpatient clinics. Most participating sites are located in academic institutions, which collectively sponsor about two-thirds of the medical toxicology training programs for physicians in the country. The database template includes de-identified demographic, clinical and toxicological data on patients cared for by the medical toxicology service at each center. The ToxIC Case Registry functions under the Western Investigational Review Board (IRB) approval, however, each site is responsible for satisfying IRB requirements at its own institution. By 2018, 65 hospitals representing 40 medical centers (in 47 cities and 23 states and 10 Federal districts) were contributing cases to the ToxIC registry. By then, the registry contained exposure data on over 1100 different toxicological agents.

Origins of physician training in medical toxicology

It was recognized by pediatricians and other primary care physicians in the 1960s that there was a curriculum to be mastered in attaining the required competencies of medical knowledge recognized as the field of medical toxicology. By the 1970s, there were PhD-oriented graduate programs in toxicology offered by many American schools of medicine (Anonymous, 1975), but these did not necessarily emphasize clinical applications. Most PhD programs in toxicology are basic science oriented and are located in the graduate schools, rather than the hospitals and medical schools, at most universities.

However, 1 or 2-year training programs in clinical toxicology had also been established in academic centers, often affiliated with PCCs, in cities like Boston, San Francisco, New York City, Denver, and Phoenix. These trainings were sometimes offered within the framework of a clinical pharmacology as well as a toxicology curriculum, and usually included opportunities to carry out research (Lovejoy Jr et al., 1979; Done, 1979). Dr. Eric Comstock published an outline for a curriculum in clinical toxicology in 1968, including details of content in six general areas: (1) an introduction (scope, prevention, and resources), (2) first aid for poisoning, (3) diagnosis of poisoning, (4) principles of the treatment of poisoning, (5) management of coma, and (6) clinical management of poisoning due to specific substances (Comstock, 1968).

The advent of a new physician-oriented medical subspecialty, medical toxicology, focused on the diagnosis, management, and prevention of human poisoning/toxicity from drugs, chemicals, occupational and environmental substances, and other hazards. Opportunities for physician training in medical toxicology became more widespread and formalized during the 1960s and 1970s as the fundamentals and scope of the specialty were defined. While the poison control movement was originally championed by pediatricians and almost half of PCC calls concerned children, a growing number of calls involved serious poisonings among adolescents and adults. These patients often presented to emergency departments in a serious or life-threatening condition, due to toxic effects of substance and alcohol use or overdoses taken in suicide attempts. Coincident to the growth of the poison control movement in the 1970s was the professionalization of the new field of Emergency Medicine as a defined specialty, culminating with its recognition by the American Board of Medical Specialties. This new Emergency Medicine specialty asserted its prominent role in the training and credentialing of physicians in medical toxicology.

American Board of Medical Toxicology

Academic hospitals and PCCs began to offer fellowships and/or preceptorships to physicians who wished to gain added expertise in clinical toxicology in the 1970s. To fill the gap in recognition of those who has mastered the fundamentals of the field, in 1974 the AACT organized within its own society a new, independent subspecialty board: the American Board of Medical Toxicology (ABMT) comprised only of physicians (Aldrich, 1998). Its first president was Dr. Daniel Teitelbaum. This new Board administered its own certifying exam. The initial ABMT board used a random number generator to determine who would take the exam in 1975 and who would give it. It was then reversed and those who had taken it, gave it to the others the next year, 1976. The first few years were only oral exams with two examiners for each hour, lasting 2 hours divided into two segments. There were three questions per hour.

After a few years, the process was modified—a written test was first given which, if passed, allowed the candidate to take an oral examination. Those who passed these hurdles were declared board-certified in medical toxicology. The general qualifications for sitting for the exam were (Lovejoy, 1979):

1. Graduation from an approved medical school.
2. A license to practice medicine in any jurisdiction.
3. Board eligibility in a recognized medical specialty.
4. High standards of professional conduct and ethical considerations similar to those required by any medical licensing board.
5. Until 1984: either 5 years of experience in the practice of medicine with emphasis on clinical toxicology (no specified minimum percentage time), or completion of 2 years of formal training in clinical toxicology in a training program approved by the board.
6. After 1984: each candidate must have completed an approved 2-year post-graduate training program in clinical toxicology.

The first certifying exam was administered in Kansas City, Missouri, in 1975 (Thoman, 1998). By 1978, there were 31 charter diplomates certified by the ABMT (Anonymous, 1979).

ABMT continued to certify medical toxicologists until the early 1990s when there was a drive by its leadership to have the specialty recognized as one of equal standing to others within medicine by the American Board of Medical Specialties (ABMS). The essential ingredients for such recognition included a body of specialized knowledge, the existence of definitive texts covering the field, and the growing number of health professionals whose career directions were defined by their identity as medical toxicologists. The ABMT was dissolved as an independent certifying board in 1992 and was subsequently transformed into a new professional society: the American College of Medical Toxicology.

ABMT board certification

Through the years, as the science improved, the new specialty of medical toxicology redefined its curriculum to include those topics considered essential for the practice of medical toxicology. Physicians were passionate about the field and recognized their unique role as experts to whom other health care providers could turn for advice. By the 1970s, the ABMT had expanded the curriculum to include: (1) acute pediatric and adult drug ingestion, (2) drug abuse and addiction, (3) chemical poisoning (e.g., heavy metals, hydrocarbons, insecticides, pesticides, plastics, gases, vapors, acids, and bases), (4) environmental hazards and pollutants (e.g., lead, carbon monoxide, and ozone), (5) occupational toxicology (e.g., solvents, metals, metalloids, and dusts), (6) biological poisons (e.g., food poisoning, ingestion of poisonous plants, or mushrooms, and envenomation), (7) basic concepts of toxicology, and (8) basic principles of poison prevention (Lovejoy, 1979). The curriculum was intended to prepare the physician to take the written examination for board certification in the specialty. The drive for specialization was also propelled by the publishing of excellent, comprehensive textbooks that became the standard references for those studying in the specialty. Such texts included *Casarett & Doull's Toxicology: The Basic Science of Poisons* (The McGraw-Hill Companies, Inc. New York, NY 1975), *Goldfrank's Toxicologic Emergencies* (Appleton & Lange Publishers, New York, NY 1978), Haddad & Winchester's *Clinical Management of Poisoning and Drug Overdose* (WB Saunders Company, Philadelphia PA 1983) and Ellenhorn and Barceloux's *Medical Toxicology: Diagnosis and Treatment of Human Poisoning* (Elsevier Publishers, New York, NY 1988). These references and others signified the growth and formalization of the new subspecialty.

Fellowship training programs in medical toxicology were centered in the new academic departments of emergency medicine, in collaboration with PCCs. While the ABMT allowed board eligibility after an "apprenticeship" period of practice and preceptorship under the guidance of an individual with clinical toxicology expertise, toward the end of the 1980s the only pathway to board certification in medical toxicology was by completing a formal fellowship. Between 1970 and 1997, 147 physicians had received fellowship training at one of 21 recognized medical toxicology training programs (Wax and Donovan, 2000).

ABMS board certification

In 1992, the American Board of Medical Specialties (ABMS) formally approved subspecialty board credentialing in medical toxicology, which completed its recognition as an American medical specialty. Medical toxicology certification was offered by the Medical Toxicology Sub-Board, administered by the American Board of Emergency Medicine (ABEM) and jointly sponsored by ABEM, American Board of Pediatrics, and American Board of Preventive Medicine. Eligibility to take the new board examination could be satisfied by several routes: fellowship completion, prior ABMT certification, an "apprentice"-like preceptorship, or a combination of preceptorship–fellowship. All but one of these choices were phased out by 2002; thereafter, only those physicians who had completed a fellowship recognized by the ABMS were eligible for board certification. The first ABMS examination in medical toxicology was administered in 1994. Board-certification is time-limited, requiring re-certification every 10 years. By 2007, there were 287 ABMS diplomates of the Medical Toxicology subboard (primary board certification: emergency medicine 82%, preventive medicine 10%, pediatrics 8%) (White et al., 2010).

During the transition from ABMT to ABMS test administration, a new Medical Toxicology Core Content, consisting of some 22 content areas, was developed to prepare applicants. It was revised in 2004 and again in 2012. In the 2012 revision, major content categories now included (1) principles of toxicology, (2) toxins and toxicants (drugs, drugs of abuse, industrial, household and environmental toxicants, natural products, warfare and terrorism, and radiological), (3) clinical assessment, (4) therapeutics, (5) assessment and population health, and (6) analytical and forensic toxicology (Nelson et al., 2012). Since year 2000, the proliferation of Internet-based learning platforms, interactive social media, and other resources have all presented opportunities to offer new methods of teaching medical toxicology. Simulated cases, case experience, tutorials, podcasts, blogs, "microblogging," video presentations, and interactive Twitter forums (tweetchats and tweetorials) can all complement the clinical learning environment. Synchronous or asynchronous "virtual" educational opportunities address the learning needs of both physicians in medical toxicology training as well as those in practice (Chai, 2015; Kim et al., 2016; Vo et al., 2019; Chary and Chai, 2020).

ACGME training program accreditation

By 1996, there were 26 academic center-based programs offering training in the specialty of medical toxicology in the United States (Anonymous, 1997). In 2000, the Accreditation Council of Graduate Medical Education (ACGME) recognized that fellowship training in medical toxicology had met its rigorous standards so as to be recognized and credentialed as a medical subspecialty. By 2002, there were 20 ACGME-certified 2-year training programs in the US. Fellowship applicants typically have already completed a residency in emergency medicine, internal medicine, family medicine, pediatrics, or preventive medicine. In 2020, the 26 ACGME-accredited programs had 46 applicants for their 51 available training positions (NRMP, 2020).

Toxicology treatment centers

Since the 1960s, the history of clinical toxicology in the United States has included the recognition of needed toxicology expertise in direct patient care—both for in-patient services and consultations, as well as ambulatory services (Inniss, 1970). Such toxicology treatment centers would complement, not replace, the daily work of PCCs. With the certification of medical toxicologists by the ABMT beginning in 1975, a few clinicians devoted their time solely to the practice of clinical toxicology. Dr. Eric Comstock described 212 cases referred to his practice from plaintiff attorneys (37%), employers, insurance companies, and defense attorneys (26%), and physicians (24%) (Comstock, 1979). By the 1990s, medical toxicologists were advocating for broader recognition of "Regional Toxicology Treatment Centers" (RTTC) to support and complement the role of PCCs while providing advanced toxicology services in both hospital and ambulatory clinic settings (Banner et al., 1993; Krenzelok, 1993). They cited instances involving serious poisonings that were either not reported to a PCC and mishandled by hospital staff, or those cases where PCC advice was offered but not followed, resulting in increased morbidity and mortality. They noted that the earliest certification criteria for PCCs set forth by the AAPCC included a requirement for access to advanced toxicological services.

Criteria for operating a high quality RTTC were offered: a staff of board-certified medical toxicologists, the availability of comprehensive specialty consultants, an intensive care unit capable of advanced therapies such as hemodialysis, an analytical toxicology laboratory, and the stocking of required antidotes (Krenzelok, 1993). Since that time, some hospitals have established multidisciplinary toxicology admitting and consultation services, which might include not only board-certified medical toxicologists but also physician trainees, nurse specialists, clinical pharmacologists, and pharmacists. Patient referrals most commonly come from three sources: the emergency department, one of the hospital general or specialty services, or the collaborating PCC (Wang et al., 2015). Such consultations are billable services and generate revenue for the emergency department or other sponsoring division, but have also been shown to lower hospitalization costs by improving management, lowering morbidity, and decreasing length of stay (Curry et al., 2015; King et al., 2019; Parish et al., 2019).

References

ACMT ToxIC. American College of Medical Toxicology, Toxicology Investigators Consortium (ToxIC), https://www.acmt.net; 2020. [Accessed 5 May 2020].

Aldrich FD. Looking back. J Toxicol Clin Toxicol 1998;36(5):397–8.

Anonymous. American Association of Poison Control Centers. N Engl J Med 1962;267(26):1371–2.

Anonymous. American Association of Poison Control Centers. AAPCC membership list 1968–1969. Clin Toxicol 1970;3(2):308–28.

Anonymous. American Academy of Clinical Toxicology membership roster 1972. Clin Toxicol 1972;5(4):585–98.

Anonymous. Schools of medicine offering training in toxicology. Clin Toxicol 1975;8(1):125–31.

Anonymous. Certified charter diplomates of the American Board of Medical Toxicology. Clin Toxicol 1979;12(4):413–6.

Anonymous. Directory of toxicology fellowships. J Toxicol Clin Toxicol 1997;35(7):773–5.

Arena JM. The pediatrician's role in the poison control movement and poison prevention. Am J Dis Child 1983;137:870–3.

Banner W, Brent J, Garrettson LK, Lawrence RA, Rodgers GC, Shannon MW, Spyker DA, Tenenbein M, Vale JA, Weisman RS. What's in a name?—regional toxicology treatment centers. J Toxicol Clin Toxicol 1993;31(2):219–20.

Chai PR. Enriching the toxicology experience through Twitter. J Med Toxicol 2015;11:385–7.

Chary MA, Chai PR. Tweetchats, disseminating information, and sparking further scientific discussion with social media. J Med Toxicol 2020;16:109–11.

Comstock EG. The treatment of poisoning: a program for the medical curriculum. Clin Toxicol 1968;1(1):49–56.

Comstock EG. The practice of medical toxicology. Clin Toxicol 1979;15(1):1–11.

Curry SC, Brooks DE, Skolink AB, Gerkin RD, Glenn S. Effect of a medical toxicology admitting service on length of stay, cost, and mortality among inpatients discharged with poisoning-related diagnoses. J Med Toxicol 2015;11:65–72.

Done AK. Design of a clinical toxicology training program in conjunction with clinical pharmacology in a children's hospital. Clin Toxicol 1979;15(4):387–92.

Inniss CN. A poison consultation system: University of Michigan Medical Center. Clin Toxicol 1970 1970;3(2):205–9.

Kim H, Heverling H, Cordeiro M, Vasquez V, Stolbach A. Internet training resulted in improved trainee performance in a simulated opioid poisoned patient as measured by checklist. J Med Toxicol 2016;12:289–94.

King AM, Danagoulian S, Lynch M, Menke N, Mu Y, Saul M, Abesamis M, Pizon AF. The effect of a medical toxicology inpatient service in an academic tertiary care referral center. J Med Toxicol 2019;15:12–21.

Krenzelok E. Facility assessment guidelines for regional toxicology treatment centers. J Toxicol Clin Toxicol 1993;31(2):211–7.

Lavergne V, Nolin TD, Hoffman RS, Roberts D, Gosselin S, Goldfarb DS, et al. The EXTRIP (*Extracorporeal TReatments In Poisoning*) workgroup: guideline methodology. Clin Toxicol 2017;50(5):403–13.

Lovejoy FH. The American Board of Medical Toxicology of the American Academy of Clinical Toxicology: requirements for certification. Clin Toxicol 1979;15(4):499–503.

Lovejoy FH, Robertson WO, Woolf AD. Poison centers, poison prevention and the pediatrician. Pediatrics 1994;94(2):220–4.

Lovejoy Jr FH, Edlin A, Goldman P. Utilization of the poison center for the teaching of clinical toxicology to medical students, house-staff, and health care professionals. Clin Toxicol 1979;15(4):393–400.

Mofenson HC. The American Association of Poison Control Centers. Clin Pediatr 1974;13:305–6.

National Resident Matching Program (NRMP). Results and data: specialties matching service 2020 appointment year. Washington, DC: National Resident Matching Program; 2020. Available at: https://www.nrmp.org/fellowship-match-data/. [Accessed 25 May 2020].

Nelson LS, Baker BA, Osterhoudt KC, Snook CP, Keehbauch JN. The 2012 core content of medical toxicology. J Med Toxicol 2012;8(2):183–91.

Parish S, Carter A, Liu YH, Humble I, Trott N, Jacups S, Little M. The impact of the introduction of a toxicology service on the intensive care unit. Clin Toxicol 2019;57(9):778–83.

Thoman M. The American Academy of Clinical Toxicology: a historic pediatric perspective. J Toxicol Clin Toxicol 1998;36(5):399–400.

Vo T, Ledbetter C, Zuckerman M. Video delivery of toxicology educational content versus textbook for asynchronous learning, using acetaminophen overdose as a topic. Clin Toxicol 2019;57(10):842–6.

Wang GS, Monte A, Hatten B, Brent J, Buchanan J, Heard KJ. Initiation of a medical toxicology consult service at a tertiary care children's hospital. Clin Toxicol 2015;53(4):192–4.

Wax PM, Donovan JW. Fellowship training in medical toxicology: characteristics, perceptions, and career impact. J Toxicol Clin Toxicol 2000;38(6):637–42.

White SR, Baker B, Baum CR, Harvey A, Korte R, Avery AN, et al. 2007 survey of medical toxicology practice. J Med Toxicol 2010;6:281–5.

Section 5

Clinical toxicology and poison information in Europe, Scandinavia, and Israel

D. Nicholas Bateman

Honorary Professor of Clinical Toxicology, University of Edinburgh, Edinburgh, United Kingdom

Although there had been expertise in Europe in the 19th century, notably Orfila in Paris who developed experimental toxicology and Christison in Edinburgh who was a forensic and experimental pharmacologist, the development of poisons centers came after World War Two. Some articles on the management of poisoning, particularly those from Denmark in the early 1950s, affected the approach of some clinicians to the management of barbiturate poisoning (Clemmesen and Nilsson, 1961).

The first poison center in Europe is generally considered to have been Dutch, founded in 1959, shortly followed by France and many other countries (Persson, 2004). In some countries such as the United Kingdom, Italy, France and Germany, there were several centers which were developed independently and merged into national networks or were conceived initially as a national system.

Clinical toxicology was often conducted as a specialty away from the poison center as part of emergency medicine, intensive care, clinical pharmacology, forensic medicine or public health, depending on the country and interests of clinicians in those specialties. Use of poison gas in the First World War and its threat in World War Two had resulted in specialist medical expertise in poisoning in the armed services in many countries. Approaches to the co-location of poison centers and treatment facilities varied across the continent. This section will show the different approaches to the specialty in a range of different European countries, Israel, and the World Health Organization.

References

Clemmesen C, Nilsson E. Therapeutic trends in the treatment of barbiturate poisoning: the Scandanavian method. Clin Pharmacol Ther 1961;2:220–9.

Persson H. European Association of Poisons Centres and Clinical Toxicologists EAPCCT 1964–2004 a perspective over four decades. EAPCCT Archive. Available on request from https://www.eapcct.org; 2004. accessed on January 5, 2020.

Chapter 5.1

United Kingdom and Ireland

D. Nicholas Bateman[a] and Alex Proudfoot[b]

[a]*Honorary Professor of Clinical Toxicology, University of Edinburgh, Edinburgh, United Kingdom*
[b]*Former Physician Royal Infirmary of Edinburgh and Director Scottish Poisons Information Bureau, Edinburgh, United Kingdom*

Origins

The origins of poisons information services in the United Kingdom date to the 1950s and 1960s, when a large increase in acute poisoning was becoming apparent. For example, in 1900 the Royal Infirmary of Edinburgh admitted less than 20 poisoned patients; by 1950 it was approximately 100 and by 1970 more than 2000 (Matthew and Lawson, 1975; Proudfoot et al., 2013). In England and Wales in 1951 deaths from poisoning averaged 65 per week but by 1957 had reached 91 per week (The Atkins Report, 1962). The social upheaval during and after World War II, the rapidly increasing availability of potentially toxic pharmaceuticals and the increasing exposures to carbon monoxide from increased use of coal gas as an agent for self-harm may have all played a role.

The first major drug poisoning problem in the United Kingdom was due to barbiturates. This led, in the 1950s, to the opening of a specific unit in Oldchurch Hospital, Romford, Essex, the North-East Thames Regional Barbiturate Unit, which provided information on the best management of this particular poisoning to clinicians who telephoned them (Locket, 1957, 1970). In the early 1960s, the pharmacy department of Leeds General Infirmary developed written protocols on the management of poisoning and operated a poisons information service from August 1961; the majority of inquiries concerned children under the age of 15. This service became well-known, receiving calls from across the United Kingdom and some from Europe (Ellis, 1964; Ellis and Blacow, 1965). Also, at the end of 1962, the American Air Force Hospital at RAF Burderop in Wiltshire (its UK poison control center) offered to provide poisons information to local doctors until it closed in 1965 (Freeman, 1965).

History of Modern Clinical Toxicology. https://doi.org/10.1016/B978-0-12-822218-8.00019-3

1962 Report

The key development was the response of the then Ministry of Health (now Department of Health (DoH)) to the poisoning "epidemic"—the establishment of a committee under the chairmanship of Professor Sir Hedley Atkins, a surgeon at Guys Hospital London. His report [Emergency Treatment in Hospital of Cases of Acute Poisoning (The Atkins Report), 1962] recommended:

1. Hospital accident and emergency departments should have textbooks on poisoning diagnosis and management.
2. One general hospital in an area should be designated as the preferred receiving center (the "District Center") for cases of poisoning.
3. Each District Center should have an adequate laboratory service.
4. Regional poisoning treatment centers should be established with specific physician expertise and techniques such as dialysis available.
5. A network of information services should be set up.
6. There should be a national center for academic research into poisoning.

The objectives of the information services included helping doctors "identify rapidly and with certainty the properties or ingredients of a substance" and "the establishment of a service which could at any time give uniform information to inquirers could be of invaluable assistance." Half a century later it is interesting to note the stress on uniformity of information as problems soon occurred. Importantly, unlike many other countries the National Poisons Information Service (NPIS) was never commissioned to answer public calls.

Four information centers

The United Kingdom had regional governments in Northern Ireland, Scotland, and Wales although DoH policies were generally implemented across the whole United Kingdom, as they were with poisoning. Four information centers were established, in London (England) at Guy's Hospital; in Belfast (Northern Ireland), at the Royal Victoria Infirmary; and in Edinburgh (Scotland), at the Royal Infirmary; all in 1963. Wales joined with a center in Cardiff Royal Infirmary in 1964 established by Dr. J.D.P. Graham, a member of the Atkins Committee. These hospitals all offered specialized treatments such as hemodialysis and, later, charcoal perfusion. Some did much research as they also cared for poisoned patients, but no true academic center was established. The Leeds poisons information database was acquired and, after being put into a standard format in London, was distributed to the centers in Belfast, Cardiff, and Edinburgh and subsequently updated.

The NPIS established

The London Center was named the National Poisons Information Center (Anonymous, 1963) but by early 1965 its director, Dr. Roy Goulding, who as a Senior Medical Officer (Toxicology) in the Ministry of Health had served as secretary to the Atkins Committee, was using National Poisons Information

Service as its title, which caused confusion among users outside England (Goulding, 1965). It was only in the 1990s that the title included the regional centers and incorporated Leeds and, later, Newcastle and Birmingham.

In the 1960s staffing of the individual centers was determined by regional governments. Cardiff was the only one with 24-h coverage. The others had office staff 9 am–5 pm, Monday–Friday, and used doctors and nurses with experience of managing poisoned patients after hours (Goulding and Watkin, 1965). In London, medical students were used to staff the after-hours service in the late 1960s until increasing numbers of "poisons information officers" were recruited and trained in house, as they were in the other units across the United Kingdom.

Regional centers join NPIS

In 1973 Noel Wright, an Edinburgh trainee, established a regional poisons information service and laboratory in Birmingham as the West Midlands Poisons Unit in Dudley Road Hospital (later renamed City Hospital). After Wright's departure Allister Vale, who had been in Guy's from the Unit's inception as a medical student information provider, moved to Birmingham in 1982 as the new director. Like Cardiff, Edinburgh, and Newcastle, this center had the major advantages of dedicated beds for poisoned patients and served a large population.

In 1974, only a year after the Birmingham Center was established, Michael Rawlins joined Newcastle University Medical School as professor of clinical pharmacology and, working with Dr. D.M. Davies, amalgamated the Regional Drug Information Unit into the Wolfson Unit of Clinical Pharmacology. This became the Northern (later Northern and Yorkshire) Regional Drug and Therapeutic Unit. It provided poisons information using pharmacists in hours, and clinical pharmacologists after-hours via the hospital switchboard. In 1983, six beds in the new Freeman Hospital in Newcastle-upon-Tyne opened for management of poisoned patients. These two new centers and Leeds joined the national network in the 1980s.

A poisons center continued to be run from the pharmacy department at Leeds General Infirmary until National Health Service (NHS) reorganization in the 1990s merged the Northern and Yorkshire Regions. The Leeds information service soon closed, as its service was now run from the Regional Center in Newcastle, though its staff continued to provide educational support to the NPIS.

In 1993 Guy's Hospital was merged with St. Thomas's Hospital and acute services moved to the latter site. New accommodation for the London information center had been built at New Cross Hospital in 1967, some miles from the main Guy's site, where it remained until 2008. It was linked to a laboratory expert in chemical and toxicological analyses not generally available in NHS hospitals. Since it had no beds, patients with suspected nonacute poisoning were seen on an outpatient basis. This was rectified when a clinical service was developed at St. Thomas's by Paul Dargan and colleagues in collaboration with the emergency department.

Service volume challenges

Individual UK centers were managed locally by clinical toxicologists everywhere but Leeds (pharmacists). Loose higher management was by regional government departments. Inquiries to the NPIS increased; those to London far outnumbered those to the others, doubling between 1971 and 1981 (Volans et al., 1981) and doubling again in the 6 years 1991–1997 to reach over 200,000 annually. In comparison, Edinburgh had 5410 inquiries in 1981 (Proudfoot and Davidson, 1983). These disparities created political and practical difficulties. Funding continued to be provided by regional governments, but the London center obtained greatly increased budgets from the DoH as well as generating funds itself. A paper record of all calls was kept (later placed in a computer record). Updating of the poisons database by the London center fell behind. There were some duplicate index entries and some containing contradictory information. As a result different information was occasionally provided to the same caller about the same patient. The workload in London created difficulties. Despite increased staffing and introduction of a telephone management system, calls were held in a queue for long periods at very busy times, which was deemed unacceptable by the DoH.

TOXBASE

The Edinburgh Center responded to the rising call load in the early 1980s when director Alex Proudfoot computerized information on poisoning with a grant from the Scottish Home and Health Department into a new database which he named TOXBASE. TOXBASE made poisons information available to distant emergency departments by means of Viewdata©teletext (Proudfoot and Davidson, 1983). By modern standards this technology was extremely slow; the screen allowed only 20 lines with approximately 10 words per line. The information presented, therefore, had to be concise, accurate, and concentrate on simple, effective treatment advice. The written poisons information database was used to insure comprehensiveness of poisons content, but not to provide the data for the TOXBASE entries, most of which were individually written by staff in Edinburgh. The system was remarkably successful and by the mid-1990s was receiving around 100,000 accesses annually, particularly from Scotland, northern England, and Northern Ireland. It was not widely promoted in the rest of England since the center in London was heavily focused on telephone answering supported by its paper poisons information database. TOXBASE was offered to the London center but not adopted as they preferred the paper system for local operational reasons.

NPIS reorganization: UK health departments plan—1997

By the mid-1990s, it was clear to the DoH that poisons advice was not consistent across centers. A distinguished clinical pharmacologist, Professor Paul

Turner, was appointed to chair meetings of the centers' directors, including Birmingham, Leeds and Newcastle. This was the real beginning of the integrated NPIS, although funding pressures remained, caused by the increasing call numbers. The London Center had expanded to providing veterinary information (for which it was not paid by the DoH and separately funded) and had other specialist services (e.g., on Chinese medicines). External consultants were called in 1997 to advise the DoH. Their report advised a complete reorganization of the service. No units were closed, but better distribution of the work-load was planned with a single telephone number for inquiries from the whole of UK. TOXBASE was adopted as the primary information source to insure that advice to clinicians was standardized and was to be provided on the Internet to all UK emergency departments as the first point of information to reduce telephone calls, particularly after hours. Centers were to be given individual areas of responsibility within the service.

A further complication at this time was the decision by DoH in 1997 to launch health information telephone lines, NHS Direct in England and Wales and NHS 24 in Scotland (later all NHS 111), as the public's first point of contact for advice on health emergencies. This was done to try to manage after-hours general practitioner call loads and hospital emergency department attendances. A pilot site was in Newcastle, and the poisons service director there, Nick Bateman, was approached when it was realized that this service would attract poisons information calls from the public. The NHS Direct pilot service was given access to the computer-based TOXBASE, which became a core component of NHS Direct. NPIS units across the United Kingdom became heavily involved in training NHS Direct and NHS 24 staff in its use. Calls from these services are still a significant part of NPIS workload (NPIS, 2017–2018 Annual Report).

The UK DoH's plan required TOXBASE to be modernized as it had used the same platform since its inception. Alex Proudfoot had retired and the first task for Nick Bateman, recruited from Newcastle, was to put TOXBASE into a modern Internet format with funding provided by the Scottish government. TOXBASE was re-launched in 1999 (Bateman et al., 2002a, 2002b).

Health Protection Agency—2002

Circumstances changed again in 2002, with the publication by the Chief Medical Officer of England, Liam Donaldson, of the monograph: *Getting Ahead of the Curve: A strategy for combating infectious diseases (including other aspects of health protection)* (Donaldson, 2002). This contained a policy to establish a new agency, the Health Protection Agency, which would be responsible for managing poison information services, as well as advising on chemical and radiation exposures. A public health physician, Professor Stephen Palmer, was appointed to the chemical and poisons component. He appointed another public health physician, Dr. Elaine Lynch-Farmery, to undertake management responsibility for the poisons service. Her task was to fully implement the policies established by the DoH in the late 1990s and early 2000s. She instituted a single national telephone number with technology that automatically directed calls to centers with free telephone lines.

A number of working groups were set up: a Management Group chaired by Farmery, included all the UK center physician directors together with the director of the Dublin Unit, information staff and public health representatives; a Clinical Standards Group of clinicians, chaired by an NPIS director; and a TOXBASE Editing Group of clinicians and information staff, chaired by the Edinburgh director in view of the key importance of TOXBASE. A new name for the information centers was also adopted, "NPIS Units," and named for the city in which they were based.

The role of the Management Group was to set policy, and the Standards Group to agree, by consensus, to any clinical protocols that might be controversial. The TOXBASE group oversaw the authoring and reviewing of TOXBASE content. At this stage, TOXBASE contained over 13,000 entries; an ambitious program of regular review of all entries was initiated. Every entry would be reviewed by every Unit; Units would all contribute new entries to the database, using an agreed upon format. To unify the clinical information collected by NPIS Units from telephone inquiries, all centers adopted UKPID (UK Poisons Information Database), the computer system developed by Cardiff, while information on commercial products was collected in Birmingham and placed in an NPIS database.

Teratology information service

In an earlier attempt to manage funding, the Teratology Information Service which had been established at Guy's in the 1970s was transferred under contract to the Newcastle poisons unit in 1995 where it ran as a sub-component of the NPIS. The teratology database was placed on TOXBASE and also had a separate website (UKTIS; http://www.uktis.org) and a public facing one (BUMPS; https://www.medicinesinpregnancy.org).

On-call responsibilities

Another challenge faced by the NPIS was the introduction of the European Working Time Directive which legally limited the total hours doctors could be on call. Before this, local physicians had covered poisons inquiries after hours and, in the case of the directors, this often meant 1 in 2 nights on-call. This situation was not sustainable; directors determined that a single national on-call rota would service the whole United Kingdom. A rota of Poisons Units on call for poisons information calls was also instituted, with staff available 24 h daily, and at least two Units being available for most of this time. This was supported by an on call out-of-hours consultant named in the clinical toxicology national rota.

The London Unit declined to join either of those rotas, leaving the other units to provide 24-h coverage. As Edinburgh information staff were not on-call, due to staffing levels and demands of TOXBASE authorship and editing, the rota comprised the three remaining Units: Birmingham, Cardiff, and Newcastle-upon-Tyne, with specialist clinician support from all four Units. The Unit in Belfast had already closed due to staffing problems and Northern Ireland was covered from the United Kingdom.

The London Unit closed after more than 40 years of operation (Oral answers to questions - Health, 2005; Guys and St Thomas' NHS Trust, 2007). The clinical service continued at St. Thomas's Hospital and, fortunately, was subsequently re-incorporated into the NPIS as part of the specialist clinician on-call rota. A Veterinary Poisons Information Service (VPIS) continues, independently funded by subscription (Annual Report VPIS, 2017).

The present NPIS

There are currently four NPIS Units (Birmingham, Cardiff, Edinburgh, and Newcastle) supported by a rota of 16 consultant clinicians with expertise in clinical toxicology, most being accredited clinical pharmacologists. The UK service answers most inquiries online; in the financial year 2017–2018 TOXBASE had 733,351 user sessions to 2,126,690 product pages (64% hospital, 23% public health telephone services) and 40,466 telephone calls (27% hospital, 37% public health telephone services). In recent years, a TOXBASE App (Android and Apple) has been available, by which there were 152,469 accesses from 15,469 users. There were 1994 referrals to NPIS consultants: 1757 from hospitals and 30 from Ireland. TOXBASE and NPIS conduct quality assurance regularly, and the ratings show high levels of service satisfaction. Full details of NPIS activity are published online (Annual Report - NPIS, 2017–2018). The service has expert pediatric advice from within its consultant staff and accesses external advice from designated toxinologists and mycologists and Public Health England for radiation and environmental hazards (Fig. 5.1.1).

NPIS also supports poisons information services overseas, TOXBASE being available under contract to poisons centers in over 50 countries and more than 150 clinicians. Brazil is the largest overseas user after the United Kingdom with 79,000 database accesses annually.

Training and accreditation

Since the 1970s training of NPIS clinicians has generally been through the discipline of Clinical Pharmacology and Therapeutics in the United Kingdom and they remain involved in direct patient care, unlike in some other countries. There is a clinical toxicology training module within the higher professional training curriculum in clinical pharmacology and therapeutics provided by the British Pharmacological Society, overseen by the Royal Colleges of Physicians. Trainees

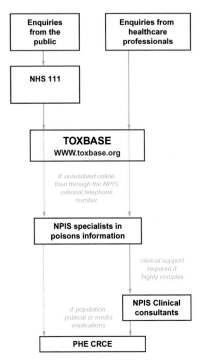

FIG. 5.1.1 Current NPIS structures. *(Courtesy of PHE CRCE: Public Health England Centre for Radiation Chemical and Environmental Hazards.)*

from other disciplines (e.g., emergency medicine) can also undertake training in clinical toxicology. Since clinical pharmacology is a research-based discipline, this approach to training has led to a continuation of the United Kingdom's record for innovative research, dating back to the 1960s and 1970s when key advances were made by clinical pharmacologists, particularly in Edinburgh (Proudfoot et al., 2013). For example, the concepts that underlie the Matthew-Rumack nomogram for managing paracetamol poisoning were developed in Edinburgh in the early 1970s, when Rumack was a visiting fellow (Proudfoot et al., 2013).

There is no standard accreditation system for poisons information staff, other than that provided within the NPIS. However, there is a training program within each poison center which is supervised by the senior information officer and medical director. Three full-day meetings annually provide continuing professional education and staff unable to attend can access lectures online.

Educational outreach

A series of "outreach" educational electronic modules hosted on TOXBASE were developed particularly for the nurses staffing public health telephone lines. TOXBASE is also freely available to UK medical schools as a learning tool for clinical students. Clinical and public health education outreach programs are undertaken. Regular training programs for NHS clinicians are provided locally by NPIS educational outreach and online training modules.

The service collaborates with other academic organizations in the United Kingdom (e.g., the Association of Clinical Biochemists and Royal College of Emergency Medicine) to develop guidelines on appropriate toxin and biochemical analysis availability for managing specific poisonings, and antidotes that should be stocked (Thompson et al., 2014; Royal College of Emergency Medicine and NPIS, 2017). It also contributes to government advisory bodies such as the Medicines and Healthcare products Regulatory Agency (MHRA), the Advisory Committee on Pesticides, and the Advisory Committee on the Misuse of Drugs (Annual Report NPIS, 2017–2018).

Future challenges

In common with many other NHS services, the NPIS is heavily dependent on central funding for its core budget. Small amounts of money are also raised by the lease of TOXBASE. The NPIS retains its reputation for accuracy of information and quality of advice when managing complex clinical cases. As resources become increasingly limited, quality may be threatened in the future, as it was in the 1990s. However, early evidence indicated that provision of poisons information was associated with reduced admissions for children locally (Graham and Hitchens, 1977). More recently, reductions in emergency department visits were observed after primary healthcare use of the UK NPIS (Elamin et al., 2018). It is therefore likely that provision of poisons information is a cost-effective use of NHS resources.

NPIS faces problems in providing up-to-date information, particularly on newer drugs of abuse that may be chemically unidentified. It also provides information generically, rather than linking to commercial products with active ingredients. For example, all dishwasher tablets tend to be similar in composition. Rather than attempting to produce individual entries for every marketed product, it concentrates on the expected effects of key active ingredients. Its lack of a direct interface with the public may also hide the full profile of its activities from the population and affect the extent of political will for funding in times of austerity.

Ireland

A poisons information center (PIC) was founded in Dublin, Ireland, in 1966 by the Irish Medical Association and the Irish Health Department under an anesthetist, Dr. Joe Woodcock, and one clerical officer, in Jervis Street Hospital, as it had a dialysis unit (Woodcock, 1968). They received support from Dr. Goulding in London and had access to the UK poisons data sheets. By 1988 the service had expanded to its current five information staff, and in 1987 relocated to Beaumont Hospital. It has always been run by anesthetists with an interest in toxicology, and since its inception has worked closely with the UK service.

Unlike the United Kingdom, the PIC serves both the public and health professionals. In 1998, calls from Ireland at night and on weekends were transferred by agreement to the NPIS Cardiff Unit. Since 2001, TOXBASE has been Ireland's main information system and since 2005, out-of-hours medical coverage has been provided by NPIS clinical toxicologists. Ireland has had a proportionally smaller workload with 10,144 telephone inquiries in 2017, of which 4221 were from the public (Poisons Information Centre of Ireland Annual Report, 2017). TOXBASE was accessed 54,000 times from Ireland: 17,000 from the PIC and 37,000 from hospitals.

Acknowledgments

We acknowledge with grateful appreciation the contributions of Prof. Philip Routledge (Wales), Ms. Joanna Tempowski (WHO), Dr. Joseph Tracey (Ireland), and Prof. Allister Vale (Birmingham), who provided expert consultation and peer-review of the text.

References

Anon. Information on poisoning. Brit Med J 1963;ii:515.

Bateman DN, Good AM, Kelly CA, Laing WJ. Poisons information in Scotland: delivery of TOXBASE on the internet. Heal Inform J 2002a;8(2):67–72.

Bateman DN, Good AM, Laing WJ, Kelly CA. TOXBASE: poisons information on the internet. Emerg Med J 2002b;19(1):31–4.

Donaldson LJ. Getting Ahead of the Curve. A Strategy for Combating Infectious Diseases (Including Other Aspects of Health Protection), https://webarchive.nationalarchives.gov.uk/+/http://www.dh.gov.uk/en/Publicationsandstatistics/Publications/PublicationsPolicyAndGuidance/DH_4007697; 2002.

Elamin MEMO, James EDA, Holmes P, Jackson G, Thompson JP, EA ES, Bradberry SM, SHL T. Reductions in emergency department visits after primary healthcare use of the UK National Poisons Information Service. Clin Toxicol 2018;56(5):342–7.

Ellis M. Poisons information centres. BMJ (Online) 1964;1:627–8.

Ellis M, Blacow NW. Poisons information Bureau at Leeds: an account of 3 Year's work. BMJ (Online) 1965;2:198–200.

"Emergency Treatment in Hospital of Cases of Acute Poisoning. (The Atkins Report)." 1962.

Freeman AG. Poisons information centre. BMJ 1965;2:482.

Goulding R. The role of poisons information Centres. Practitioner 1965;120–5.

Goulding R, Watkin RR. National poisons information service. Mon Bull Minist Health Public Health Lab Serv 1965;24:26–32.

Graham JDP, Hitchens RAN. The National Poisons Information Service and hospital admissions for children—the experience in Wales of the Cardiff Centre. Br Med J 1977;2(6098):1339–40.

Guys and St Thomas' NHS Trust. Consultation Paper on the Future Options for the Guy's and St Thomas' Poisons Information Service, https://moderngov.lambeth.gov.uk/documents/s4622/; 2007.

Locket S. Clinical toxicology. Henry Kimpton; 1957.

Locket S. Haemodialysis in the management of acute poisoning. Proc Roy Soc Med 1970;63:427–30.

Matthew H, Lawson AAH. Treatment of common acute poisonings. 3rd ed. Churchill Livingstone; 1975.

NPIS. Annual Report, https://www.npis.org/Annualreports.html; 2017–2018.

Oral answers to questions - Health. Poisons Unit (Guy's and St Thomas' Hospital Trust) in the House of Commons 11:30 Am 20 Dec, https://www.theyworkforyou.com/debates/?id=2005-12-20b.1703.1; 2005.

Poisons Information Centre of Ireland Annual Report, https://www.poisons.ie/About-Us/Annual-Reports; 2017.

Proudfoot AT, Davidson WSM. A Viewdata system for poisons information. BMJ (Online) 1983;286:125–7.

Proudfoot AT, Good AM, Bateman DN. Clinical toxicology in Edinburgh, two centuries of progress. Clin Toxicol 2013;51(6):509–14.

Royal College of Emergency Medicine and NPIS. Royal College of Emergency Medicine and National Poisons Information Service Guideline on Antidote Availability for Emergency Departments (January 2017), https://www.rcem.ac.uk/docs/College Guidelines/RCEM NPIS Antidote Guideline List.pdf; 2017.

Thompson JP, Watson IDD, Thanacoody HKRK, Morley S, Thomas SHL, Eddleston M, Vale JA, Bateman DN, Krishna CV. Guidelines for laboratory analyses for poisoned patients in the United Kingdom. Ann Clin Biochem 2014;51(Pt 3):312–25.

Volans GN, Mitchell GM, Proudfoot AT, Shanks RG, Woodcock J. National Poisons Information Services; report and comment 1980. BMJ (Online) 1981;1:1613–5.

VPIS. Annual Report; 2017. https://www.vpisglobal.com/wp-content/uploads/2019/01/vpis-annual-report-2017.pdf.

Woodcock JA. The poisons Information Service. J Ir Med Assoc 1968;61:439–41.

Chapter 5.2

Czech Republic and other Central European and Eastern European countries

Daniela Pelclova

Toxicological Information Centre, Department of Occupational Medicine, First Faculty of Medicine, Charles University in Prague and General University Hospital Prague, Czech Republic

Origins

The Czech Toxicology Information Center (TIC) was established at the Department of Occupational Medicine of the General University Hospital in Prague in 1961 by Professor Jaroslav Teisinger. Acute intoxications that were not occupational, including self-harm, had been treated at this 27-bed in-patient department, with oxygen supplied to every bed, since its founding in 1947. In the late 1950s, with the development of the chemical and pharmaceutical industry, the number of chemical and pharmaceutical products on the domestic market increased rapidly. Professor Karel Rejsek started a small paper file of the most common chemical products that caused occupational poisoning during their manufacture or misuse. This file included their composition and toxicity. Manufacturers' data had to be kept secret and could only be provided to hygienists and physicians for managing occupational intoxications or allergies.

In 1961, after returning from the United States, where poison control centers (PCCs) already existed, Teisinger decided to develop a similar center in Prague. Occupational physician Jarmila Filipová and pharmacist Dana Šedivcová processed the data, stored it, and informed healthcare facilities in Czechoslovakia of its existence. The PCC was officially opened in 1962, and it participated in 1964 in the establishment of the EAPCCT. Professor Teisinger was a member of the first EAPCCT board. Initially the Czechoslovak PCC was financed by the Hospital and the City of Prague. Later, it was also supported financially by the Ministry of Health. Two toxicologists created the basis of a comprehensive data-file of thousands of chemicals, pharmaceuticals, plants, fungi, and poisonous animals. The Czech toxicological database now contains data on 70,000 potentially toxic agents. The original paper file was digitized at the turn of the 1990s and remains in the TIC as a historical document. Further heads were the

History of Modern Clinical Toxicology. https://doi.org/10.1016/B978-0-12-822218-8.00048-X

author (Prof. Pelclova) (1991–1994), who then went on to head the Department of Occupational Medicine for the next 22 years, followed by RNDr. Ludmila Pavlíková (1994–1995), Dr. Jarmila Filipová (1996–1997), Dr. Hana Rakovcová (1998–2011), and Associate Professor Sergej Zacharov (2011–2017). The author again became head of the PCC in 2017.

Organization of PCCs across Central and Eastern Europe

Poison centers have developed across other countries taken under the influence of the old Soviet Union at different rates, as shown in Table 5.2.1. Czech, Polish, and Slovak centers date to the 1960s. In contrast, PCCs in Belarus and in Moldova are being created at the time of this writing. Most Central European (CE) and Eastern European (EE) countries have one PCC. Only Poland has more than one PCC, and these share that country's population. PCCs in all countries except Slovenia answer calls from the public. They all operate 24 h a day except Georgia, which is open 09.00–23.30. The PCCs were established in different types of departments (Table 5.2.1). The majority of them work with a clinical department, generally at a university hospital in the capital. In contrast to some other parts of the world, medical staff specialized in internal and emergency medicine and clinical toxicology often answer calls. The departments may be able to transfer and admit severely poisoned patients, with a range of facilities including intensive care units (ICU), extracorporeal renal replacement therapy, and hyperbaric chambers. These larger clinical departments are self-sufficient for night and weekend services.

About one-third of PCCs who participated in this survey work as independent units. As in the Czech Republic, they started as Departments for Occupational Medicine but lost their beds because of the successful prevention of life-threatening occupational diseases. These smaller PCCs are assisted by physicians from other departments, who provide clinical or out-patient coverage 24/7, and their staffs may include pharmacists. None of the PCCs employ veterinarians, although they provide information on the treatment of animal poisoning to veterinary surgeons and the lay public.

Daily operations

Telephone calls on acute human poisonings come from the public, ambulances, local community medical centers, and large hospitals. Some stand-alone PCCs consult local experienced clinical toxicologists about complex cases, and also use specialists in botany, toxic mushrooms, toxic snakes, and spiders. Chronic poisonings are more commonly managed by the departments of occupational medicine, industrial hygienists, or local medical centers.

A number of databases are used. About one-half of the centers maintain their own national toxicological database. The data stored usually includes information on the formula or chemical composition, use, properties, kinetics, biotransformation, mechanism of action, toxicity, symptoms of acute poisoning, and treatment. The basis for pharmacological drug information is generally the National

TABLE 5.2.1 Characteristics and staff of the Poison Control Center (PCC) in Central European and Eastern European countries and Kazakhstan.

	Country	City	PCC established (year)	No. of calls in 2019	Population served (million)	Type of the department	Patients treated (yes, no)/ no. of beds	Director	Antidote stocks	PCC/TIC web
1	Azerbaijan	Baku	1982	12,230	10.0	Clinical Toxicology	Yes/50	Assoc. Prof. Ismayil Afandiyev, MD PhD	Y	No
2	Belarus	Minsk	2020	Data not available	9.5	Being formed	Yes/30	Ihar Hrihorieu, MD	N	No
3	Croatia	Zagreb	1971	2400	4.1	PCC (Occupational and environmental)	No	Rajka Turk, MSc	N	www.imi.hr
4	Czech Republic	Prague	1962	21,000	10.7	PCC (Occupational Medicine)	No	Prof. Daniela Pelclová, MD PhD	Y	www.tis-cz.cz
5	Estonia	Tallinn	2008	3000	1.3	PCC (Chemical safety)	No	Mare Oder, MSc	Y	www.16662.ee
6	Georgia	Tbilisi	1998	200	3.7	PCC	No	Assoc. Prof. Teimuraz Kobidze, MD PhD	Y	No
7	Hungary	Budapest	Data not available	6800	3.0	Emergency and Toxicology	Yes/50	Csaba Pap, MD	Y	No
8	Kazakhstan	Almaty	Data not available	400	18.6	Clinical Toxicology	Yes/47	Gulmira Taybaeva, MD	N	No

TABLE 5.2.1 Characteristics and staff of the Poison Control Center (PCC) in Central European and Eastern European countries and Kazakhstan—cont'd

	Country	City	PCC established (year)	No. of calls in 2019	Population served (million)	Type of the department	Patients treated (yes, no)/ no. of beds	Director	Antidote stocks	PCC/TIC web
9	Lithuania	Vilnius	2002	2914	2.8	Clinical Toxicology	Yes/43 beds	Robertas Badaras, MD PhD	Y	http://www.rvul.lt/rvul-central/toksikologijoscentras/
10	Moldova	Chisinau	2020	Data not available	4.0	Just being formed	Data not available	Iurie Pinzaru, PhD	N	No
11	North Macedonia	Skopje	1995	180	2.1	Clinical Toxicology	Yes/29	Assoc. Prof. Zanina Pereska, MD PhD	Y (limited)	toxicocenter.com.mk
12	Poland	Gdańsk	1972	About 3000	5.0	Clinical Toxicology	Yes/17	Prof. Jacek Sein Anand, MD PhD	Y	http://www.pctox.pl/new/
13	Poland	Łódź	1967	About 1000	2.5	Clinical Toxicology	Yes/26	Anna Piekarska-Wijatkowska, MD PhD	Y	No
14	Poland	Poznań	1967	3000	6.0	Clinical Toxicology	Yes/21	Magdalena Łukasik-Głębocka, MD PhD	Y	No
15	Slovakia	Bratislava	1968	6300	5.4	PCC (Occupational Medicine)	No	Silvia Plačková PharmDr, PhD MPH	Y	www.ntic.sk
16	Slovenia	Ljubljana	1973	2000	2.1	Internal Medicine	Yes/21	Miran Brvar, MD PhD	Y	www.ktf.si

Information System of Medicinal Products and individual drug Summary of Product Characteristics. Toxicological data on chemicals, poisonous fungi, plants, and animals were originally obtained from toxicological literature. Most also use globally recognized toxicological databases including TOXBASE, TOXINZ, and POISINDEX. In addition, free sources are used to search missing data: TOXBASE (free for economically challenged centers in the region), the National Institute for Occupational Safety and Health (NIOSH), National Library of Medicine (NLM) (earlier TOXNET), German GIZ-NORD, the WikiTox electronic database or the International Programme on Chemical Safety (IPCS) INCHEM (no longer up-dated). PCCs in CE and EE countries also collect Material Safety Data Sheets (MSDS) of local and imported chemical products, including a large range of cleaning products that may be involved in accidental or intentional exposures. Thus the Czech MSDS database includes more than 200,000 products.

All CE and EE countries keep a database of archived calls. In the early years, these were only briefly handwritten notes on treatment recommendations and the nature of the poisoning. Over the years, records have been refined into more detailed forms, complemented by full text. These databases are also used for the statistical evaluation of the trends in poisoning, severity of intoxication and treatment recommendations. In the Czech Republic and some other countries, the recording of telephone calls enables auditing of the quality of the information offered. Most countries also keep a stock of rare antidotes that are not commonly available on the market for less common poisonings. The Czech Republic is the only one maintaining a stock of drugs for the treatment of radiological emergencies, financed by the Ministry of Health.

Country-specific information

Nineteen countries with a total 29 PCC were identified, but data could not be obtained from all of them. Countries that may have PCCs but from whom data could not be obtained by the author include Albania, Armenia, Bulgaria, Latvia, Romania, Serbia, and Ukraine. In total, information from 14 countries, including 16 PCCs is presented in summary below and in Table 5.2.1.

Azerbaijan

The PCC is in the process of transition. It will be financed by the government until 2021, after which PCC costs will be covered by health insurance. Facilities of the Toxicology Department for Children and Adults include the State Health Aviation Services, treatment on site of poisoned patients, or transport to health care facilities capable of advanced treatment for medical, intensive care unit, and hyperbaric therapy.

Belarus

The PCC in Belarus is just being formed at the Minsk City Emergency Hospital. At present, the clinical toxicological departments (Minsk region and Brest) give advice to physicians and to the public on how to treat acute intoxication. The PCC collects data, such as numbers and the epidemiology of poisoning. The head of the PCC is an employee of the Ministry of Health of the Republic of Belarus.

Croatia

The PCC of the Occupational and Environmental Health Unit of the Institute for Medical Research and Occupational Health in Zagreb employs four occupational medicine physician–epidemiologists and three pharmacists. The recent research focus has been on occupational toxins (Turk et al., 2007) and e-cigarettes (Vardavas et al., 2017). The PCC is financed from resources of the department, except for answering calls during out of office hours, which is covered by local health insurance schemes.

Czech Republic

The nature of the services provided by TIC has changed during its history. While at the beginning the annual acute consultations were a few dozen, all from physicians, in 2019 more than 21,000 calls were received, the majority from the public. The Czech Department of Occupational Diseases reduced its beds to 15 in 1999 and closed them finally in 2011. Today the hospital has two poison treatment beds available for the PCC. The PCC employs three physicians and one pharmacist. One of approximately nine occupational physicians answer calls overnight and during weekends. Health insurance companies cover costs for inquiries about insured patients. The main toxicological interests are chemicals, such as mercury (Pelclová et al., 2002), thallium (Pelclová et al., 2009), cobalt released from a hip transplant (Pelclová et al., 2012), and solvents: ethylene glycol (Křenová and Pelclová, 2007) and methanol (Zakharov et al., 2016). Workers intoxicated with 2,3,7,8-tetrachlorodibenzo-p-dioxin have been followed-up for 50 years (Pelclová et al., 2018).

Estonia

The PCC is located at the Department of Chemical Safety, Estonian Health Board, which is a competent authority in the field of chemical and product safety. The database of toxicological information (1600 monographs) is constantly updated. There are two half-time physicians and five emergency nurses answering all calls and a second tier of consulting physicians, if needed. The PCC provides educational activities for the public, hospitals, and ambulance services. It is led by a nursing specialist (emergency nurse, MSc). All activities of the PCC are paid from the state budget, including preventive measures. Estonia has established a co-operation with the Nordic Association of PIC (https://www.nordic-apc.org/). Publications are centered on poisoning prevention, substance abuse and the consequences of methanol ingestion (Paasma et al., 2009).

Georgia

The PCC for Georgia at the Clinic of Tbilisi State Medical University is in the process of a prolonged reorganization and many issues are not clarified yet. In Georgia, most patients with acute poisoning are admitted to emergency departments of regional hospitals (Kobidze et al., 2009; Afandiyev et al., 2019). Difficult cases are transported by the Disaster Medicine Center to four specialized toxicology departments in Tbilisi, served by 26 physicians and clinical toxicologists. Georgia uses free databases such as TOXNET and Pubmed, in addition to Georgia's monographs of toxicology.

Hungary

There are two independent units in Budapest—one is the National PCC, the National Institute of Chemical Safety (NICS, www.okbi.hu), providing information and storing data of archived calls. This PCC did not answer in this survey. A second unit, the Department of Emergency Medicine and Clinical Toxicology provides toxicological advice for a part of Hungary, although, since 1949, its main task has been the local management of poisoning. This department is paid to treat poisoned patients (11,000 patients a year). This clinical center does not maintain any toxicological or archived calls database.

Kazakhstan

The Kazakhstan PCC was started in Almaty, the former capital of Kazakhstan, in Soviet times, probably in the 1990s. It was related to an intensive care and toxicology unit for patient rehabilitation. After Nur Sultan (previously known as Astana or Celinograd) became the capital of Kazakhstan, the PCC was moved there. Finally, it was decided in November 2019, that the Department of Toxicology of Almaty City would become the Kazakhstan PCC and was called the Republican Coordination Center for Toxicological Service. It also monitors and analyzes national toxicological data. Toxicology physicians from Kazakhstan receive additional toxicology education in Moscow and they use the Poizon-1 and Poizon-3 databases created by Russian colleagues. In addition, a free database in English (INCHEM) is used. The clinical toxicology departments in Nur Sultan, Shymkent, Karaganda, and Ust-Kamenogorsk treat patients. A database of archived calls was started in December 2019.

Lithuania

There are two separated services in Lithuania with very close cooperation. In 2019, the PCC with telephone services became a part of the State Medicines Control Agency. The clinical services are supported by the Clinical Toxicology Department (started in 1991), of the Republic of Vilnius University Hospital Toxicology Center, consisting of three separate departments: Acute Poisonings,

Toxicology ICU, and Psychiatry departments. They manage all types of poisoning (Dragelytė et al., 2014; Badaras et al., 2016; Vardavas et al., 2017).

Moldova

According to information provided by Raisa Sircu, PhD, and Tatiana Tonu, MD, from the National Agency for Public Health of Ministry of Heath, Labor and Social Protection, the PCC of the Republic of Moldova in Chisinau is in the process of formation of a poison information service.

North Macedonia

The PCC in North Macedonia was first established in 1995 at the Clinic of Toxicology of the University St. Cyril and Methodius in Skopje, but there was no recording of any data. As part of the project "Chemical Risk Management in Macedonia" (2009–2011), with the assistance of the Swedish PCC, a modern concept of a working PCC was introduced and an electronic database for archived calls started. It contains a total of 13,600 records, including hospital discharge and outpatient records. Additionally, the PCC works as a poisons registry for the country (Pereska et al., 2019).

Poland

Polish PCCs were started in the 1960s. There is no central unit in Poland, but 10 independent units (Gdańsk, Kraków, Lublin, Łódź, Poznań, Rzesów, Sosnowiec, Tarnów, Warszawa, and Wroclaw) situated at clinical toxicology departments (Sein Anand et al., 2005; Kabata et al., 2015). They are coordinated by a General Consultant in Toxicology from the Nofer Institute of Occupational Medicine in Łódź (Krakowiak et al., 2017). Polish PCCs are not paid either for providing toxicological information or for database creation and update. There is thus no common Polish toxicological database. Each PCC keeps a limited toxicological database and some are shared.

Slovakia

The National PCC of Slovakia at the University Hospital in Bratislava was initiated within the Department of Occupational Medicine by the pharmacist Olga Horáková in 1968, and the toxicological database extended by 12,000 photocopies of the Prague toxicological file cards. After the split of the Federal Republic of Czechoslovakia in 1993, this PCC has operated for the Slovak Republic. It is financed by the Ministry of Health with four pharmacists covering the work during the day. The PCC co-operates with the Department of Occupational Medicine, and during their other clinical duties, its staff, two internists and four occupational physicians, answer the phone. Their research focus is on accidental corrosive ingestions (Cagáňová et al., 2017) and e-cigarettes (Vardavas et al., 2017).

Slovenia

The PCC in Slovenia is located within the Division of Internal Medicine of the University Medical Center Ljubljana, with its intensive care unit, treating all types of acute and chronic poisoning (Brvar et al., 2004; Brvar et al., 2017). There are six physicians and two pharmacists. Only call answering costs are covered by health insurance, resulting in budgetary challenges.

Poisoning prevention

Only Estonia and Lithuania receive money for poisoning prevention, meaning elsewhere any such activities must be financed from grants. The PCCs in the region often use local media for public information; for example, giving warnings and first aid information during the methanol outbreak in the Czech Republic in 2012–2013 (Zakharov et al., 2016), or taking action in North Macedonia in 2014–2015 which led to the Ministry of Health banning production and sales of 80% acetic acid to consumers, and requiring replacement of these products with 20%–25% concentrations. CE and EE PCCs also publish information brochures for the public and provide information on their PCC websites (Table 5.2.1).

Staffing and professionalism

In a majority of countries, telephone services are provided by specialists with practical knowledge of clinical toxicology. In severe poisoning cases, experienced physicians in intensive care, otorhinolaryngology, toxic mushroom, plant or snake bite exposure are contacted. Occupational medicine specialists working with PCCs are consulted in cases of chronic intoxications with toxic metals, organic solvents, pesticides, or exposure to toxic gases. For feedback, PCCs ask hospitals for discharge summaries for novel intoxications or unusual cases. All PCCs also teach toxicology to medical students and/or physicians specializing in internal, emergency, or occupational medicine. Most PCCs also publish research studies, surveys, or case reports.

Challenges

In the majority of CE and EE countries, there are many everyday challenges, most often related to the weak economic situation of the country. The staffing of all PCCs is limited by available budgets. Research grants in some countries enable toxicologists to cover conference fees and travel to congresses. This is crucial as it works as a motivation to undertake academic work and submit manuscripts to quality journals. PCCs elsewhere cannot afford travel or registration costs to such congresses. As these are of key importance for toxicologists' continuing education and development, this has local implications.

The challenge for PCCs is the small budget on the one side, and the ambitious need to continuously update their national toxicological databases.

In countries that have a tradition of quality foreign language teaching, use of English databases without translation is possible. However, this is a not a solution for all countries.

Cooperation

The ICPS INTOX Project, launched in 1988, was a joint venture of the World Health Organization (WHO), the United Nations Environment Program (UNEP), and the International Labor Organization (ILO). Its main objective was to promote sound management of chemicals in countries. The Project also provided a forum for collaboration between experts in the continuous development of poisons control. It included the IPCS/EC Evaluation of Antidotes Series and WHO new guidelines for poison control, and representatives of several CE and EE countries participated in these ventures.

Later, there was further collaboration in European Union projects. These included the Alerting System for Chemical Health Threats (ASHT) I (2005–2008), ASHT II (2008–2011), and ASHT III (2012–2014). This was coordinated by the UK Health Protection Agency and both Lithuania (ASHT I–III) and the Czech Republic (ASHT II–III) participated. Additionally, PCCs collaborated in other projects, such as DeNaMiC (Description of the Nature of the Accidental Misuse of Chemicals and Chemical products) or collection data on e-cigarette exposure incidents (Vardavas et al. 2017). The EU collaboration of the CE and EE countries continues in the frame of the Scientific Committee on Health, Environmental and Emerging Risks (SCHEER) and the European Union Rapid Alert System for Chemicals (RAS-CHEM). Cooperation between PCCs in the Region has been facilitated by the EAPCCT through its Eastern European Working Group. Several EAPCCT Board members have also come from the Region, further strengthening international links.

Conclusions

In the countries behind the old "iron curtain," PCCs have been active in working to save lives and reduce the cost of treating poisonings with both man-made chemicals and natural toxins. They have a role in the management and prevention of poisonings. They save time and money of the healthcare sector by reducing unnecessary visits to doctors and hospitals in the case of toxicologically insignificant cases. In addition, they provide important information on the prevention and management of toxic exposures, and carry out toxicovigilance, research, analytical support, education, and training. The budgets they receive do not reflect the value they provide to the healthcare sector, but it seems that there is increasing recognition of their importance by governments as PCCs are now working in most CE and EE countries.

Acknowledgments

I thank Professor Yuri Ostapenko from Russia, Dr. Raisa Sircu from Moldova, Dr. Gabija Laubner-Dragelytė, head of Acute Poisonings and Toxicology ICU departments in Vilnius,

Lithuania, Associate Professor Ismayil Afandiyev from Azerbaijan; Dr. Ihar Hrihorieu from Belarus; MSc. Rajka Turk from Croatia; MSc. Mare Oder from Estonia; Associate Professor Teimuraz Kobidze from Georgia; Dr. István Elek from Hungary; Associate Professor Zanina Pereska from North Macedonia; Professor Jacek Sein Anand, Dr. Anna Piekarska-Wijatkowska, and Dr. Magdalena Łukasik-Głębocka from Poland; PharmDr. Silvia Plačková from Slovakia; Dr. Miran Brvar from Slovenia; and Dr. Galina Bashynskaya from Kazakhstan, for their important help to complete the data. This work was supported by Progres Q25/LF1 and Q29/LF1 of the Charles University in Prague.

References

Afandiyev I, Kobidze T, Kereselidze M, Tsetskhladze N, Ahmadov R, Hajizada N. The comparative structure of acute poisonings in two capital cities of the South Caucasus Region. Georgian Med News 2019;287:105–10 [Russian].

Badaras R, Jovaisa T, Judickas S, Ivaskevicius J. Changes in potassium concentration during opioid antagonist induction: Comparison of two randomized clinical trials. J Addict Med 2016;10(4):244–7.

Brvar M, Mozina H, Osredkar J, Mozina M, Noc M, Brucan A, Bunc M. S100B protein in carbon monoxide poisoning: a pilot study. Resuscitation 2004;61(3):357–60.

Brvar M, Kurtović T, Grenc D, Lang Balija M, Križaj I, Halassy B. Vipera ammodytes bites treated with antivenom ViperaTAb: a case series with pharmacokinetic evaluation. Clin Toxicol (Phila) 2017;55(4):241–8.

Cagáňová B, Foltánová T, Puchoň E, Ondriašová E, Plačková S, Fazekaš T, Kuželová M. Caustic ingestion in the elderly: influence of age on clinical outcome. Molecules 2017;22(10).

Dragelytė G, Plenta J, Chmieliauskas S, Jasulaitis A, Raudys R, Jovaiša T, Badaras R. Myocardial rupture following carbon monoxide poisoning. Case Rep Crit Care 2014;2014:281701.

Kabata PM, Waldman W, Sein Anand J. Toxicological consultation data management system based on experience of Pomeranian Center of Toxicology. Med Pr 2015;66(5):635–44 [Polish].

Kobidze TS, Gerzmava OK, Areshidze TK, Tsintsadze MA, Dikhamindzhiia OB. Most common poisonings and their management-data from Tbilisi. Georgian Med News 2009;166:85–8.

Krakowiak A, Piekarska-Wijatkowska A, Kobza-Sindlewska K, Rogaczewska A, Politański P, Hydzik P, Szkolnicka B, Kłopotowski T, Picheta S, Porębska B, Antończyk A, Waldman W, Sein Anand J, Matuszkiewicz E, Łukasik-Głębocka M. Poisoning deaths in Poland: types and frequencies reported in Łódź, Kraków, Sosnowiec, Gdańsk, Wrocław and Poznań during 2009–2013. Int J Occup Med Environ Health 2017;30(6):897–908.

Křenová M, Pelclová D. Does unintentional ingestion of ethylene glycol represent a serious risk? Hum Exp Toxicol 2007;26(1):59–67.

Paasma R, Hovda KE, Jacobsen D. Methanol poisoning and long term sequelae - a six years follow-up after a large methanol outbreak. BMC Clin Pharmacol 2009;27(9):5.

Pelclová D, Lukáš E, Urban P, Preiss J, Ryšavá R, Lebenhart P, Okrouhlík B, Fenclová Z, Lebedová J, Stejskalová A, Ridzoň P. Mercury intoxication from skin ointment containing mercuric ammonium chloride. Int Arch Occup Environ Health 2002;75(Suppl):S54–9.

Pelclová D, Urban P, Ridzoň P, Šenholdová Z, Lukáš E, Diblík P, Lacina L. Two-year follow-up of two patients after severe thallium intoxication. Hum Exp Toxicol 2009;28(5):263–72.

Pelclová D, Sklenský M, Janíček P, Lach K. Severe cobalt intoxication following hip replacement revision: clinical features and outcome. Clin Toxicol (Phila) 2012;50(4):262–5.

Pelclová D, Urban P, Fenclová Z, Vlčková S, Ridzoň P, Kupka K, Mecková Z, Bezdíček O, Navrátil T, Rosmus J, Zakharov S. Neurological and neurophysiological findings in workers with chronic 2,3,7,8-tetrachlorodibenzo-p-dioxin intoxication 50 years after exposure. Basic Clin Pharmacol Toxicol 2018;122(2):271–7.

Pereska Z, Chaparoska D, Bekarovski N, Jurukov I, Simonovska N, Babulovska A. Pulmonary thrombosis in acute organophosphate poisoning-case report and literature overview of prothrombotic preconditioning in organophosphate toxicity. Toxicol Rep 2019;6:550–5.

Sein Anand J, Chodorowski Z, Burda P, Twardowska M. Toxicological information conducted by Polish Poison Information Centres based on selected cases of acute intoxication. Przegl Lek 2005;62(6):561–3.

Turk R, Varnai VM, Bosan-Kilibarda I. Gas poisoning: respiratory irritants and axphyxiants. Lijec Vjesn 2007;129(Suppl 5):119–23 [Croatian].

Vardavas CI, Girvalaki C, Filippidis FT, Oder M, Kastanje R, de Vries I, Scholtens L, Annas A, Plackova S, Turk R, Gruzdyte L, Rato F, Genser D, Schiel H, Balázs A, Donohoe E, Vardavas AI, Tzatzarakis MN, Tsatsakis AM, Behrakis PK. Characteristics and outcomes of e-cigarette exposure incidents reported to 10 European Poison Centers: a retrospective data analysis. Tob Induc Dis 2017;15:36.

Zakharov S, Pelclova D, Urban P, Navratil T, Nurieva O, Kotikova K, Diblik P, Kurcova I, Belacek J, Komarc M, Eddleston M, Hovda KE. Use of out-of-hospital ethanol administration to improve outcome in mass methanol outbreaks. Ann Emerg Med 2016;68(1):52–61.

Websites

European Association of Poison Centres and Clinical Toxicologists http://www.eapcct.org/.

WHO Directory of Poison Centres https://apps.who.int/poisoncentres/.

International Programme on Chemical Safety "IPCS INTOX PROJECT" https://www.who.int/ipcs/poisons/intox/en/.

International Programme on Chemical Safety "INCHEM Internationally Peer Reviewed Chemical Safety Information" http://www.inchem.org/pages/pims.html.

Centers for Disease Control and Prevention "The National Institute for Occupational Safety and Health" https://www.cdc.gov/niosh/topics/chemical.html.

National Library of Medicine "TOXNET information" https://www.nlm.nih.gov/toxnet/index.html.

WikiTox "WikiTox Home Page" http://www.wikitox.org/doku.php?id=wikitox:wikitox_home.

Chapter 5.3

Russia

Yu. S. Goldfarb[a,b] and Yu. N. Ostapenko[a,b,c]

[a]N.V. Sklifosovsky Research Institute for Emergency Medicine (RIA) of the Moscow Health Department, Moscow, Russia, [b]Federal State Budgetary Educational Institution of Additional Professional Education "Russian Medical Academy of Continuous Professional Education" of the Ministry of Healthcare of the Russian Federation, Moscow, Russia, [c]Research and Applied Toxicological Center of the Russian Federal Medical and Biological Agency, Moscow, Russia

Origins

The organization of clinical toxicology in the USSR and Russia began in the second half of the 20th century. Much credit for this belongs to the research begun in the therapeutic clinic of the N.V. Sklifosovsky Emergency Medicine Research Institute (RIA), established in 1923 at the Sheremetev Hospital. This hospital had been providing emergency medical care for more than 100 years, and the Emergency Medicine Research Institute had been originally established in the 1820s.

In the 1950s–1970s widespread use of chemicals began in industry, agriculture, and home in the USSR. This was associated with the development of the chemical industry and the creation of new medicines and was accompanied by an increase in the incidence of acute poisoning and their adverse outcomes. The inadequate treatment of poisoning in hospitals became obvious and required new therapeutic and organizational approaches. In the N.V. Sklifosovsky RIA, patients with acute poisoning were hospitalized in the 2nd therapeutic clinic. The head of this clinic, Professor Pavel Sukhinin, repeatedly raised the issue of organizing a toxicology department. He sent a memorandum to the director of the Institute and submitted a report to its Scientific Council on the organization of a toxicology laboratory. As a result, he was instructed "… to carry out work on the organization of this center."

In 1962, the first toxicological department in the country was opened at the Institute, making it possible to adopt new approaches to managing acute poisoning. Particular attention was paid to the then frequent acute poisonings with mercury, arsenic, and caustic agents. The work of this new department attracted great interest from intensive care physicians. As a result, in 1968, the N.V. Sklifosovsky RIA held the first All-Russian Conference on Clinical Toxicology.

History of Modern Clinical Toxicology. https://doi.org/10.1016/B978-0-12-822218-8.00003-X

As a result of the success of this meeting, the government decided to contribute to the formation of clinical toxicology as a scientific and medical specialty and distribute the experience of the Moscow Center on treating poisoning throughout the country. This was supported by the USSR Ministry of Health (MoH). Largely in connection with this, the Collegium of the MoH organized a formal network of toxicology centers (TCs) in the Russian Soviet Federative Socialist Republic (RSFSR) and the Kazakh Soviet Socialist Republic (SSR) (Collegium of the USSR MoH, 1969).

Expansion of clinical toxicology

In 1964, a pediatric center was started at the Children's City Hospital No. 13, "N.F. Filatov," in Moscow for the treatment of poisoning in children younger than 15 years (now up to 18 years). Subsequently, in 1970, the Republican Center for the Treatment of Poisoning (RCTP) was created, organized at the N.V. Sklifosovsky RIA (MoH of the Russian Federation (RSFSR) order No 70, 1970). The RCTP was tasked with the monitoring, prevention, and treatment of acute poisoning and charged with organization, research, poisons information, and educational functions. Associate Professor Evgeny A. Luzhnikov, Candidate of Medical Sciences and head of the toxicology department of the N.V. Sklifosovsky RIA, was appointed as the head of the RCTP.

To perform these tasks, the following divisions were deployed within RCTP:

1. The main academic and research subdivision of the Center, which was first led by Victor N. Dagaev, and then Vladimir N. Aleksandrovsky. This included three research groups to organize specialized care: (1) information and prevention of acute poisoning, (2) statistics, (3) training of medical specialists in clinical toxicology. Training was carried out by travelling to territorial centers nationwide to give seminars on poisoning treatment. In 1986, the Department of Clinical Toxicology, organized at the Central Institute of Advanced Training of Doctors in Moscow (now the Russian Medical Academy of Continuing Professional Education), began to train doctors in clinical toxicology. Professor E.A. Luzhnikov was founder and the first head of the Department of Clinical Toxicology until 2016. It now regularly trains first responders, anesthesiologists, emergency physicians, pediatricians, toxicologists, and nurses.

2. Clinical facilities: 25 beds within the intensive care unit; a 25-bed psychiatric department; the dialysis department for performing extracorporeal techniques; research department for assessing new treatment methods for poisoning.

3. The forensic chemical toxicological laboratory for urgent analysis in acute poisoning and biochemical studies during various types of treatment.

Among the legal documents supporting the changes in clinical toxicology, the three most important were the MoH order no. 1527 which required the implementation of artificial detoxification methods in acute poisoning through specialized hospital departments with facilities for hemadsorption and hemodialysis (MoH of the USSR No. 1527, 1986); an MoH letter (MoH of the USSR letter No. 02-14/118-4, 1987); and No. 02–14/61–14 (February 15, 1988), allowing the creation of such wards as part of the acute poisoning treatment units.

By 2000, poisoning services in the Russian Federation consisted of a network of 44 TCs, each for a population of 500,000 or more. This was created in multidisciplinary and emergency hospitals in accordance with the 1980 MoH order No. 475, resulting in a total of 1235 toxicological beds (MoH 475). Today, this network provides specialized assistance and advanced therapies to the population of 50% of the territory of the Russian Federation. Financing of TC and clinical departments is from the national compulsory medical insurance fund.

National Service Development

The 1970 order No. 70 also established 13 inter-regional TCs in large cities with a sufficient base to support management of acute poisoning (Vladivostok, Volgograd, Voronezh, Gorky [Nizhny Novgorod], Irkutsk, Leningrad [St. Petersburg], Novosibirsk, Omsk, Perm, Sverdlovsk [Yekaterinburg], Stavropol, Khabarovsk, and Chita). The MoH established the post of Chief Clinical Toxicologist, responsible for overseeing the activities of these TCs. This position was taken by the head of the RCTP: Evgeny A. Luzhnikov, who played an outstanding role in the formation of clinical toxicology as a new specialty in medicine and created a scientific school of clinical toxicologists. At the local level, the TC is administered by the head physician of the hospital where it is located.

Communication between centers is through the MoH's Chief Clinical Toxicologist. In addition, the TCs contact each other to discuss aspects of care during scientific conferences and practical workshops. The RCTP takes the lead in poisons prevention by liaisons with public health and epidemiology departments. Actions include, for example, prohibition of the free sale of household chemicals containing highly toxic substances (e.g., dichloroethane, a component of plastic glues) or their removal from household products. The prevention of occupational poisoning in Russia is the responsibility of institutes of occupational pathology, not TCs.

The most important result of the RCTP's work was MoH order No. 475 signed by Academician Boris V. Petrovsky who was interested in this development of a new branch of clinical medicine (MoH of the USSR order No. 475, 1980). This completed the first stage of the development of national toxicological services. It established clear regulations for the creation and operation of TCs not only in the Russian Federation, but throughout the USSR, with the introduction of a toxicologist post and approval of the principle of creating departments in cities with populations of 500,000 and above.

In the Soviet period, work in acute poisoning was also carried out by the All-Union Center for the Treatment of Acute Poisoning, created by order No. 1598 (MoH of the USSR order No. 1598, 1985). The N.V. Sklifosovsky RIA has continued to expand and is currently a scientific department (headed by Mikhail M. Potskhveriya) with 73 beds, tripling in size since 1965, including (1) treatment of acute poisoning, (2) diagnostics, resuscitation, and intensive care including emergency detoxification, (3) poisoning recovery, (4) psychiatric beds, and (5) a chemical-toxicological laboratory.

Poisons information

In the early days, the N.V. Sklifosovsky RIA provided poisons information and advisory support to health care professionals and the general population. Initially, this work was the responsibility of the department's clinicians—both by telephone consultations and travel to the site of emergency toxicological situations as part of a specialized emergency team from the intensive care and treatment departments of Moscow. For cities away from Moscow, air transport was provided by the Public Health Service of the RSFSR.

Research and Applied Toxicology Center of the Medical and Biological Agency

Following this early work at N.V. Sklifosovsky RIA, the MoH issued order No. 319 (MoH RSFSR order No. 319, 1992). This institution was organized by Viktor N. Dagaev who was appointed the Institute's head. After 2011, the Research and Applied Toxicology Center of the Medical and Biological Agency (RTIAC), headed by Yuri Ostapenko (from 2015, Pavel Rozhkov) began to play a larger role in addressing organizational and other aspects of clinical toxicology. RTIAC provides 24 h daily information (using chemical safety data sheets) and advice on acute chemical exposure to the general public and health professionals by a single national telephone number. It also provides information on the treatment on animal poisoning. Regional TCs can, if necessary, use online communication; an online interactive database has been specially developed for this purpose.

Call volumes

The RTIAC provides advice throughout the Russian Federation, but the majority of calls come from Moscow, the Moscow Region, and neighboring territories of Russia with 11.98 million inhabitants. In some large cities, toxicological information and advisory groups have been organized as part of poisoning treatment centers, covering 4.7 million people in the Sverdlovsk region, 4.3 million in Rostov on Don, and 3.38 million in Omsk. All of these informational and advisory groups work 24 h daily. Some patients are transferred from other locations as a result of telephone consultations. The number of calls to these groups per 100,000 population per year was RTIAC—97.95; Sverdlovsk—11.02; Rostov—8.64; and Omsk—3.38. Patients with poisoning are hospitalized in therapeutic TCs at the following rates: in Moscow and surrounding region per 100,000 population are: 125.6 at the N.V. Sklifosovsky RIA, 168.7 at Rostov and 139.3 at Sverdlovsky.

Information sources

For general inquiries TC employees obtain data on the toxicity of drugs and chemicals from the Russian Register of potentially hazardous chemical and biological substances as well as various reference books and monographs, including standard western texts such as: "Ellenhorn's Medical Toxicology," "Goldfrank's Toxicologic Emergencies," and the IPCS INCHEM website.

In addition, a special computerized information retrieval toxicological system "POISON," developed by the staff of the N.V. Sklifosovsky RIA under the leadership of Viktor N. Dagayev, is used to provide advice to health professionals and the public (Litvinov et al., 1996). This system contains data on 1040 drugs and chemical and biological substances, set out as computerized toxicology monographs (Poison Information Monograph - PIM), and is funded from the federal budget.

Case records

A national poisons telephone consultation record card is used, developed following the template recommended in the "Guidelines for Poison Control," (IPCS, WHO, Geneva 1997) and approved by the MoH. The recording of patient information is then entered into a computer database of telephone consultations. Following the admission of a patient to the hospital, an MoH-approved hospital patient form is used.

Local TCs

One of the main functions of RTIAC is the coordination of TCs throughout the country, as well as monitoring poisoning epidemiology, analyzing and disseminating this information, and preparing instruction manuals. In severe cases of poisoning regional TCs may consult the RTIAC by phone or online, and a joint consultation is held including leading specialists of the medical TC of the N.V. Sklifosovsky RIA, as well as with the Chief Clinical Toxicologist of the MoH. Local administration of TCs is carried out by the chief physician of the hospital in which the TC operates, based on MoH order No. 925n (MoH of Russia order No. 925n, 2012) and No. 152 of February 21, 2005, of the MoH. The basis for these documents is Federal Law No. 323 FZ (Federal Law No. 323 FZ, 2011).

Research

The accumulated experience of the N.V. Sklifosovsky RIA led to a systematic approach to improving the treatment of acute and subacute poisoning, using both specific and nonspecific decontamination treatments and rehabilitation. Studies included complex detoxification approaches studying novel (e.g., magnetic, ultraviolet, and laser) therapies of blood to extract or alter the chemical structures of circulating toxins (Goldin et al., 2004). An important contribution to the development of intestinal detoxification methods was made by basic research carried out jointly with clinicians in the experimental laboratory of the Institute, headed by Professor Galperin.

The use of the new treatment algorithms was accompanied by a sharp decrease in mortality among the most severely poisoned patients. Institute staff also studied new forms of acute poisoning with substances used in production and in everyday life and the possibility of rehabilitation of toxicological patients. This success was facilitated by the introduction of modern methods of analysis (i.e., chromatographic, immune, mass spectrometric) to the N.V. Sklifosovsky RIA. It also performed urgent analyses 24 h daily for the poisoning center and other hospitals in Moscow to assist in the diagnosis of acute poisoning.

This research served as the basis of publications in Russian (Ostapenko et al., 2001a,b). The first Russian National Guide to Clinical Toxicology "Medical Toxicology" (2012), editor E.A. Luzhnikov, with input from the country's leading specialists from St. Petersburg (Professor Georgy A. Livanov) and Yekaterinburg (Professor Valentin G. Sentsov), gave advice on topics including emergency in situ diagnosis and care, and the treatment of acute poisoning. The National Emergency Medical Care Manual (2017) was created by specialists from St. Petersburg, edited by Sergei F. Bagnenko, Academician of the toxicological section of the Russian Academy of Sciences.

The development and widespread introduction of new medical technologies, created on a sound theoretical base, facilitated improvements in the diagnosis and treatment of acute poisoning. This was also promoted by the formation of the new, enlarged E.A. Luzhnikov Scientific School in Clinical Toxicology in Moscow. This school had the priority of scientific research to create an independent toxicological service in Russia for the overall improvement of treatments at the regional level. The scientific ideas of Academician E.A. Luzhnikov continue to be developed by his closest students employed in the N.V. Sklifosovsky RIA as well as colleagues in Yekaterinburg.

Much scientific and organizational work was also carried out by the leading Russian territorial TCs (Ostapenko et al., 2005, 2011). New information on the diagnosis and treatment of acute poisoning with cardiotoxic drugs was obtained in Yekaterinburg under the guidance of Professor V.G. Sentsov. The epidemiology and organization of toxicological services, as well as prevention of acute poisoning, are other topics now being addressed. In St. Petersburg, Professor Georgy A. Livanov headed research on new approaches to poisoning-induced respiratory disorders, methods of artificial detoxification, acute poisoning syndromes and the organization of the outpatient toxicological service (Berezina et al., 2017). In addition, the study of multiple poisoning and its epidemiology is currently ongoing.

Training and standards

To train specialists in the field of clinical toxicology and conduct scientific research within the Russian system of postgraduate education, departments have also been created for teaching clinical toxicology at leading universities. There are two departments in Moscow (Professor Yuri S. Goldfarb, Professor Salavat H. Sarmanaev), and in St. Petersburg (Professor Viktor V. Shilov), Yekaterinburg (Professor Valentin G. Sentsov), Ufa (Professor Zakia S. Teregulova), Khabarovsk (Associate Professor Alexander Yu. Shchupak), and Khanty-Mansiysk (Associate Professor Boris B. Yatsinyuk).

Physicians with a basic medical education and a higher diploma work in TC's with clinical toxicologists or anesthesiologists in treatment centers. The requirements are the same for physicians working in a treatment center and those working in a poisoning information center. A specialist certificate is obtained after graduating from a medical school. It requires ICU training and 504 academic hours in toxicology. There is mandatory re-accreditation every 5 years. Specialists providing poisoning information and the treatment of poisoning are trained in line with MoH order No. 707n (MoH order No. 707n, 2015). Once trained, no further special authorization is required to work in a poison information center. All regulatory documents on toxicology were prepared on the basis of Federal Law No. 323 FZ (Federal Law No. 323 FZ, 2011).

Conclusion

In Russia, toxicological assistance from TCs in large cities has been available to the population for over 50 years. The organization of TCs was initially carried out by the efforts of the RCTP with assistance provided by local health authorities, as well as the MoH in the form of formal orders and information letters. TCs were organized as part of general hospitals, which made it possible to perform emergency care for resuscitation and treatment, including intensive care, diagnostic investigations, and laboratory studies.

Informational services were subsequently organized by the Scientific and Practical Toxicological Center of the Federal Medical Biological Agency of Russia (RTIAC). These services are intended to provide standard advice on poisoning throughout the Russian Federation. RTIAC is funded from the federal budget. In addition to information and advisory functions, it coordinates the activities of poison information centers and departments throughout the country, monitors poisons epidemiology, collects and disseminates information, and prepares information monographs. In recent years, a formal regulatory framework for the country's toxicological service has also been formed. Employees of the

RTIAC and TC at the N.V. Sklifosovsky RIA in Moscow have had a leading role in these changes.

The main toxicological institution in the Russian Federation has studied and applied modern methods of the diagnosis and treatment of poisoning and completed a large amount of research in the field of enteral detoxification. The introduction of modern technologies for the treatment of acute poisoning and the preparation of regulatory documents has made it possible to standardize the working and organization of toxicological departments.

References

Berezina IY, Badalyan AV, Sumsky LI, Goldfarb YS. Dynamics of EEG and psychophysiological indicators of acute poisoning neurotoxicants on the stage of rehabilitation on the background of different methods of treatment. Zh Nevrol Psikhiatr Im S S Korsakova 2017;117:53–63 [in Russian].

Collegium of the USSR MoH. On the state and measures for the further development of toxicology. 10 April; 1969.

Federal Law No. 323 FZ. On the Basics of Health Protection of Citizens in the Russian Federation. 21 November; 2011.

Goldin MM, Volkov AG, Goldfarb YS, Luzhnikov EA. Electrochemical generation of active oxygen into aqueous solutions for organism detoxification. Toxicol in Vitro 2004;18:791–5.

Litvinov NN, Ostapenko YN, Kazachkov VI. Information technologies for clinical toxicology in Russia. Clin Toxicol 1996;34:665–8.

MoH of Russia order No. 925n. On approval of the procedure for providing medical care to patients with acute chemical poisoning. 15 November; 2012.

MoH of the Russian Federation (RSFSR) order No 70. On measures to further strengthen the toxicological service of the health authorities of the Russian Federation. 26 March; 1970.

MoH of the USSR letter No. 02-14/118-4. On the creation of resuscitation and intensive care wards as part of the departments (centers) of acute poisoning. 16 December; 1987.

MoH of the USSR No. 1527. On measures to improve specialized medical care in acute poisoning. 20 November; 1986.

MoH of the USSR order No. 1598. On measures for the further development and improvement of specialized medical care in acute poisoning. 12 December; 1985.

MoH of the USSR order No. 475. On the improvement of inpatient specialized medical care in acute poisoning. 5 June; 1980.

MoH order No. 707n. On approval of qualification requirements for medical and pharmaceutical workers with higher education – toxicology. Health and Medical Sciences; 2015. 8 October.

MoH RSFSR order No. 319. On the establishment of an information and consultation toxicological center of the Ministry of Health of the Russian Federation. 7 December; 1992.

Ostapenko YN, Luzhnikov EA, Nechiporenko SP, Petrov AN. Clinical and institutional aspects of antidote therapy in Russia. Przegl Lek 2001a;58(4):290–2.

Ostapenko YN, Matveev SB, Gassimova ZM, Khonelidze RS. Epidemiology and medical aid at acute poisoning in Russia. Przegl Lek 2001b;58(4):293–6.

Ostapenko YN, Lisovik ZA, Belova MV, Luzhnikov AE, Livanov AS. Comparative assessment of blood and urine analyses in patients with acute poisonings by medical, narcotic substances and alcohol in clinical toxicology. Przegl Lek 2005;62:591–4.

Ostapenko YN, Brusin KM, Zobnin YV, Shchupak AY, Vishnevetskiy MK, Sentsov VG, Novikova OV, Alekseenko SA, Lebed'ko OA, Puchkov YB. Acute cholestatic liver injury caused by poly-hexamethyleneguanidine hydrochloride admixed to ethyl alcohol. Clin Toxicol 2011;49:471–7.

Chapter 5.4

Germany

Herbert Desel[a] and Andreas Stürer[b]

[a]German Federal Institute for Risk Assessment, Berlin, Germany, [b]Mainz Poison Centre, University Medical Center of the Johannes Gutenberg University Mainz [JG|U], Mainz, Germany

Origins

As in other countries many new pharmaceuticals, pesticides and other chemicals became available in the workplace and at home in Germany in the 1950s and 1960s. Health risks from these agents were not as comprehensively studied as today, leading to an increasing number of new poisonings requiring treatment by medical services. Physicians had limited experience in the management of such new diseases at that time.

Soon a range of new medical options for treatment of poisonings became available. In the early years after their introduction some of these were regarded as applicable for almost all poisonings, particularly methods for enhancing toxin elimination, starting with hemodialysis in 1955 (Jaeger, 2004). Experience with these invasive treatments was limited and treatment sometimes caused severe complications. Other new treatments, in particular antidotes, were appropriate for selected poisonings. Laboratory investigations were recognized as another important aspect of appropriate poison management and important new analytical methods, based on chromatographic separation techniques, were developed for routine use.

These new poisonings and options for diagnosis and treatment required a new expert knowledge, ideally available to support the management of all poisoned patients. Thus starting in the 1960s, Departments of Clinical Toxicology for specialized treatment were founded at several major German hospitals and combined with advanced toxicological laboratory services. These centers carried out many scientific studies on the improvement of the diagnosis and treatment of intoxications (Solfrank et al., 1977; Keller et al., 1981; Besser et al., 1989). The Munich Department was outstanding in this regard, and with other centers carried out an important research project on the antidote: obidoxime in organophosphate poisonings. This study was undertaken in cooperation with the Institute for Pharmacology and Toxicology of the German military (Bundeswehr) (Eyer et al., 2009). In recent years, the frequency of severe poisoning requiring long-term

History of Modern Clinical Toxicology. https://doi.org/10.1016/B978-0-12-822218-8.00029-6

expert medical treatment has substantially decreased. All but one Department of Clinical Toxicology were closed, with only Munich remaining.

Development of poisons centers (Giftnotruf)

Not all patients could be treated in a specialized center; access to clinical toxicological information needed to be made available for other hospitals. This need led to the introduction of telephone services provided by expert toxicologist-clinicians. The first were in Munich (West Germany) and Leipzig (East Germany) in 1963. One year later the Berlin Poison Centre started, focusing on pediatric poisonings. The Mainz Poison Centre, integrated in an internal intensive care unit, started its service. These services were initially only offered to medical staff and focused on severe poisoning (Hahn, 2019). In West Germany, the services were soon opened to the general public, recommending the best first aid measures and avoiding unnecessary use of emergency medical services in cases with a low risk of poisoning. In Germany, this is an almost unique service, due to professional regulations. With very few exceptions, physicians are not allowed to treat a patient without personal contact.

By the 1980s there were about 25 poisons centers (PCs), most using toxicology monographs and knowledge of a few experienced physicians. Availability and quality of advice was very variable in some centers, depending on availability of experienced staff members and their other duties. Information on product composition and toxicologically important features of products were collected on index cards but infrequently used in daily practice. A case database system—INDEX LINE—was developed by the Munich center in the 1970s and was implemented at the German Institute for Medical Documentation and Information (DIMDI) (Clarmann et al., 1978). Cases from most other centers were documented on paper and stored locally.

Toxicological analysis

Rapid analytical laboratory investigations for the diagnosis of poisoning were developed and improved in sensitivity and specificity in the 1970s and 1980s. In West Germany, the development of standardized methods was coordinated and substantially sponsored by the German Research Foundation (DFG), the country's most important research funding organization. Germany became one of the leading countries in the science of toxicological analysis. The German-speaking Society of Toxicological and Forensic Chemistry (Gesellschaft für Toxikologische und Forensische Chemie, GTFCh) was founded as an independent association of scientists and physicians working in this field in 1978. Toxicological screening analyses, intended to detect as many agents taken by the poisoned patient as possible, became important, since leading experts in the field in Germany were convinced that a comprehensive analysis was as important for poisoning as an X-ray for bone fracture (von Meyer, 2006).

National coordination

West Germany's Federal Health Office (Bundesgesundheitsamt, BGA) coordinated the work of experts from toxicological medical treatment centers, laboratories, and PCs; experts from Austria and Switzerland were also included. A Committee for Diagnosis and Treatment of Poisonings (Kommission zur Erkennung und Behandlung von Vergiftungen, Giftkommission, GiKo) was formed in 1965 and continues to meet twice a year. GiKo discusses scientific developments in clinical toxicology and trends in poisoning epidemiology. The committee also focuses on improving safety measures to prevent poisoning, especially among children. Another important task of GiKo is the development of standardized substance-related monographs in German summarizing all properties of a substance that are important for poisoning advice. These include—among other items—synonyms, identifying codes, symptoms, specific laboratory analyses, and treatment options.

GiKo was the main forum for clinical toxicology in West Germany. Nevertheless, because of the increasing role and a raised political awareness of PCs, a national association was formed: a subgroup of GiKo members founded the National Working Group on Poisons Centers (Arbeitsgemeinschaft Giftnotruf, AGGN). The national working group was registered in 1985 to represent all German PCs in political discussions.

In 1981, East Germany changed its PC system to a central service located in Berlin. This national PC offered reliable 24-h service, had its own staff and access to all formulas of products marketed in the country—an outstanding feature, difficult to obtain today (Hahn, 2019). However, the service was only available for medical professionals.

Following German re-unification in 1990 the majority of laboratories providing a high-quality 24/7 toxicological analytical service formed a national forum: the "Scientific Committee on Clinical Toxicology" (Arbeitskreis Klinische Toxikologie) in 1997. This forum was established within the Society of Toxicological and Forensic Chemistry (GTFCh).

Organization of poisons centers in Germany

In 2020, 8 PCs serve Germany's 83.1 million inhabitants (Table 5.4.1). Their organizations and roles have developed during the decades.

All PCs are within hospitals, most within university hospitals, with different degrees of organizational and economic independence. Initially, all services were provided by hospital staff in limited slots of working time. Increasing inquiry frequency and the need for high quality evidence-based advice, IT support and accurate case recording, meant all centers started hiring staff working exclusively for them. Most now have their own staff and provide a 24/7 service. Staff covering both patient care and PC services still exist but are now unusual. Night shifts present a challenge, and some centers transfer the telephone service to hospital duty-physicians, who can find it difficult to manage both tasks. Other

TABLE 5.4.1 Poisons centers in Germany in 2020.

Location	"Länder" (federal states) served	Population in 2019[a] (millions)
Bonn	North Rhine-Westphalia	17.9
Göttingen	Bremen, Hamburg, Lower Saxony, Schleswig-Holstein	13.4
Munich	Bavaria	13.1
Freiburg	Baden-Württemberg	11.1
Mainz	Rhineland-Palatinate, Hesse	10.4
Erfurt	Mecklenburg-West Pomerania, Saxony, Saxony-Anhalt, Thuringia	10.0
Berlin	Berlin, Brandenburg	6.2
Homburg (Saar)	Saarland	1.0
	Germany	83.1

[a] *Statistisches Bundesamt (2020) GENESIS-Online: Bevölkerung: Bundesländer, Stichtagam 31. Dezember 2019, https://www-genesis.destatis.de/genesis/online?operation=abruftabelleBearbeiten &levelindex=2&levelid=1595934440415&auswahloperation=abruftabelleAuspraegungAuswaehlen& auswahlverzeichnis=ordnungsstruktur&auswahlziel=werteabruf&code=12411-0010&auswahltext=& werteabruf=Werteabruf#abreadcrumb accessed: July 28, 2020.*

centers share night call duties or combine poison center service with tasks in pharmacovigilance or toxicovigilance for third parties.

Up to the 1980s PCs mainly provided advice on the care of patients. A substantial percentage of all consultations involved asymptomatic children and adults with suspected poisoning. Supported by discussions in the national poisoning committee (GiKo) and other networks, PCs developed an important role in poisoning prevention. They accomplished this by systematic case analysis and identification of undetected risks that indicated a need for new safety measures, such as the introduction of child-resistant closures for corrosive household products.

Legal duties

In the 1980s, there was increased recognition of environmental pollution and its potential human health impact. An amendment of the national Chemicals Act (Chemikaliengesetz) established a role for PCs in medicine and public health in 1990 and provided a legal basis for their operations. In the same year, East and West Germany were reunited and structures and duties were established in the whole country, without significant subsequent change. There are 16 federal states (Länder) of (formerly East and West) Germany. States have the duty to enforce the majority of laws and organize the medical system in their area. They were legally required to nominate at least one PC (Informationszentrum für Vergiftungen) to the Competent Federal Governmental Authority. Initially BGA was the Competent Authority, followed by the Bundesinstitut für gesundheitlichen Verbraucherschutz und Veterinärmedizin (BgVV). The German Federal Institute for Risk Assessment (Bundesinstitut für Risikobewertung [BfR]) has been in charge since 2004.

Key duties of the nominated PCs in the legal text (literally translated from the German) are to:

(a) collect and evaluate knowledge on health effects of hazardous substances or hazardous mixtures
(b) provide help by giving advice in case of substance-related illnesses
(c) report to the Competent Authority about insights derived from their activities that are of general importance for poisoning advice.

Finally, the Chemicals Act requires that industry submit detailed information, including a full formula on a subset of consumer products classified as hazardous to the Competent Authority (today BfR) which has to make this confidential business information available to all nominated PCs. Implementation led to substantial changes in the PC system in the 1990s. The states became responsible for financing PCs adequately so they could perform a fully harmonized professional service that could handle and use the product information. A professionalization and concentration process followed, so that by 2020 there were eight independent PCs (Table 5.4.1), all with 24/7 service (4 PCs serve more than one state).

Further poisons center activities

Other tasks are performed by German PCs today. As described by a committee of PC directors within the Society of Clinical Toxicology in 2017, German PCs have important roles in the management of chemical outbreaks, medical education, postgraduate trainings, pharmacovigilance, and poisons prevention (GfKT, 2017).

Funding of poisons centers

PC activities were initially limited to a small number of calls per day and no full-time staffs were needed. At that time funding was based on hospital budgets—transiently supported by externally funded scientific income. After an amendment of the Chemicals Act in 1990 the states were expected to provide PC budgets. Despite this legal basis, few financed their nominated PC adequately. PCs are still dependent on their hospital's support, and this support has been affected negatively by stricter cost-control of financial reimbursement for all hospital services.

The situation became worse in the 2000s, leading to increased financial pressure on PCs. PC costs were reduced (e.g., by sharing night shifts) and additional income was generated from contracts with third parties. Today, almost all PCs are managed as profit centers within their hospitals. A substantial part of most German centers' budgets (in some, greater than 50%) is generated via industry contracts and by charging for hospital consultations. Prices for services are not harmonized, leading to economic competition between PCs.

National poisoning registries

Another duty described in the amended Chemicals Act of 1990 was that all physicians treating a poisoning or having submitted an expert opinion on a (lethal) poisoning should report to the Federal Authority (BfR) on each case in a standardized and detailed manner. This has led to a national registry of notified poisonings. Unfortunately, only a small minority of cases are reported (~3%). A potential reason is that reporting is not rewarded, and failure to report not penalized. The completeness is much higher for occupational cases, reported by the Institution for Statutory Accident Insurance and Prevention.

Only a very small subset of case reports created by PCs have been submitted to BfR and included in the national registry as required by the German Chemicals Act. BfR, GiKo, and PCs have spent much time producing a more complete national poisoning registry during the past decade. However, as there is no legal basis for comprehensive national case data collection, there is no public funding for this additional PC workload. The German Federal Government's coalition agreement of 2018 includes the implementation of a national registry of poisonings at BfR as a political objective, and this has stimulated public discussion. A legal basis for the registry now needs to be established, with funding divided between the German Federal Government and the governments of the 16 states. This will need to comply with European Union data protection legislation.

National cooperation today

As mentioned earlier, representatives from PCs of Germany (supported by one expert from the Netherlands) formed the national working group, AGGN, in 1985. AGGN was renamed to "Society for Clinical Toxicology" (Gesellschaft für Klinische Toxikologie, GfKT) in 2000. This has increased scientific progress in clinical toxicology—and experts from Switzerland and Austria have joined. The Society became a member of the Association of the Scientific Medical Societies in Germany (Arbeitsgemeinschaft der Wissenschaftlichen Medizinischen Fachgesellschaften e.V., AWMF) in 2015. Both toxicological societies have organized annual clinical toxicology meetings in German since the 1990s, with increasing numbers of participants and content. Since 2004, five working groups have existed: analysis of cases with drug exposures; development of quality standards; cooperation with the mushroom expert network; harmonization of case documentation; and maintenance of the national product category system (TKS). They have about 60 active members and each meets twice a year. In the 2010s, GfKT acted as study lead for many third-party sponsored studies collecting cases from all German, Austrian, and Swiss PCs; for example, the MAGAM study (Stürer et al., 2010) and MAGAM II DEAT study (Hermanns-Clausen et al., 2019). Both focused on eye effects caused by cleaning products and detergents and both were referenced in an OECD Document (OECD, 2017). Furthermore, systematic analysis of cases of specific pharmaceuticals collated from all German, Austrian, and Swiss PCs is performed by a working group of GfKT (Prasa et al., 2013), leading to substantial national harmonization of poisoning advice.

In 2018, the BfR was appointed as the body responsible for harmonized product notification by an amendment of the Chemicals Act, legally based on Article 45 and Annex VIII of the EC Regulation No. 1272/2008 on classification, labeling and packaging. European regulation is widening and harmonizing duties of the 1990 Chemicals Act for industry. GiKo is active at BfR, serving as an information exchange forum for BfR, PCs, industry and other stakeholders on poisoning risk assessment. It also supports BfR in improving the national case registry.

Publicly funded national research projects

Based on the early GiKo network, German PCs and the BfR (or its predecessor authorities) were involved in three publicly funded research projects that aimed to facilitate and improve cooperation within the legal frame of the German Chemicals Act.

The *EVA Project* (registration and evaluation of poisoning [Erfassung von Vergiftungen und ihre Auswertung]) in the early 1990s formed the basis for harmonized and computerized case-data collection leading to a prototype of a case registry database and a product category system, components of which are still in use today.

The *TDI Research Project* (toxicological network for documentation and information [Toxikologischer Dokumentations- und Informationsverbund]) ran from 1998 to 2006. TDI focused on the development of a national product information network to handle the increasing volume of product data voluntarily and legally submitted by industry. Its purpose was to provide rapid access to product data retrieval and display for emergency advice and case documentation. Additionally, an improved product category system (TKS) was developed that is now maintained by GfKT. It served as a model for the European product category systems for cosmetic products (an integral part of the EU Cosmetic Products Notification System, CPNP) and for the European Product Category System (EuPCS) as part of the harmonized product data notifications based on Article 45 of CLP.

The *PiMont Project* (pilot project on national monitoring of poisonings [Pilotprojekt zum nationalen Monitoring von Vergiftungen]) (2017–2019) piloted a comprehensive national registry of poisonings intended to combine a substantial subset of all poisoning cases registered in all German PCs and in the BfR. The project tested organizational and technical aspects and concluded with an expert opinion covering options for the legal foundation and financing of the registry (discussed earlier).

Current operations

Today, all PCs in Germany answer calls from medical staff and from the public. The majority of cases relate to acute substance exposure in humans. Animal poisonings and calls without a specific exposure contribute little (well below 10%) to the total number of 250,000 calls per annum. Information related to exposures is only provided by direct telephone contact. Only very general treatment advice is provided online (e.g., the AACT/EAPCCT position statements of gastro-intestinal decontamination measures). Information on toxic hazards in households or on poisonous plants, is disseminated by many different channels by PCs and by BfR to aid in poisons prevention. Websites, personal presentations and flyers for parents of small children are most frequently used, the latter via kindergartens or pediatric wards.

Databases

Most PCs in Germany use complex, but easy-to-retrieve custom-made database systems, combining product information, toxicological information and access to the PC's own case registry. Some PCs use separate systems for different subsets of data.

The group of PCs sharing their services at night uses a WIKI database (GIZWIKI) to ensure harmonized advice from all group member PCs. Although databases differ, substantial parts of the data are shared between most German PCs, including medical drug monographs created by a GfKT working group based on: the experience of all PCs, toxicological substance fact sheets developed by GiKo, and external sources, like Poisindex and TOXBASE.

Case registration

All PCs register calls in local databases. After the EVA Project in the early 1990s some database systems are shared, but PC datasets remain separate. Most PCs have had access to electronic records since 2000 or earlier. The frequency of PC calls is rising, indicating the continuing acceptance of PC services as the first contact point for all cases of poisoning and poisoning concerns in Germany. On average about 40% of all calls come from medical staff and 60% from the general public.

Staffing and professionalism

Originally all calls were answered by physicians with professional experience in intensive care, emergency medicine, internal medicine, pediatrics, clinical pharmacology, surgery, occupational medicine, and other specialties. In 2010, other professions joined the telephone service, mainly pharmacists and nurses. Nurses only answer calls from the public. GfKT has established three postgraduate educational programs in clinical toxicology for different professions: Clinical Toxicologist GfKT, Human Toxicologist GfKT, and Specialist Consultant in Human Toxicology GfKT (Fachberater Humantoxikologie GfKT), for physicians with extended experience in the treatment of poisoned patients, other physicians and scientists and nurses, respectively. Requirements for acceptance are 3 years of PC working experience, a minimum number of registered consultations, and scientific publications (see GfKT Website www.klinitox.de/281.0.html for details [in German]). The majority of PC staff members are involved in these training programs. Almost all experienced and executive staff members have passed the final oral exam and participate in continuing education in clinical toxicology. GfKT training programs were developed in the 2010s using a training program of GTFCh for laboratory specialists in toxicology (Clinical Toxicologist, GTFCh) as a model.

In the 1980s, some PCs became better staffed, especially the West Berlin Poisons Center. This opened the opportunity to develop better working procedures. Exposures to selected agents with insufficient toxicological data or few published poisoning reports were systematically followed up and documented by senior experts. The importance of exact agent identification was recognized. Detailed knowledge of mixture formulas was considered important for case analysis. Based on this systematical review of cases, monographs for risk assessment and treatment advice were developed, continuously maintained and used for improved routine service. Many documents were published, the most important by Mühlendahl et al. (2003) and used as standard references in all centers. As reported earlier, a working group of GfKT still continues case analyses at the national level (Prasa et al., 2013).

In recent years, contributions from Germany to annual congresses of the EAPCCT and to the journal *Clinical Toxicology* have increased. German PCs have been involved in several projects funded by the European Commission since 2007 (ASHT Phase I to III, ECHEMNET) (GIZ-Nord Poisons Centre, 2018a, 2018b).

Conclusions

PCs are well-established in Germany and respected stakeholders of medical specialties, particularly emergency, internal, and pediatric medicine. PCs play an essential role in local and national toxicovigilance, scientific clinical studies, and poisons prevention. Although the important role of poisons reporting is recognized for improved product safety and poisons prevention, implementation of a national registry of poisonings is still pending.

References

Besser R, Gutmann L, Dillmann U, Weilemann LS, Hopf HC. End-plate dysfunction in acute organophosphate intoxication. Neurology 1989;39:561–7.

Clarmann MV, Mathes G, Solfrank G, Bystrich E. The index line as a new aid in clinical and forensic toxicology. Arch Toxicol 1978;40:125–9.

Eyer F, Worek F, Eyer P, Felgenhauer N, Haberkorn M, Zilker T, Thiermann H. Obidoxime in acute organophosphate poisoning: 1 - clinical effectiveness. Clin Toxicol 2009;47(8):798–806.

GfKT (2017) Leiterinnen und Leiter der Giftinformationszentren der Länder Deutschland, Österreich und der Schweiz in der Arbeitsgruppe II der Gesellschaft für Klinische Toxikologie (2017) Aufgaben der Giftinformationszentren, Version 20 wwwklinitoxde/100html (https://www.klinitox.de/fileadmin/DOKUMENTEPUBLIC/ARBEITSGRUPPEN/AG-II/GfKT_Aufgaben-GIZ_v2-0_s20170302_b20170901.pdf, accessed 2020-05-30).

GIZ-Nord Poisons Centre (2018a) The ASHT Public Health Projects. https://www.giz-nord.de/php/index.php/akademische-aktivitaeten/laufende-studien#3-the-asht-public-health-project (accessed 2021-03-25).

GIZ-Nord Poisons Centre (2018b) ECHEMNET - European Chemical Emergency Network. https://www.giz-nord.de/php/index.php/akademische-aktivitaeten/laufende-studien#3-the-asht-public-health-project (accessed 2021-03-25).

Hahn A. Giftinformationszentren in Deutschland - Historie. Arbeitsweise Bedeutung Bundesgesundheitsbl 2019;62(11):1304–12.

Hermanns-Clausen M, Desel H, Färber E, Seidel C, Holzer A, Eyer F, Engel A, Prasa D, Tutdibi E, Stürer A. MAGAM II – prospective observational multicentre poisons centres study on eye exposures caused by cleaning products. Clin Toxicol 2019;57(9):765–77.

Jaeger A. Changes in the approaches to drug elimination in poisoning over the last 40 years. J Toxicol Clin Toxicol 2004;42(4):412–4.

Keller F, Koeppel C, von Keyserling HJ. Schultze G (1981) Hemoperfusion for organic mercury detoxication? Klin Wochenschr 1981;59:865–6.

von Meyer L. Personalia - in memoriam prof. Dr Max von Clarmann. Toxichem Krimtech 2006;73(2):88.

Mühlendahl KEV, Oberdisse U, Bunjes R, Brockstedt M. Vergiftungen im Kindesalter. 4th ed. Stuttgart: Thieme; 2003. ISBN: 3-13-129814-6.

OECD (2017) Guidance documentation an integrated approach on testing and assessment (IATA) for serious eye damage and eye irritation. Series on Testing & Assessment no. 263. (http://www.oecd.org/officialdocuments/publicdisplaydocumentpdf/?cote=ENV/JM/MONO(2017)15&docLanguage=En accessed 2020-07-04).

Prasa D, Hoffmann-Walbeck P, Barth S, Stedtler U, Ceschi A, Färber E, Genser D, Seidel C, Deters M. Angiotensin II antagonists - an assessment of their acute toxicity. Clin Toxicol 2013;51(5):429–34.

Solfrank G, Mathes GV, Clarmann M, Beyer KH. Haemoperfusion through activated charcoal in paraquat intoxication. Acta Pharmacol Toxicol (Copenh) 1977;41(Suppl 2):91–101.

Stürer A, Seidel C, Sauer O, Koch I, Zilker T, Hermanns-Clausen M, Hruby K, Hüller G, Tutdibi E, Heppner HJ, Desel H. Poisons centres' data for expert judgement within classification, labelling and packaging regulation: solid household automatic dishwashing products do not cause serious eye damage. Clin Toxicol (Abstract) 2010;48:245.

Chapter 5.5

The Netherlands

Irma de Vries and Antoinette van Riel

Dutch Poisons Information Center, University Medical Center Utrecht, Utrecht University, Utrecht, The Netherlands

Origins

The exact date of origin of the Dutch Poisons Information Center (DPIC) is lost in the archives of the National Institute for Public Health and the Environment (RIVM). The first archive documents in the RIVM referring to this concept are in 1960; after this, the DPIC was slowly established. As in other Western countries, the number of poisonings in the Netherlands increased in the 1950s. The introduction of many new medicines, household products and pesticides resulted in a rise in accidental and intentional intoxications with these products. Accidental exposures of young children caused the most concern.

In the early 1950s, following a lead from colleagues overseas (most notably Chicago), Dutch pharmacists, united in the Royal Dutch Society for the Promotion of Pharmacy (established 1842), developed a card system with treatment information about various poisonings for its members. At the same time, the Laboratory of Pharmacology (established 1909) of the National Institute of Health (RIV, from 1984 the National Institute for Public Health and the Environment, RIVM), headed by Prof. W. Lammers, developed a similar card system for its own use. Prof. Lammers had a keen interest in clinical toxicology; many pharmacists called him and his staff for advice on various medication errors and poisonings. In the late 1950s, both documentation systems were combined. Prof. Lammers and the Dutch public health authorities both felt there was a need for an information center where Dutch pharmacists and physicians could obtain information on poisonings around the clock, 7 days a week. In 1960, Prof. Lammers visited some early poisons information centers (PIC) in the United States and brought back guidelines to set up a Dutch Poisons Information Center, similar to the American National Clearing House for Poison Control Centers. This early center was set up as a unit within the Pharmacology Laboratory of the National Institute of Health (Lammers and Cohen, 1960; Pikaar and van Heijst, 1979).

History of Modern Clinical Toxicology. https://doi.org/10.1016/B978-0-12-822218-8.00047-8

First challenges

In the early 1960s, the number of consultations about nonpharmaceutical products rose, as well as the number of requests for information from doctors. More specific medical treatment advice had to be provided and required a next step. Providing information was already helpful but combining this with the clinical toxicological experience of physicians would be a major improvement. This experience was found in the person of Prof. Ad N.P. van Heijst, head of the Department of Intensive Care (Reanimation) of the Medical Faculty of the University Utrecht. It was Prof. van Heijst, with his love for France, who insisted on the French name "Service de Réanimation" for his Intensive Care Department. As in the Dutch language this stands for resuscitation, this sometimes caused confusion among patients who had not been resuscitated and consequently refused to pay their hospital bill! It took well over 30 years before the name was changed into the Department of Intensive Care and Clinical Toxicology, which later merged into a larger Intensive Care Center.

In 1962, the DPIC was linked to this Department and became an individual entity within the RIV, as was the Laboratory of Pharmacology. With this change, the DPIC found new accommodations within the Academic Hospital of the University of Utrecht (now the University Medical Center Utrecht). Prof. van Heijst became its Director (De Wilde, 1987). As part of the then RIV, the DPIC was under the jurisdiction of and funded by the Ministry of Health. Until the 1980s, the RIV, University Hospital and DPIC were all situated in Utrecht's city center. After that the RIV moved to Bilthoven, some 5 km outside Utrecht on the eastern outskirts and was renamed the National Institute for Public Health and the Environment (RIVM). The DPIC moved with the University Hospital to the newly built university campus. In 2011 the DPIC would become an official department of the UMC Utrecht, but its projects remained part of the RIVM programs.

Organization

A 24-h daily service was, and is, provided to physicians, pharmacists, and veterinarians but not to the public. The decision not to provide information to the public was very different from how most toxicological units and poisons centers worldwide operated. The Dutch view is that a poisons information center needs to be positioned within the existing health care system of a country. In the early 1960s, the Netherlands had a population of around 12 million people (in 2020: 17.5 million people). The health care system was well-organized and health care insurance was available to all. This system offered quick and easy access to the general practitioner (GP), and after referral by the GP, to the next echelon of medical care in a hospital. In medical emergencies, acute assistance could be offered by ambulance services and self-referral to emergency departments was possible. Because of the relatively short distances in a small country, the (potentially) poisoned patient could be examined rapidly. With this additional medical information, including information on the medical history of the patient, the GP would consult the DPIC. Providing information from professional to professional has several advantages. For example, the history is taken by the consulting medical professional, who actually sees the patient and information can be given in medical terms, rendering relatively efficient calls. There are also fewer calls, because medical professionals can handle mild exposures without consulting the DPIC. It was therefore decided that the DPIC would take calls from professionals only and this is still the case.

Initially, employees of the DPIC only provided information during office hours (Monday to Friday); out-of-office hours were covered by the staff and doctors in training at the Intensive Care Unit. In the beginning of the 1980s the number of information requests had risen to about 17,000 calls per year (Van Heijst, 1981). Literature research and answering the telephone became separate functions; telephone personnel were all nurses, and literature researchers were academics. From 2000 on, with a call volume of around 25.000 calls/year, the entire 24-h daily information service was handled by the DPIC, without further assistance of ICU fellows. In 2000, the DPIC telephone staff increased to seven full-time employees. Literature research and answering the telephone were again combined to improve monographs, making them better tailored to answering telephone inquiries. Today, these functions are still largely combined, which greatly benefits the quality of the monographs.

The Documentation Department of the DPIC was headed by Mrs. S.A. Pikaar. With incredible energy, she extended the existing documentation into an enormous card file system with information on all kinds of substances and products. The information on product compositions was provided by manufacturers on a voluntary basis. After every information request a follow-up form was sent, asking for the course and outcome of the poisoning. This information was fed back into the documentation system, thus improving the quality of the documentation.

In the late 1970s a response rate of approximately 80% was achieved (Van Heijst et al., 1979). In later years this response rate dropped, and the follow-up information provided was mostly inadequate and not informative on the circumstances of the exposure. This last issue is the disadvantage of not having direct contact with the public. Standard follow-up requests were abandoned and from the year 2000, DPIC researchers started organizing formal follow-up studies into the causes of poisoning, by means of standardized interviews by telephone with doctors and/or patients. Studies into the utility of using online questionnaires are ongoing. To improve trend monitoring dedicated software was developed. An automated Early Warning System is currently operational within the DPIC, giving daily signals on substantial increases in the number of poisonings with certain products, product groups, or substances (Van Zoelen et al., 2014).

Scientific research

At the end of the 1970s the Department of Intensive Care and Clinical Toxicology—its new name to stress the importance of clinical toxicology—treated about 400 acutely poisoned patients per year. From the beginning, the DPIC established good contacts with the hospital's pharmacy laboratory, with 24-h availability of toxicological analytical services. Prof. van Heijst had a specific interest in pathophysiological mechanisms of acute intoxications. Due to the unique position of the DPIC within the RIV, with its many laboratories, animal research, already occasionally carried out by Prof. Lammers for specific intoxications, was now focused on cardiovascular effects of poisons. With this initiative, Prof. van Heijst bridged the gap between animal research and clinical toxicology. This led to a series of PhD theses, initially with a focus on the cardiovascular effects of tricyclic antidepressants, the anti-Parkinson drug: orphenadrine, and cardiovascular drugs (De Wilde, 1987).

Trained by Prof. van Heijst, Prof. Bart Sangster succeeded him in 1985 as the new director of the DPIC (1985–1989). He, in turn trained the next director, Prof. Jan Meulenbelt, who took over in 1989 and remained the director until his untimely death in 2015. With him, a new period of clinical research projects started within the DPIC. He realized the importance of human volunteer studies in toxicology, again trying to bridge the gap between animal toxicology and clinical toxicology. For the majority of nonpharmaceuticals there were limited data on human metabolism and toxicity. Results of in vitro and animal studies are not always directly relevant to the patient. The dose–effect relationships for a given substance may be different for humans. Human volunteer research can contribute essential data for human risk assessment (Meulenbelt et al., 1998). A highlight among these research projects was the cannabis study. It characterized the pharmacokinetics of tetrahydrocannabinol (THC) and its metabolites after smoking a combination of tobacco and cannabis (the usual way of smoking cannabis in the Netherlands) containing low to high THC doses. Even today publications resulting from this study are frequently cited (Hunault et al., 2009, 2014). The next logical research step was the development of kinetic models and physiologically based pharmacokinetic models (PB-PK), for THC as well as for several other chemicals. However, research in the laboratory was not abandoned: Prof. Meulenbelt had his chair with the Institute for Risk Assessment Sciences (IRAS, Utrecht University). The IRAS Neurotoxicology Research Group had a specific focus on the effects of drugs of abuse on neurotransmission in the central nervous system. The important connection between *in vitro* research and clinical toxicology continues to stimulate research projects.

Chemicals in the Environment: A new category of information requests

In 1980, the realization that chemicals in the environment could pose a threat to human health became very clear to the Dutch. The "town of Lekkerkerk" affair began: a residential area was built on the heavily contaminated soil of an illegal chemical dumpsite. This caused great concern within the population and the involvement of the DPIC, in particular Prof. Sangster, in the Lekkerkerk health investigations. Several more of these incidents would follow. The DPIC started providing toxicological information by mailed letters to individual doctors who were confronted with patients exposed in such circumstances and worrying about their health.

When the National Institute for Public Health (RIV) became the National Institute for Public Health and the Environment (RIVM) in 1984, the consequences of chronic exposure due to environmental pollution became another target for DPIC research. This included study of both acute incidents leading to environmental contamination and potential health effects of exposure. National and international networks of experts were set up to perform risk assessments and deal with the immediate consequences of acute environmental incidents. After the 1986 Chernobyl disaster, expertise on the health effects of accidental radiation exposure was also developed within the DPIC and is still operational today.

From the beginning, the DPIC has always been an important partner in these networks. The current network of national scientific institutes, called the Crisis Expert Team, dates back to the 1990s. The network is facilitated by the Ministry of Infrastructure and Water Management, which is responsible for disaster management. The experts in the network are able to generate integrated advice on the handling of major chemical incidents within a few hours, using Interrnet-based communication tools. This advice is directed to the local disaster management team. It contains measures local authorities can take early on to reduce health and environmental impacts of the incident immediately and minimize long-term effects. Assistance with modeling of the spread of the chemical(s) released, environmental sampling and laboratory analysis is also possible. The role of the DPIC in this network is to advise on the prevention of exposure and the medical treatment of any persons already exposed, including decontamination and antidotal treatment if available. The DPIC will also advise on and if necessary, participate in, follow-up studies into long-term health effects related to the chemical disaster.

Information technology developments

In the 1980s the development of computer technology accelerated, offering great potential for support in the provision of toxicological information. Within the DPIC the first version of the Toxicological Information and Knowledge Bank (TIK) was developed (Reinders and Bourgeois, 1988). An advanced version of this same database is still being used today. It was a period of intense work, developing the database and transforming the card system into substance monographs that were uploaded into it. In 1994, the first version of the DPIC database was launched.

All monographs are written by the literature researchers of the DPIC and checked for clinical relevance by the medical specialists. Based on literature reviews and data from the DPIC, human dose-effect relations in mg/kg are determined for all compounds (4 levels: no poisoning, mild, moderate, severe). The database contains a unique severity calculation tool. Based on the dose ingested of a certain compound and the body weight of the patient, the system presents the expected severity of the poisoning for that patient. Based on this severity estimation, the symptoms that are expected to develop are presented on the screen. This is done with easy color coding, making the main risks for the patient very clear at a glance. Using such a system greatly adds to uniformity in poisons information advice by the various staff members. With this tailor-made information, a better and more uniform triage of patients is possible at three levels: (1) the patient can stay at home safely; (2) hospital observation; and (3) further treatment required. Obviously, this calculation tool is an aid; specific circumstances and the medical history of the patient need to be taken into consideration for a final decision. In 2007, the web application of this system became available in Dutch (www.vergiftigingen.info). For internal use within the DPIC, this database also includes a differential diagnostic system. After the input of a patient's symptoms, the system produces a list of potential causative agents (De Vries et al., 2004). In 2020, there were 47,235 telephone consultations (only health professionals) and 139,347 consultations of the web application.

Staffing

Since the beginning, the DPIC has been funded by the Dutch government, which realized the benefits and savings of having a poisons center on a national level. Although there have been heated discussions in the past on budgets, the general insight still is that the DPIC saves the community money and yields health benefits by signaling trends in poisonings that help subsequent prevention.

The staffing has increased since the 1960s and today there are approximately 30 whole time equivalents (wte) (40 people) in four groups:

- Physicians: 3.1 wte in specialties: intensive care medicine (2 doctors, 1.0 wte), acute internal medicine (2 doctors, 0.6 wte), anesthesiology (1 doctor, 0.4 wte), emergency medicine (0.26 wte), and nuclear and environmental medicine (0.8 wte). These seven doctors are second on-call for telephone information and for the management of chemical disasters. Another (1.0 wte) is a GP and epidemiologist by training and is dedicated to research with a special interest in statistics and modeling.
- Specialists in poisons information (SPIs). There are 16 SPIs (around 13.0 wte) with one team leader and two sorts of positions. Six work a combination of SPI-rota (usually 0.2–0.3 part of one's appointment) and scientific work. The major part of their appointment is conducting literature searches and preparing database monographs and/or research projects. These six have academic backgrounds in biology, biomedicine, health sciences, and/ or chemistry. The other 10 work solely as SPIs, handling telephone calls,

product information, assistance in follow-up projects and so forth. This job requires a higher education level (backgrounds such as laboratory training, pharmacist assistant, nursing, etc.) or a university level of preparation.

- Scientific literature researchers. 12 people (10.0 wte) university level staff without SPI tasks.
- 10 European Registered Toxicologists (SPI's, researchers, and medical doctors)
- 4 registered radiation experts (2 researchers and 2 medical doctors)
- Administrative/IT support (around 3.0 wte)

Management is done by people who also have scientific tasks and consists of the head of the Poisons Center (Prof. Dr. Dylan de Lange), a location manager/senior toxicologist, an ICT/financial coordinator, a quality officer, a medical specialist, and the SPI team leader.

The DPIC has its own training program for new colleagues and for continuing education. Participation in national and international toxicology courses and congresses is supported financially by the Center. The total annual budget for the DPIC is around 4.4 million Euros. The major part of this comes from the Ministry of Health, with smaller amounts from the Ministry of the Environment and the Food and Consumer Product Safety Authority.

International involvement

The staff of the DPIC has always recognized the importance of international collaboration and from its inception established a very close relation with the European Association of Poisons Centres and Clinical Toxicologists (EAPCCT) as well as with other toxicology associations. Several members have served and still serve on the EAPCCT Board, the Scientific Committee, or working in Poisons Centers Activity Working Groups. Notably, three Directors of the DPIC became President of the EAPCCT: Prof. Ad van Heijst was the third president (1974–1986); Prof. Jan Meulenbelt from 2002 to 2004, and Irma de Vries (Director of the DPIC 2015–2018) from 2012 to 2014.

Conclusion

The DPIC has now been in existence for 60 years and is consistently supported by the Dutch government. The DPIC has developed into a well-established component of the Dutch health system, contributing to individual healthcare as well as to public health in the Netherlands. It is funded by three government ministries, reflecting its areas of activity. It has an established staffing structure, operating a 24-h daily information system by telephone and its own online Dutch poisons information system. It has close links with the intensive care and internal medicine department in its base hospital in Utrecht, stimulating joint research projects. It plays a role in chemical incident management.

Challenges for the future include maintaining its monitoring function, especially with a rising number of Internet consultations. More emphasis needs to be put on electronic follow-up studies into newly emerging poisonings. As there is only one PIC in the country, interaction with other PIC's abroad is essential to exchange knowledge and experiences and to advance clinical toxicology and poisons centers for future generations.

References

De Vries I, Los PM, Brekelmans PJAM, van Riel AJHP, van Zoelen GA, Mensinga TT, et al. Early warning in terrorist chemical attacks. Experience with a computer-based differential diagnostic system. Clin Toxicol 2004;42(5):440–1.

De Wilde DJ. Cardiovascular and respiratory toxicity of drugs in overdose. Proceedings of the symposium "25 years clinical toxicology" on the occasion of the retirement of Prof. Dr. A.N.P. van Heijst from the National Institute of Public Health and Environmental Hygiene; 1987. p. 23–7.

Hunault CC, Mensinga TT, Böcker KB, Schipper CM, Kruidenier M, Leenders MEC, et al. Cognitive and psychomotor effects in males after smoking a combination of tobacco and cannabis containing up to 69 mg delta-9-tetrahydrocannabinol (THC). Psychopharmacology (Berlin) 2009;204(1):85–94.

Hunault CC, Böcker KB, Stellato RK, Kenemans JL, de Vries I, Meulenbelt J. Acute subjective effects after smoking joints containing up to 69 mg Δ9-tetrahydrocannabinol in recreational users: a randomized, crossover clinical trial. Psychopharmacology (Berlin) 2014;231(24):4723–33.

Lammers W, Cohen EM. Hulpverlening bij acute vergiftigingen. Ned Tijdschr Geneeskd 1960;104:1665–72 [in Dutch].

Meulenbelt J, Mensinga TT, Kortboyer JM, Speijers GJA, de Vries I. Healthy volunteer studies in toxicology. Toxicol Lett 1998;102-103:35–9.

Pikaar SA, van Heijst ANP. The National Poisons Information Center. Vet Hum Toxicol 1979;21:76–81.

Reinders A, Bourgeois FC. Definitiestudie toxicologische kennis- en informatiebank. RIVM-rapport 238707001; 1988. 59p. [in Dutch].

Van Heijst ANP. Activities of the national poisons control center in the Netherlands. Some remarks on data collection. J Toxicol Med 1981;1:69.

Van Heijst ANP, Douze JMC, Sangster B, En Pikaar SA. Het Nationaal Vergiftigingen Informatie Centrum; van vóórkomen tot voorkómen. In: Proceedings of the Dr. J. Spaander symposium 11–13 December; 1979. p. 113–9 [in Dutch].

Van Zoelen GA, van Riemsdijk TE, van Riel AJHP, de Vries I, Meulenbelt J. Computerized early warning system for emerging poisonings threatening public health. Clin Toxicol 2014;52(4):296–7.

Chapter 5.6

Belgium

Anne-Marie Descamps[a,b] and Dominique Vandijck[a,b]
[a]*Belgian Poison Center, Brussels, Belgium,* [b]*Faculty of Medicine and Health Sciences, Ghent University, Ghent, Belgium*

Origins

The Belgian Poison Center (BPC) was founded in 1963. This was at a similar time to other European centers. The driving force behind this was Dr. Monique Govaerts. She had graduated in pediatrics at the Free University of Brussels (ULB) and obtained a scholarship, which led her to obtain a Masters in Science and Hygiene in the Harvard School of Public Health in Boston. Her visits to several pediatric wards in the United States made her aware of the existence of poison centers and their important role in management of child poisoning and in public health. The idea to create a BPC came quickly on her return to Europe, when Dr. Govaerts, assisted by her husband Dr. André Govaerts, professor of immunology and microbiology and director of the blood transfusion center of the Belgium Red Cross, successfully persuaded their network of scientists and politicians to establish a poison center in Belgium. Cooperation with, among others, Prof. Corneel Heymans, Nobel Laureate in Medicine, Prof. André Lilar, lawyer, senator and former Minister of Justice, Dr. Christine Hendrickx-Duchaine, vice-president of the National Children's Charity (Oeuvre Nationale de l'Enfance, ONE), Prof. Paul Spehl, chairman of the Red Cross Medical Committee, Prof. Jean Van Beneden, president of the National Health Council, and Edouard Vekemans, director of the Belgian pharmaceutical and chemical company Union Chimique Belge (UCB), led to the publication on September 28, 1963, of the statutes of the BPC, which was called "Centre national de prévention et de traitement des intoxications, Centre Antipoisons." The choice for an independent structure was mainly driven by the aim of serving the entire population with no direct link or affiliation with one particular hospital or university. Immediately after its foundation, three physicians were recruited to develop an information system, writing toxicological information cards based on available data on chemicals, pharmaceuticals, and drugs of abuse. Information on the composition of commercial products available on the Belgian market

History of Modern Clinical Toxicology. https://doi.org/10.1016/B978-0-12-822218-8.00035-1
421

was gathered. In the spring of 1964, the emergency telephone line became operational, initially for medical professionals but soon also for the general public. A Royal Decree of October 9, 2002, added the BPC to the list of Belgian emergency services.

Mission of the BPC

The main mission of the BPC, as initially formulated, is still applicable today: to provide information to the general public and healthcare professionals in cases of acute poisoning, and to guide them to the appropriate level of care. Physicians, and since 2016 pharmacists, provide 24/7 toll-free telephone advice via an emergency number that has changed more than once in its history (currently +32 70,245,245). The BPC covers Belgium and since 2015 the Grand Duchy of Luxembourg (total population: about 12 million). Risk assessment is carried out by BPC staff, who then advise patients to (1) stay at home and take first aid measures, (2) consult a family physician, or (3) go to the hospital. Patients advised to go to the hospital are first assessed in the emergency department. For patients who are already in the hospital, the BPC receives calls for advice in most cases from the treating physician, but occasionally from a patient or their family. The number of calls has steadily increased from 964 in 1964, to 33,091 in 1984, 51,962 in 2004, and 60,668 in 2019, of which 52,211 calls were relating to exposures, and 8457 calls were for information. Twenty-two percent of calls now come from healthcare professionals (Antigifcentrum (BPC), 2020, 11–22). The center provides responses in two languages, Dutch and French. In addition, many academic meetings are conducted in English for political neutrality, so most poison center staffs are bilingual or trilingual.

Operations

Database on toxic substances

Initially obtaining commercial product information for nonpharmaceutical products was a major challenge. In the 1960s, product data were not widely available, and product composition was a trade secret. Nevertheless, access to product data was important to provide assistance in case of a poisoning accident and contacting a manufacturer on a case by case basis was time-consuming. As a result, Dr. Govaerts explained the role of the BPC to the Federation of the Belgian Chemical Industry and obtained their cooperation. The Federation encouraged its members to provide the composition of their products to the BPC on a voluntary basis. The BPC guaranteed strict confidentiality of the data. Most Belgian consumer product manufacturers were prepared to cooperate with the BPC. This collaboration with industry, before any legal requirements, subsequently proved to be useful when in 1993 the BPC became the Belgian designated contact point when the first European directive on dangerous preparations came into force.

Antidotes

On December 3, 1990, the Council and the representatives of the governments of the European Member States adopted a Resolution on improving the prevention and treatment of acute human poisoning. Member States were invited to take measures, such as providing availability of antidotes (European Commission, 1991). This was the first sign of recognition of poison centers by the European Commission. Facilitating access to antidotes for hospital emergency services became an important mission for the BPC which now maintains a stock of less common and expensive products, organizing transport to the point of care if necessary.

Toxicovigilance

Toxicovigilance by the BPC contributes to public health by detecting new risks and by monitoring some types of products or accidents at the request of public health authorities. A memorable example of a toxicovigilance action occurred in April 1981. The BPC received three calls about three children with nausea and hypotension after having played with the same sneezing powder. After contact with the German manufacturer, it appeared that the common name "sneezing root" used to order the main ingredient had resulted in the use of *Veratrum album* instead of *Helleborus niger.* The Ministry of Health was informed, and the product was withdrawn from the market (Mostin and Van Tittelboom, 1984). The BPC has registered carbon monoxide poisonings since 1995, an example of long-term surveillance that demonstrates the public health impact of regulatory measures (Anonymous, 1996).

Toxicological laboratory

Between December 1, 1972, and December 31, 1976, the BPC ran a toxicological laboratory. When legislation changed in 1976, only funding laboratories linked to a hospital, the laboratory was split off from the BPC, finally closing in 2000.

The executive board

The election of the first executive board followed the publication of the BPC statutes. Under the presidency of Professor André Lilar (1963–1966), it consisted of the nine funding members, representing the main Belgian universities, and Mr. Vekeman, director of the Belgian pharmaceutical and chemical company: Union Chimique Belge (UCB).

   The presidents of the executive board were Corneel Heymans (1966–1968), Paul Spehl (1968–1969), Jean-François Goossens (1969–1973), Paul Cornil (1974–1979), Frédéric Thomas (1979–1984), Camille Pirson (1984), Raymond Vermeylen (1985–2002), and Daniël Van Daele (2002–2009), successively. Since 2009, Alain Dewever, emeritus professor in health economics, hospital governance and honorary director of Brugmann Hospital, and Erasmus Hospital (Belgium), has been the president of the board.

Management

Dr. Govaerts, who was the first general manager of the BPC, ran the BPC for 27 years. She was succeeded by Dr. Martine Mostin in 1991, who joined the medical staff in November 1979, and devoted her career to the BPC. She developed the documentation system, organized a permanent medical literature survey and prepared the informatization of the BPC. In 1993 she ensured that the BPC was designated as the appointed body to receive the composition of dangerous products on the Belgian market, and she also strengthened pharmacovigilance and toxicovigilance activities. Dr. Mostin retired on October 1, 2019, and was succeeded by Dr. Anne-Marie Descamps (doctorate in health sciences and biomedical sciences). In January 2020, Prof. Dominique Vandijck (doctorate in medical sciences), an expert in healthcare policy, economics, innovation, and quality management, joined the management team.

Clinical toxicology in Belgium

While only a few doctors were interested in clinical toxicology in the 1960s, this changed in the 1970s and 1980s. Prof. Paul Mahieu, an intensivist at the Université Catholique de Louvain (UCL) spent time learning toxicology at the Fernand Widal Hospital in Paris under the supervision of Prof. Chantal Bismuth. At that time the French school of toxicology was famous and most of the toxicological cases in UCL were discussed once a month at Fernand Widal. Other physicians also developed an interest in toxicology. For example, Prof. Agnes Meulemans, an emergency physician at the Katholieke Universiteit van Leuven (KUL) participated in many European Association of Poisons Centres and Clinical Toxicologists (EAPCCT) congresses. At the Université Libre de Bruxelles (ULB), Prof. Philippe Lheureux, another emergency physician was also involved in the scientific activities of the EAPCCT. Ghent University also had an interest in clinical toxicology, based primarily around its emergency department physicians: Prof. Walter Buylaert and Prof. Peter De Paepe.

When UCL built a new hospital in 1976, it included a seven-bed intensive care unit (ICU) dedicated to neurocritical care and acute poisoning. This was the only ICU dedicated to acute poisoning in Belgium. After the retirement of Prof. Paul Mahieu, Prof. Philippe Hantson became head of this unit. In the 1980s a Center for Clinical Toxicology was formed by clinician experts in the management of acute poisoning, pharmacists specialized in laboratory investigations and specialists in environmental and occupational medicine. Since the 1990s the UCL has also offered a Master's Degree in Biomedical Sciences, with a subspecialty in toxicology.

Most developments in clinical toxicology were on an individual basis in universities; it is still not a medical specialty in Belgium. There is, however, a Belgian Society of Toxicology (BLT) with approximately 80 members, mostly pharmacists working for industry or in toxicological laboratories.

BPC staffing 2020

The staff of the BPC currently consists of 27 employees, of which 14 are physicians or pharmacists. New employees are given an intensive training in toxicology by the BPC. Continuing education for staff includes participation in national and international conferences, study-time, and in-house discussions on scientific literature. Staff have access to internal and external databases. Internal databases include product information, data on previous cases and journal articles; external databases include Drugdex, Poisindex, Toxbase, and Toxinz. Written protocols are available for paracetamol, toxic alcohols, and antidote administration. When a mushroom needs identification, a countrywide network of mycologists is available to help.

Until 2017, telephone call information was initially recorded on paper forms and stored on microfilms. These were later scanned, to obtain a digital version. On the first of January 2018, the BPC switched from paper to electronic data forms, filled in by the information specialist during the call. Changes were made to the form to enable optimal data collection, now linked to a detailed categorization system which facilitates data analysis.

Resources

The financing of the BPC has always been an issue, not only in the start-up phase, but also later, with periods of severe financial difficulty. Initially funding was provided by the association of the pharmaceutical industry, chemical companies, banks, and private donors. The Red Cross offered to house the new service in a small flat in Brussels. Recruitment of a small staff became possible and it was decided to hire medical professionals. These initial resources rapidly ran out, but to obtain government funding it was necessary to become a public interest organization. More than a year after the founding of the BPC, the Belgian Ministry of Health agreed to fund half of the operational cost, and from 1968 onwards, a more substantial part. A representative of the Minister of Health was appointed to the executive board to ensure appropriate use of resources. Since 2001, funds allocated to the BPC are determined by the Federal Minister of Public Health and paid by the National Lottery (De Cock, 2019). The "Friends of the Poison Center," a non-profit sister organization founded in 1982, organizes the "Monique Govaerts Prize," a reward for valuable scientific work in the field of toxicology (BPC, n.d.).

Cost-effectiveness

Funding is dependent on showing cost-benefit of the poison center. The BPC undertook cost-benefit analyses by assessing the link between characteristics, associated factors, compliance, and costs of patients with poisoning advised to go to the hospital (Descamps et al., 2019a). In the absence of the BPC, patients with unintentional poisoning would use medical services, such as physician consultation and hospital attendance, with an estimated cost-benefit ratio for the BPC of 5.70.

Other BPC studies analyzed the characteristics, direct cost and cost components charged by a university hospital to the government in 1214 cases of acute poisoning (Descamps et al., 2019b,c). The mean cost per episode was $1558 (Standard Deviation: $3212), while the mean cost for a call to the BPC was $30 (US dollars). The mean time of a call to the BPC is less than 3 min, and these figures demonstrate its benefit. In 2018, the BPC studied the compliance of patients the BPC advised to go to hospital. Follow-up revealed 58.0% were compliant with the advice, while 31.7% decided to stay at home (care on site), and 10.3% went to a family physician.

Evolution in toxicological inquiries

There has been little change in the proportion of accidental exposures in adults and children since 1964. The main changes are in the nature of toxic agents involved and in the management approach to poisoning. Pharmaceuticals, more specifically analgesics, hypnotics and sedatives, have always appeared as the top agents involved in poisoning. In the 1960s Belgian pharmacies had an impressive range of active ingredients with high toxicity and/or abuse potential available, often without prescription. These older drugs, including barbiturates, carbromal, alpha-chloralose, glutethimide, meprobamate, and methaqualone, caused severe effects in overdose. Placing them on prescription and the introduction of benzodiazepines and nonbenzodiazepine sedative-hypnotics (such as zopiclone) led to a decrease in acute poisoning hospitalizations. They were gradually replaced by drugs with a better safety profile. Similar improvements have been seen with newer, safer drugs for psychiatric disease.

Important changes also affected analgesics. Phenacetin nephropathy was regularly seen until its withdrawal in 1983. Large packages of raspberry-flavored aspirin tablets made salicylate poisoning in children a common cause of admission to pediatric wards. Anaphylactoid reactions due to the NSAID, glafenine, were common before its withdrawal. Withdrawal of pyrazolyne derivatives, the decreased use of salicylate, withdrawal of dextropropoxyphene (2011) and increased use of paracetamol and tramadol have affected the profile of analgesic poisoning. Corrosives, toxic alcohol-based preparations and, to a lesser extent, petroleum distillates remain products of concern. New formulations of laundry detergents in pods altered the accident profile of those products resulting in calls to the BPC, highlighting acute respiratory problems and corneal injuries after exposure. Their actions triggered regulatory measures at a European level.

While European regulations have improved product safety, through harmonization of requirements for the evaluation of drugs and pesticides, poison centers and public health authorities in Belgium still face the problem of Internet trade that makes identification and control of products coming from all parts of the world particularly challenging.

Evolution in the treatment of the poisoned patient

In Belgian hospitals, poisoning casualties usually underwent gastric lavage and administration of activated charcoal. In pediatric wards, ipecac syrup was largely used to provoke emesis. The BPC regularly informed medical professionals of the contraindication of gastric decontamination in ingestion of petroleum distillates, corrosives or convulsive agents, and the importance of airway protection. Domestic use of ipecac syrup was never encouraged in Belgium. The BPC recommended families with young children to keep activated charcoal at home and to contact the BPC before using it. Until April 2018, each pharmacy in Belgium had to have activated charcoal available.

The publication in 1992 of a consensus statement on gastric decontamination by the French society of intensive care and emergency medicine followed in 1997 by joint position statements of the American Academy of Clinical Toxicology (AACT) and EAPCCT on ipecac syrup, gastric lavage, activated charcoal and cathartics strongly limited the use of gastric decontamination in poisoning.

Pharmacokinetic studies also demonstrated the limited usefulness of forced diuresis, urine alkalinization, and extracorporeal elimination techniques in the majority of poisonings.

The use of antidotes has also seen major progress. In 1979 nalorphine, an agonist/antagonist used in the treatment of opiate-induced respiratory depression was replaced by naloxone which was devoid of agonist effect and safer to use (see Chapter 3.6). Digoxin fab antibodies became commercially available in 1985 and improved the prognosis of digoxin poisoning.

The use of ethanol as an alcohol dehydrogenase inhibitor in the treatment of methanol and ethylene glycol poisoning was efficient and affordable but presented several drawbacks. Maintenance of the appropriate ethanol level to achieve enzyme inhibition required intensive monitoring. The introduction of 4-methylpyrazole, a potent and well-tolerated alcohol dehydrogenase inhibitor was a great progress, despite its high cost (see Chapter 3.2). It became available in Belgium in March 2002.

International profile

From the beginning, Dr. Govaerts perceived the importance of giving international visibility to the work of poison centers. When the "Association Européenne des centres de lutte contre les Poisons," later renamed EAPCCT, was created in Tours (France) in 1964, the statutes of the Association were published in the Belgian official journal and the EAPCCT is still officially registered in Belgium. Dr. Govaerts served as treasurer until her retirement and developed close relationships with her European colleagues. Her successor Dr. Mostin took over her function as treasurer and was actively involved in the discussions between the EAPCCT and the European industry to harmonize data transmission from the industry to poison centers. Further international activities include the participation of the BPC in the International Programme on Chemical Safety (IPCS) Intox Program of the World Health organization (WHO) and currently in the discussions with the European Chemical Agency (ECHA) on data transmission about dangerous mixtures to poison centers.

Communication and prevention

Prevention has always been key for the BPC. Inspired by the example of the US, "anti-poison weeks" were organized between 1969 and 1973 resulting in positive exposure and brand recognition. Campaigns have been launched on first aid in case of poisoning, including educational packages for different types of organizations, schools, medical professionals, and hospitals, with information on how to recognize, prevent, and treat poisonings. Traditional communication tools continue to be used, while electronic communication tools are becoming more and more important. Since 2015, content from the BPC website (https://www.centreantipoisons.be) is used for prevention messages on social media.

Challenges

The BPC was created with the goal of improving the care of poisoned patients and prevention. Several decades later, it is still recognized for these traditional key activities but faces new challenges. The development of many toxicological databases on the Internet has changed the needs of both public and health professionals to call a poison center, reducing the number of inappropriate inquiries but potentially increasing the need for PC-expertise in hospital care.

The general concern about the cost-effective use of scarce healthcare resources should further enhance the role of poison centers by reducing unnecessary referrals to general practitioners and hospitals. Health authorities are now interested in continuous surveillance systems for potential toxic events of public health importance, including terrorism. It has been recognized that poison centers are in a unique position to monitor patterns, incidence and severity of exposures and hence detect new trends. In this way, the BPC should be able to better contribute to the accuracy of risk assessment and assist in the identification of a priority list of chemicals for assessment and monitoring.

From the perspective of using poison center data for global risk assessment and public health, another challenge is the development of international harmonization of human poisoning data collection to allow comparison (Descamps, 2019; Descamps et al., 2020). European poison centers will have to work more closely together to face these challenges, which are often common and cannot be met organizationally or financially by a single center. A European example of cooperation is the "European Product Categorisation System" for dangerous mixtures developed by ECHA in the context of Annex VIII of the Classification, Labeling, and Packaging (CLP) Regulation, and the creation of a unique identification number (UFI) for dangerous mixtures. Although a very noble objective, work is still required to create a useful tool in the context of emergency medical advice.

The BPC continues to play an important role in health protection, including prevention, health promotion and screening. To achieve this, it will be necessary to initiate new activities, acquire new toxicological skills, methodologies and quality assurance that are in alignment with a fast-evolving healthcare landscape. This will entail recruitment and training of different types of staff and adequate funding to sustain and expand BPC operations.

Acknowledgments

The authors acknowledge the contributions from Dr. Martine Mostin, Prof. Dr. Philippe Hantson, and Patrick De Cock.

References

Anonymous. Nationaal Register van de CO-vergiftigingen. Brussel: BPC; 1996.

Antigifcentrum (BPC). Activiteitenverslag 2019: 1 januari - 31 december. Brussel: BPC; 2020. https://www.antigifcentrum.be/sites/default/files/imce/2019%20jaarverslag%20NL.pdf. Accessed on 08/18/2020.

BPC. n.d. Prijs dr. Monique Govaerts voor Nelly Saenen. https://www.antigifcentrum.be/nieuws/nieuw-prijs-dr-monique-govaerts-voor-nelly-saenen. Accessed on 08/18/2020.

De Cock P. Pillen en Producten: Geschiedenis van het Belgische Antigifcentrum. 1st ed. Brussel: BPC; 2019. p. 150–2.

Descamps A. Patient profile and cost of acute poisonings. A comparative study of emergency department admissions versus poison Centre consultations. 1st ed. Asse: A. Descamps; 2019.

Descamps A, De Paepe P, Buylaert W, Mostin M, Vandijck D. Belgian poison centre impact on healthcare expenses of unintentional poisonings: a cost-benefit analysis. Intl J Pub Heal 2019a;64(9):1283–90.

Descamps A, De Paepe P, Buylaert W, Mostin M, Vandijck D. Adults with acute poisoning admitted to a university hospital in Belgium in 2017: cost analysis benchmarked with national data. Clin Toxicol 2019b;58(5):406–13.

Descamps A, Vandijck D, Buylaert W, Mostin M, De Paepe P. Characteristics and costs in adults with acute poisoning admitted to the emergency department of a university hospital in Belgium. PLoS One 2019c;14(10), e0223479.

Descamps A, Vandijck D, Buylaert W, Mostin M, De Paepe P. Hospital referrals of patients with acute poisoning by the Belgian poison Centre: analysis of characteristics, associated factors, compliance, and costs. Emerg Med J 2020. https://doi.org/10.1136/emermed-2019-209202.

European Commission. 1991. The prevention and treatment of acute human poisoning. https://cordis.europa.eu/article/id/181-the-prevention-and-treatment-of-acute-human-poisoning. Accessed on 08/17/2020.

Mostin M, Van Tittelboom T. Toxicité des poudres à éternuer. Partie II. Expérience du Centre Belge Anti-Poisons. J Pharm Belg 1984;39(39):380–2.

Chapter 5.7

France

Robert Garnier[a] and Bruno Mégarbane[b]

[a]*Paris Poison Control Centre, Federation of Toxicology, Fernand-Widal Hospital, University of Paris, Paris, France,* [b]*Department of Medical and Toxicological Critical Care, Federation of Toxicology, Lariboisière Hospital, University of Paris, Paris, France*

Origins

The founder of French medical toxicology, Mathieu-Joseph-Bonaventure Orfila, was born in Minorca, in the Balearic Islands, in 1787. He arrived in Paris at the age of 20. Eight years later, in 1818, he published the book that founded modern medical toxicology, the "Traité des poisons tirés des règnes minéral, végétal et animal, ou Toxicologie générale." He was a forensic pathologist and nearly 150 years later Michel Gaultier, another forensic pathologist, founded French clinical toxicology. In the 1940s, he focused his forensic activity toward toxicology. In the early 1950s, he became head of the department of internal medicine and forensic medicine at the Fernand-Widal Hospital in Paris. He guided department activity toward toxicology and forensic and clinical toxicology and from the end of the 1950s, toward the management of acute poisonings. In the early 1960s the Fernand-Widal Hospital Toxicology Clinic, its name at that time, included four medical intensive care beds. The poisonings managed at that time were mainly due to carbon monoxide, barbiturates, trichloroethylene, then ethylene glycol, carbamate, digitalis, first-generation antipsychotics and tricyclic antidepressants (Gaultier et al., 1968a,b; Gaultier et al., 1969; Gaultier et al., 1970; Fréjaville et al., 1970).

1950s and 1960s: The first poison control center

The toxicological specialization of the department headed by M. Gaultier began to be known by all Parisian hospital doctors. Thereafter, in the mid-1950s, he and his first students and later assistants, Etienne Fournier and Pierre Gervais started to respond increasingly to telephone requests to assist poisoned patient diagnosis and management. Over the years, the demand increased exponentially, extending to Parisian doctors working in outside hospitals, then to provincial doctors and finally to the public. In 1959, this situation justified the creation of the Telephone Information Service in the Toxicological Clinic, the embryo of the first French poison control center (PCC). In the mid-1960s, the Toxicological Clinic included a medical intensive care unit dedicated to life-threatening acute poisonings, a hospital unit to treat less severely intoxicated patients, patients leaving intensive care and patients with subacute and chronic intoxications, a PCC as well as a professional and an environmental toxicology consultation service. Raymond Bourdon set up a toxicological analysis laboratory in adjoining premises at the Toxicological Clinic. Michel Gaultier was responsible for teaching toxicology at the Paris University of Medicine while Raymond Bourdon did this at the Paris University of Pharmacy. Thereafter the second generation of Michel Gaultier's students came to the Toxicological Clinic. This complete organization quickly developed its activity. In the mid-1960s, the Paris PCC managed approximately 10,000 exposures per year and the Toxicological Intensive Care Unit managed approximately 1000 acute poisonings per year (Fréjaville et al., 1970). In parallel, in the early 1960s, Louis Roche created a Centre for Toxicological Pathology in Lyon, in a medical emergency department. Next to this center, he funded a telephone toxicological information service, entrusted to Véronique Vincent in 1965. Louis Roche was also a forensic physician as was Jacqueline Jouglard who founded the Marseille PCC in 1967.

The group for combating poisoning and EAPCCT

In 1962, the "Groupement de lutte contre les intoxications" was created. This scientific society brought together practitioners working in PCCs and departments focused on treating poisoning in France (Sunshine et al., 1966). This organization was the ancestor of the current French Society of Clinical Toxicology (STC), funded in the early 1980s with new statutes allowing all medical, veterinary and analytical toxicologists to become members. The European Association of Poisons Centres and Clinical Toxicologists (EAPCCT) was founded in Tours, France, in September 1964 (see the EAPCCT Chapter 5.14 in this book). Michel Gaultier was its first president. In the following decades, several other French toxicologists became presidents including Albert Jaeger and Bruno Mégarbane.

1970s: Rise of the French PCCs

From the late 1960s to the mid-1970s, PCCs developed extensively in France. In 1975, there were 17 French PCCs in Angers, Bordeaux, Clermont-Ferrand, Grenoble, Lille, Lyon, Marseille, Montpellier, Nancy, Nantes, Paris, Reims, Rennes, Rouen, Strasbourg, Toulouse and Tours and almost as many toxicological intensive care units, on the same sites. These units, initially functional units of the same department, started to be individualized in the beginning of the 1970s. In Paris, Marie-Louise Efthymiou directed the PCC. It became an independent department in 1971 with Georges Lagier and later Robert Garnier as its head. A few years later, the toxicological intensive care unit was headed by

Chantal Bismuth. During the 1970s and 1980s, major centers of medical toxicology were also set up in several major provincial cities: in Strasbourg with Albert Jaeger, in Nancy with Henri Lambert then Jacques Manel, in Marseille with Jacqueline Jouglard, in Lyon with Jean-Claude Evreux then Jacques Descotes and in Angers with Patrick Harry. Under the direction of Jean-Pierre Fréjaville and Chantal Bismuth, the first edition of "Toxicologie Clinique" was published in 1971. It became the primary reference book in the field in the French-speaking community and is now in its 6th edition (Fréjaville et al., 1971).

Mission

Until the mid-1970s, the organization of clinical toxicology departments in France was not regulated. In 1976, the organization and missions of the French PCCs were defined for the first time by the national regulation authorities based on a circular issued by the General Directorate for Health (DGS-1976-257). According to this circular, the French PCCs were requested to provide toxicological information 24 h a day. They had to be located in a hospital, associated with a specialist care unit; and they had to undertake pharmacovigilance. A clinical toxicology physician should direct each PCC, while PCC staff could include physicians, pharmacists, and librarians. PCCs had to develop a database focused on the end-use product composition. They had to constitute a database of cases using a common software and be able to provide epidemiological information required by public health authorities on request. In 1973, the PCCs of Lyon, Marseille and Paris adopted a common electronic system, recommended to be generalized to all French PCCs by the governmental circular. Once published, the circular indicated that only Lyon, Marseille, and Paris PCCs fulfilled the required conditions for recognition. During the 1970s, French PCCs focused their work on the determination of prognostic factors and treatments of poisonings such as colchicine, digitalis, and ethylene glycol (Bismuth et al., 1973, 1977; Gaultier et al., 1977).

1980s: Toxicovigilance

In the 1970s, PCCs participated in the creation and development of the French pharmacovigilance system; Lyon, Marseille, and Paris PCCs became the first three French pharmacovigilance centers. On April 10, 1980, a decree reorganized French pharmacovigilance and created a toxicovigilance system for the first time in Europe and the world, dedicated to collect, preserve, and analyze adverse reactions related to nonpharmaceuticals of natural or synthetic origin. PCCs represented the basis of this new system. A decree of January 20, 1988, created the National Toxicovigilance Commission to coordinate all toxicovigilance activities.

The main PCC missions during this decade were focused on:

- Investigation of the presence of highly concentrated chlorinated hydrocarbons, including carbon tetrachloride and 1,2-dichloroethane, in the technical trichloroethylene available to the population on the French market as impurities causing liver damage (Conso et al., 1982).
- Critical review of sneezing powder marketing that contained *Veratrum album* root at risk of causing harm to users (Carlier et al., 1983).
- Identification of prognostic factors in paraquat poisoning following the rapid increase in its incidence (Bismuth et al., 1982).
- Determination of prognostic factors and treatment principles for chloroquine poisoning due to its exponential increase, following publication of a book recommending its use for suicidal purposes (Riou et al., 1988).
- Use of fomepizole rather than ethanol for ethylene glycol poisoning management (Baud et al., 1988).

1990s and early 2000s: Reorganization of the PCC network

A March 30, 1992-decree redetermined PCC missions and attributions, stating that PCCs were responsible for toxicovigilance, pharmacovigilance, and addiction monitoring. They had to contribute to the prevention of intoxication, health education, and the teaching of clinical toxicology. They were requested to use a common electronic file system accessible to all network participants and suitable for the establishment of a national exposure database. The March 23, 1993-decree set out the first official French PCC list reduced to 11: Angers, Bordeaux, Grenoble, Lille, Lyon, Marseille, Nancy, Paris, Rennes, Strasbourg, and Toulouse. Seven PCCs were also the head of regional toxicovigilance networks (Lille, Lyon, Marseille, Nancy, Paris, Rennes, and Toulouse). A technical committee was set up at the national level, the "National Toxicovigilance Commission" to coordinate the PCC network. Thereafter the September 17, 1996, and the November 29, 1996, decrees restated the PCC missions and defined the conditions for being officially listed. A new decree on June 1, 1998, established a list of 10 PCCs, resulting in the closure of Grenoble PCC. However, the Grenoble center as well as Clermont-Ferrand, Reims, and Rouen PCCs were temporarily maintained with toxicovigilance activity until their definitive disappearance between the late 1990s and the early 2010s. The Grenoble toxicovigilance center was the last to close.

In 1999, the PCCs changed their electronic systems. This modification of computerized medical records was endorsed by the decree of June 18, 2002, which indicated that the PCC information system should rely on two major databases: the National Database of Exposure Cases (BNCI) and the National Database of Product Composition (NBCP). During these two decades, PCC major contributions included the extension of fomepizole use to acute poisoning by other glycols and alcohols (Mégarbane et al., 2001, 2005); the validation of the

preferential use of hydroxocobalamin to treat cyanide poisoning, especially after fire smoke inhalation (Borron et al., 2007a,b); the use of dimercaptosuccinic
acid to treat various metals and metalloids poisonings (Fournier et al., 1988);
the validation of immunotherapy to treat digitalis poisoning; and the development of immunotherapy to reverse colchicine poisoning (Taboulet et al., 1993;
Baud et al., 1995).

PCCs 2010–2020

Over the past decade, Rennes and Strasbourg PCCs closed. There are now eight
French PCCs: Angers, Bordeaux, Lille, Lyon, Marseille, Nancy, Paris, and
Toulouse. In addition, a specific organization for toxicovigilance has been set
up overseas, with La Reunion and Mayotte on one hand and with La Martinique,
Guadeloupe, St Martin, St Barthélémy, Guyana and St. Pierre and Miquelon on
the other. The first organization is attached to the Marseille PCC; the second to
the Paris PCC.

ANSES, CCTV, SICAP

In 2005, the coordination of toxicovigilance was entrusted to a national public
health agency called the Institut de Veille Sanitaire (Institute of Health Watch).
In 2016, this coordination was taken over by the National Agency for Food,
Environment and Work (ANSES). Under these successive changes, the French
PCCs carried out several surveys and preventive actions (see http://www.cen-
tres-antipoison.net/CCTV/index.html). Among these were: persistent paraquat
poisoning in certain French overseas departments after its ban in Europe; the
little-known neurotoxic syndrome occurring after the consumption of morels;
poisoning resulting from the proliferation of cyanobacteria in surface waters;
factors of acute colchicine poisoning determining toxicity; adverse effects of dimethyl fumarate-treated items; adverse effects caused by the consumption of energy drinks; Asian hornet stings; acute toxicity and fatalities attributed to level-2
analgesics including dextropropoxyphen; acute intoxications with buflomedial,
baclofen, diquat, clenbuterol, trimeboutin, methocarbamol, alphachloralose-
based raticides; phosphides; accidental methadone poisoning; addiction to
Datura stramonium; eye disorders associated with "popper" (amyl nitrate)
consumption; dysgeusia associated with the consumption of certain pine nuts;
the adverse effects of iodoformed wicks; accidental ingestion of water-soluble
laundry pods; respiratory disorders associated with the use of water proofing
products; and gastrointestinal disorders caused by certain squash considered
edible. These working groups were chaired by the Coordination Committee
of ToxicoVigilance (CCTV) and the Strategic Committee for PCC Activities
(SICAP), under the responsibility of the ANSES. The CCTV (which included
one representative of each PCC) worked with the Directorate-General for Health
(DGS) and the different French health agencies [e.g., ANSES, the Agence

Nationale de Sécurité du Médicament et des Produits de Santé (ANSM) and the Santé Publique France]. The CCTV's main missions included the following:

- investigate health signals and alerts transmitted by the PCCs or any other sources including health authorities from France or any other countries, automated detection, spontaneous reports, monitoring of indicators;
- respond to specific requests from the Ministry of Health or other public health authorities; and
- provide expertise and contribute to the monitoring of toxic effects of manmade products, natural substances or pollution.

SICAP, established in 2017, had the task of issuing an opinion on the general organization of PCC activities, on the necessary developments in terms of surveillance, expertise and management of the toxic risks, and on the strategic orientations of the PCC information system. This committee consisted of representatives from the General Directorate of Health (DGS), the General Directorate of Health Offer (DGOS), the National Agency for Food, Environment and Work (ANSES), the National Agency for Medicines and Health Products Safety (ANSM), the National Agency of Public Health (ANSP), the Digital Health Agency (ANS or ASIP Santé), the French National Research and Safety Institute for the Prevention of Occupational Accidents and Diseases (INRS), and four PCC members, including two representatives from SICAP. ANSES was responsible for the coordination and the CCTV scientific board, the toxicovigilance operational cell, and the strategic committee for PCC activities. Four working groups were coordinated by ANSES: (1) vigilance for chemicals; (2) toxicovigilance of controlled products; (3) vigilance for natural toxins; and (4) methods of PCC database utilization. SICAP management, including the decision-making system, national exposure database, and national commercial mix composition information database was taken up in 2017 by the ANSES, which provided PCC with electronic support. At present, French PCCs are open 24 h a day. Approximately 300,000 calls regarding 200,000 cases per year are received from health professionals and the public (Sinno-Tellier et al., 2017).

Clinical toxicology departments

In parallel with the decrease in PCC number, the number of French centers specialized in the treatment of acute poisonings gradually decreased from 1990 to 2000. The only French critical care department now dedicated to poisoning management is the Department of Medical and Toxicological Critical Care (called "RMT") in Lariboisière Hospital, previously headed by Frédéric Baud and currently by Bruno Mégarbane. This department was created in 1998 with the move of the former toxicological clinic of Fernand-Widal Hospital directed by Chantal Bismuth to Lariboisière Hospital. In 2017, the Federation of Toxicology of Assistance Publique-Hôpitaux de Paris was created gathering the Department of Medical and Toxicological Critical Care (headed by Bruno

Mégarbane), the Emergency Department (headed by Patrick Plaisance), the Laboratory of Toxicology (headed by Laurence Labat), the Paris PCC (headed by Jérôme Langrand), and the Center of evaluation and information on drug dependence (headed by Samira Djezzar). The aim of this federation was to promote the development of research, education and patient management in the field of clinical toxicology. Several research projects were conducted over the last decade to improve poisoning management, including the use of extracorporeal oxygenation membrane to treat cardiotoxicity due to poisoning, the optimization of hemodialysis in lithium poisoning and the confirmation of fomepizole safety (Mégarbane et al., 2007; Vodovar et al., 2016; Rasamison et al., 2020). A research team dedicated to experimental investigations (UMRS-1144) was funded by the National Institute of Medical Research (Inserm). Several studies were performed using rodent animal models to improve the understanding of the neuro-respiratory effects of psychotropic drugs, the addiction to stimulant drugs including new psychoactive substances and the mechanisms of lithium-related toxicity (Alhaddad et al., 2012; Hanak et al., 2015; Lagard et al., 2018; Chartier et al., 2018; Mégarbane et al., 2020).

Conclusion

The French school of clinical toxicology is one of the most famous worldwide. Many important clinicians and biologists contributed to the progress of the science and the improvement of poisoned patient management. Despite current threats to PCC organization and hospital finances, the French school should remain as an example for the promotion of clinical toxicology.

References

Alhaddad H, Cisternino S, Declèves X, et al. Respiratory toxicity of buprenorphine results from the blockage of P-glycoprotein-mediated efflux of norbuprenorphine at the blood-brain barrier in mice. Crit Care Med 2012;40:3215–23.

Baud FJ, Galliot M, Astier A, Bien DV, Garnier R, Likforman J, Bismuth C. Treatment of ethylene glycol poisoning with intravenous 4-methylpyrazole. N Engl J Med 1988;319:97–100.

Baud FJ, Sabouraud A, Vicaut E, Taboulet P, Lang J, Bismuth C, Rouzioux JM, Scherrmann JM. Brief report: treatment of severe colchicine overdose with colchicine-specific fab fragments. N Engl J Med 1995;332:642–5.

Bismuth C, Gaultier M, Conso F, Efthymiou ML. Hyperkalemia in acute digitalis poisoning: prognostic significance and therapeutic implications. Clin Toxicol 1973;6:153–62.

Bismuth C, Gaultier M, Conso F. Medullary aplasia after acute colchicine poisoning. 20 cases. Nouv Press Med 1977;6:1625–9.

Bismuth C, Garnier R, Dally S, Fournier PE, Scherrmann JM. Prognosis and treatment of paraquat poisoning: a review of 28 cases. J Toxicol Clin Toxicol 1982;19:461–74.

Borron SW, Baud FJ, Mégarbane B, Bismuth C. Hydroxocobalamin for severe acute cyanide poisoning by ingestion or inhalation. Am J Emerg Med 2007a;25:551–8.

Borron SW, Baud FJ, Barriot P, Imbert M, Bismuth C. Prospective study of hydroxocobalamin for acute cyanide poisoning in smoke inhalation. Ann Emerg Med 2007b;49:794–801.

Carlier P, Efthymiou ML, Garnier R, Hoffelt J, Fournier E. Poisoning with Veratrum-containing sneezing powders. Hum Toxicol 1983;2:321–5.

Chartier M, Malissin I, Tannous S, Labat L, Risède P, Mégarbane B, Chevillard L. Baclofen-induced encephalopathy in overdose - modeling of the electroencephalographic effect/concentration relationships and contribution of tolerance in the rat. Prog Neuropsychopharmacol Biol Psychiatry 2018;86:131–9.

Conso F, Souquière JP, Bismuth C, Efthymiou ML, Fournier E. Valence B.[Hepatonephritis and hepatitis due to fraudulent trichlorethylene]. Gastroenterol Clin Biol 1982;6:539–41.

Fournier L, Thomas G, Garnier R, Buisine A, Houze P, Pradier F, Dally S. 2,3-Dimercaptosuccinic acid treatment of heavy metal poisoning in humans. Med Toxicol Adv Drug Exp 1988;3:499–504.

Fréjaville JP, Gorin N, Gaultier M. Acute poisoning by phenothiazine amines. (apropos of 152 cases). Ann Med Interne 1970;121:1057–64.

Fréjaville JP, Bourdon R, Christoforov B, Bismuth C, Pebay-Peyroula F, Nicaise AM, Pollet J. Toxicologie clinique et analytique. Paris: Flammarion-Médecine-Sciences; 1971. 243p.

Gaultier M, Fournier E, Efthymiou ML, Frejaville JP, Jouannot P. Dentan M.89. [acute digitalis poisoning (70 cases)]. Bull Mem Soc Med Hop Paris 1968a;119:247–74.

Gaultier M, Fournier E, Bismuth C, Rapin J, Fréjaville JP, Gluckman JC. Acute poisoning by meprobamate. Apropos of 141 cases. Bull Mem Soc Med Hop Paris 1968b;119:675–705.

Gaultier M, Kanfer A, Bismuth C, Crabié P, Fréjaville JP. Current data on acute colchicine poisoning. Apropos of 23 cases. Ann Med Interne 1969;120:605–18.

Gaultier M, Pebay-Peyroula F, Rudler M, Leclerc JP, Duvaldestin P. Acute ethylene glycol poisoning. Eur J Toxicol 1970;3:227–34.

Gaultier M, Conso F, Bismuth C, Leclerc JP, Mellerio F. Ethylene glycol acute poisoning. Acta Pharmacol Toxicol 1977;41(Suppl 2):339.

Hanak AS, Chevillard L, El Balkhi S, Risède P, Peoc'h K, Mégarbane B. Study of blood and brain lithium pharmacokinetics in the rat according to three different modalities of poisoning. Toxicol Sci 2015;143:185–95.

Lagard C, Malissin I, Indja W, Risède P, Chevillard L, Mégarbane B. Is naloxone the best antidote to reverse tramadol-induced neuro-respiratory toxicity in overdose? An experimental investigation in the rat. Clin Toxicol 2018;56:737–43.

Mégarbane B, Borron SW, Trout H, Hantson P, Jaeger A, Krencker E, Bismuth C, Baud FJ. Treatment of acute methanol poisoning with fomepizole. Intensive Care Med 2001;27:1370–8.

Mégarbane B, Borron SW, Baud FJ. Current recommendations for treatment of severe toxic alcohol poisonings. Intensive Care Med 2005;31:189–95.

Mégarbane B, Leprince P, Deye N, Résière D, Guerrier G, Rettab S, Théodore J, Karyo S, Gandjbakhch I, Baud FJ. Emergency feasibility in medical intensive care unit of extracorporeal life support for refractory cardiac arrest. Intensive Care Med 2007;33(5):758–64.

Mégarbane B, Gamblin C, Roussel O, Bouaziz-Amar E, Chevillard L, Callebert J, Chen H, Morineau G, Laplanche JL, Etheve-Quelquejeu M, Liechti ME, Benturquia N. The neurobehavioral effects of the designer drug naphyrone - an experimental investigation with pharmacokinetics and concentration/effect relationship in mice. Psychopharmacology 2020;237:1943–57.

Rasamison R, Besson H, Berleur MP, Schicchi A, Mégarbane B. Analysis of fomepizole safety based on a 16-year post-marketing experience in France. Clin Toxicol 2020;58:742–7.

Riou B, Barriot P, Rimailho A, Baud FJ. Treatment of severe chloroquine poisoning. N Engl J Med 1988;318:1–6.

Sinno-Tellier S, Djaoudi J, Manel J. Epidémiologie des intoxications en France. Etude des cas d'exposition enregistrés par les centres antipoison français en 2013. In: Baud F, Garnier R, editors. Toxicologie Clinique. 6th ed. Lavoisier Médecine Paris; 2017. p. 112–32.

Sunshine I, Govaerts A, Gaultier M, Roche L, Vincent V. Les centres anti-poisons dans le monde. Paris: Masson; 1966. 200 p.

Taboulet P, Baud FJ, Bismuth C. Clinical features and management of digitalis poisoning-rationale for immunotherapy. J Toxicol Clin Toxicol 1993;31:247–60.

Vodovar D, El Balkhi S, Curis E, Deye N, Mégarbane B. Lithium poisoning in the intensive care unit: predictive factors of severity and indications for extracorporeal toxin removal to improve outcome. Clin Toxicol 2016;54:615–23.

Chapter 5.8

Spain and Portugal

Ana Ferrer Dufol[a,b] and Santiago Nogué Xarau[b]
[a]*Unit of Clinical Toxicology, Clinic University Hospital, Zaragoza, Spain,* [b]*Spanish Foundation of Clinical Toxicology, Barcelona, Spain*

Clinical toxicology in Spain

Clinical toxicology in Spain developed at a slower rate than in some other European countries. This was related to the development of Spanish health care institutions, scientific associations dealing with poisoning, epidemiological changes in poisoning and the resulting requirement for new medical treatments, and the development of university programs in toxicology.

Health care institutions

Two different systems are involved in the prevention, diagnosis, and treatment of human poisoning in Spain: the Toxicological Information Service (TIS) and public hospital emergency departments and intensive care units (ICU).

Toxicological information

The Spanish poison control center (PCC), known as the Toxicological Information Service, is a center within the National Institute of Toxicology and Forensic Sciences (NITFS) which is within the portfolio of the Justice Ministry, and fully independent of the health care system which is managed by the Health Ministry. This anomaly is due to historical reasons. The NITFS was created in 1935 by merging three forensic laboratories set up in 1887 in Madrid, Barcelona, and Seville. It was intended to assist the Justice administration in guaranteeing the best quality of the scientific expertise in the field of forensic sciences. Their main functions were analytical, and specific sections of biology, histopathology, and chemistry were created in 1967.

The TIS started in 1971 in the Madrid NIFTS headquarters to cover one of the NIFTS's objectives: to disseminate knowledge in toxicological matters, contribute to the prevention of poisonings, and attend to any questions asked about them. It is currently one of the six services integrated within the NIFTS.

History of Modern Clinical Toxicology. https://doi.org/10.1016/B978-0-12-822218-8.00032-6
441

The TIS is the only Spanish PCC. It answers phone inquiries on toxic exposures coming from the whole country 24/7, 365 days a year. Referrals, dealt with by general practitioners and forensic specialists, come from the general population (70%) and health professionals (30%). The inquiries are mainly related to actual poisonings and potential toxic exposures (~ 80%) and, secondarily, to more general information requests (e.g., medicinal adverse effects, chemical exposure, and pregnancy). Responders have no direct contact with the patient and clinical advice on an exposure is provided by the caller. The TIS gets around 80,000 phone calls per annum. The number of calls increased in 1999 when the TIS phone number was formally added to the labels of household products (Royal Decree 770/1999). Subsequently the TIS phone calls have stabilized and have then reduced slightly in recent years.

The staff of the TIS comprises an integrated medical service with 20 physicians in charge of phone information, a documentation service with five physicians and pharmacists who update the PCC database and nine civil servants as administrative support. In addition to phone consultations, the staff are involved in the production of expert reports for the different parts of the administration of Justice in toxicological matters. Following the European directive on dangerous substances, the TIS has kept information on the composition and formulation of regulated chemicals.

Medical care assistance

The relationship between toxicology and forensic medicine, typical of the 19th century, which broke down decades earlier in other countries, proved persistent in Spain. The Spanish TIS is still part of the Justice Ministry structure and the link at the university level with programs of legal medicine and toxicology persisted until 1996. This, and the absence of a medical specialty recognized by the National Health Service, prevented the implementation of hospital wards for poisoned patients linked to PCCs as established in neighboring countries such as France, the United Kingdom, or Germany.

In common with other European countries, medical treatment of acute poisoning in Spain is provided by the emergency departments and intensive care units (ICUs) of general hospitals. Both were part of the services established in the 1960s and provided by public and private hospitals. The introduction of the National Health Service (NHS) that currently covers the whole population of Spain, originated in the NHS legislation (1944) that stablished a compulsory health insurance system. During the 1960s large public hospitals first complemented and then replaced smaller health institutions funded by local corporations, medical academic faculties, or the Church. They controlled the introduction of emergency departments and out-of-hospital points of care in 1964. The first ICU was created in the Concepción Clinic in Madrid in 1966.

Since the beginning of the 1980s, professionals coming from different medical and biological fields such as forensic medicine, internal medicine, intensive care, pharmacology and biochemistry started training and research centered on the diagnosis and treatment of poisoned patients. This led to the creation of Clinical Toxicology Units (CTU) in some Spanish Hospitals. The first CTUs were related to the emergency departments at the Clinic Hospital in Barcelona, the Clinic University Hospital in Zaragoza, and the Rio Hortega University Hospital in Valladolid.

We have defined a CTU (FETOC, 2020c) as a location where two or more hospital professionals combine their efforts to improve the treatment of poisoned patients who go to their hospital for management of acute or chronic exposures. The services offered by a CTU include treatment guidelines, control of antidote availability, epidemiological surveillance of acute and chronic poisonings, interpretation of analytical toxicology, and collaboration in teaching and research in clinical toxicology. These CTUs which originally developed spontaneously have also been promoted by scientific societies, but most lack institutional support or regulation. Therefore they are quite heterogeneous regarding their service portfolios. An area of weakness in most Spanish hospitals is analytical toxicology. Some of these units offer also phone information on toxicological consultations from health care professionals and a few provide out-patient consultation in their health area. None of them is open to calls from the general public. There are now eight hospitals with a CTU; the other five are sited in Catalonia, Aragon, Baleares, Castilla, and Madrid.

Spanish scientific societies

The Spanish Association of Toxicology (AETOX, 2020) was founded in 1980 with the aim of gathering professionals from different fields of toxicology, at that time principally from the forensic, academic, and pharmaceutical settings. The Association gained momentum when NITFS organized National Toxicological Conferences in 1971, 1974, and 1979 at their regional departments in Barcelona and Seville. AETOX currently has 400 members and is affiliated with EUROTOX and IUTOX. A Clinical Toxicology Section was created in 1997 and first met at the Clinical University Hospital in Zaragoza to bring together the members whose professional activities centered on poisoned patients.

The Spanish Foundation of Clinical Toxicology (FETOC, 2020a) was added to the Spanish Register of Foundations in 2010. The aims of FETOC are to promote optimum care and increase knowledge of acute and chronic human poisoning. Their members carry out prevention, provide poisons information, clinical care, teaching, and research in clinical toxicology. These activities are intended to benefit health professionals, health institutions, and the general population.

Other general scientific societies in the fields of emergency medicine, intensive care and pediatrics also deal with the diagnosis and treatment of poisoning and include toxicological aspects in their meetings and journals. Some of them incorporate working groups on clinical toxicology. Among them are the Spanish Society of Emergency Medicine (SEMES, 2020) with its toxicology working group, the Spanish Society of Intensive Care and Coronary Units (SEMICYUC, 2020), and the Spanish Society of Pediatric Emergencies (SEUP, 2020). The problem of addiction is addressed by other Spanish societies (Sociodrogalcohol, 2020). These societies and their working groups have promoted the development of research in multicenter studies on different aspects of poison treatment. Their work provides an overview of the profile of clinical toxicology in Spain, and provides information on the epidemiology and future trends in poisoning (Burillo-Putze et al., 2003; Azkunaga et al., 2011; Puiguriguer et al., 2013).

Epidemiology of human poisoning in Spain

The pattern of human poisoning has evolved in Spain similar, but not identical, to that observed in other countries. Interestingly, there are differences in this pattern when comparing TIS cases with the epidemiology recorded in a hospital. The three main situations leading to acute poisoning that we have analyzed are self-harm, poisoning by drugs of abuse and accidental poisoning.

Cases of self-harm involving medicines changed rapidly from severe barbiturate poisoning, mainly phenobarbital, to the benzodiazepine overdoses that are now common (Caballero Vallés et al., 2008; Monteis, 1990). The pattern of antidepressant overdose followed the evolution of psychiatric prescriptions, so tricyclic antidepressants, prevalent in the 1980s, were replaced by lower risk selective serotonin reuptake inhibitors (SSRIs). Unlike Anglo-Saxon countries, analgesic overdose has never been very prevalent in Spain. Aspirin cases gave way to paracetamol and other antipyretic-analgesics in the 1980s but in total never exceeded 10% of cases. Despite the rise in the prescription of opiates for the treatment of chronic pain from the mid-90s, there has not been a clear shift to uncontrolled abuse nor a significant number of intentional or accidental overdoses (Caparrós et al., 2019).

Overdoses by drugs of abuse also show large variations. The most common agent producing acute poisoning presenting at the EDs has always been ethanol but the second place has markedly changed from the 1980s. What can be described as an epidemic of heroin overdoses afflicted Spain for 15 years, until the end of the 1990s. It produced around 25,000 deaths in a young population (PNSD, 2020b). Since 2000 cases have fallen rapidly, initially replaced by cocaine and then cannabis. Novel psychoactive substances have not reached more than an anecdotal level in terms of consumption and emergency presentations. This evolution is illustrated in annual reports of the Health Ministry's Spanish National Plan on Drugs (PNSD, 2020a).

In the group of hazardous chemicals, carbon monoxide and caustics were the main agents producing severe poisoning in the 1950s (Nolla, 1956). In 1981 the Toxic Oil Syndrome broke out in Spain, producing the largest food toxicity epidemic in modern times in Europe. It was caused by the manipulation of non-food grade rapeseed oil and its fraudulent distribution for human consumption

(Posada de la Paz et al., 2001). The precise chemical involved was never discovered [Editor's Note: See Chapter 1.5 in this book for details].

The strict regulations implemented in the past decades have drastically reduced chemical risks and lowered the incidence of emergency presentations. They are the object of a Toxicosurveillance Program launched in 1999 by the Health Ministry (Ferrer et al., 2000), designed as a multicenter prospective study: in the EDs of public hospitals, which is coordinated by the FETOC. The participants report on a voluntary basis all cases of poisoning due to household, agricultural, or industrial chemicals treated in their emergency departments. This system has collected over 20,000 cases in 20 years from a total of 20 hospitals, some of which now have clinical toxicology units. The main chemicals involved are toxic gases, principally carbon monoxide exposures, followed by caustic cleaning agents and irritant gases, with a mean age of 38 years and a mortality of approximately 1% (FETOC, 2020b).

By comparing the data collected on chemical poisoning in acute hospital emergency department data and the cases reported to the TIS, it is possible to compare different patterns of poisoning seen in different systems in Spain. Seventy-five percent of the cases the TIS deals with come from the general population, 90% of which are accidental exposures. This pattern affects the severity of TIS cases. The main agents involved are medicines and cleaning agents; 50% involve children and 80% have mild or no symptoms. Poisoning accounts for 1% of total emergency cases in Spanish emergency departments: 50% involve drugs of abuse, mainly ethanol, followed by cases of cannabis abuse; approximately 30% are prescription drug overdoses, mainly self-harm with benzodiazepines; and 15% cases are due to deliberate or accidental exposure to chemical agents. The mean age is 35 years and mortality is under 0.1%. Severe cases have fallen due to several factors, including the prescription of safer medicines such as the replacement of barbiturates by benzodiazepines and tricyclic antidepressants by SSRIs. Another major factor has been controls introduced by the European Union regulation of drugs and poisons.

Educational syllabus

Administrative decentralization in Spain affects the coherence of university programs. Owing to the multidisciplinary aspects of toxicology, its content is addressed in different faculties, including medicine, pharmacy, veterinary science, biology, and biochemistry. Toxicology remained formally linked to legal medicine in Spanish universities until 1996 but since then it has been recognized as a specific area of study. In medical schools, clinical toxicology is still taught in different departments. The syllabus in different Spanish regions is not harmonized, resulting in teaching by different disciplines and to a different extent and content in different universities.

At universities where teaching of clinical toxicology is prominent, their medical schools are linked to teaching hospitals in which there is a clinical toxicology unit with staff working part-time or, very exceptionally pursuing full-time teaching and doing research in clinical toxicology. However, clinical toxicology is not yet recognized as a medical specialty by the Spanish National Health Service, and hence educational activities aimed at professionals involved in the diagnosis and treatment of poisoned patients remain mainly restricted to the voluntary activity of scientific societies.

Clinical toxicology in Portugal

Portuguese poison control center

Portugal has a single PCC located in Lisbon (CIAV, 2020). The center was created on June 16, 1982, at the National Institute of Medical Emergencies (INEM), although its origin was a poison information center founded as a private service in 1963. The CIAV is a medical telephone consultation center in the field of toxicology and is responsible for providing information to health professionals or the general public, with the aim of offering an effective approach to poisoned patients. The CIAV provides toxicological information on all existing products, from medicines to products for domestic or industrial use, natural products, plants, or animals. It operates 24 h daily, 7 days a week. The service is offered by specialized medical personnel and is available through an exclusive free telephone line (800250250). The connection to the Instituto Nacional de Emergência Médico (INEM) "Urgent Patient Orientation Centers" (CODU) also allows easy access through the European Emergency Number (112). The CIAV also answers e-mail inquiries (ciav.tox@inem.pt).

During 2019 the CIAV received 30,076 calls (2506/month, 82/day). The last published statistics from 2016 show that 41% of calls came from the general population and 46% from health care providers. Agents involved were medicines (75%), domestic products (16%), pesticides (5%), and abused drugs (4%). Data published in a 2010 PhD dissertation (Loureiro-Cardoso, 2011) revealed that 77.9% of consultations were related to human or animal poisoning, 7.9% were requests for information on prevention of poisoning, and requests for articles or statistical data, and 14.2% were "void calls." Fifty-four percent of inquiries were related to poisonings in adults 16 years or older (63.2% female), 42% in children, and 4% in animals. When analyzing the types of toxin involved in the cases attended by the CIAV in that year, drug poisonings were most prevalent, followed by household products, pesticides, industrial products, cosmetic or hygiene products, substances of abuse and, finally, poisonings of animal origin.

The CIAV provides information on acute or chronic poisoning: on the diagnosis, clinical manifestations, therapeutic options, and prognosis after exposure to toxic products. It also collaborates in training activities, develops preventive measures and, based on permanently available and updated information, provides support for research or statistical analysis of the incidence of the varied products causing poisoning in Portugal.

The CIAV has a website (https://www.inem.pt/category/servicos/centro-de-informacao-antivenenos/) providing a checklist of questions to ask in case of poisoning, and first aid response in case of an exposure to a toxic product. CIAV also has specific advice, such as on detergent capsules or the bite of the Portuguese Caravel "Portuguese Man-of-War" (*Physalia physalis*), preventive measures to avoid poisoning, the meaning of hazard warning symbols, product notifications, legislation on the different types of agents, consultation statistics, links with scientific societies in the field of toxicology, and means of contact with the CIAV.

Currently a group of 10 doctors work at this Center; 5 belong to the INEM board and work full time at the poison center. The other five are hospital doctors who collaborate with the CIAV on a shift basis to insure the telephone answering service and are specialized in a range of disciplines (pulmonology, anesthesiology, general practice, and public health). No particular specialty is required, but it is essential that they are engaged in active clinical activity. Among INEM doctors, some have the Emergency Medical Competency from the Portuguese Medical Association. Clinical toxicology is not a specialty in Portugal and the doctors who work at CIAV all undergo a period of training in the service before beginning their duties. In terms of assistance of poisoned patients, they work, as in Spain, in the EDs and ICUs of general hospitals. There is nothing similar to Spain's CTUs.

Analytical toxicology is performed by the National Institute of Legal Medicine and Forensic Sciences, which has three units: Lisbon, Coimbra, and Porto. They deal predominantly with analytical requests from forensic cases and provide this service for poisoned patients admitted to the hospital. The Coimbra unit has established this type of collaboration with the University Hospital Center.

Several research teams from clinical and forensic settings have studied specific poisoned populations (Brandão et al., 2011; Costa et al., 2019; Ferreira et al., 2008; Teixeira et al., 2004) but there is no epidemiological surveillance or research network in the field of clinical toxicology at the national level other than the CIAV. There are seven medical schools, whose programs have complete autonomy. Toxicology contents appear linked to legal medicine; specific clinical toxicology topics used to be linked to other medical contents. In Coimbra's medical school, clinical toxicology is included as an optional subject. It is not included in the catalogue of postgraduate medical specialties.

Portuguese Toxicology Association

The Portuguese Toxicology Association (APT) is a non-profit institution that aims to promote and develop the areas of toxicology, environmental health and occupational health (AP Tox, 2020). It was founded in 2009 in response to the need to create a space for debate and the exchange of knowledge between professionals in the areas of toxicology, environmental health, and occupational health in Portugal. To strengthen this integration, APT supports interprofessional relations and the creation of networks and associations with other organizations.

The APT is open to all professionals with an interest in toxicology, environmental health, and occupational health. Its associates belong to industry, are academics or belong to government organizations. The APT keeps its members up to date on toxicology issues, disseminates relevant information, and regularly organizes thematic meetings. APT also has a mission to carry out activities that raise public awareness about toxicology and risk assessment for human health and the environment. There is not a specialty section on clinical toxicology.

References

AETOX. Spanish Association of Toxicology (AETOX), https://www.aetox.es/; 2020. [Accessed 1 June 2020].

AP Tox. Portuguese Society of Toxicology, https://www.aptox.pt/; 2020. [Accessed 1 June 2020].

Azkunaga B, Mintegi S, Bizkarra I, Fernández J, Intoxications Working Group of the Spanish Society of Pediatric Emergencies. Toxicology surveillance system of the Spanish Society of Paediatric Emergencies: first-year analysis. Eur J Emerg Med 2011;18(5):285–7.

Brandão JL, Pinheiro J, Pinho D, Correia da Silva D, Fernandes E, Fragoso G, Costa MI, Silva A. Mushroom poisoning in Portugal. Acta Medica Port 2011;24(Suppl 2):269–78.

Burillo-Putze G, Munne P, Dueñas A, Pinillos MA, Naveiro JM, Cobo J, Alonso J, Clinical Toxicology Working Group, Spanish Society of Emergency Medicine (SEMESTOX). National multicentre study of acute intoxication in emergency departments of Spain. Eur J Emerg Med 2003;10(2):101–4.

Caballero Vallés PJ, Dorado Pombo S, Díaz Brasero A, Eugenia García Gil M, Yubero Salgado L, Torres Pacho N, Ibero Esparza C, Cantero Bengoechea J. Epidemiologic survey of acute poisoning in the south area of the community of Madrid: The Veia 2004 Study. An Med Int (Madrid, Spain:1984) 2008;25(2):67–72.

Caparrós S, Pallas Villaronga AO, Cirera Lorenzo I. Epidemiología de las intoxicaciones en un servicio de urgencias hospitalario. In: Xarau SN, editor. Toxicología Clínica. Bases Para El Diagnóstico Y Tratamiento De Las Intoxicaciones En Servicios De Urgencias, Áreas De Vigilancia Intensiva Y Unidades De Toxicología. Barcelona: Elsevier España; 2019. p. 13–8.

CIAV. Centro De Informaçao Antivenenos, https://www.inem.pt/category/servicos/centro-de-informacao-antivenenos/; 2020. [Accessed 12 March 2020].

Costa M, Silva BS, Real FC, Teixeira HM. Epidemiology and forensic aspects of carbon monoxide intoxication in Portugal: a three years' analysis. Forens Sci Int 2019;299:1–5.

Nolla R. Estudio estadístico de los intoxicados ingresados en el Hospital Clínico y Provincial de Barcelona en el quinquenio de 1951-1955. Arch Esp Med Int 1956; II: 283-288.

Ferreira AMR, Borges A, Ranges R, Monsanto P, Dias MJ, Carvalho M. Avaliação das intoxicações medicamentosas em Portugal. Rev Faculd Ciênc Saúde 2008;5:94–100.

Ferrer A, Nogué S, Vargas F, Castillo O. Toxicovigilancia: una herramienta útil para la salud pública. Med Clin 2000;115(6):238.

FETOC. Spanish Foundation of Clinical Toxicology, http://www.fetoc.es/; 2020a. [Accessed 1 July 2020].

FETOC. Spanish Foundation of Clinical Toxicology. Toxicovigilancia, http://www.fetoc.es/toxicovigilancia/toxicovigilancia.html; 2020b. [Accessed 15 July 2020].

FETOC. Units of Clinical Toxicology, http://www.fetoc.es/unidades/unidades.html; 2020c. [Accessed 30 June 2020].

Loureiro-Cardoso N. Casuística Das Intoxicações Clínicas Em Portugal: Perfil Das Intoxicações no Serviço De Urgência Geral do Hospital De São Teotónio – Viseu, E.P.E. Universidade da Beira Interior; 2011. https://ubibliorum.ubi.pt/handle/10400.6/912.

Monteis J. Evolución epidemiológica de las urgencias toxicológicas. Rev Toxicol 1990;7(2):101–12.

PNSD. National Plan AntiDrugs. Annual Reports, https://pnsd.sanidad.gob.es/pnsd/memorias/home.htm; 2020a. [Accessed 15 June 2020].

PNSD. National Plan AntiDrugs. Report 2007, https://pnsd.sanidad.gob.es/profesionales/sistemasInformacion/informesEstadisticas/pdf/oed-2007.pdf; 2020b. [Accessed 15 June 2020].

Posada de la Paz M, Philen RM, Borda AI. Toxic oil syndrome: the perspective after 20 years. Epidemiol Rev 2001;23(2):231–47.

Puiguriguer J, Nogué S, Echarte JL, Ferrer A, Dueñas A, García L, Córdoba F, Burillo-Putze G. Mortalidad hospitalaria por intoxicación aguda en España (EXITOX 2012). Emergencias 2013;25:467–71.

SEMES. Spanish Society of Emergency Medicine, https://semes.org/; 2020. [Accessed 30 June 2020].

SEMICYUC. Spanish Society of Intensive Care and Coronary Units, https://semicyuc.org/; 2020. [Accessed 15 June 2020].

SEUP. 2020 Spanish Society of Paediatric Emergencies. Accessed 06/15/2020 https://seup.org/.

Sociodrogalcohol. Accessed 06/30/2020, https://socidrogalcohol.org/; 2020.

Teixeira H, Proença P, Alvarenga M, Oliveira M, Marques EP, Vieira DN. Pesticide intoxications in the centre of Portugal: three years analysis. Forens Sci Int 2004;143(2–3):199–204.

Chapter 5.9

Italy

Carlo Alessandro Locatelli

Toxicology Unit, Pavia Poison Centre and National Toxicology Information Centre, Laboratory of Clinical and Experimental Toxicology, IRCCS Hospital of Pavia, Istituti Clinici Scientifici Maugeri, Pavia, Italy

Origins

It was after World War II that the increased frequency of human exposure to chemicals and drugs in Italy led to the development of clinical toxicology and Poison Information Services/Centers (PICs). Although Prof. Aiazzi-Mancini created a Division of Clinical Toxicology at the Pharmacology Institute of the University of Florence in 1917 (Aiazzi-Mancini, 1921), the development of modern academic toxicology dates to 1955–1970, originally as a part of pharmacology. At that time, the need to optimize the treatment of increasing numbers of poisoned patients in intensive care units (ICUs) became clear (Introna, 1967; Santi, 1970).

The origins of PICs can be dated to 1967, which was the key year for clinical toxicology in Italy. In Pavia, on October 20, 1967, Prof. Mascherpa (Director of the Institute of Pharmacology of the University of Pavia, School of Medicine), Prof. Benzi and Prof. Berté founded both the first post-graduate school for specialist training in toxicology, and the Italian Society of Toxicology (SITOX, formerly SIT). Immediately after this, the first Italian PIC was established in Milan. SITOX was officially recognized by the President of the Republic on May 16, 1972. It promotes scientific and professional aspects of toxicology and is the scientific society for Italian clinical toxicologists, some of them contributing as board members and presidents.

The Italian National Health Service

The Italian National Health Service (NHS) was established in 1978, revised in 1992–1993 and again in 1999. These revisions gave each Italian region more power, autonomy and responsibility for the management of their Regional Health Services (RHS), coordinated and supervised by the central government and the Ministry of Health (MoH) (Marinovich et al., 2020). The MoH is the central

History of Modern Clinical Toxicology. https://doi.org/10.1016/B978-0-12-822218-8.00033-8

body that organizes the NHS and determines its targets. It is supported by scientific and technical organizations and agencies, of which the National Institutes for Care and Scientific Research Hospitals (IRCCS-Istituti di Ricovero e Cura a Carattere Scientifico) are most relevant to PICs and clinical toxicologists. The IRCCS, governed by Law 33 of 2/12/1978, DPR 617/1980 and by Legislative Decree 269/1993, play a major role providing NHS health care. They carry out research and training, and provide technical and operational support to NHS research targets.

The Permanent Conference for Relations between the State and the Regions (Conferenza Permanente Stato-Regioni-Provincie Autonome) is the most important link between the MoH and regional governments, insuring uniformity, and facilitating subsidiary functioning among the 21 Italian RHSs, which serve different populations and therefore have different levels of facilities (Marinovich et al., 2020). The Italian NHS provides uniform publicly financed health care via a core benefit package of health services across the country, called the "Essential Levels of Care" (LEA, Livelli Essenziali di Assistenza), free to all citizens. In 2017 the LEA were updated (Presidency of the Ministry Council Decree, January 12, 2017) to include PIC activities.

When Italian PICs first started, most poison admissions involved neuropsychiatric and anticholinergic drugs (mostly barbiturates), ethanol, carbon monoxide, viper bites, poisonous mushrooms, solvents (e.g., trichloroethylene), drugs of abuse and occupational exposures. This pattern has changed over the years: while in the 1960s–1970s poisoned patients were mainly admitted to ICUs (23%–70% of ICU patients), today only 2% of poisoned patients admitted to the hospital end up in the ICU. In contrast, emergency department (ED) presentations are high and increasing. Acute poisoning (excluding adverse drug reactions) is recorded by the National Information System for Monitoring Emergency Assistance (EMUR). MoH admission data shows it among the main problems causing ED presentations.

Initial PIC development

The Italian PICs (*Centri Antiveleni*—the Italian term that emphasizes the "counteraction" of poisons) originated in a variety of clinical departments, including the ICU, ED, and pediatric wards, with considerable heterogeneity in structure and organization. The first medical services that developed a PIC were in Milan (Prof. Bozza-Marrubini, Niguarda Hospital, 1967) and Rome (Prof. Magalini, Gemelli Hospital, 1971; Prof. Malizia, Umberto I Hospital, 1972). They were located in ICUs to which poisoned patients were frequently admitted and treated, and started to provide information on the diagnosis and treatment of poisoned patients to other hospitals, general practitioners, and citizens (De Francisci et al., 1977; Bozza-Marubini, 1978). A few physicians (mostly anesthesiologists) were commissioned to initiate PIC activities (e.g., Dr. Ghezzi in Milan), assisted in on-call by colleagues working in ICUs.

Between the 1970s and 1990s, other PICs opened in Italy, starting their service with the collaboration of medical personnel operating in different clinical units:

- Naples and Bologna (in EDs)
- Genoa, Turin, La Spezia, Palermo, Catania, Lecce, Pordenone, Cesena, Chieti, Reggio Calabria (in ICUs)
- Genoa and Trieste (in pediatric hospital EDs)
- Padua (in a university department of pharmacology)
- Pavia (in the clinical unit and PIC activities of an IRCCS Hospital)
- Florence (in the Division of Clinical Toxicology alongside clinical activities)

As in other countries, all PICs had the same basic activities (poisons advice), but differed in other characteristics. Several PICs were born as a marginal activity within clinical units devoted to other priorities. These were not really PICs but hospital inpatient units in which a physician dealt specifically with poisoned patients. Only seven services had characteristics corresponding to those of a PIC, and a progressive reduction of the smallest services occurred.

Toxicological information available in the first PICs was very limited, including data on a few hundreds of potentially toxic substances and commercial products. Thanks to the collaboration with industry, as no legal obligations to provide data then existed in Italy, the databases in some PICs improved, with data collection, verification, and storage carried out independently in each service.

In the 1970s, another important development was Prof. Montagna's establishment of the first 24-h laboratory service for toxicological emergencies. This laboratory (IRCCS Policlinico S. Matteo, Pavia) remains the national reference for most urgent toxicological analyses. At the same time, another laboratory, initially structured for environmental toxicological analyses (ICS Maugeri IRCCS Hospital, Pavia), was equipped and accredited for the detection of environmental xenobiotics in biological matrices in poisoned and occupationally exposed patients.

Following European Resolution (90/C 329/03 CEE), WHO-IPCS guidelines (WHO-IPICS, 1997), and scientific society documentation on quality and standards for accreditation (Persson and Tempowski, 2004) published in the 1990s, Italian PICs improved their performance, function, and organization. Nevertheless, there was no clear funding system, still an issue today. Despite these problems, PICs continued to provide information, refer cases to outpatient facilities, and treat patients in clinical toxicology units (Florence, Pavia). All calls were recorded on paper by PICs in the 1990s and some RHSs began to accredit their PICs (e.g., Naples, Rome, Florence), but in a diverse way.

Government recognition of Italian PICs

After 2000, the need to improve and consolidate PIC activities into the NHS/RHS was obvious if they were to fulfill public health roles (e.g., homeland security). Five crucial steps led to the legal recognition of PICs in the Italian NHS/RHSs:

1. In 1999–2000 the Istituto Superiore di Sanità (ISS, scientific/technical agency of the MoH) asked that PICs be accredited for the operational access (24 h daily) to the "Dangerous Preparation Archive," a national database created to meet the requirements of European Directives 88/379/EEC and 1999/45/EC (now included in CLP Regulations, 2008). As this includes data on hazardous commercial products, it was no longer necessary for each PIC to collate its own proprietary database. PIC accreditation was necessary to ensure both 24-h daily access to confidential data on compositions and to ensure necessary clinical-toxicological skills. Accreditation of PICs for "quality and confidentiality criteria" for access to this database was included in Italian legislation (MoH Decree April 19th, 2000, and Legislative Decree N. 65, March 14th, 2003). From 2002 the Department of Civil Protection-Presidency of the Council of Ministers has given the Pavia PIC national responsibility for planning and operation of a toxicological terrorism response.

2. In September 2004, SITOX asked the MoH to recognize PIC activities in the NHS. After 20 days, this suggestion was accepted; the MoH established it was necessary to create a network for the "prediction, surveillance and rapid alert, control and coordinated management of events" to provide timely indications on possible natural or deliberate epidemic events and acute diseases with a high impact on public health. This involved PICs and other emergency services. A national commission (MoH, RHSs, SITOX-PICs; and some officials) started to work on these specific tasks.

3. After this, the MoH activated a "poisoning surveillance network" through PICs into the National Health Plan 2006–2008, with identification of toxicological syndromes and notification of consequent alerts. This was first tested during the 2006 Winter Olympiad in Turin, the first Olympic event subject to toxicological surveillance. The surveillance was activated in three PICs in Lombardy (Bergamo, Milan, Pavia), in collaboration with an office for statistical evaluation in Piedmont (Epidemiological Consultation Team et al., 2006).

4. Spurred by requests made by Dr. Locatelli (SITOX Vice-President in 2006), the MoH established a program to recognize the role of PICs in the NHS and to integrate these activities into the "Essential Levels of Care" (LEA). Dr. Vellucci (MoH), Dr. Fanuzzi (RHSs), Dr. Locatelli (SITOX-PICs), and officials worked to complete the "Italian State-Regions agreement regarding the definition of activities and the fundamental functions, roles, and requirements for PICs in Italy." Published in 2008 by the Italian Conference

Box 5.9.1 Summary of activities/functions of PICs required in Italy by Legal Act (Accordo Stato-Regioni 56/CSR, February 28, 2008).

- Provide specialist consultation to health professionals for the management of patients with any toxicological problem
- Guarantee availability of specialist consultation to the population to help manage poisoned patients
- Ensure availability of consultation to hospital units
- Improve availability of analytical–toxicological testing
- Implement and update toxicological databases
- Conduct epidemiological evaluation of intoxications
- Conduct joint surveillance activities with the MoH, Regional Governments, and others
- Monitor the availability and use of antidotes in the NHS
- Supply toxicological expertise in the management of chemical emergencies
- Support Civil Protection and Defense
- Contribute in the preparation of emergency plans for chemical risks
- Provide toxicological collaboration with and consultation to the NHS
- Support education and training in clinical toxicology for NHS health professionals
- Conduct poisoning prevention educational activities
- Conduct research activities on poisonings
- Maintain and improve a national network, integrated with both EDs and prevention departments
- Interface with other European PICs

between the Central and the Regional Governments (Accordo Stato-Regioni 56/CSR, February 28, 2008) (Locatelli, 2009), this requires PICs to perform 17 functions and activities in the NHS/RHSs (Box 5.9.1). This Act emphasizes the roles and functions of PICs:

- PICs are autonomous services recognized through an accreditation process that must comply with requested functions 24 h daily.
- Their medical-specialist activity is exclusive and essential in the NHS, and is not expertly addressed by other existing medical services.
- Toxicological advice on clinical care must be provided by physicians with specialization in clinical toxicology.

Technical details of the Act included the minimum dataset established to facilitate PIC data sharing, and syndromes for inclusion in the national surveillance system, using a tentative system of coding signs/symptoms/diagnosis of poisoning in ICD-9/ICD-10.

Three major benefits were expected by NHS/RHSs: (1) better management and appropriate care of poisoned patients; (2) reduction of improper access to EDs, unnecessary hospital admissions and inappropriate diagnostic investigations; (3) specialized support to governmental agencies in the management of chemical and toxicological emergencies, and in surveillance and poisoning prevention.

5. The last, very important step, stimulated by the SITOX President (Dr. Locatelli) in 2013 was the Decree of the President of the Council of Ministers (Definition and consequent updating of the essential assistance levels—Livelli essenziali di Assistenza-LEA, January 12, 2017) that stated PICs activities were indispensable in the NHS.

These milestones resulted in rapid development and regulatory compliance of PICs, to respond effectively to emergency calls and increasing requests for documentation and epidemiological data from national and international agencies and organizations. Although some initial approaches to computerized call recording had already been implemented, it was only after 2000 that PICs developed electronic recording of calls, although in different ways in each PIC.

Present status

Despite legal recognition of the functions and importance of PICs in the NHS (Accordo Stato-Regioni 56/CSR/2008) by the Presidency of the Ministry Council Decree, January 12, 2017 (LEA, 2017) and the certification of specialists in clinical toxicology, there are still some organizational and administrative aspects that need improvement in some PICs to insure optimal functioning.

Differences among PICs and their staff

Italian PICs potentially serve 60.5 million people without geographical or RHS limitation: every PIC can be called from anywhere in Italy. This allows the more effective services to substitute for those that are less efficient, busy, or in difficulty, but there is no single telephone number that covers the country.

PIC telephone advice is provided by physicians (helped by nurses in some PICs with limited activity). Since 2008, Italian law has strongly recommended that PIC physicians should preferably be specialists in clinical toxicology.

Although PICs need to fulfill the 17 functions listed in Box 5.9.1, this has not yet been universally achieved. Nine PICs in Italy are recognized by the MoH: Bergamo, Milan, Pavia, Florence, Rome (three PICs in Umberto I, Gemelli and Pediatrico Bambino Gesù [OPBG] Hospitals), Naples, Foggia (Table 5.9.1). To date, only four (Bergamo, Florence, Milan, and Pavia) are organized as autonomous services with a dedicated trained staff of full-time physicians specialized in medical/clinical toxicology available 24 h daily. The remaining PICs have insufficient toxicology-specialized medical staff to cover all shifts, and must resort to the use of nursing staff, graduates in other disciplines (e.g., biologists), or nontoxicologist physicians simultaneously carrying out other activities in their clinical units (e.g., ICU) to answer calls.

All Italian PIC physicians are involved in direct clinical care and remote consultancy for the diagnosis and treatment of poisoning, including veterinary poison information. Some PICs have other specific core activities: the PIC in Rome, OPBG works exclusively on pediatric toxicology; Bergamo and Florence are mostly involved in the Teratology Information Service (TIS); Pavia is commissioned by government departments for chemical, biological, radiation, or nuclear (CBRN) events and major chemical accidents, industrial and environmental toxicology, novel psychoactive substances (National Early Warning System), and management of the national antidote stockpile. This development of specific skills has been a powerful driving force in stimulating the scientific and operative interests of PIC physicians.

Italian PICs answer approximately 200,000 information requests annually, all of which are audio-recorded. As not all the PICs are operational 24h daily with a dedicated staff, and some stop activity during night and holiday shifts, the consultations in 2019 varied from 2000 for the smallest and youngest services, up to more than 65,000 and 85,000 for Milan and Pavia, respectively. Except for Pavia for which 85% of calls come from hospital departments, most inquiries to other PICs are from the general public. Peer review of calls and complete follow-up of cases represent a further workload, and are currently only done in well-structured PICs.

All the PICs collaborate with the MoH and national agencies in epidemiological surveys, allowing identification of products that have safety problems and unexpected effects of drugs and chemicals.

Clinical units

Some PICs lack a specialist clinical unit; they refer patients to other clinical departments. This is a problem that needs to be solved, as ideally, in a modern and "needs adapted" NHS, severely poisoned patients with rare poisons should be treated by specialists in the discipline.

Clinical toxicology laboratories (ToxLabs)

Research ToxLabs are present in some university and/or IRCCS hospitals (Florence, Pavia), whereas clinical ToxLabs are present only in the Pavia PIC. Pavia also hosts the national reference clinical toxicology laboratory (Foundation IRCCS Policlinico San Matteo) linked to the PIC. It can perform most analytical tests required for urgent diagnosis of poisoned patients and management of toxicological emergencies. The lack of a country-wide network of clinical toxicology laboratories is partially off-set by rapid transport to the Pavia laboratories and by use of local forensic laboratories.

TABLE 5.9.1 Activities and main structural/personnel characteristics of PICs recognized by the Italian Ministry of Health.

PIC (region, year of origin)	MDs dedicated full-time to PIC	MDs collaborating part-time and/or from other units	MD residents	MD fellows
			Staff number	
Bergamo (Lombardy, 1999)	5	2	–	–
Milan (Lombardy, 1967)	9	4	1	4
Pavia[a] (Lombardy, 1992)	7	–	3	–
Florence (Tuscany, 1990)	7	–	11	–
Rome Umberto I[c] (Lazio, 1972)	7	–	4	
Rome Gemelli[c] (Lazio, 1971)	2	6		
Rome Bambino Gesù[c] (Lazio, 2012)	1	5 MD	N.A.	1
Naples[c] (Campania, 1975)	1	7	N.A.	N.A.
Foggia[c] (Puglia, 2005)	4	–	N.A.	N.A.

[a] Formalized assignments for special tasks (National Early Warning System for New Psychoactive Substances, chemical terrorism and major toxicological emergencies, National Antidotes Stockpile) by Italian Government/Agencies (Presidency of the Council of Ministers; Ministry of Health).
[b] Staff dedicated to Laboratories (clinical and research).
[c] These PICs are a part of other hospital units (all ICUs).
2019 data, with rounding of calls to the nearest.
Data provided by each PIC in July 2020 (personal communication).
Data refer to PIC consultancies, excluding hospital inpatient consulting and outpatient visits.
IRCSS, Scientific Institute for Research, Hospitalization and Healthcare; TIS, Teratology Information Service; Y, yes; N, no; N.A., not available; U, University Hospital.

Non-MD staff dedicated full-time to PIC	No. of calls			PIC characteristics		
	PIC toxicological consultancies (% from public)	TIS calls	Autonomous service	IRCCS and/or University Hospital (U)	Toxicology laboratory of PIC (Staff)	
1 nurse 1 Biologist 1 secretary	10,000	41,000	Y	N	N	
1 biologist 2 pharmacists 1 IT technician 1 secretary	67,000 (50%)	N.A.	Y	N	N	
4 pharmacists 1 IT technician 2 secretaries	84,000 (15%)	1000	Y	IRCCS/U	Y (4 biologists 1 chemist 1 Lab technician)[b]	
1 nurse	6000 (33%)	10,000	Y	U	N	
1 secretary	6500	450	Y	U	N	
1 Biologist	6000 (70%)	N.A.	N[c]	U	N	
–	1500	N.A.	N[c]	IRCCS	N	
5 nurses	3300	N.A.	N[c]	N	N	
5 nurses 1 pharmacist	3000 (66%)	3000	N[c]	U	N	

Networking

Italian PICs operate separate information systems. A single national telephone number has never been used in Italy. The main reasons are as follows: (1) different RHSs in which the PICs operate have different accreditation and quality assurance rules: only one Italian PIC is certified ISO 9001:2015 (2) variability in operations and activities in each service (e.g., exclusive pediatric activity, CBRN-related responsibility), (3) funding level, and (4) different workloads.

Data collection

Each PIC stores all inquiries on a proprietary database developed according to local needs (e.g. research). There is no national report of Italian PICs activities: the last data collection was published in 2006 (Mucci et al., 2006), although cumulative data on specific problems have been provided to authorities on several occasions (e.g., poisonings due to dangerous chemicals) (Draisci et al., 2018).

Antidotes and rare drug availability

The majority of PICs have a stockpile of some antidotes in amounts adequate for the treatment of a few patients. Pavia PIC stocks all antidotes in high quantities together with drugs for nontoxicological diseases (e.g., rabies immunoglobulins and diphtheria antitoxin), and some orphan drugs that may be lacking in Italy (Locatelli et al., 2006). Specific procedures are available for rapid countrywide mobilization. Since 2004, a series of national surveys in EDs, ICUs and hospital pharmacies has enabled construction of a National Database of Antidote Availability regularly updated online on the Pavia PIC website and freely accessible by all Italian hospitals (Anonymous, 2020). The Pavia PIC is also designated by the MoH to provide specialist advice in case of terrorist events and to develop, manage and maintain the National Antidote Stockpile (Civil Defense) for CBRN and major toxicological emergencies.

Teaching and research activities

Some PICs (Pavia, Florence, and the 3 PICs in Rome) operate in university hospitals and/or in IRCCS (Pavia and Rome Bambino Gesù). The latter two are required to carry out research activities in the field of clinical toxicology on projects that are promoted by national agencies and the EU. Teaching is regularly performed in university-linked PICs, and a variety of teaching activities are regularly organized locally by all PICs.

Education for clinical toxicologists: A degree of medical specialty in clinical toxicology

Clinical toxicology has expanded since the 1970s and has become an independent discipline in the past two decades (Wax et al., 2000). While specific educational programs in clinical toxicology have been established internationally, a specific qualification in clinical/medical toxicology, overseen by a university, scientific society, or official medical organization is not available in many European Union (EU) countries. In Italy a specific 4-year full-time postgraduate educational program, regulated by the laws of the Ministry of University, Education and Scientific Research had led the EU to recognize the title of "specialist in clinical/medical toxicology." In Italy, clinical toxicology is an obligatory part of the pharmacology course within the undergraduate curriculum in medicine and surgery (Manzo, 2006).

At its inception in 1967 in Pavia, the specialty in clinical toxicology developed with a 3-year postgraduate course. Courses have spread to approximately 15 universities. Between 1980 and 2014 the specialty course's name varied, sometimes being known as "medical toxicology"; its duration was 3–4 years. Since 2015, the specialty course of "pharmacology and clinical toxicology" has been 4 years. Eight schools are active today in Italian universities, with Pavia, Florence, and Rome Umberto I being only for physicians, as they have local PICs as operational headquarters, while those in other locations also admit pharmacists.

Specialist training covers the entire field of clinical toxicology, including acute and chronic intoxications, drug addiction, effects of workplace chemical exposure, and chemical emergencies. It includes basic and preclinical toxicology and pharmacology, carcinogenesis, teratology, environmental toxicology, regulatory toxicology, the conduct of clinical studies, and research. Physicians who train in schools with associated PICs are obliged to train in these, and may have other opportunities. For example, those who attend the Pavia and Florence schools also have the opportunity for professional internships in other hospitals/ services/units (e.g., adult and pediatric EDs, ICUs, dialysis units, and addiction services) both in Italy and abroad.

Training in clinical toxicology is quite widespread in Italy, with increasing numbers of physicians and pharmacists becoming specialists in the discipline. In addition, PhD programs (3–4 years in length), research fellowships (2–4 years), and training courses in clinical toxicology, supported by SITOX and with other scientific societies, are also available to physicians working in EDs and ICUs, as well as to pediatricians and psychiatrists.

Role of SITOX

The Italian Society of Toxicology (SITOX) has had a key role in putting requests to the MoH and participating in MoH commissions on the legal recognition of PIC activities. SITOX also organizes courses, meetings, congresses (the MoH continuing medical education program), and study groups for PICs. It sponsors the *Emergency Care Journal* (the reference *Italian Journal for Clinical Toxicologists*), and, in collaboration with other scientific societies and academic bodies, develops guidelines and operational procedures.

Challenges

The workload of some Italian PICs is greater than that of others. Calls may be in a queue at busy times and the standard of service may suffer. Advice given to inquirers by PICs is not uniform, which is related to local expertise and the experience and specialization of physicians in different centers.

Three things are needed to address these issues: (1) adaptation to the regulations established by Italian legislation, (2) sufficient resources to allow change, and (3) a central (MoH) observatory that quality-assures the system. This may also impact the national system for the accreditation of clinical toxicologists, the qualification required for full-time physicians in PICs, and agreements on core functions and roles of PICs at national and regional levels.

Funding is currently adequate only for PICs operating in public hospitals, where the staff budget is supported by the NHS/RHS. It is insufficient in those operating in private hospitals, where personnel costs are not reimbursed by the NHS/RHS. Despite these differences, PICs do the same job of providing public health services in the emergency system.

Conclusions

Italian PICs developed in three phases (1967, 2008, and 2017) and are established in a clear legal framework. Although the service performs important functions supported by evidence of health benefits and of cost-effectiveness, full accreditation of all centers has not yet been completed. PICs are now a key component of public health services, performing specific functions not performed by other parts of the Italian NHS. They are seen as one of the most efficient NHS services.

Clinical toxicologists now have specific accredited skills supported by specialist postgraduate schools and the SITOX continuing education program. Although there are only a small number of specialists, no other public health services in Italy allow 24-h daily direct access to this level of expertise across a range of medical emergencies nationally. The Italian model is a good example of how PICs can be integrated into a national framework; it may serve as a useful example for others.

References

Aiazzi-Mancini M. Clinical-toxicological statistics collected in Florence in the triennium 1917-1918-1919. Giorn Clin Med 1921;1:25–30.

Anonymous. Banca dati nazionale degli Antidoti, http://www-9.unipv.it/reumatologia-tossicologia/cav/CAV/index.php; 2020. [Accessed 7 April 2021].

Bozza-Marubini M. Current therapeutic aspects in toxicology. Brux Med 1978;12:621–35.

De Francisci G, Addario C, De Giacomo M, Magalini SI. Epidemiological study of acute poisoning assisted by the anti-poison centre in the A Gemelli hospital. Acta Pharmacol Toxicol (Copenh) 1977;41(Suppl 2):522–7.

Draisci R, Giordano F, Malaguti Aliberti L, Rubbiani M, Marano M, et al. Esposizione a sostanze e miscele pericolose: risultati preliminari del progetto pilota multicentrico basato su dati provenienti da Centri Antiveleni. Notiz Istit Super Sanità 2018;31(11):13–8.

Epidemiological Consultation Team, Demicheli V, Raso R, Tiberti D, Barale A, Ferrara L, Lombardi D, et al. Results from the Integrated Surveillance System for the 2006 Winter Olympic and Paralympic Games in Italy. Euro Surveill 2006;11(8):E060817.5.

Introna F. On the necessity for a campaign against poisonings according to the operational directives of the centers for social diseases (regulation of 11 February 1961, no. 249). Minerva Med 1967;58(63):2789–95.

LEA 2017. http://www.salute.gov.it/portale/lea/menuContenutoLea.jsp?lingua=italiano&area=Lea &menu=leaEssn.

Locatelli CA. National integration of poison control centres: the Italian experience. Clin Toxicol 2009;47(suppl):464–5.

Locatelli C, Petrolini V, Lonati D, Butera R, Bove A, Mela L, et al. Antidotes availability in emergency departments of the Italian National Health System and development of a national databank on antidotes. Ann Ist Super Sanita 2006;42(3):298–309.

Manzo L. Medical toxicology - regulations, quality of care and licensing practitioners across Europe. Clin Toxicol 2006;44(suppl):437–8.

Marinovich M, Della Seta M, Locatelli CA, Attias L, Rubbiani M, Marcello I. Italy. In: Wexler P, Gilbert SG, Mohapatra A, Bobst S, Hayes A, Humes ST, editors. Information Resources in Toxicology. Volume 2: The Global Arena. 5th ed. London: Academic Press, Elsevier; 2020. p. 265–88.

Mucci N, Alessi M, Binetti R, Magliocchi MG. Profile of acute poisoning in Italy. Analysis of the data reported by poison Centres. Ann Ist Super Sanita 2006;42(3):268–76.

Persson H, Tempowski J. Developing and maintaining quality in poisons information centers. Toxicology 2004;198(1–3):263–6.

Santi R. Poison control centers: considerations and perspectives. Acta Anaesthesiol 1970;21(1):115–9.

Wax PM, Ford MD, Bond GR, Kilbourne EM, Walter FG, Avery AN, et al. The core content of medical toxicology. Ann Emerg Med 2000;43:209–14.

WHO-IPICS. Guidelines for poison control. Geneva: World Health Organization; 1997.

Chapter 5.10

Switzerland

Hugo Kupferschmidt

Poisons Centre, Charité-Universitätsmedizin Berlin, Berlin, Germany

Origins

Tox Info Suisse, originally the Swiss Toxicological Information Center, was established in 1962 by the Swiss Society of Pharmacists (today *pharmaSuisse*) in cooperation with the University of Zurich as the national poisons information center for Switzerland (Anon. 2020). To secure funding for the service, a foundation was created in 1965. By the end of March in 1966, the service started with availability 24 h daily. Some 1923 calls were answered in that first year (Fig. 5.10.1). An opening ceremony took place in May 1966.

With an increasing number of inquiries to the service, additional funding was necessary and was found in the contribution of the Swiss Society of Chemical Industry (SGCI, today "scienceindustries") as a co-founder of the organization. Ten different organizations together established a foundation and subsequently have contributed to the funding of Tox Info Suisse during the more than 50 years it has existed (Table 5.10.1). To be able to maintain its activities, Tox Info Suisse also depends on donations from private individuals, companies, and organizations.

Presidents of the Foundation were Attilio Nisoli (1967–1989), Franz Merki (1989–2011), and Elisabeth Anderegg-Wirth (since 2012). Medical Directors of the poisons information service were Franz Borbély (1967–1974), Josef Velvart (1974–1989), Peter Meier-Abt (1989–2003), and Hugo Kupferschmidt (2004–2021). Administrative Directors were Hans Peter Jaspersen (1967–1983), Jean-Pierre Lorent (1983–2003), and Hugo Kupferschmidt (2004–2021).

From its beginning, Tox Info Suisse has been located in Zurich, the largest city in Switzerland. Initially, it was housed by the Institute of Legal Medicine of the University of Zurich. Since that time, the center has moved twice because of increasing demand: in 1976, half a mile from its original location and again in 1999, to its current location, to be close to the University and University Hospital of Zurich for strategic reasons. On the occasion of the celebration of its 50th year of existence in 2016, it changed its name from the original *Swiss Toxicological Information Center* (STIC) to the more convenient *Tox Info Suisse*.

History of Modern Clinical Toxicology. https://doi.org/10.1016/B978-0-12-822218-8.00013-2

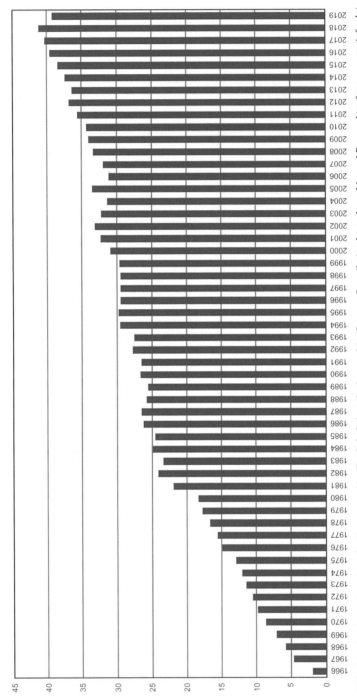

FIG. 5.10.1 Annual number of calls answered by Tox Info Suisse (in thousands). (*Source: Compilation by author of Annual Report data from www.toxinfo.ch.*)

TABLE 5.10.1 Organizations contributing to the funding of Tox Info Suisse.

- pharmaSuisse (formerly Swiss Society of Pharmacists)
- scienceindustries (formerly Swiss Society of Chemical Industry SGCI)
- Cantons (Swiss Conference of Cantonal Directors of Public Health, GDK)
- Swiss Federal Office of Public Health (FOPH)
- Swissmedic (Swiss Agency of Therapeutic Products)
- santésuisse (for the Swiss health insurance companies)
- Association of public and private hospitals (H+)
- Swiss National Accident Insurance Fund (SUVA)
- Swiss Insurance Association (SVV) (until 2010)
- Swiss Medical Association (FMH) or the Conference of the Cantonal Medical Associations (KKA)

Organization

Tox Info Suisse has always been the only poisons information center for Switzerland and the Principality of Liechtenstein, covering a population of approximately 8.6 million. It takes inquiries 24 h daily from members of the public, as well as from medical professionals and organizations, covering mostly acute human toxic exposures and some animal inquiries. In recent years, call numbers have been in the region of 40,000 per annum. In 2019, 36,340 calls were related to exposures (34,843 human; 1497 veterinary), while 2869 calls were asking for advice on poison prevention.

As a foundation, Tox Info Suisse is a stand-alone institution, having its own organization and budget. It is managed by its medical and administrative director(s) and is supervised by the foundation council composed by representatives of the supporting bodies. The foundation council meets twice per year.

The service is funded by public (governmental) sources as well as by private or semi-private organizations (Tox Info Suisse Annual Report, 2020), partly in the form of noncontractual annual contributions (pharmaSuisse, scienceindustries, santésuisse, SUVA, KKA) and partly as compensation for services delivered based on service level agreements (Cantons, FOPH, H+, Swissmedic). The latter have become more important during the past 15 years, while the former tend to increasingly taper. Veterinarians pay individually for their calls, as no organization is willing to cover the cost of this service.

Since November 2003, Tox Info Suisse has used the national emergency (albeit not entirely toll-free) phone number 145 for its calls. For calls from outside Switzerland/Liechtenstein, the standard phone number +41 44,251 51 51 is used.

Daily operations

During office hours, calls are triaged into medical or administrative services, according to the degree of clinical urgency, by specially trained non-medical personnel, with routing of all calls to an appropriate specialist. During office hours, medical calls are normally answered by physicians and public calls by pharmacists or nurses. During out-of-office hours, the calls are taken directly by physicians. A specific feature of the service is that there is no waiting time for callers; every call is taken immediately, irrespective of whether other calls are being answered concurrently. At all times, a senior officer (clinical toxicologist) is either in-house or on-call. The senior officers supervise the service and discuss difficult cases; they also, if necessary, take calls at peak times. In addition, these senior officers check and sign-off call reports which are then sent to the physicians who called the service. The purpose of these reports is to provide a document to the inquirer, and to ask for a medical follow-up of the cases. Approximately 70% of physicians respond and return clinical follow-ups. Since 1995, both call documentation and follow-up information is recorded in an in-house database and information system specifically developed and maintained by Tox Info Suisse (older information is still available in a paper database with some of the data having been digitalized). This information system not only contains case data but also product data and specific information on agents. Thus this database, in addition to online sources such as Poisindex, is an important source of information for poisons information. Based on its status as an associated institute of the University, Tox Info Suisse has online access to medical literature via the library of the University of Zurich.

Other Tox Info Suisse services

Tox Info Suisse serves the Swiss Federal Office of Public Health (FOPH) as the official poisons center under a service level agreement based on the Swiss federal law on chemicals. As such it is legally granted full access to the FOPH Register of Chemical Products (RPC), including information on product composition. In Switzerland and Liechtenstein, Material Safety Data Sheets (MSDS) carry the Tox Info Suisse emergency phone number in case of medical incidents with the products. For MSDS circulating internationally, companies can use this service on a contractual basis. Similarly, Tox Info Suisse provides 24-h emergency consultation for the transportation of hazardous goods outside Switzerland for a small fee. In that case, after an advance agreement is signed, its emergency phone number is printed on the transportation documents. For many years, Tox Info Suisse has offered out-of-office hours telephone coverage for pharmaceutical companies on a contractual basis.

Tox Info Suisse provides a number of additional services closely related to poisons information: senior medical staff carry out clinical consults at the University Hospital Zurich under an agreement with its Department of Clinical Pharmacology and Toxicology. Tox Info Suisse contributes case notifications to the national pharmacovigilance system and provides toxicovigilance reports to authorities and manufacturers. In addition, there is a pill identification system (identipharm) in place, which also includes older medications no longer marketed.

Antidotes

Since its beginnings, Tox Info Suisse has cooperated with hospital pharmacies to guarantee the antidote supply in Switzerland. Initially, this was an initiative of the center, but after the 1980s, this has been an official function under a mandate of the Swiss Conference of Cantonal Directors of Public Health. The important work is carried out by a working group staffed by delegates of the Swiss Association of Public Health Administration and Hospital Pharmacists (GSASA), the Swiss Army Pharmacy, and Tox Info Suisse. Its work results in the publication of the *Swiss Antidote List* in the Bulletin of the FOPH and online (www.antidota.ch).

Staffing and professionalism

Poisons information at Tox Info Suisse is largely provided by physicians. They are supported by a professional staff (nurses and pharmacists) and a veterinarian in answering public calls during peak-times. Senior officers are all physicians. Tox Info Suisse is accredited by the Swiss Society of Clinical Pharmacology and Toxicology (www.clinpharm.ch) as a site for postgraduate training for physicians in the specialty of clinical pharmacology and toxicology (category B, i.e., only for the toxicology part of the training program). At the beginning of their employment, prior to be included in the general poisons information schedule, all staff undergo a specific training program for several months. After having worked several years as a poisons information specialist, members of the staff can obtain a certificate as a Poisons Information Specialist issued by the Association of German Speaking Poisons Information Centers (Gesellschaft für klinische Toxikologie e.V., GfKT, https://www.klinitox.de/3.0.html).

For clinical issues and pharmacovigilance, Tox Info Suisse closely collaborates with the Department of Clinical Pharmacology of the University Hospital of Zurich which is in close walking distance; its Institute of Clinical Chemistry serves as the analytical laboratory. Until 2020 the director of Tox Info Suisse served as a clinical consultant in the University Hospital in the departments of Clinical Pharmacology and Toxicology in internal medicine, intensive care, and emergency medicine.

Research and scholarly activities

Tox Info Suisse is engaged in research and education as an associated institute at the University of Zurich Faculty of Medicine. All of these activities are under the responsibility of the head of the Tox Info Suisse Department of Science. The focus of the clinical toxicology research group at Tox Info Suisse includes (1) investigating the acute toxicity of xenobiotics, (2) describing the clinical effects in specific types of poisoning, (3) investigating the dose–effect relationship and the epidemiology of acute human poisoning. The faculty members at Tox Info Suisse offer and supervise master's degree level theses for medical and pharmacy students, and M.D. level theses.

Faculty members at Tox Info Suisse have active research collaborations with many national university and regional hospitals, and with national and international academic institutions including the Institute of Pharmaceutical Sciences at the Federal Institute of Technology (ETH) Zurich.

The professional network of Tox Info Suisse extends to the cantonal laboratories for analytical issues and to the Spiez Laboratory and the Federal Office for Civil Protection in the field of chemical, biological, radiation, and nuclear (CBRN) threats. Senior staff are instructors of the Advanced Hazmat Life Support (AHLS) courses held annually in German and English. Tox Info Suisse is represented in the Foundation Council of the Swiss Center for Applied Human Toxicology (SCAHT www.scaht.org), which is supported by the Swiss Confederation and the Universities of Basel, Geneva and Lausanne.

International ties

Strong professional ties exist internationally to the European Association of Poisons Centres and Clinical Toxicologists (EAPCCT), the American Academy of Clinical Toxicology (AACT), and the Association of the Poisons Information Centers in Germany, Austria, and Switzerland [Gesellschaft fur klinische Toxikologie (GfKT)], all of which hold an annual scientific meeting.

Challenges

After more than 50 years of successful funding by the public and the private sector in Switzerland, the conception that poison information is a responsibility of public health becomes increasingly evident. Thus, in the years to come, the challenge will be to replace the decreasing contributions of the private sector by increasing funding by the cantons and the federation.

References

Tox Info Suisse short portrait. https://toxinfo.ch/portrait_en (accessed Oct 30, 2020).

Tox Info Suisse annual reports: 2001–2020. https://www.toxinfo.ch/jahresberichte-neu_en (accessed Oct 28 2020).

Swiss Society of Clinical Pharmacology and Toxicology (SSCPT). www.clinpharm.ch (accessed Oct 29 2020).

Gesellschaft für Klinische Toxikologie e.V. (GfKT). https://www.klinitox.de/3.0.html (accessed Oct 28 2020).

University of Zurich Faculty of Medicine. https://www.med.uzh.ch/en.html (accessed June 15 2021).

University Hospital Zurich. www.en.usz.ch (accessed Oct 28 2020).

Swiss Centre for Applied Human Toxicology. www.scaht.org (accessed Oct 28 2020).

Chapter 5.11

Scandinavia

Lotte C.G. Hoegberg

Department of Anesthesiology and The Danish Poisons Information Centre, Copenhagen University Hospital Bispebjerg, Copenhagen, Denmark

Introduction

Clinical toxicology in Scandinavia has a strong history and dates back to 1961 where Clemmesen and Nilsson focused on poisonings in their presentation of the "Scandinavian method" of treating barbiturate poisoning (Clemmesen and Nilsson, 1961). Their basic principle—supportive care—continues to be a key factor in present day management of all poisoned patients (Graudins, 2019). Today, each of the Scandinavian countries has a national poisons information center, but they are closely connected in the Nordic Association of Poisons Centers (NAPC). The NAPC counts Denmark, Norway, Sweden, Finland, Iceland, Estonia, and Lithuania. This chapter focuses on the first four countries. The NAPC gathers for an annual meeting in one of the membership countries for a 3-day conference that includes academic presentations within research and educational topics, everyday poisons center operation developments and challenges as well as field work.

Denmark

Origins

The current Danish Poisons Information Center (DPIC) was established in 2006 at the Copenhagen University Hospital Bispebjerg. Back then, the Ministry of Health supported the need of a formal national poisons information center, and its establishment was prioritized with governmental financial support. It was established as a collaboration of three hospital departments: the Department of Anesthesiology, the Department of Clinical Pharmacology, and the Department of Occupational and Environmental Medicine. The DPIC serves Denmark and two Danish independent territories: Greenland and the Faroe Islands, and the service is available to the public and to health care services. The key concepts are: to provide risk assessment and treatment guidelines; to conduct research within medical and clinical toxicology; to provide education of health care staff; and to pursue prevention measures within all topics of clinical and medical toxicology.

History of Modern Clinical Toxicology. https://doi.org/10.1016/B978-0-12-822218-8.00014-4

Before the current DPIC was established, a poisons information service had been established in 1972 in the Department of Occupational Medicine. It only took calls from health care staff related to chemical exposure, both industrial and from household products (Fogh, 1994). Advice on pharmaceutical poisonings and those involving substances of abuse was provided by Steno Pharmacy, a large 24-h public pharmacy situated in central Copenhagen. In the few years before the establishment of DPIC, pharmaceutical poisonings were evaluated by a collaboration between the Departments of Anesthesiology and Clinical Phamacology.

Organization

The basic structure of DPIC has essentially remained unchanged since its establishment. The service is accessible 24-h daily. Incoming calls are received by specially trained nurses. They are supported by physicians specialized in anesthesiology, clinical pharmacology or occupational medicine, or a pharmacist, all with medical/clinical toxicology expertise, who are on-call for severe poisoning or challenging situations. The service is managed by a senior physician from each of the departments of anesthesiology, clinical pharmacology, and occupational medicine and a senior nurse. The political and economic aspects of the service are managed by the chief physicians from each of the departments of anesthesiology, clinical pharmacology and occupational medicine and a senior nurse.

Daily operations

The DPIC provides advice to both the public and to health care staff. There are two telephone numbers, one for the public and one reserved for health care staff. Calls entering the health care staff line are prioritized to the public line if there are several calls creating a queue. Acute and chronic poisonings are triaged based on the same algorithm. Risk assessments are in-house treatment guidelines based on the international literature and toxicological database information from the Swedish poisons information center, and database information from the US. Treatment advice to the public differs from that for health care staff, depending on the nature of the xenobiotic. The in-house treatment guidelines are divided in two types—action cards, which are short 1-page information materials, primarily for an initial risk assessment by the nurses receiving the primary call. The action cards cover all topics, including medication overdoses, medication errors, chemicals, toxins of biological origin, and drugs of abuse. The second type of guidance consists of detailed monographs covering advanced treatment modalities and antidotes. The guidelines are prepared by the academic staff (physicians and pharmacist) at the DPIC.

Another of the functions of DPIC is to provide health advice to reduce the risk from accidental overdose and poisoning. This poisoning prevention advice includes reducing the risk of medication errors; poison prevention by the safe storage of both prescription and over-the-counter medicines such as paracetamol or antihistamines; information about strong household chemicals such as drain cleaners; and warnings on wild mushrooms, wild plants, herbs, and berries sometimes harvested by the public for cooking.

Calls to the DPIC are recorded, archived, and saved for 10 years according to current Danish law. Patient information and case descriptions are archived in an internal patient database. In 2019, the number of calls received was approximately 34,000. The approximate yearly increase in calls was around 30% in the first years (Bøgevig et al., 2011) and today the yearly increase continues to be approximately 10%. The current population served is approximately 5,906,000 people (Greenland 56,000, Faroe Islands 50,000, and Denmark 5,800,000) (Statistics Denmark, 2021; Naalakkersuisut, 2021; Føroya landsstýri, 2021).

Staffing and professionalism

DPIC nurses have special training on the risk assessment of poisonings. In severe, unusual cases the nurse can either discuss the case with, or hand over the original call to a physician trained in clinical toxicology (and with a primary specialty background within anesthesiology, clinical pharmacology or occupational and environmental medicine) or a pharmacist specialized in clinical toxicology. Initially, the physician on call during evenings, nights, and weekends was also covering the intensive care unit (ICU) at the hospital. As the number of poison center calls increased and the number of ICU beds doubled, in 2019 the service changed such that a dedicated team of physicians are now on call. They have all received special toxicology training prior to taking on this service function.

The poisons information specialists are nurses with a background in emergency medicine, anesthesiology, or post-operative care. They receive specialized training for 2 months before they are allowed to handle poison center calls on their own. The training is provided as side-by-side training by the colleague nurses as well as training from the medical and pharmaceutical staff of the DPIC. There is no formal medical or clinical toxicology education in Denmark, either for nurses or for clinical staff. Danish clinical toxicologists were originally self-trained, or did courses provided by universities in other countries. Subsequently, they trained new colleagues one-to-one.

Challenges

The number of calls to the DPIC continues to increase. The complexity and severity of cases has also increased for a significant number of calls. This results in a greater demand for specialized advice, and higher requirements for staff expertise, both in the handling of the initial call and from the clinicians on call. Increasing numbers of available chemical products and a greater variation in registered pharmaceuticals challenge the production of accurate guideline material. The production of good, high level guidance materials including thoughtful toxicological evaluations is time-consuming, and the background materials available for the guidelines are sparse. At the same time, the staff-number working at the DPIC has not increased. This situation challenges the balance between acceptable waiting times experienced by callers to the DPIC, the documentation of calls, the completeness of the guideline material available for the management of poisonings, and the promotion of prevention measures, including education of the public and health care staff.

Norway

Origins

The Norwegian Poisons Information Center (NPIC) was stablished in 1961 as a response to the increasing need for a national or regional knowledge-based center to consult in cases of poisonings. It was founded by pharmacist Elsa Wickstrøm as *Giftkartoteket* (The Archives of Poisons) and was initially located on the premises of the Institute of Pharmacology at the University in Oslo (Wickstrøm, 2000; Jacobsen et al., 2011). To insure a close relation to the medical professionals, a cooperation with professor of nephrology Erik Enger at Ullevål Hospital in Oslo was initiated. He later became physician manager. This cooperation with specialists at Ullevål has been continued and developed further, as described later.

For the first years, *Giftkartoteket* was only open during daytime working hours. To meet the need for advice from hospitals during the night, a copy of the archive was placed at Ullevål Hospital. Doctors on call for the hospital took turns answering calls from other hospitals at night from 1964, in addition to their own clinical work (Wickstrøm, 2000). In 1980, the name was changed to *Giftinformasjonssentralen* (The Poisons Information Center) to match the names used in other countries. From 1991, the number of calls increased markedly, and the numbers outside working hours became too much for on-call physicians at Ullevål to handle. The need for specially trained personnel with access to more than an archive to answer calls was acknowledged. In 1993, funding was granted to increase the staff and opening hours, to insure a service available 24 h daily to both the public and healthcare services.

Organization

The NPIC serves the whole country of Norway and is based solely on governmental funding. Initially, in 2001, it was directly under the Department of Health, but it has since been part of the Norwegian Directorate of Health. From 2015, the NPIC has been a department of the Norwegian Institute of Public Health.

Daily operations

The main role of NPIC is to provide telephone advice to health care professionals and the public on the prevention, diagnosis, and management of poisoning. Inquiries about exposure to medical products, biological toxins and chemicals, including household products, natural toxins, pesticides and industrial chemicals are answered 24 h daily. The center also provides limited information on chronic exposures, interactions, adverse effects, and exposure during pregnancies and lactation. The calls are manually registered in an internal database, which has toxicological information incorporated. While it is an unusual occurrence, the service is required to provide advice to anonymous callers.

In addition to counseling by telephone, the center works on surveillance, revision of advisory documentation and quality assurance thereof. Poisoning prevention in the form of lectures, information brochures, web pages, and social media is also done. The poison center is a vital part of the preparedness organization of the Institute of Public Health for major chemical events.

There is no registration of products/mixtures directly to NPIC. The poison center has access to information in the Norwegian Product Register. In the future, information according to CLP Regulation Annex VIII though ECHA (European Chemicals Agency) will also be available. These two registers serve different purposes and co-exist, meaning that a product/mixture on the Norwegian market may have to be entered both in the Product Register and in the ECHA registry. According to CLP article 45, in Norway the appointed body is The National Institute of Public Health, represented by NPIC and The Norwegian Environment Agency (Product Register).

Number and characterization of inquiries

In 1995 NPIC received approximately 18,000 calls. This number has increased steadily since then, passing 35,000 calls in 2005 and more than 40,000 calls in 2015. From 2015 to 2019, the number remained stable at approximately 42,000–43,000 calls per year, but call volume is estimated to increase in 2020. The 2020 population of Norway is around 5,400,000 (Statistisk sentralbyrå, 2021).

In 2019, NPIC received 42,992 calls. Ninety-two percent of the calls concerned acute or chronic exposures. Thirty-three percent of the calls came from the health care system, 62% from the general public, and the rest from schools or kindergartens, workplaces, public offices, media, fire department or police, and others. A slight increase in calls from the healthcare system has been seen in recent years. In 2019, 41% of the exposures concerned chemicals/products/substances, 34% of exposures involved pharmaceuticals, and 25% involved plants and berries, mushrooms, and other/miscellaneous agents.

Since 2016, human exposures have been prioritized, and calls from owners about animal exposures are increasingly referred to veterinarians. From 2016 to 2019, this approach reduced the number of calls on animal exposures from more than 3100/year to less than 1500/year.

Staffing and professionalism

In 2020, the poison center has a total of 24 full-time equivalent (FTE) staff, including a director, and an administrator. The academic background of the specialists in poisons information includes pharmacology, veterinary medicine, medicine, and toxicology. A training period of approximately 3.5–4 months is required before newly hired personnel are allowed to answer calls without supervision. Outside daytime working hours, a senior consultant is on call if needed in difficult cases. In addition, 5 medical intensivists with a broad experience in the treatment of poisoning are hired part-time and serve as on-call clinical consultants with 24-h daily availability.

Challenges

Both the general public and medical professionals have easier access to information and treatment recommendations from online sources than before. Nevertheless, NPIC handles an increasing number of inquiries. A greater proportion of the calls require assistance from the clinicians on call. The variety of products available are also increasing, together with an increase in questions about unknown substances, and a need for the toxicological evaluation of those. The balance between enough people answering calls to insure an acceptable waiting time and time to work on functions such as documentation and poisons prevention can be difficult. Remaining a service where people can seek advice anonymously, while staff still fulfill their ethical requirements as healthcare workers is challenging. A general cut-back in funding of the health management in Norway may affect operations of the poison center as well, as part of cuts to the Institute of Public Health. But up to now, NPIC has been spared large budget cuts, and it is still a preferred source of information on acute poisonings in Norway.

Sweden

Origins

The origins of poisons information services in Sweden date back to a Sunday in 1957 at the Crown Princess Lovisa's Children's Hospital in Stockholm when the pediatrician on call, Dr. Bengt Karlsson, was compelled to perform gastric lavage in 13 small children arriving together at the emergency care facility. The children came from all around the municipality of Stockholm and they had all been drinking fluids of unknown origin at home. In most of these cases, it was not possible to know the content of the products and thereby the risks were difficult to assess. Observation at the hospital turned out to be event-free, with no corrosive damages or constitutional symptoms. All the physician colleagues of Dr. Karlsson thought that it was now time to establish a specific unit for taking care of poisoned patients.

In 1958, the pharmacy at the Karolinska Hospital started to collect toxicological data supported by the pharmacist: Per-Åke Wikander. In 1959, Dr. Bengt Karlsson moved from Crown Princess Lovisa's Children's Hospital to the Karolinska Hospital. This made it possible to start a cooperation in 1959 between the pediatric department at Karolinska, the pharmacy, and the government, leading to a nationwide unit for advice on diagnosis and treatment of poisoned patients under the name of *Giftinformationscentralen* (GIC), the Swedish Poisons Information Center. Initially, this was not easy, since a number of doctors opposed the idea. A "trial unit" was allowed, financed by the National Swedish Board of Health with a small group of one physician, one pharmacist and a secretary. This was probably Europe's first national medical unit, focusing only on poisonings and open both for the general public and health care personnel. Luckily, this unit was supported by the director-general and a professor in pediatrics of the Karolinska. It was not until July 1, 1964, that the poisons center, based at the pediatric clinic at Karolinska Hospital, first became a formally established organization, with full-time offices, after an institute staff vote of 71 in favor and 66 against. The negative voices against its establishment gradually disappeared and today the poisons center remains a well-established essential governmental service and the first on call service for health care staff funded in Sweden. In the period 1967–1982 the poisons information center was led by a pediatrician and associate professor at the pediatric clinic at Karolinska Hospital. During this period, the poisons center developed rapidly but pediatric inquiries became less frequent. A national antidote program was also started and the integration of educational efforts for medical personnel was included in the work program.

Information data bank

The collection of usable toxicological data was started in 1958. This accumulation has been continued and updated over the years both from academic literature and clinical data from hospital discharge summaries. All this together created a database which now includes documents covering 3500 chemical substances, pharmaceutical substances, plant toxins, other biological toxins, and other entries. Swedish industry, importers, and distributors were asked to send information regarding the content of chemical products. These contributions added up to more than 100,000 product information data entries today, with an annual incoming number of 20,000.

Organization

Guidelines, assessment of product toxicity, processing of patient case reports, and prevention brochures are prepared by the pharmaceutical staff. The physicians are responsible for the medical adaptation of the guideline database. To maintain their clinical competence, doctors periodically participate in the work at one of the Stockholm region's intensive care units (Persson and Personne, 2001). The Swedish poisons information system answers calls from both health professionals and the general public. It has its own internal database on poisons information developed by its staff.

Daily operations

In 1961 the number of calls to the poisons center was about 1000, after which there was a constant increase, and in 2016 more than 90,000 calls were received. The current population in Sweden is approximately 10,400,000 people (Statistikmyndigheten SCB, 2021).

Staffing and professionalism

The poisons center is a service available 24 h daily, and is staffed by specially trained pharmacists, most with many years of experience in providing toxicological advice. In severe poisonings and when additional clinical competence is required, the call is transferred to a physician who is part of the center's emergency call system. The physicians are specialized in anesthesiology or internal medicine, with experience in intensive care.

Finland

Origins

Child mortality from poisonings in Finland was substantial in the 1940s and peaked at the end of 1950s. In 1959, the Finnish Pediatric Society appointed a committee to improve the treatment and prevention of poisoning accidents. As a result, a nationwide Finnish Poison Information Center (FPIC) was founded in 1961. In the beginning, pediatricians from the Helsinki Children's Hospital answered the phone on a voluntary basis. The first pharmacist was hired in 1966 and first physician in 1974. From 1974 on, FPIC staff in permanent positions answered poisons center calls during the daytime and the pediatricians continued to be on call during out-of-office hours. This changed in 1995, when FPIC staff began answering calls full-time.

Organization

The FPIC is now part of the services of the Helsinki University Hospital (HUS), in the Department of Emergency Medicine. FPIC works in close collaboration with various institutions in order to provide efficient and cost-effective services to Finnish citizens. In 2018, the poison center phone number became toll-free. FPIC is very active on social media (Facebook, Twitter, and Instagram), and started a Podcast series in 2019, to deliver toxicological information to health care professionals. The FPIC operates in close conjunction with the Finnish

Teratology Information Service; both use the same operational systems, thus producing synergy between the two services.

Daily operations

During the first year of FPIC operation, in 1961, the pediatricians received 60 calls on child exposures. This number has increased steadily and now covers all ages. FPIC call volumes reached 4,467 calls in 1975, 26,520 calls in 1990, and peaked in 2005 with 41,460 calls. Since 2012, annual call numbers have stabilized at around 37,000 (e.g., 37,139 calls in 2015). The population of Finland in 2020 was approximately 5,530,000 people (Tilastokeskus, 2021).

Staffing and professionalism

The FPIC staff presently includes a chief physician, two other physicians, a senior pharmacist, and 11 pharmacists. None of these medical staff are on call outside of weekday office hours, but the Department of Emergency Medicine of Helsinki University Hospital provides medical back-up for difficult consultations after hours.

Acknowledgment

The author thanks Mari Tosterud and Jatrud W. Skjerdal for providing the information on the Norwegian Poisons Information Center, and to Peter Hultén from the Swedish Poisons Information Center for providing data from the Swedish and Finnish Poisons Information Centers.

References

Bøgevig S, Hoegberg LC, Dalhoff KP, Mortensen OS. Status and trends in poisonings in Denmark 2007-2009. Dan Med Bull 2011;58:A4268.

Clemmesen C, Nilsson E. Therapeutic trends in the treatment of barbiturate poisoning. The Scandinavian method. Clin Pharmacol Ther 1961;2:220–9.

Fogh A. Giftinformationscentraler. Organisation - rådgivning - internationalt netværk [Danish]. Månedsskr Prakt Lægegern 1994;967–73.

Føroya landsstýri, The Government of the Faroe Islands. Accessed on 2021-04-06, https://www.government.fo/en/foreign-relations/about-the-faroe-islands/; 2021.

Graudins A. Therapeutic trends in the treatment of barbiturate poisoning: the 'Scandinavian method'. Emerg Med Australas 2019;31:893–4.

Jacobsen D, Rygnestad T, Muan B, Andrew E. Giftinformasjonen 50 år - forgiftningsbehandling før og nå. Tidsskr No Lægeforen 2011;13:1915–7.

Naalakkersuisut, Government og Greenland. Accessed on 2021-04-06, https://naalakkersuisut.gl/en/About-government-of-greenland/About-Greenland/Facts-about-Greenland; 2021.

Persson H, Personne M. Toxicologic information through four decades [Swedish]. Lakartidningen 2001;98:2921–5.

Statistics Denmark. Accessed on 2021-04-06, https://www.dst.dk/da/Statistik/emner/befolkning-og-valg/befolkning-og-befolkningsfremskrivning/folketal; 2021.

Statistisk sentralbyrå, Statistics Norway. Accessed 2021-04-06, https://www.ssb.no/befolkning/faktaside/befolkningen; 2021.

Statistikmyndigheten SCB, Statistics Sweden. Accessed on 2021-04-06, https://www.scb.se/hitta-statistik/sverige-i-siffror/manniskorna-i-sverige/sveriges-befolkning/; 2021.

Tilastokeskus, Statistics Finland. Accessed on 2021-04-06, https://www.stat.fi/til/vrm_en.html; 2021.

Wickstrøm E. Giftinformasjonssentralen (GIS). Om oppbyggingen av en ny helsetjeneste 1961–98. Cygnus - en norsk farmacihistorisk skriftserie 2000;5:9–26.

Chapter 5.12

Israel

Yedidia Bentur

Israel Poison Information Center, Rambam Health Care Campus, The Rappaport Faculty of Medicine, Technion-Israel Institute of Technology, Haifa, Israel

Origins

The rapid expansion of the young State of Israel (established in 1948) was associated with an increasing number of poison exposures and poisonings. Therefore in 1964 the Israel Ministry of Health (MOH) decided to establish a national poison information center. By doing so, Israel followed the North American and Western European poison centers initiatives. Dr. Naftali Hertz was chosen for this mission, as he was well known for his wide knowledge in medicine and chemistry, and his considerable management skills. The Israel Poison Information Center (IPIC) was established in Rambam Hospital (now Rambam Health Care Center) in Haifa, the tertiary care hospital for northern Israel, where Dr. Hertz served as the head of the Laboratory of Biochemistry. Since then, the IPIC has remained the only national provider of clinical toxicology services for both the public and health care system 24 h/day, 7 days/week (24/7) in Israel and has been mainly funded by the MOH.

Organization

The IPIC staff positions have been funded by the Israel MOH. The physical plant, accommodation, utilities and administrative costs are funded by the Rambam Health Care Campus hosting the Center. No other governmental or nonprofit organizations have contributed financial support to the IPIC, although many professional collaborations were established and sustained.

The initial mission of the IPIC was to provide emergency departments (EDs) throughout the state with an updated card-index of toxic commercial products and medications available in Israel. Each card contained essential details, including the product's name, manufacturer/importer/distributor, ingredients, main clinical manifestations expected, most essential treatments, and toxicity grading according to LD_{50} values. For each ingredient, a numbered folder with

History of Modern Clinical Toxicology. https://doi.org/10.1016/B978-0-12-822218-8.00051-X

articles, a material safety data sheet, and many others, was created, and referenced in the product card-index. The entire task was performed by Dr. Hertz and his secretary Mrs. Lea Matri.

After very few years, it was clear that the updates could not keep up with the magnitude and rate of accumulated new information. In addition, more hospital physicians called in with patient-specific questions. In the late 1960s the IPIC was mandated to provide telephone consultations on poison-exposure cases to the health system. Provision of the product card-index to EDs was discontinued. The MOH funded a pediatrician and a PhD-trained staff member (biochemistry) for the IPIC, and more clinical-oriented consultations became possible. A medical record form with limited information was created and the existing commercial product database continuously updated.

In 1977 Dr. Hertz retired, and Dr. Uri Taitelman, an expert in internal medicine and intensive care medicine replaced him. The IPIC approach now was to provide tailored patient-oriented consultations, 24/7. As hospital physicians became familiar with the IPIC service, they began referring patients and families directly to the Center. It became evident that many cases did not require referrals to EDs, and that there was a need for IPIC service to be expanded to include phone consultations to the public. The commercial products card-index was expanded to include more chemical information and some clinical data, and clinical management protocols were written. All calls to the IPIC and the consultations provided were documented in the medical record database. The number of calls to the IPIC steadily increased, and in the early 1980s more physician posts were funded by the MOH. It should be noted that at this point in time training and hiring nurses as specialists in poisons information (SPI) was not approved by the MOH because of the concept that only physicians can consult physicians. In addition, there was a growing need to absorb physicians immigrating to Israel from Eastern Europe and the Soviet Union.

In the late 1980s the IPIC databases were computerized using Informix Software, mainly to include the commercial product card-index, and to a lesser extent the medical records database. In addition, the IPIC subscribed to Micromedex, at that time a microfiche database. The number of calls continued to increase, from 5992 in 1981 [84% from physicians, penetrance (calls/1000 population) 1.5] (Aloufy et al., 1983), to 12,153 in 1988 (72% from physicians, penetrance 2.7) (IPIC Database, Table 5.12.1). However, in 1989 the MOH began charging health care organizations for the consultations provided by the IPIC; revenues were used primarily for database subscription. The result of this action was a decrease in the number of calls (mainly from physicians) to 9971 in 1993 (penetrance 2.1). As part of national preparedness for a multicasualty toxicological incident, an additional on-call physician 24/7 was approved. In 1993–1994 the MOH decided to cut the IPIC staff, from six to four physicians.

TABLE 5.12.1 Annual distribution of Israel Poison Information data: Calls, population served, penetrance, and callers.

Year	Poison exposures reported	Calls from the public	Calls from physicians	Population served[a]	Penetrance (exposures reported per 1000 population)
1981	5992	599 (10%)	5033 (84%)	3,977,700	1.5
1982	6350	–	–	4,063,600	1.6
1983	7324	–	–	4,118,600	1.8
1985	8478	–	–	4,266,200	2
1986	9568	–	–	4,331,300	2.2
1988	12,153	2540 (21%)	8717 (72%)	4,476,800	2.7
1989[b]	11,508	2893 (25%)	7790 (68%)	4,559,600	2.7
1990	11,694	3008 (26%)	7938 (68%)	4,821,700	2.4
1991	10,151	3148 (31%)	6821 (67%)	5,058,800	2
1992	9971	3295 (33%)	6432 (65%)	5,195,900	1.9
1993	11,090	3667 (33%)	7003 (63%)	5,327,600	2.1
1994	12,325	4437 (36%)	7272 (59%)	5,471,500	2.2
1995	12,235	4338 (35%)	7395 (60%)	5,619,000	2.2
1996	13,695	3089 (39%)	7952 (57%)	5,759,400	2.4
1997	14,792	5547 (37%)	8457 (58%)	5,900,000	2.5
1998	15,712	6508 (41%)	8471 (54%)	6,041,400	2.6
1999	15,729	7675 (49%)	7338 (47%)	6,209,100	2.5
2000	16,687	8451 (51%)	7570 (45%)	6,369,300	2.6
2001	17,035	9166 (54%)	7256 (43%)	6508,800	2.6
2002	18,775	10,842 (58%)	7243 (39%)	6,631,100	2.8
2003	19,582	11,827 (60%)	7115 (36%)	6,748,400	2.9
2004	22,602	14,577 (64%)	7263 (32%)	6,869,500	3.3
2005	24,605	16,905 (69%)	7052 (28%)	6,990,700	3.5

TABLE 5.12.1 Annual distribution of Israel Poison Information data: Calls, population served, penetrance, and callers—cont'd

Year	Poison exposures reported	Calls from the public	Calls from physicians	Population served[a]	Penetrance (exposures reported per 1000 population)
2006	24,218	16,975 (70%)	6760 (28%)	7,116,700	3.4
2007	26,738	19,471 (73%)	6824 (26%)	7,242,200	3.7
2008	28,198	20,834 (74%)	6947 (25%)	7,412,200	3.8
2009	29,042	21,706 (74%)	6973 (24%)	7,552,000	3.8
2010	26,981	20,389 (76%)	6244 (23%)	7,695,100	3.5
2011	30,137	23,059 (76%)	6831 (23%)	7,836,600	3.8
2012	31,519	23,225 (74%)	7462 (24%)	7,984,500	3.9
2013	30,640	22,983 (76%)	7166 (24%)	8,059,500	3.8
2014[c]	36,740	28,731 (78%)	7744 (21%)	8,215,700	4.4
2015	35,616	27,399 (77%)	7508 (21%)	8,380,100	4.3
2016	36,751	29,470 (79%)	7070 (19%)	8,546,000	4.3
2017	39,928	32,083 (80%)	7119 (18%)	8,797,900	4.5
2018	39,985	31,985 (80%)	7344 (18%)	8,967,600	4.6
2019	38,948	30,991 (80%)	6992 (18%)	9,138,400	4.3

Sources: Aloufy et al., 1983, Bentur et al., 2008a,b,c, 2014, 2019; manual counting of records (1981–1988), computerized queries, and annual reports to the Israel MOH (1989 onwards).
[a] According to the data of the Central Bureau of Statistics, Israel.
[b] 1989—the year the MOH began charging health care organizations for medical toxicological consultations provided by the IPIC.
[c] 2014—the year when SPIs (nurses) joined the IPIC team and began providing consultations.

In 1994 Dr. Taitelman was appointed director of the Intensive Care Unit of Rambam Health Campus, and Dr. Yedidia (Didi) Bentur replaced him as director of the IPIC. Dr. Bentur was trained in intensive care medicine and internal medicine in Rambam, as well as in clinical pharmacology and toxicology in the Hospital for Sick Children, Toronto, Ontario. A year later, a new, detailed, designated toxicological medical record database was developed that could serve clinical, medicolegal, epidemiological, and research purposes. In addition, a new computerized commercial product database that could be incorporated into the toxicological medical record database and provide an extensive rapid view on products' categories, ingredients, and hazards was developed. These databases used MS Access on a SQL server; updating and de-bugging were done periodically. In 2014 a new computerized database was developed by the information technology (IT) team of Rambam Health Care Campus using Java Software and Oracle Database (Oracle Corporation, Redwood Shores, CA, USA). This database has enabled online data entering, and more updated and comprehensive queries, information searches, data analyses, and research. These databases have been used for numerous studies, for example, dipyrone poisoning (Bentur and Cohen, 2004), *Vipera palaestinae* bites (Bentur et al., 1997, 2004a), Lessepsian migration (Bentur et al., 2008a, 2018), atropine and atropine-TMB4 auto-injectors distributed to the Israeli population since the 1991 Gulf War (Amitai et al., 1992; Kozer et al., 2005; Bentur et al., 2006), medication errors (Lavon et al., 2014), drugs of abuse (Bentur et al., 2008b; Sznitman et al., 2020), pediatric poisonings (Bentur et al., 2010), deliberate self-poisoning (Bentur et al., 2004b), poison exposures in military personnel (Lavon and Bentur, 2017), and annual IPIC reports (Bentur et al., 2008c, 2014, 2019).

New management protocols were written, and the old ones updated. The IPIC has encouraged physicians (hospital and community) as well as health maintenance organizations (HMOs) call centers to refer exposed patients directly to the IPIC, thus minimizing "second hand" consultations, misunderstandings, and mistakes. Drug and reproductive toxicology services have been expanded to advise an increasing number of physicians and patients. IPIC physicians began providing a growing number of bedside clinical toxicology consultations in Rambam Health Care Campus, mainly to the ED. This move increased the quality of patient care and the professional level of the IPIC, as well as trust in its consultations.

In 2011 the number of calls increased to 30,137 and penetrance to 3.8 (172% and 81% increases, respectively, compared with 1993). This large call volume load together with having only one consultant at any given time, resulted in blocking the available hotline, precluding further increase in call volume (Table 5.12.1).

Training

Although the IPIC together with the Clinical Pharmacology Unit of Rambam Health Care Campus were accredited for providing a residency in Clinical

Pharmacology, it was very hard to recruit new physicians. After a long, serious, and constructive discussion with senior MOH officials, it was decided to launch a program for training nurses as SPIs, and their integration in the routine IPIC work, initially as a pilot. The two positions allocated by the MOH were staffed by five nurses who were trained by the IPIC clinical toxicologists according to a program consisting of theoretical lectures and practical experience specifically designed for this purpose. In January 2014, the nurses joined the IPIC and began answering calls from the public, under the supervision of the clinical toxicologists; a second 24/7 hotline could then be opened.

At the end of the first year of physicians–nurses' joint operation (2014), it was clear the project was a great success; the annual number of calls increased to 36,740, penetrance to 4.4 (20% and 16% increases, respectively) (Table 5.12.1). The number of calls from the public increased, as well as prevention of unnecessary referrals to the ED. The SPI nurses went on to answer calls from community physicians and later on from hospital physicians. The number of calls continued to increase and reached 39,928 in 2017 (penetrance 4.5) similar to those in 2019. In about 89% of the calls coming from the public, referral to an ED was deemed unnecessary, and patients could stay home with poison center or community clinic follow-up. Given this success, its impact on ED load across the country and the saturation of the two phone hotlines available, the MOH approved two more positions for SPI nurses. A more extensive training program was designed, in which the senior and experienced nurses also participated. The new nurses started routine IPIC work in June 2020, thus enabling the use of 3–4 hotlines simultaneously. During this period, the MOH and Rambam Health Care Campus also funded upgrades of the working stations (e.g., computers, monitors, and telephones), workload monitoring system, and computerized database support.

IPIC staff has contributed extensively to teaching clinical toxicology and clinical pharmacology to residents, practicing physicians medical students, nurses and pharmacists, in Rambam Health Care Center and other centers and universities.

National services

The IPIC has been involved in national activities and poisoning prevention efforts. Involvement has increased over the years, particularly after the early 1990s. Collaboration and joint efforts have included the following agencies: Israel Institute of Standards (safe packaging and content of commercial products, mainly cleaning agents; carbon monoxide detectors for home gas operating heating and cooking systems), MOH (drug registration, generic medications, over-the-counter medications for general sale, list of teratogenic agents, stocking antidotes, writing guidelines on multicasualty toxicological incidents for EDs, ad hoc consultations), Ministry of Environmental Protection (registration of insecticides for domestic use), interministerial committees (e.g., water safety), National Councils (home and leisure safety, suicides prevention), and child safety (e.g., BETEREM - Safe Kids Israel, National Council for the Child). In addition, the IPIC has been heavily involved in preparedness efforts for multicasualty toxicological incidents, chemical warfare agents and chemical terrorism, collaborating mainly with the Emergency Division of the MOH, and Medical Corps of the Israel Defense Forces. In these collaborations, the IPIC provides its data, experience and knowledge to the decision-making process.

The IPIC is directly subordinate to the Senior Director General of the MOH; annual working plans and budget requirements are submitted to and approved by him and by the Chief Financial Officer.

The IPIC has been the only national center providing clinical toxicology consultations to both public and health care professionals 24/7. Over the years, several clinical toxicology units were established in a few medical centers (Carmel, Sheba, Sorasky, Shamir). These units serve their hospitals; three of them practice also clinical pharmacology and reproductive toxicology. Two of the directors of these units were trained in Toronto, one in Toronto and Denver and one in the IPIC. Funding is provided to these units by their hospitals, not by the MOH. These units occasionally consult the IPIC.

Daily operations

The IPIC responds to inquiries from the public as well as health care professionals from hospitals, community clinics, pre-hospital emergency medical services and the Israel Defense Forces. Acute exposures constitute the majority of IPIC inquiries but all types of exposures are handled similarly. The consultant on call obtains exposure details, clinical manifestations, and treatment that has already been given; directed questions complement history-taking. After identifying life-threatening conditions, rational first aid and decontamination advice is given followed by triage recommendations. Triage of acutely exposed patients includes: stay on-site, go to a community clinic clinic, or go to an ED. Patients who are advised to stay on-site are encouraged to call the IPIC if any change occurs. Calls from community clinics are handled the same way, with additional evaluation and follow-up. Triage of patients who are already in the ED includes: discharge home, discharge to community physician follow-up, observation in the ED or admission to a ward or an ICU; consultation also includes evaluation and management recommendations. Pro-active follow-up is done in severe, complicated or unclear cases, and when compliance is questionable. For chronic exposures, the consultant verifies whether a referral to the ED is required. If not, referral is made to a community or occupational physician, whenever relevant. In any of these cases, the patient is encouraged to provide the physician with the IPIC phone number, enabling a dialog. A senior staff clinical toxicologist is available 24/7 to assist and backup the consultants.

All IPIC consultations are provided directly to the caller during a phone conversation. When the call is received from a call center of a health maintenance organization (HMO), a conference call is set up and the consultation is provided directly to the patient or caregiver. The IPIC assisted in writing triage protocols for the call center of the major HMO in Israel and these emphasize the importance of direct communication of the IPIC with the patient or caregiver.

The IPIC uses Micromedex poison, drug and reproductive toxicology databases, and the RightAnswer database (formerly Tomes Plus and Chemknowledge). The subscription started in 1980s, funded by the MOH. Other information sources include leading textbooks in clinical toxicology, clinical pharmacology and reproductive toxicology, and online databases such as Toxnet. Other information sources include the web sites of the MOH, and the Ministries of Environmental Protection and Agriculture. In addition, the IPIC staff have in house management protocols, including acetaminophen, drugs to treat attention deficit hyperactivity disorder, hydrogen peroxide, methanol, ethylene glycol, and snake bites.

The IPIC uses its own toxicological medical record database, which is generally completed online during the consultation. All calls are recorded, and all data entries are stored in servers of the IT Unit of Rambam Health Care Campus, with backup. Queries can be made according to any combination of any field in the medical record. Archiving of consultations began in the late 1970s as hard copies and since the early 1990s data are additionally stored digitally. The commercial product database designed and updated by the IPIC staff is extensively used. This database contains information on products available in Israel (locally manufactured or imported). Transfer of data from the old computerized database (MS Access) to the new one (Oracle) is intended.

Annual reports of the IPIC data are periodically published (Aloufy et al., 1983, Bentur et al., 2008a,b,c, Bentur et al., 2014, 2019). Table 5.12.1 shows annual distribution of some IPIC data since 1981. Over the past 10 years the main causative agents were pharmaceuticals (~50%), chemicals (~37%), and poisonous plants and venomous animals (~5%). The age groups most affected were children 5 years and younger (0–5 years ~45%; 6–12 years ~6%; 13–18 years ~4%). Most patients were asymptomatic (~53%), incidence falling with increasing severity (minor ~29%, moderate ~3%, major ~0.6%, and death ~0.01%). Most fatalities were intentional exposures; causes included substance abuse, corrosives, organophosphate insecticides, carbon monoxide, colchicine, cyclic antidepressants, neuroleptics, paracetamol, and opioids. It is interesting to note that the number and severity of exposures to organophosphate insecticides has greatly decreased in the past 10 years (80% reduction) after banning their use as over-the-counter insecticides, and the introduction of pyrethrins and pyrethroids for domestic and agricultural uses.

Staffing and professionalism

The IPIC is managed by 6 physicians staffing 4 positions. The IPIC director was trained in intensive care medicine and clinical toxicology, and is board certified in internal medicine and clinical pharmacology (Israel). His deputy is board certified in internal medicine and clinical pharmacology, one senior staff member is board certified in pediatrics, and another one in internal medicine.

Two other physicians joined the IPIC after gaining clinical experience, but they are not board certified in a core medical discipline. All clinicians but the Director were trained in clinical toxicology and pharmacology at the IPIC.

Prerequisites for the nurse SPIs who joined in 2013 included an academic degree in nursing and registered nurse certification, at least five years of experience in an active hospital ward, graduation of an intensive care or emergency medicine course, and preferably also having an M.Sc. degree in nursing. After an interview, the selected nurses were trained in clinical toxicology. At the end of the course, the nurses had to successfully pass theoretical and practical examinations. The practical part included cases evaluation in rotating stations. The first group of nurses did the course in 2013, two more courses were given in 2015 and 2019. The senior nurses participated in all courses and examinations and were involved in the practical teaching in the last course. A physician backup is readily available to the nurses 24/7. The new nurses that joined the IPIC in mid-2020 will follow the same process of integration into the IPIC work; supervision and teaching will also be provided by the senior SPI nurses. There are no SPIs in other hospitals, or a training program outside of the IPIC.

Besides the clinical arm, the IPIC has also an adjacent clinical toxicology and pharmacology laboratory. The services provided include drug monitoring, urine screens (drugs of abuse, opioids, and psychiatric medications), occupational toxicology (metals and organic solvents), and special toxicological assays (e.g., acetylcholinesterase, paraquat, cyanide, sulfonylureas, formic acid, and glycolic acid). Equipment includes an immunochemistry auto-analyzer, HPLCs, LS-MS/MS, GC, and an atomic absorption spectrophotometer. Recently the laboratory has been expanded to include pharmacogenetic tests. A PhD-trained director runs the laboratory (position funded by the MOH), with the aid of four experienced technicians (funded by the revenue generated by the laboratory); the IPIC director is in charge of the laboratory.

Clinical toxicology is not an accredited medical specialty in Israel. Clinical toxicologists are trained mainly in the IPIC. In the few hospitals that have an accredited clinical pharmacology residency program, the trainees get their clinical toxicology education as part of this program. The Israeli clinical pharmacology board examination includes a chapter on drug overdoses and poisonings.

Israel Society of Toxicology

The Israel Society of Toxicology was established in 1996 by a group of clinical toxicologists. Past presidents (in chronological order) were Yona Amitai, Yedidia (Didi) Bentur, Matityahu Lifshitz, and Eran Kozer; the present chairman is Ophir Lavon. The Society is a scientific organization within the Israel Medical Association. Owing to the small number of clinicians practicing clinical toxicology in Israel, especially those who devote their entire time to this specialty, the Scientific Council of the Israel Medical Association decided not to recognize clinical toxicology as an accredited medical specialty.

The Society has focused mainly on clinical scientific meetings. Some of them were joint conferences with the Israeli Associations of Emergency Medicine and Clinical Pharmacology. A smaller part of the actions was devoted to participation in regulatory and preparedness activities and issuing position statements. Throughout the years, the IPIC played an important role in the Society's activities. In 2010, 2013, and 2019 joint conferences were held together with the American College of Medical Toxicology in Rambam Health Care Campus, Haifa, Israel, where the IPIC is located. The organizing committees included the IPIC director, and leaders of the Israel Society of Toxicology and the American College of Medical Toxicology. These conferences included 2 days of clinical and basic research presentations and keynote lectures, and observation of a chemical warfare agent drill organized by the Emergency Division, MOH (1 day, 2013 and 2019).

Challenges

The main challenges that clinical toxicology in Israel and the IPIC face include the following:

1. Establishing an accredited training program aiming to staff each hospital with a clinical toxicologist. By this initiative, poisoned patient care will improve, as well as preparedness for and management of multicasualty toxicological incidents.
2. Increasing teaching time devoted to clinical toxicology in faculties of medicine, nursing, and pharmacy schools, and EDs across Israel.
3. Increasing call volume to the IPIC, thus further reducing unnecessary referrals to EDs and reducing their load.
4. Increasing involvement in poison prevention education in the community.
5. Continuing research and initiating multicenter joint research.
6. Creating a national registry for poison exposures and poisonings admitted to EDs.
7. Establishing a national toxicological authority which will guide and support regulatory governmental and nongovernmental decisions and actions.
8. Planning and implementing a toxicovigilance program.
9. Obtaining increased and steady funding from the government (mainly MOH), HMOs, and industry to support and maintain required IPIC activities.

References

Aloufy A, Raikhlin-Eisenkraft B, Taitelman U. Poisoning in Israel 1981. Harefuah 1983;105(7):155–8 [Hebrew].

Amitai Y, Almog S, Singer R, Hammer R, Bentur Y, Danon YL. Atropine poisoning in children during the Persian Gulf crisis. A national survey in Israel. JAMA 1992;268(5):630–2.

Bentur Y, Cohen O. Dipyrone overdose. J Toxicol Clin Toxicol 2004;42(3):261–5.

Bentur Y, Zveibel F, Adler M, Raikhlin B. Delayed administration of *Vipera xanthina palaestinae* antivenin. J Toxicol Clin Toxicol 1997;35(3):257–61.

Bentur Y, Raikhlin-Eisenkraft B, Galperin M. Evaluation of antivenom therapy in *Vipera palaestinae* bites. Toxicon 2004a;44(1):53–7.

Bentur Y, Raikhlin-Eisenkraft B, Lavee M. Toxicological features of deliberate self-poisonings. Hum Exp Toxicol 2004b;23(7):331–7.

Bentur Y, Layish I, Krivoy A, Berkovitch M, Rotman E, Haim SB, Yehezkelli Y, Kozer E. Civilian adult self-injections of atropine-trimedoxime (TMB4) auto-injectors. Clin Toxicol 2006;44(3):301–6.

Bentur Y, Ashkar J, Lurie Y, Levy Y, Azzam ZS, Litmanovich M, Golik M, Gurevych B, Golani D, Eisenman A. Lessepsian migration and tetrodotoxin poisoning due to *Lagocephalus sceleratus* in the eastern Mediterranean. Toxicon 2008a;52(8):964–8.

Bentur Y, Bloom-Krasik A, Raikhlin-Eisenkraft B. Illicit cathinone ("Hagigat") poisoning. Clin Toxicol 2008b;46(3):206–10.

Bentur Y, Lurie Y, Cahana A, Lavon O, Bloom-Krasik A, Kovler N, Gurevych B, Raikhlin-Eisenkraft B. Poisoning in Israel: annual report of the Israel Poison Information Center, 2007. Isr Med Assoc J 2008c;10(11):749–56.

Bentur Y, Obchinikov ND, Cahana A, Kovler N, Bloom-Krasik A, Lavon O, Gurevych B, Lurie Y. Pediatric poisonings in Israel: National Poison Center data. Isr Med Assoc J 2010;12(9):554–9.

Bentur Y, Lurie Y, Cahana A, Kovler N, Bloom-Krasik A, Gurevych B, Klein-Schwartz W. Poisoning in Israel: annual report of the Israel poison information Center, 2012. Isr Med Assoc J 2014;16(11):686–92.

Bentur Y, Altunin S, Levdov I, Golani D, Spanier E, Edelist D, Lurie Y. The clinical effects of the venomous Lessepsian migrant fish *Plotosus lineatus* (Thunberg, 1787) in the Southeastern Mediterranean Sea. Clin Toxicol 2018;56(5):327–31.

Bentur Y, Lurie Y, Cahana A, Bloom-Krasik A, Kovler N, Neuman G, Gurevych B, Sofer P, Klein-Schwartz W. Poisoning in Israel: annual report of the Israel Poison Information Center, 2017. Isr Med Assoc J 2019;21(3):175–82.

Kozer E, Mordel A, Haim SB, Bulkowstein M, Berkovitch M, Bentur Y. Pediatric poisoning from trimedoxime (TMB4) and atropine automatic injectors. J Pediatr 2005;146(1):41–4.

Lavon O, Bentur Y. Poison exposures in young Israeli military personnel: a National Poison Center Data analysis. Clin Toxicol 2017;55(5):322–5.

Lavon O, Ben-Zeev A, Bentur Y. Medication errors outside healthcare facilities: a national poison Centre perspective. Basic Clin Pharmacol Toxicol 2014;114(3):288–92.

Sznitman SR, Pinsky-Talbi L, Salameh M, Moed T, Bentur Y. Cannabis and synthetic cannabinoid exposure reported to the Israel poison information Center: examining differences in exposures to medical and recreational compounds. Int J Drug Policy 2020;77:102711. 32126489.

Chapter 5.13

Contribution of the World Health Organization to toxicology and poisons centers

John Haines and Joanna Tempowski
Formerly International Programme on Chemical Safety, World Health Organization, Geneva, Switzerland

Background

The World Health Organization (WHO) is a specialized agency of the United Nations (UN), established in 1948. It has a decentralized structure with a headquarters in Geneva, Switzerland, and six regional offices covering Africa, the Americas and the Caribbean, eastern Mediterranean, Europe, south-east Asia, and the western Pacific. Staff in 150 WHO country offices provide technical cooperation and advice, and work to implement WHO programs at the national level.

The WHO mandate encompasses communicable diseases, noncommunicable diseases, diseases of environmental origin, including those caused by chemicals and toxins, emergencies, and social determinants of health. Its work is carried out at global, regional, and country levels and frequently involves collaboration with partners who may be intergovernmental or civil society organizations.

Early work on the toxicological assessment of chemicals

During its first two decades, WHO's work on chemicals was associated with its long-term priority policy areas for the promotion and protection of public health: environmental sanitation (including vector control), food safety, health risks associated with the use of pesticides, occupational exposures to chemicals, and the standardization of pharmaceuticals.

Concern about the possible health implications of the increasing use of chemicals in the food industry and of pesticide residues in food and feedstuffs led to the establishment of the Joint Food and Agriculture Organization (FAO)/ WHO Expert Committee on Food Additives (JECFA) in 1956 and the Joint

History of Modern Clinical Toxicology. https://doi.org/10.1016/B978-0-12-822218-8.00043-0

493

FAO/WHO Meeting on Pesticide Residues (JMPR), which first met in 1961. In both cases, WHO carries out the toxicological evaluation of the specific chemicals of concern.

In 1965 WHO established the International Agency for Research on Cancer (IARC) to coordinate and conduct research on the causes of human cancer, the mechanisms of carcinogenesis, and to develop scientific strategies for cancer prevention and control. IARC convenes interdisciplinary scientific working groups to review published data and assess the strength of the available evidence that an agent can cause cancer in humans. These reviews are published as IARC Monographs (IARC, 2019).

Consolidation of work on chemical safety

Prior to the 1970s, both national and international action on the control of chemicals was piecemeal, being directed toward specific chemicals that caused health problems. There was, however, growing concern about the increasing number and types of chemicals in use for which information was largely lacking on their potential effects on human health and the environment. The UN Conference on the Human Environment, held in Stockholm in 1972, marked the start of the environmental governance movement. One of its recommendations was for programs to be established for the early warning and prevention of the harmful effects of chemicals and for the assessment of their potential risks to human health (UN, 1973). This led to the establishment of the International Programme on Chemical Safety (IPCS) by WHO (WHO, 1978) and the development of chemical safety programs in the six WHO regions.

In anticipation of the 1972 Conference, the 23rd World Health Assembly in 1970 reaffirmed WHO's leading role in the prevention and control of environmental factors adversely affecting human health (WHO, 1970). This resulted in the establishment of the Environmental Health Criteria (EHC) program in 1973 to provide health and environmental risk assessments of potentially toxic chemicals (WHO, 1973).

In 1992, the UN Conference on Environment and Development held in Rio de Janeiro, recognized that the environmentally sound management of chemicals was an important component of sustainable development. It adopted Agenda 21, Chapter 19 as an international strategy for action on chemical safety into the 21st century (UN, 1992). This strategy addressed among other things the need for action to prevent poisonings, undertake toxicovigilance, and prevent chemical accidents. Governments, with the support of international organizations, were recommended to promote the establishment and strengthening, as appropriate, of national poisons centers to insure prompt and adequate diagnosis and treatment of poisonings. Subsequent intergovernmental environmental meetings have reiterated these same needs and WHO was given the mandate to support countries in these endeavors. More recently the revised International

Health Regulations (2005) (IHR) have highlighted poisons centers as an important component of a public health program (WHO, 2015a).

International Programme on Chemical Safety (IPCS)

IPCS was formally launched in 1980 as a joint undertaking of WHO, the International Labour Organization (ILO), and United Nations Environment Programme (UNEP). WHO was responsible for the overall management of the Programme. In more recent times, IPCS has operated solely as a WHO program; collaboration with ILO and UNEP continues on specific projects.

The two main roles of IPCS are to provide the scientific basis on which governments can establish the safe use of chemicals, and to strengthen capabilities and capacities in countries for chemical safety. IPCS has six main objectives: risk evaluation of priority chemicals; development of methodologies for health risk assessment; technical cooperation among Member States; management of chemical emergencies; prevention and treatment of chemical poisonings; and human resource development.

Production of EHC documents became IPCS's responsibility, and these were followed by the Concise International Chemical Assessment Documents, which have largely replaced EHCs. IPCS jointly with ILO, also produces the multilingual International Chemical Safety Cards (WHO and ILO, 2020).

Most of the scientific work of IPCS is undertaken through working groups of experts chosen for their independence and competence in the field and endeavoring to insure a balanced geographical and gender participation. This work is supported by a global network of WHO Collaborating Centres and by scientific bodies designated as nonstate actors in official relations with WHO, such as the International Union of Toxicology (IUTOX). Projects may also be undertaken with international scientific organizations, other intergovernmental organizations, such as the Organisation for Economic Co-operation and Development (OECD), and relevant professional bodies (such as clinical toxicology associations).

In 1997 the IPCS INCHEM databank was established in partnership with the Canadian Center for Occupational Health and Safety (CCOHS), a WHO Collaborating Centre (IPCS, 2020a, 2020b). This databank is freely available on the Internet, offering rapid access to thousands of searchable full-text documents produced by WHO and other agencies on chemical risks and the sound management of chemicals. The databank is also accessible through the OECD eChemPortal (OECD, 2020).

IPCS INTOX project

To address the expressed need for progress in the prevention and treatment of poisonings, IPCS organized a consultation with relevant professional associations, in particular the World Federation of Associations of Clinical Toxicology

Centers and Poison Control Centers. In 1984–1986 a global survey of poisons centers was carried out by IPCS jointly with the World Federation and the European Commission, with the support of the Belgian National Poisons Center. This revealed that there were only 11 developing countries with well-established poisons centers (Haines et al., 1988).

The INTOX Project was launched in 1985 with the aim of strengthening capacities in countries to prevent and respond to toxic exposures through: (a) the development of guidance and training materials; (b) the preparation and dissemination of internationally peer reviewed, evaluated information; (c) the provision of information management tools and promotion of harmonized international data exchange; and (d) networking. Over 100 professionals from over 70 poisons information, clinical and analytical toxicology units and related facilities from all regions of the world have participated in the project and contributed to the development of materials and tools. These are briefly described later. The project launch was enabled, in part, by a grant from the International Development Research Centre of Canada (IDRC), which was itself supporting the establishment of poisons centers in Cairo (Egypt), Colombo (Sri Lanka), Manila (Philippines), and Montevideo (Uruguay). These centers were all active in the INTOX project.

Guidance and training materials

Guidelines for poison control (IPCS, 1997). Available in English, French, Russian, and Spanish, this unique guidance provides a policy overview of a poison control program and describes the necessary facilities and technical resources for a poison center. This book has now been extensively updated to reflect new developments and is published under the title: *Guidelines for establishing a poison centre* (WHO, 2020a).

Basic analytical toxicology (Flanagan et al., 1995). This manual provides information on simple laboratory techniques, such as thin layer chromatography and spot tests, for use in hospitals to support the diagnosis and treatment of toxic exposures. It is available in English, French, and Thai.

Management of poisoning (Henry and Wiseman, 1997). This was a handbook for health care workers on diagnosis and treatment of toxic exposures in settings without access to advanced hospital facilities. It is now out of print. Updated information on the management of selected poisonings has been published by WHO in the *IMAI district clinician manual: hospital care for adolescents and adults*, which provides guidelines for the management of illnesses where resources are limited (WHO, 2012).

Guidelines on the prevention of toxic exposures: education and public awareness activities (IPCS, 2004). These guidelines were developed to help governments, national agencies and communities plan, carry out and evaluate education campaigns to promote the prevention of poisoning.

Poisons center training manual: Training materials for poisons information staff (IPCS, 2013). This is available in a trainer's and trainee's version. It provides an overview of training methods for poisons information staff and materials on specific aspects of poisons center operations.

Evaluated information

At the launch of the INTOX project, an important need was identified for a package of evaluated information on the toxicity of chemicals and toxins, and on the diagnosis and management of poisoning (IPCS, 1989). A series of international working groups was convened by IPCS to identify the priority substances and then to develop and review these information materials. Three types of materials were developed: poisons information monographs (PIMs), treatment guides, and antidote evaluations.

Poisons information monographs (PIMs) were published on 294 chemicals, pharmaceuticals and venomous or toxic animals, plants, fungi, and bacteria. For each agent, the documents summarized the physicochemical and toxicological properties, toxic effects, patient management, and supporting analytical investigations. The monographs were published in the INTOX (discussed later) and INCHEM databanks. Production of the monographs stopped in 2002.

Treatment guides dealt with specific clinical features of toxic exposures, such as methemoglobinemia and acute anticholinergic syndrome. Over 40 treatment guides were developed, some of which were translated into French, Portuguese, and Spanish. The guides were included in the INTOX Databank.

Antidote evaluations were developed in a joint project with the European Commission. An expert group identified the antidotes and ancillary agents routinely used in the management of poisoning, categorized by strength of evidence for efficacy and the urgency of use (Pronczuk de Garbino et al., 1997). For each antidote, information was presented on its clinical use, mode of action, administration, contraindications, and precautions. Three volumes were published as books: (1) naloxone, flumazenil and dantrolene; (2) antidotes for poisoning by cyanide; and (3) antidotes for poisoning by paracetamol, and 3 electronically; atropine, diazepam, and deferoxamine. All are in the INCHEM databank.

As was usual at the time, these evaluations were developed by one or two authors by literature review, followed by peer review by an international group of experts in clinical toxicology. This procedure was relatively low cost and enabled a large amount of material to be developed over a fairly short period of time. Since 2008, WHO has required a more systematic procedure for the development of treatment guidelines, using guideline methodologists; standard tools for synthesis and evaluation of evidence quality; and the use of a transparent and documented process (WHO, 2014). While this has undoubtedly assured the quality and reliability of treatment guidelines published by WHO, it has also increased the cost and time involved. It is no longer possible to produce the same volume of treatment guidance materials as were developed during the 1990s. In parallel the need for WHO to produce such material has decreased due to extensive development of electronic clinical toxicology databases, available for use by poisons centers around the world, albeit sometimes for a fee. There has also been a huge growth in the amount of good quality peer-reviewed information on chemicals freely available on the Internet.

Information management tools

In the 1990s a data management package was developed with the technical assistance of the Canadian Centre for Occupational Health and Safety (CCOHS) and the Quebec Toxicology Centre to assist poison center establishment. The INTOX Data Management System comprised an electronic tool for collecting and managing data on toxic exposures and a mechanism for uploading PIMs. The data collection component was available in English, French, Portuguese, and Spanish and could be used to document and retrieve inquiries to the poisons information service and to generate statistics. The system included controlled, defined terminology (authority lists) for routinely collected types of information, and classification schemes for substances and products. It also incorporated the poisoning severity score (PSS), a harmonized severity grading scheme for use by poisons information services, developed in cooperation with the European Association of Poisons Centres and Clinical Toxicologists and with the support of the Swedish Poisons Information Centre (Persson et al., 1998). Although work was undertaken to develop and test a harmonized system for describing clinical features of cases, resources were not available to complete and incorporate a clin-tox score into the INTOX system.

These components were intended to promote the collection of comparable data within the poisons center itself, within a country or region, and internationally with the goal of assessing poisoning cases and toxic risks in different regions, promoting toxicovigilance and poisons prevention. To encourage the use of the INTOX Data Management System by poisons centers, there was the possibility of customization. Ultimately, however, this limited the degree to which harmonized data could be aggregated.

The INTOX Data Management System was eventually used by around a dozen poisons centers, including in Australia, Brazil, Chile, India, Malaysia, Morocco, the Philippines, and South Africa. As it was never financially self-sustaining, the system was terminated around 2016. The data collection format, authority lists and classifications have, however, been used as the basis for poison center databases in other countries, and have informed discussions within the European Commission about harmonized poisons center reporting.

The INTOX Data Management System included the INTOX Databank, with PIMS, treatment guides, antidote monographs, the books *Management of Poisoning* and *Basic Analytical Toxicology*, International Chemical Safety

Cards, Environmental Health Criteria documents, and CCOHS CHEMINFO databases and other chemical information. As there was overlap in INTOX and INCHEM databank content, due to financial pressures the INTOX Databank was terminated.

Networking

Networking between poisons centers is facilitated through international working groups and training activities, and through the maintenance of a Listserv called INTOX-General through which information can be shared and questions answered. WHO also publishes an interactive map and database of poisons centers (WHO, 2021). INTOX meetings have stimulated formation of regional networks and associations, such as the Asia-Pacific Association of Medical Toxicology.

Some WHO regional offices have established their own networks of poisons centers. The Regional Office for the Americas (also known as the Pan-American Health Organization) maintains two long-standing networks of clinical toxicologists and toxicology centers (RETOXLAC), and toxicology laboratories (Red de Laboratorios en Toxicología). The African Regional Office established the African Network of Poison Control Centers in 2018. The Eastern Mediterranean Regional Office established its poisons center network in 2019.

Other work on poisons centers

With the support of its clinical toxicology network, IPCS and the WHO regional offices have carried out training activities on poisons centers and management of poisoning in countries. In 2012–2013, IPCS conducted a study into the feasibility of establishing a subregional poisons center to serve countries in east Africa (WHO, 2015b).

Chemical incidents

In parallel with the INTOX project, IPCS started a project to improve the public health management of chemical incidents, working with the WHO Regional Office for Europe, OECD and UNEP. IPCS contributed to guidance published by these organizations and also published its own guidance on the public health management of chemical incidents (WHO, 2009). It has also contributed to WHO guidance on exposure to chemical weapons (WHO, 2004).

Other WHO work relating to toxicology

There are some specific toxicological issues where WHO carries out work, involving IPCS, the regional chemical safety units, other WHO programs and other intergovernmental organizations. These are described briefly later.

Toxicity and safe use of pesticides

During the period 1998–2003, IPCS and the chemical safety units in the regional offices for south-east Asia and the Americas worked on a number of projects to improve data collection on pesticide exposure using community-based studies (WHO Regional Office for South-East Asia, 2001; Henao and Arbelaez, 2002). To standardize data collection and improve comparability, a pesticides exposure record was developed, providing a standard format for collecting a core dataset on human exposures to pesticides (IPCS, 2020b).

WHO, in partnership with UNEP and the University Sains Malaysia, developed a training package on pesticide poisoning called *Sound management of pesticides and diagnosis and treatment of pesticide poisoning* (WHO, 2006).

WHO has had a long-standing program to evaluate the safety of pesticides used for vector control, provide guidance on their use, and promote the development of safer products and approaches to pest control (WHO, 2020b).

IPCS maintains the *WHO Recommended Classification of Pesticides by Hazard* (updated 2019), which categorizes pesticide formulations according to their acute risk to human health (WHO, 2019a). The classification is widely used by pesticide regulators to support decisions on pesticide registration and use, and on banning or restricting highly hazardous pesticides.

Pesticide ingestion is a common means of suicide in rural areas in many countries. Therefore, in the early 2000s the WHO Department of Mental Health and Substance Misuse launched a global public health initiative to reduce morbidity and mortality related to pesticide poisoning. Activities included coordination of community-based projects to restrict access to pesticides through safe storage (WHO, 2016), and the development of a resource guide for pesticide regulators (WHO, 2019b). A short guide on the clinical management of acute pesticide poisoning was also developed (WHO, 2008).

Prevention and management of snakebite

Snakebite has long been recognized as a serious public health problem in many countries in Africa, Asia, and Latin America. Regional guidelines have been published on the prevention and management of snakebite in Africa (WHO Regional Office for Africa, 2010) and south-east Asia (WHO Regional Office for South-East Asia, 2016). The major challenge, however, is in accessing antivenom for treatment. Snakebite was first recognized by WHO as a neglected tropical disease in 2008. But without a clear mandate to address this issue, it was difficult to mobilize resources and establish a program. In 2018, however, there was sufficient support from Member States for a World Health Assembly resolution, resulting in the launch of a WHO strategy on the prevention and management of snakebite in 2019 (WHO, 2019c). One of the objectives is to improve the availability of antivenoms in countries where snakebite is a problem.

Improving the availability of antidotes

The lack of antidotes and antitoxins presents a challenge for the management of poisoning cases in many low and middle-income countries. The WHO Model List of Essential Medicines provides a guide to countries about the medicines that should be included in national formularies and it includes selected antidotes (WHO, 2019d). Antidote cost is a major hurdle to purchase and use by hospitals. To address this problem, in 2019 the WHO Regional Office for South-East Asia, in collaboration with the Ministry of Health of Thailand started piloting the regional procurement of selected antidotes (WHO Regional Office for South-East Asia, 2019).

Challenges

Although much has been achieved, a key problem for the WHO is its requirement for formal mandating of activities by its governing body, the World Health Assembly (WHA), and the fact that a significant part of the WHO budget is for programs specified by donors. There was a high level of interest in funding poisons center activities in the 1980s and 1990s, which then tailed off. Moreover, WHO can only do so much—the governments of countries wishing to establish poisons centers must commit long-term funding for premises, personnel, equipment, and so on, and this can be difficult.

As of 2019, the majority of countries still did not have a poisons center. There is, however, a stronger WHO mandate to support countries in establishing centers. This comes from the International Health Regulations (IHR) which identify poisons centers as a core capacity for the detection, alert and response to public health events caused by chemicals (WHO, 2015a). Furthermore, the establishment and strengthening of poison centers is a priority action for governments in the *WHO Chemicals Road Map,* which was endorsed by the 70th WHA (WHO, 2017). This reinforces the role of the health sector in reaching the goals of the Strategic Approach to International Chemicals Management.

Conclusions

Since its first decades, WHO has had programs for evaluating the toxicity of chemicals to assist regulatory authorities in protecting the population from harmful exposures. The growing movement for international environmental governance, led by the UN, gave WHO additional mandates to strengthen capacities for the prevention and management of chemical exposures and poisoning. By the 1980s, WHO recognized the important role that poisons centers could play in both chemical safety and public health. WHO developed a program to support the establishment and strengthening of these services, particularly in low- and middle-income countries. Much was achieved in terms of developing information management tools, harmonization of data collection, and providing access to poisons information materials. Participation in working groups and training activities has benefited professionals by providing opportunities for sharing experiences and knowledge. A reduction in donor support for the some of the above activities, coupled with the development of alternative sources of poisons information has resulted in a refocusing of WHO's work toward training, policy development, and improving the availability of existing information.

References

Flanagan RJ, Braithwaite RA, Brown SS, Widdop B, de Wolff FA. Basic analytical toxicology. Geneva: World Health Organization & International Programme on Chemical Safety; 1995. Accessed 21 September 2020 https://apps.who.int/iris/handle/10665/37146.

Haines JA, Berlin A, van der Venne MT, Govaerts M, Roche L. Report of the survey of poison control centres and related toxicological services 1984–1986. J Toxicol Clin Exp 1988;8:313–71.

Henao S, Arbelaez MP. Epidemiological situation of acute pesticide poisoning in the central American isthmus, 1992-2000. Epidemiol Bull 2002;23:5–9.

Henry JA, Wiseman HM. Management of poisoning: A handbook for health care workers. Geneva: World Health Organization & International Programme on Chemical Safety; 1997.

IARC. IARC Monographs on the identification of carcinogenic hazards to humans: questions and answers [online]. Lyon: International Agency for Research on Cancer; 2019. Accessed 21 September 2020 https://monographs.iarc.fr/wp-content/uploads/2018/07/QA_ENG.pdf.

IPCS. Record of the first meeting of the poison centre working group for the project to develop a poisons information package for developing countries, 7–11 March 1988, London. Geneva: World Health Organization & International Programme on Chemical Safety; 1989. Accessed 21 September 2020 https://apps.who.int/iris/handle/10665/62276.

IPCS. Guidelines for poison control. Geneva: World Health Organization & International Programme on Chemical Safety; 1997. Accessed 21 September 2020 https://apps.who.int/iris/handle/10665/41966.

IPCS. Guidelines on the prevention of toxic exposures: Education and public awareness activities. Geneva: World Health Organization & International Programme on Chemical Safety; 2004. Accessed 21 September 2020 https://apps.who.int/iris/handle/10665/42714.

IPCS. Poisons Centre training manual: Training materials for poisons information staff: trainer's version. Geneva: World Health Organization & International Programme on Chemical Safety; 2013. Accessed 21 September 2020 https://apps.who.int/iris/handle/10665/329502.

IPCS. INCHEM Databank. Accessed 21 September 2020 http://www.inchem.org/#/search; 2020a.

IPCS. Improving availability of information about human exposures to pesticides [online]. World Health Organization & International Programme on Chemical Safety; 2020b. Accessed 21 September 2020 https://www.who.int/ipcs/poisons/pesticides/en/.

OECD. eChemPortal. Accessed 21 September 2020 https://www.echemportal.org/echemportal/; 2020.

Persson HE, Sjöberg GK, Haines JA, de Garbino JP. Poisoning severity score. Grading of acute poisoning. J Toxicol Clin Toxicol 1998;36:205–13.

Pronczuk de Garbino J, Haines JA, Jacobsen D, Meredith T. Evaluation of antidotes: activities of the international programme on chemical safety. J Toxicol Clin Toxicol 1997;35:333–43.

UN. Report of the United Nations conference on the human environment, Stockholm, 5-16 June 1972. New York: United Nations; 1973. Accessed 21 September 2020 https://digitallibrary.un.org/record/523249?ln=en.

UN. United Nations Conference on Environment and Development, Agenda 21, Rio de Janeiro, 3–14 June 1992: paragraph 19.49(f). New York: United Nations; 1992. Accessed 21 September 2020 https://sustainabledevelopment.un.org/content/documents/Agenda21.pdf.

WHO. Human environment. World Health Assembly, 23. Geneva: World Health Organization; 1970. Accessed 21 September 2020 https://apps.who.int/iris/handle/10665/91738.

WHO. WHO's human health and environment programme. World Health Assembly, 26. Geneva: World Health Organization; 1973. Accessed 21 September 2020 https://apps.who.int/iris/handle/10665/92151.

WHO. Evaluation of the effects of chemicals on health. World Health Assembly, 31. Geneva: World Health Organization; 1978. Accessed 21 September 2020 https://apps.who.int/iris/handle/10665/93426.

WHO. Public health response to biological and chemical weapons: WHO guidance. 2nd ed. Geneva: World Health Organization; 2004. Accessed 21 September 2020 https://apps.who.int/iris/handle/10665/42611.

WHO. Sound management of pesticides and diagnosis and treatment of pesticide poisoning. Geneva: World Health Organization & United Nations Environment Programme; 2006. Accessed 9 April 2021 https://www.who.int/publications/i/item/WHO-PCS-94.3-Revision-2006.

WHO. Clinical management of acute pesticide intoxication: prevention of suicidal behaviours. Geneva: World Health Organization; 2008. Accessed 21 September 2020 https://apps.who.int/iris/handle/10665/44020.

WHO. Manual for the public health management of chemical incidents. Geneva: World Health Organization; 2009. Accessed 21 September 2020 https://apps.who.int/iris/handle/10665/44127.

WHO. IMAI district clinician manual: hospital care for adolescents and adults. Volume 1. Geneva: World Health Organization; 2012. Accessed 21 September 2020 https://apps.who.int/iris/handle/10665/77751.

WHO. WHO handbook for guideline development. 2nd ed. Geneva: World Health Organization; 2014. Accessed 21 September 2020 https://apps.who.int/iris/handle/10665/145714.

WHO. International Health Regulations (2005) and chemical events. Geneva: World Health Organization; 2015a. Accessed 21 September 2020 https://apps.who.int/iris/handle/10665/249532.

WHO. Improving the availability of poison centre services in Eastern Africa: highlights from a feasibility study for a subregional poison centre in the Eastern Africa subregion. Geneva: World Health Organization; 2015b. Accessed 21 September 2020 https://apps.who.int/iris/handle/10665/183149.

WHO. Safer access to pesticides: experiences from community interventions. Geneva: World Health Organization; 2016. Accessed 21 September 2020 https://apps.who.int/iris/handle/10665/246233.

WHO. Road map to enhance health sector engagement in the Strategic Approach to International Chemicals Management towards the 2020 goal and beyond. Geneva: World Health Organization; 2017. Accessed 21 September 2020 https://apps.who.int/iris/handle/10665/273137.

WHO. World directory of poison centres [online]. World Health Organization; 2021. Accessed 9 April 2021 https://www.who.int/data/gho/data/themes/topics/indicator-groups/poison-control-and-unintentional-poisoning.

WHO. The WHO recommended classification of pesticides by hazard and guidelines to classification 2019. Geneva: World Health Organization; 2019a. Accessed 21 September 2020 https://www.who.int/publications/i/item/9789240005662.

WHO. Preventing suicide: a resource for pesticide registrars and regulators. Geneva: World Health Organization & Food and Agriculture Organization of the United Nations; 2019b. Accessed 21 September 2020 https://apps.who.int/iris/handle/10665/326947.

WHO. Snakebite envenoming - A strategy for prevention and control. Geneva: World Health Organization; 2019c. Accessed 21 September 2020 https://www.who.int/snakebites/resources/9789241515641/en/.

WHO. The selection and use of essential medicines: report of the WHO Expert Committee on Selection and Use of Essential Medicines, 2019 (including the 21st WHO Model List of Essential Medicines and the 7th WHO Model List of Essential Medicines for Children). Geneva: World Health Organization; 2019d. Accessed 21 September 2020 https://apps.who.int/iris/handle/10665/330668.

WHO. Guidelines for establishing a poison centre. Geneva: World Health Organization; 2020a. Accessed 9 April 2021 https://apps.who.int/iris/handle/10665/338657.

WHO. Technical guidance for management of public health pesticides [online]. World Health Organization; 2020b. Accessed 21 September 2020 https://www.who.int/neglected_diseases/vector_ecology/pesticide-management/who_fao_guidelines/en/.

WHO, ILO. International Chemical Safety Cards. Geneva: World Health Organization & International Labour Organization; 2020. Accessed 21 September 2020 https://www.ilo.org/safework/info/publications/WCMS_113134/lang--en/index.htm.

WHO Regional Office for Africa. Guidelines for the prevention and clinical management of snakebite in Africa. Brazzaville: World Health Organization Regional Office for Africa; 2010. Accessed 21 September 2020 https://apps.who.int/iris/handle/10665/204458.

WHO Regional Office for South-East Asia. Pesticide poisoning database in SEAR countries. New Delhi: World Health Organization Regional Office for South-East Asia; 2001. Accessed 21 September 2020 https://apps.who.int/iris/handle/10665/205615.

WHO Regional Office for South-East Asia. Guidelines for the management of snakebites. 2nd ed. New Delhi: World Health Organization Regional Office for South-East Asia; 2016. Accessed 21 September 2020 https://apps.who.int/iris/handle/10665/249547.

WHO Regional Office for South-East Asia. Access to medical products in the South-East Asia region 2019: review of progress. New Delhi: World Health Organization Regional Office for South-East Asia; 2019. Accessed 21 September 2020 https://apps.who.int/iris/handle/10665/326829.

Chapter 5.14

The European Association of Poisons Centres and Clinical Toxicologists (EAPCCT)

D. Nicholas Bateman
Honorary Professor of Clinical Toxicology, University of Edinburgh, Edinburgh, United Kingdom

Although many medical and scientific societies existed when poison centers (PC) were established in Europe in the 1960s, there was no natural academic home for them to present and discuss their activities. Both the editors and societies sponsoring specialist journals were less interested in publishing material about the activity of poison centers rather than cases of poisoning. In the 1960s the fledgling poisons information centers across Europe came together to form an association (Person private communication, 2004; Persson and Hulten, 2014). Precise details of who made the first initiatives are lost in time, however, there is no doubt that the French were a driving force in the association's formation. The individual then appointed as the treasurer and conference editor for the first event, Louis Roche, was important in the early days. The first academic meeting in Tours in 1964 established the *Association Europeene des Centres de Lutte Control les Poisons* (European Association of Poisons Control Centres) and its officers were: president, Prof Gaultier, 7 vice-presidents, from Czechoslovakia (Teisnger), Belgium (Govaerts), United Kingdom (Goulding), France (Valet), Italy (Gerin), Norway (Wickstrom), and Netherlands (van Raalte). The general secretary was Prof Fournier and treasurer Prof Roche. (Person private communication, 2004) Following the Tours meeting in 1966, the original constitution set forth seven objectives:

(a) to collaborate with international organizations, and, in particular, the World Health Organization (WHO) European regional office,
(b) to establish and maintain effective collaboration with governments, governmental organizations, professional bodies, and other groups or individuals concerned with those problems, to promote in all countries of Europe, of means of research and of action appropriate to each of them,
(c) to assemble the studies, observations, and data essential to the understanding of poisoning,
(d) to promote and conduct scientific research and investigations for the study of poisoning,

History of Modern Clinical Toxicology. https://doi.org/10.1016/B978-0-12-822218-8.00056-9

505

(e) to supply information and advice in this field through information centers in Europe,

(f) to set up a Secretariat with responsibility for realizing the objectives of the Association, and

(g) to accept and administer gifts and bequests … of every kind of nature without restriction as to amount to a value and to use the same for furthering the aims of the Association.

The Association included three categories of members: founder members (those present and applying for membership at the first two congresses), regular members and associated members, all to pay an annual subscription. Rules were also set out for a General Assembly (every 2 years), voting procedure, and a quorum on decisions. The governing body included a president, a general secretary and representatives from countries across Europe. How they were selected was up to local country associations, but since many countries did not have such associations this arrangement would seem rather undemocratic from today's perspective. It also occasionally caused other problems. For example, one discussion on a country's Board membership was anecdotally settled by referring to the countries listed as members of the Union of European Football Associations (UEFA). Since the association had very limited funds, board members had to pay their own travel and accommodation when attending meetings.

Early meetings

At the first meeting in Tours in 1964 a focus on certain aspects of toxicology and PC working (i.e., toxic mushrooms, poisoning by fungicides, and the importance of liaison between PCs) was adopted as the theme for the Congress. This concept of focusing on important topics as themes continues today. There is no record of attendance by American colleagues at the first meeting in 1964, which had 47 attendees, but Americans were certainly present at the second meeting held in 1966. This was in no small part due to Roche's interest in analytical and forensic toxicology and overseas contacts. This 2nd congress had 94 participants from 24 countries. The predominant use of English in congresses followed later, and thus the 6th Congress in 1974 included abstracts in French, English, and Italian. In 1976, in Utrecht, the congress was predominantly in English, though presentations were occasionally given in French, the last being from Louis Roche in Milan in 1990. Initially, there were Congresses every 2 years, with a smaller academic meeting in the intervening year, and then the EAPCCT moved to an annual cycle of Congresses in 1998.

Progress 1964–1998

Between the formation of the association and the major change that occurred 35 years later in 1999, there were only six presidents: 1964–1966 Michel Gaultier, France; 1966–1974 Roy Goulding, United Kingdom; 1974–1986 Ad van Heijst, The Netherlands; 1986–1992 Hans Persson, Sweden; 1992–1998 Allister Vale, United Kingdom; 1998–2002 Albert Jaeger, France.

There were only five General Secretaries in this time frame: 1964–1970 Etiénne Fournier, France; 1970–1972 Pierre Gervais, France; 1972–1980 Enrico Malizia, Italy; 1980–1996 Elsa Wickstrøm, Norway; 1996–2000 Jan Meulenbelt, Netherlands. The length of service of Ad van Heijst and Elsa Wickstrøm, 12 and 16 years, respectively, is quite remarkable, bearing in mind the time frames set out in the first constitution and speaks to their enthusiasm. In 35 years, there had been only 2 treasurers, 1964–1991 Monique Govaerts, 1991–2000 Martine Mostin, both based in Belgium as that was where the EAPCCT held its bank accounts and had formally registered its constitution in 1966.

The EAPCCT became active internationally. Its officers played a key role in setting up a World Federation in 1975 in Lyon (Govaerts, 1985). At its peak the World Federation had members in 35 countries, but as the EAPCCT itself and other national societies became stronger and organized international meetings, the Federation weakened and dissolved in 1998. In 1983, the EAPCCT joined the International Union of Toxicology; it has also been a member of EUROTOX since 2011.

Official journal

In the early days, the EAPCCT did not have a formal relationship with an academic journal. Scientific abstracts from its congresses were published intermittently in scientific journals, as negotiated by the host country responsible for the Congress. Regular updates were published in French in the *Bulletin de Médcine Légale et de Toxicologie Médicale*. A newsletter for EAPCCT members was started in 1981. The journal issue was resolved in the 1990s. Following negotiations with the American Academy of Clinical Toxicology (AACT), the American Association of Poison Control Centers (AAPCC), and the publisher, the EAPCCT became formally associated with the journal, then called *Journal of Toxicology: Clinical Toxicology* (since renamed *Clinical Toxicology)* and was accorded membership on the journal's editorial board. This journal is now sponsored by three other major societies in the field: AACT, AAPCC, and the Asia Pacific Association of Medical Toxicology (APAMT).

Second constitution, renaming, and restructuring

In 1999, the name of the association formally changed to the European Association of Poisons Centres and Clinical Toxicologists (EAPCCT). The constitution was revised to set out the current society's objectives:

(a) foster a better understanding of the principles and practice of clinical toxicology to prevent poisoning and to promote better care for the poisoned patient particularly through poisons information centers and poisons treatment centers;

(b) unite into one group individuals whose professional activities are concerned with clinical toxicology whether in a poisons center, university, hospital or in government or industry;

(c) encourage research into all aspects of poisoning;

(d) facilitate the collection, exchange, and dissemination of relevant information among individual members, poison centers and organizations interested in clinical toxicology;

(e) promote training in, and set standards for the practice of, clinical toxicology and to encourage high standards in poisons centers and in the management of poisoned patients generally.

Following this reorganization, a system was established of a rotating president every 2 years. Three classes of members were agreed: member, associate member, and emeritus. The make-up of the Board was agreed as a President, President Elect and immediate Past President, the General Secretary, a Treasurer and nine elected members. A number of committees were also established, the most important being the Scientific Committee. It has the task of reviewing meeting abstracts and setting the program for each annual scientific meeting, with active input by members from other international societies. There were also publications and nominating committees, and special interest groups set up by the President, such as a group to assist the development of centers in Eastern Europe.

In addition, the EAPCCT officers took on the responsibility for organizing Congresses, at some cost and inconvenience to themselves. They negotiated contracts with hotels or congress facilities and any profit was channeled back to the Association. Only in this way did the EAPCCT become solvent, and able to pay for travel for its officials and enable a truly democratic organization to emerge nearly 40 years after its foundation. In 2016, the annual congress attracted over 400 delegates and the Board changed to using a professional congress organizer.

Louis Roche Lectureship

In 1999, the award of a named lectureship was introduced to acknowledge distinction in the specialty. It was named the Louis Roche Lectureship—an appropriate recognition. This lecture is given as a major part of the annual congress. Recipients from Europe, North America, and Australia have been so recognized, and as of 2021 there were 23 individual awardees.

Current EAPCCT activities

The EAPCCT continues to host an annual international congress in different European countries every spring. An Internet website and EAPCCT domain name (https://www.eapcct.org) were acquired in the early 2000s, promoting the organization and its activities to members, as well as providing a portal to the journal.

The website also includes an electronic alerting system so that information on toxic events or products can be rapidly disseminated. A notable early example in 2003 concerned a formulation of a waterproofing product associated with acute lung injury that resulted in rapid product withdrawal. Later events were mass methanol outbreaks in Estonia and the Czech Republic (Paasma et al., 2007).

The EAPCCT, in collaboration with the AACT, developed position statements (published in the journal *Clinical Toxicology*) on common treatments for poisoning, such as gastrointestinal decontamination methods and poison removal by urinary alkalinization in the late 1990s and early 2000s. More recently, EAPCCT is a founder member of the Clinical Toxicology Recommendations Collaborative, a new venture in establishing a unified voice to the management of poisoning across scientific societies worldwide. In 2014, EAPCCT celebrated its 50th birthday and to mark the occasion set up a Fellowship scheme to recognize its more distinguished members.

The EAPCCT has been active in the "European Community on Classification, Labeling and Packaging Regulation and later Cosmetic Regulations" to insure appropriate information is available to poison centers and clinicians treating affected patients. It maintains its relationship with the WHO and has also collaborated with the European project: "Alert System for Health Threats" (ASHT phase I–III) funded by the European Union and run by Public Health England. The EAPCCT also provides a link to educational courses relating to toxicology across its member network. It offers a number of awards at its meetings, including to abstract presenters from economically challenged countries.

Future challenges

The society has grown since its inception, and particularly over the past 20 years. Its congresses are bigger and attract members and guests from all over the world. During the COVID-19 epidemic of 2020 and 2021, the congress was moved to an exclusively Internet-based, 'virtual' format for both live and on-demand presentations of lectures, abstracts, and posters. As the cost of air travel and concerns regarding climate change affect behavior, it will be interesting to see how the model for meetings and such exchanges alters in the next decade.

References

Govaerts DM. World Federation of Associations of clinical toxicology and poison control centres. J Toxicol Clin Exp 1985;5:205–7.

Paasma R, Hovda KE, Tikkerberi A, Jacobsen D. Methanol mass poisoning in Estonia: outbreak in 154 patients. Clin Toxicol 2007;45:152–7.

Persson H. European Association of Poisons Centres and Clinical Toxicologists EAPCCT 1964–2004 A Perspective over Four Decades. EAPCCT Archive. Available on request from https://www.eapcct.org/; 2004.

Persson H, Hulten P. The European Association of Poisons Centres and Clinical Toxicologists (EAPCCT). In: Encyclopedia of toxicology. 3rd ed; 2014. p. 544–6.

Section 6

Clinical toxicology and poison control in Asia and Australia

Alan D. Woolf[a], Jou-Fang Deng[b], and Chen-Chang Yang[b,c]
[a]*Boston Children's Hospital & Harvard Medical School, Boston, Massachusetts, United States,*
[b]*Division of Clinical Toxicology & Occupational Medicine, Department of Medicine, Taipei Veterans General Hospital, Taipei, Taiwan,* [c]*Institute of Environmental & Occupational Health Sciences, School of Medicine, National Yang Ming Chiao Tung University, Taipei, Taiwan*

Introduction

The common interests of people everywhere include avoiding harm from toxins, poisons, venomous creatures, botanicals, and chemicals. There are many clinical toxicologists in Asia and many governmental agencies and non-profit, non-governmental organizations whose mission includes the promotion of a healthy environment by poisoning prevention. They advocate for safeguards against exposure to hazardous substances. In this section, authors from seven countries (Australia, Vietnam, South Korea, Taiwan, China, the Philippines, and Thailand) describe their nation's history of the development of clinical toxicology and poisons information centers.

We also describe here briefly four influential international professional societies that, along with the World Health Organization (see Chapter 5.13 in this book) have assisted countries in Asia and elsewhere achieve their goals in clinical toxicology and poison control and prevention. We apologize to those whose countries, while they may also have interesting histories of clinical toxicology and ongoing poison control, could not be included here because of space considerations.

Asia Pacific Association of Medical Toxicology (APAMT)

The Asia Pacific Association of Medical Toxicology (APAMT) sponsors a Congress each year bringing together clinical toxicologists, researchers and scientists to describe their toxicology research findings and exchange ideas and knowledge. It was founded in 1989 by Dr. Ralph Edwards of Sweden, who was its first president from 1989-1991. Since then, its presidents have included Dr. Mahdi Balali-Mood (Iran 1994–2001), Dr. Jou Fang-Deng (Taiwan 2001–2006), Professor Andrew Dawson (Australia 2006–2008), Dr. Winai Wananukul (Thailand 2008–2010), Dr. Chen-Chang Yang (Taiwan 2010–2012), Dr. Reza Afshari (Iran 2012–2014), Professor Nicholas Buckley (Australia 2015–2016), Dr. Indika Gawarammana (2017–2018), Dr. Ashish Balla (2019–2020) and Dr. Man Li Tee (2021–2022).

The APAMT encourages research collaborations and promotes interdisciplinary awareness of resources and networking between members. APAMT gives out travel awards to its annual congress and confers honorary fellowship status to reward prominent leaders in clinical toxicology. APAMT is a co-sponsor of the professional journal: *Clinical Toxicology*. Its leadership includes an elected president, secretary-general and treasurer; and a governing board of directors. https://www.apamt.org

Asian Society of Toxicology (ASIATOX)

The Asian Society of Toxicology (ASIATOX) was established in 1994 by the founding member societies of Japan, Korea, Thailand, China and Taiwan. ASIATOX was created with the main objectives to foster scientific cooperation among Asian countries and promote progress in toxicological sciences in the Asian region, in particular by sponsoring "The International Congress of ASIATOX." The first scientific congress was held in Yokohama, Japan, organized by Professor Tomoji Yanagita, the founding president of ASIATOX. The International Congress of ASIATOX was then held once every 3 years in a sequence of Korea, Thailand, China, Taiwan, Japan, Korea and Thailand. The next congress will be held in Hangzhou, China in 2021, and it then will be held every other year by different hosting country member societies. In addition to the 5 founding member societies, the Iranian Society of Toxicology, Singapore Toxicology Society, and Malaysian Society of Toxicology also have joined the ASIATOX in the past few years.

The future objectives of ASIATOX include (1) the recruitment of new member societies; (2) the provision of an education and training platform; (3) the certification and accreditation of toxicologists; (4) publication of a newsletter; (5) the establishment of awards (Merit Award, Young Toxicologist Award, Best Presentation Award), and (6) the establishment of a permanent headquarters. https://www.asiatox.com

International Union of Toxicologists (IUTOX)

The International Union of Toxicology (IUTOX) is a confederation of toxicology societies from around the world. It was founded in 1980 by 13 national and regional toxicology societies to bring together toxicologists from academia, governments, and industry. Currently, it has more than 63 contributing professional societies and agencies representing more than 25,000 toxicologists worldwide. IUTOX achieves its vision by "fostering international scientific cooperation for the global acquisition and utilization of knowledge in toxicology for improvement of the health of humans and their environment" (taken from its website). Its mission is to improve human health through the science and practice of toxicology. It achieves this vision by fostering international scientific cooperation for the global acquisition and utilization of knowledge in toxicology for improvement of the health of humans and their environment. Delegates who serve on the governing Executive Committee are elected by their member societies and change every 3 years. Leadership includes a president, vice-president, director, treasurer and secretary-general. Committees include scientific, education, nominating, finances and fundraising, developing countries and communications. IUTOX offers a variety of resources, including sponsorship of international meetings, webinars, newsletters, and shared information and meetings with other societies. It issues awards in toxicology and fosters collaboration between members on projects and promotes such activities through grants and sponsorship. https://www.iutox.org/about.asp

Middle East & North African Clinical Toxicology Association (MENATOX)*

The Middle East and North Africa Clinical Toxicology Association (MENATOX) was established and incorporated in the U.S. in 2014 by its founder and current president, Dr. Ziad Kazzi. In May 2018, MENATOX received a Federal Tax Exempt Status from the U.S. as a 501(c)(3) non-profit organization.

MENATOX is a professional organization dedicated to the care of the poisoned patient in the Middle East and North Africa (MENA) region, defined geographically as Algeria, Bahrain, Djibouti, Egypt, Iran, Iraq, Israel, Jordan, Kuwait, Lebanon, Libya, Malta, Morocco, Oman, Palestinian Authority, Qatar, Saudi Arabia, Sudan, Syria, Tunisia, United Arab Emirates, and Yemen. The purpose of MENATOX is to study of problems related to all forms of toxicological exposures. MENATOX will engage in interdisciplinary research, education, prevention and treatment of poisonings from

---

* Information obtained from its website: www.menatox.org.

chemicals, drugs of abuse, pharmaceutical agents, and other toxins in humans. MENATOX will also engage in interdisciplinary research, education, prevention and treatment of exposures to ionizing radiation. In pursuance of these objectives, MENATOX will (taken from the website):

1. Foster a better understanding of the principles and practice of clinical toxicology in order to prevent poisoning and to promote better care for the poisoned patient, particularly through poison information and treatment centers;
2. Unite individuals whose professional activities are concerned with clinical toxicology whether in a poison center, academic institution, health care facility or in government or industry;
3. Encourage basic and clinical research in all aspects of poisonings and overdoses;
4. Facilitate the collection, exchange, and dissemination of relevant information among individual members, poison centers and organizations interested in clinical toxicology;
5. Promote training in and set standards for the practice of clinical toxicology and encourage high standards in poison centers and in the management of poisoned patients generally;
6. Collaborate with international organizations including the World Health Organization, European Association of Poisons Centres and Clinical Toxicologists, American College of Medical Toxicology, American Academy of Clinical Toxicology, Asia-Pacific Association of Medical Toxicology, and others.
7. Establish and maintain effective collaborations with governmental agencies, professional bodies, nongovernmental organizations, and other relevant groups or individuals involved with the practice, education and research of clinical toxicology.

MENATOX continues to grow, remaining always adaptable, motivated and responsive to the needs of the diverse Middle East & North Africa region. The world of clinical toxicology is an exciting area in which MENATOX members continue to meet and bring inspired people together. https://www.menatox.org.

Chapter 6.1

Australia

Andrew Dawson[a,b], Nicole Wright[b], and Ian Whyte[c]

[a]Clinical Toxicology and Drug Health, Royal Prince Alfred Hospital, Sydney, NSW, Australia,
[b]New South Wales Poisons Information Centre, Children's Hospital Westmead, Sydney, NSW,
Australia, [c]Department of Clinical Toxicology and Pharmacology, Calvary Mater Newcastle,
Waratah, NSW, Australia

Poison information centers

Poisons Information Centers (PICs) started in Australia in the 1960s and by the 1970s a PIC existed in five states and one territory. Each PIC was based within a public hospital with the funding coming from within the budget of the local facility. Each state's Ministry of Health supported the facilities but with no specific budget allocation for the PICs. Budget pressure within individual hospitals contributed to the closure of PICs in South Australia and the Australian Capital Territory by the mid-1990s. States and territories without a local PIC then negotiated on a per call basis for their supply of poisons information from the remaining PICs (New South Wales, Queensland, Victoria, and Western Australia).

There are currently four PICs operating in Australia. The Victorian Poisons Information Center started in 1962 at the Royal Children's Hospital until 2008, when the center moved to the Austin Hospital to coordinate with the Austin Hospital Clinical Toxicology Service. The New South Wales (NSW) PIC, formed in 1966 at the Royal Alexandra Hospital for Children in Sydney, began as an office-hours service (Byrne, 1976). It expanded in the early 1970s to 18 h of staff coverage daily (0600 till midnight) with after-hours calls taken by medical house staff within the Children's Hospital. In 1986, NSW Health agreed to provide for 24-h coverage with Specialist Poisons Information officers (SPIs). In 1995, the service relocated to the Children's Hospital at Westmead and provided services to NSW, Tasmania and the Australian Capital Territory. The Western Australian Poisons Information Center provides telephone consultation to the public and medical professionals in Western Australia, South Australia, and the Northern Territory. It opened in the Princess Margaret Hospital for Children in 1966 and moved to the Sir Charles Gairdner Hospital, Perth, in 1999. The Queensland Poisons Center has been operating since 1973 and is in the Pharmacy Department of the Royal Children's Hospital, Brisbane.

History of Modern Clinical Toxicology. https://doi.org/10.1016/B978-0-12-822218-8.00031-4

National toll-free telephone number

A national poison center toll-free call number was established in 1991. The telephone service identifies the source of the call and connects the caller to the PIC that provides the service to that locality. PICs take calls from the public (170,000 calls per annum) and health professionals (30,000 calls per annum) (Huynh et al., 2018). There are no direct charges to members of the public or health professionals to use the PIC services. PIC services to the general public have been shown to produce healthcare savings of at least three times the cost of the PIC service (Huynh et al., 2020). From 0800 to 2200, each PIC takes calls from its own state plus those jurisdictions with whom the PIC has a contractual agreement. After 2200 h, the four PICs contribute to a roster with a single PIC providing the national service. Each jurisdiction's Ministry of Health pays the PIC for taking those calls.

PIC staffing and data collection

Originally, a card index was used for poisons information and logbooks recorded call information. By the late 1980s, PICs recorded call data in an electronic form which later developed into formal call databases. While each PIC database recorded comparable information, the databases only became congruent in 2011 when NSW, Victoria, and Queensland changed to a common database. Audio call recording has been implemented: Victoria and Queensland record SPI calls; since 2019, NSW has recorded SPI and consultant calls. All SPI calls are peer reviewed by the next shift.

Each PIC has an SPI director and a medical director. The primary call staff are SPIs, typically pharmacists or science graduates who have further in-house training in clinical toxicology before taking calls. SPIs have no defined, specific industrial award and so are contracted on various permutations of established awards such as pharmacist or hospital scientist.

Medical consultant toxicologist services

The medical consultant toxicologist service has evolved from a single center to existing in all PICs. Formal consultant medical toxicology services commenced in 1980 from the NSW PIC, initially provided by Drs. Geoffrey Duggin and William Hensley for adults and Dr. Henry Kilham for children. The consultant service was expanded in 1991 by the addition of Professor Susan Pond and further in 1993 by the inclusion of consultants from the Hunter Area Toxicology Service to provide a consultation service for all Australian PICs. The national medical consultant service delivered through the NSW PIC continued to grow with recruitment of Australian emergency physicians trained in medical toxicology in the United States, supplemented by increasing numbers of locally trained clinicians. As the numbers of clinical toxicologists increased, they provided support to their local PIC during the day and contributed to the after-hours national roster. The consultant service was an honorary service until 2011. In 2011, the NSW PIC began to pay consultants on a per call basis with subsequent cross billing to the states and jurisdictions using those services. These costs provided an economic incentive for states and jurisdictions to develop their own consultant services, resulting in paid consultant services with availability 24 h daily being established in the states of Western Australia (2019) and Victoria (2020). Records of toxicology consultations are distributed after each shift to the four PICs for handover and peer review.

Clinical toxicology training

Clinical toxicology is not a recognized subspecialty in Australia although it is a significant component of training in several specialties: clinical pharmacology and toxicology, emergency medicine and intensive care. The de facto standard for peer recognition as a clinical toxicologist and employment within a PIC is recognized postgraduate training in an appropriate specialty, successful completion of postgraduate course work, working within a recognized hospital tertiary toxicology service, and completion of a postgraduate fellowship within a PIC. Since 2004, most Australian clinical toxicologists have also completed a locally developed postgraduate degree in clinical toxicology. This distance learning course was developed under a creative commons license and was initially delivered from the University of Newcastle and then offered to a number of other institutions.

Toxicology medical services

Prior to 1987, consultation services in clinical toxicology existed in Royal Prince Alfred Hospital (Sydney), Royal Brisbane Hospital, Queensland Children's Hospital, and Melbourne Children's Hospitals. The first inpatient, tertiary clinical toxicology service was established in Newcastle in 1987. Tertiary services are characterized by specific funded appointments to run a dedicated admitting service responsible for assessment and treatment of acute toxicology patients. Newcastle provided a model of care with an economic justification and a body of research based on prospective systematic collection of detailed clinical data (Whyte et al., 1997). This, in a growing pool of clinical toxicology expertise linked by the PICs, furnished the stimulus for further clinical toxicology tertiary services and training positions (Isoardi et al., 2017; Parish et al., 2019; Lee et al., 2001).

In Australia, there are now 11 established tertiary toxicology services with a further two in development. These centers provide direct training for clinical toxicologists with a strong emphasis on bedside toxicology.

Toxicology societies

The professional society in Australia and New Zealand for clinical toxicologists and poisons information center staff and those interested in clinical toxicology is the Toxicology and Poisons Network Australasia (TAPNA). It was established in 2013 and runs an annual scientific meeting in addition to regional meetings and postgraduate training. TAPNA and poisons center staff have strong relationships with local medical specialty societies and the regional professional societies in Asia, Europe, and North America.

The major direct international activity for Australian toxicology has been in Asia, notably in research and in the development of postgraduate training. The network of PICs and tertiary clinical toxicology units have had a consistent research output since 1990. Research has been facilitated by the Australian public health system which pays the salaries of all staff. Since 2004 the Australian toxicology community has had increased support from gaining competitive research grants.

Future challenges

The continued challenge for Australian PICs is the fragility of institutionally based funding and governance. While this is unlikely to result in closures of the poisons information system, it has restricted growth in other areas apart from direct call taking. While the PICs work collaboratively, there is no government support for a national framework for clinical toxicology and poisons information.

References

Byrne M. The poisons information centre—its role and scope. Med J Austral 1976;2(1):21–2.

Huynh A, Cairns R, Brown JA, Lynch AM, Robinson J, Wylie C, Buckley NA, Dawson AH. Patterns of poisoning exposure at different ages: the 2015 annual report of the Australian poisons information centres. Med J Austral 2018;209(2):74–9.

Huynh A, Cairns R, Brown JA, Jan S, Robinson J, Lynch AM, Wylie C, Buckley NA, Dawson AH. Health care cost savings from Australian poisons information Centre advice for low risk exposure calls: SNAPSHOT 2. Clin Toxicol 2020;58(7):752–7.

Isoardi KZ, Armitage MC, Harris K, Page CB. Establishing a dedicated toxicology unit reduces length of stay of poisoned patients and saves hospital bed days. Emerg Med Australasia 2017;29(3):310–4.

Lee V, Kerr JF, Braitberg G, Louis WJ, O'Callaghan CJ, Frauman AG, Mashford ML. Impact of a toxicology service on a metropolitan teaching hospital. Emerg Med 2001;13(1):37–42.

Parish S, Carter A, Liu YH, Humble I, Trott N, Jacups S, Little M. The impact of the introduction of a toxicology service on the intensive care unit. Clin Toxicol 2019;57(9):778–83.

Whyte IM, Dawson AH, Buckley NA, Carter GL, Levey CM. Health care. A model for the management of self-poisoning. Med J Austral 1997;167(3):142–6.

Chapter 6.2

The Chinese mainland

Xiangdong Jian and Mei Zeng

Department of Poisoning and Occupational Diseases, Emergency, Qilu Hospital, Cheeloo College of Medicine, Shandong University, Jinan, Shandong, China

Origins

In the early days of its foundation, China began to take the road of industrialization. Subsequently the prevention and control of chemical poisoning became a primary task, and research on chemical toxicity testing and classification became very urgent. Thus in the early 1950s, industrial toxicology was first to develop and was the prelude to the development of modern toxicology in China.

By the early 1960s, food toxicology and dermatotoxicology were rising one after another. On May 23, 1967, China launched the "Five-Two-Three Project," in which toxicology was an important research content. By the 1980s–1990s, along with the exploitation of natural resources, the expanding scope of industrial and agricultural production activities, and the emergence of new materials and substances, toxicology entered a period of rapid development. The Chinese Society of Toxicology (CST) was established in 1993. At that time, domestic poisoning services were scattered in various departments of the state and local governments, and major poisoning events were handled by the government (Gu, 2004; Chen, 2015; Zhou, 2016).

China is a country with a large population and, as the chemical industry flourished, poisoning cases kept happening in increasing numbers. From 1985 to 1990, there were more than 12,000 acute poisoning cases and 304 poisoning deaths recorded in China. In 1992, more than 80,000 cases of pesticide poisoning occurred in 25 provinces. More importantly, some of the poisoning cases were completely preventable, such as the acute benzene poisoning in a chemical plant in Changchun, China in 1991. However, due to the lack of basic knowledge of chemical poisoning and safety measures to prevent poisoning, deaths occurred.

To disseminate chemical poisoning knowledge and strengthen poisoning prevention education, as well as change the management and evaluation of toxic chemicals, it was necessary to establish poisoning information institutions. In 1988, with the support of a World Bank loan from the Ministry of Health, the National Institute of Occupational Health and Poison Control (NIOHP, China

History of Modern Clinical Toxicology. https://doi.org/10.1016/B978-0-12-822218-8.00053-3

CDC) established the China Poison Information System (Xu et al., 1994; Jiang et al., 2016).

NIOHP, Chinese CDC

The National Institute of Occupational Health and Poison Control, Chinese Center for Disease Control and Prevention (NIOHP, China CDC) was established in 1954 (http://www.niohp.net.cn/). It was originally named the "Labor Health Research Institute of the Central Health Research Academy" (renamed the China Academy of Medical Sciences in 1956) and was the first professional academic institution for labor health and occupational disease control and prevention. Professor Zhizhong Wu, the founder of occupational medicine in China, has been a leader of the institute for a long time. With the change of institutional setup and job functions, it became affiliated with the Chinese Center for Preventive Medicine in 1983 (renamed the Chinese Academy of Preventive Medical Sciences in 1985), and then changed to the National Institute of Occupational Health and Poison Control (NIOHP), Chinese CDC in December 2001.

The NIOHP, Chinese CDC is well-known as the national base for the treatment and cure of chemical poisoning. The Chemical Toxicity Tests Center of the Ministry of Health provides doctor's and master's degrees and postdoctoral research in health-related toxicology. The affiliated unit of the industrial Toxicology Specialty Section of the Chinese Society of Toxicology also supports such activities. In addition, the Institute was qualified as a Class A institute by the State Bureau of Technical Supervision on chemical toxicity identification. Presently, its working fields cover occupational health, occupational medicine, poison control, industrial toxicology, etc. The Institute has set up several sections:

- Department of Physical and Chemical Risk Assessment
- Department of Occupational Health Protection and Ergonomics
- Department of Biomarkers and Molecular Epidemiology
- Department of Toxicology
- Department of Poison Control

and other professional departments. The Institute performs a variety of functions including:

1. Occupational health and poisoning control.
2. The management of national chemical poisoning treatment bases and teams, providing technical support for the emergency handling of major occupational health hazards and sudden poisoning incidents.
3. Chemical toxicity identification and quality control of occupational health and poisoning testing laboratories.
4. Scientific research on occupational health and poisoning control.

5. Postgraduate education, continuing education and business training related to occupational health and poisoning control.
6. International communication and cooperation in the field of occupational health and poisoning control, and many others.

The national poisoning treatment system

In 1999, the Poison Control Center of the Chinese Academy of Preventive Medical Sciences (now NIOHP, Chinese CDC) was established, and a national poison counseling hotline was opened. Since then, the national poison control center, subcenters or network hospitals have been established in 11 institutions in 8 provinces and cities. These units have played a key role in local poison prevention and poison control, and they have promoted the formation of a national poison control network.

At the beginning of the 21st century, China's labor force reached more than 740 million, 30% of whom were regularly exposed to toxic or harmful chemicals or radioactive sources. With the rapid development of science, technology and the economy, the types and quantities of harmful toxic substances were increasing. The type of chemical use was expanding rapidly, and all kinds of major acute chemical poisoning events and radiation accidents were on the rise. However, the capacity for emergency rescue was seriously insufficient (Jin and Wang, 2009).

In 2005, the National Development and Reform Commission and National Health Commission of the People's Republic of China issued a circular to build chemical poisoning treatment bases in 30 provinces, municipalities and autonomous regions. The project was carried out according to the national administrative divisions, the population within the jurisdiction, the existing facilities and conditions, the number of toxic enterprises, the number of people engaged in toxic and harmful work, and the characteristics of the production and application of chemicals, as well as the types of toxic hazards and the scope of poisoning events. The project formed a four-level medical treatment network: (1) national, (2) provincial and prefecture-level chemical and nuclear radiation poisoning treatment bases, (3) county-level general treatment institutions, and (4) special treatment points.

By 2016, there were 35 chemical poisoning treatment bases nationwide, including one at the national level and 34 at the provincial level. About 47.1% of provincial-level poisoning treatment bases were located in general hospitals, while the rest were located in specialized hospitals for occupational diseases, pulmonary diseases, and endemic diseases. Among the provincial poisoning treatment bases, 97.1% have dedicated emergency departments, 52.9% have 24-h duty calls, 69.7% use an ADSL network, 21.2% use a LAN network, and 9.1% use dedicated lines (Wang et al., 2016).

Poison information system

In 1988, the Chinese Academy of Preventive Medical Sciences established the China Poison Information System. The information used by the system is obtained partly from relevant international databases and partly from domestic data. It includes poisoning information, literature information, and some auxiliary reference information. The system consists of four parts:

1. *Poison Information Computer Retrieval System*: Including a poison identification database, a physical and chemical properties database, uses and manufacturers, a poison toxicology database, a poisoning diagnosis and treatment database, a poison analysis database, a diagnostic standard database, and a literature database.
2. *INTOX System*: Originating from the joint program activities from ICPS and CTQ.
3. *RTECS (CD-ROM) Retrieval System:* This is a compact disc (1991 version) from the American Silver Platter company, containing more than 100,000 compounds, including toxicity data, irritant data, mutagenesis data, reproductive effect data, as well as test methods, experimental animals, substance concentration and dose, etc.
4. *Chinese Document Title Retrieval System for Chemicals:* Collects domestic medicine, health, environmental protection, chemical industry, agriculture and other relevant journals and literatures.

The system provides an information consultation service about poison and lays the information foundation for the establishment of the national poison control center in China (Xu et al., 1994).

Technical assistance data system for chemical accidents

In the 1990s, with the support of the former Ministry of Chemical Industry, the Shanghai Institute of Occupational Disease for Chemical Industry organized relevant experts and established the Technical Assistance Data System for Chemical Accidents, which was regularly revised and updated. The system includes information on the medical and engineering rescue of poisoning, and involves leakage treatment, extinguishing chemical fires, international accidents, and the regulations and standards of hazardous chemical safety management.

Emergency public reporting system

The Emergency Public Reporting System is one of the subsystems of the China Information System for Diseases Control and Prevention, including acute food poisoning and occupational poisoning. The China Information System for Diseases Control and Prevention is a wide area network covering the CDC at the central, provincial, prefecture (city), county level and medical units at or above the township level. It connects the computer LAN of 31 provincial CDCs and 331 prefecture (city) level CDCs and the computer network of 2863 county (city, district) CDCs. The information system covers disease control, disaster relief and disease prevention, health resource management and other aspects. It was first put into use in 2004 (Wu et al., 2007).

Information platform for acute poisoning incidents

In 2006, the National Health Commission (formerly the Ministry of Health) began to organize the formulation of the health emergency plan for an acute poisoning incident and to develop the supporting technical scheme. To cooperate with the implementation of the program, the NIOHP developed an Internet-based information platform for emergency warning and treatment of sudden poisoning incidents (Yin et al., 2010).

Other poisoning counseling systems

The Pesticide Manual: The software for this manual is designed by experts organized by the Ministry of Agriculture. It is the pesticide database application software with the largest capacity and the most complete data in China. The software has more than 20 databases, such as a pesticide component database, pesticide product database, pesticide-related unit database, environmental toxicology and toxicity database, pesticide use database, and others. It is a reference tool for pesticide research, pesticide application, and emergency treatment of pesticide poisoning.

Other poisoning-related institutions include the National, Provincial and Municipal Medical Products Administration, provincial and municipal Emergency Medicine Storage, provincial and municipal pharmaceutical companies, provincial and municipal Epidemic Prevention Stations, provincial and municipal drug inspection institutes, Public Security Departments, Criminal Investigation Institutes (Divisions), and some professional research institutions and companies (Song and Qin, 2002).

Education, training, and certification

In the 1970s, with the rapid development of the economy, toxicologists were required to solve a series of safety problems, such as the safety evaluation of food, drugs, pesticides and chemical products. By the end of the 1980s, a small number of medical schools began to recruit graduate students majoring in toxicology, followed by undergraduate students, offering courses on "Health Toxicology Basics," and publishing textbooks, monographs, and magazines.

At present, toxicology has developed into an independent scientific system with certain basic theories and experimental means. It has gradually formed many new branches of toxicology, which are intermingled with clinical medicine, preventive medicine, environmental ecology, pharmacy, and other disciplines. At first, the Chinese Preventive Medicine Association set up a Health Toxicology Branch. Then, the Chinese Society of Toxicology (CST) was established in 1993 (http://www.chntox.org/default.aspx). Moreover, most universities actively carry out international academic exchanges and send their students overseas for part of their education (Huang, 2001).

CST is a nonprofit academic organization voluntarily formed by Chinese toxicology scientists and technicians. It is also the academic group with the highest academic level in the field of toxicology in China. In 2009, the CST officially started the work of certifying applicants for qualification in toxicology. By 2019, the CST had successfully conducted the Chinese toxicology certification for 10 consecutive years. The certification has been widely recognized by the relevant national departments and international organizations. The international union of toxicology (IUTOX) has agreed in principle that the professionals who have obtained China's toxicology qualification (DCST) can obtain the "IUTOX Recognized Toxicologist (IRT)" designation through the "green channel." At the same time, to strengthen the training of toxicology personnel, the CST founded the "Chinese Society of Toxicology Continuing Education Working Committee" in 2009 and has successfully held the "Advanced Training Class on Modern Toxicology Basis and Progress" for 10 consecutive years. These activities provide strong support for applicants wishing to qualify for certification in toxicology in China.

Future challenges

With the progress of science and technology, the kinds of poisons that people can contact are increasing day by day, and poisoning incidents happen frequently. The Chinese mainland has a large population, with a wide spectrum of acute poisoning types and a large number of poisoning cases. With a vast territory, different areas are exposed to different poisons, showing different poisoning patterns. The challenges of poisoning treatment, prevention, control and research are enormous. China has always attached great importance to the development of its integrated poisoning information system. But, as time goes by, some of the original database query functions are only single entries. The quality of useful information is low, the utilization rate is low, the application scope is limited, and the case data does not accumulate. Other shortcomings gradually emerge. It is necessary to further integrate, update or rebuild a strong poison information system that can meet the needs of clinical practice, scientific research, and governmental disease prevention and control institutions.

China is the world's largest chemical-producing country, and serious accidents happen from time to time. Our command system of emergency rescue is complex, with many treatment institutions and heavy tasks of organization and coordination. It is of great importance to establish a simple and efficient network command system for poisoning incidents.

In addition, many cities and regions in China still do not have special departments to provide poisoning information services to ordinary citizens. Most of the existing poisoning information systems are designed for the poisoning-related needs of health professionals. It is a continuing challenge to expand the poisoning information service group to meet the needs of the general population and improve their awareness and utilization rate.

References

Chen W. Current developments and future challenges in toxicology. Science Focus 2015;10(5):34–8.

Gu Z. Review and prospect on toxicology of our country. Shanghai J Prev Med 2004;16(6):253–5.

Huang X. Education in toxicology in mainland China. In: The first cross-strait toxicology symposium papers (abstract) collection; 2001. p. 3–4.

Jiang S, Zhang Y, Lang N, et al. Investigation and analysis of awareness rate and cognition status about poisoning consultation hotline. Chinese J Indust Med 2016;29(3):189–92.

Jin Y, Wang S. Problems and suggestions in the project of constructing national medical treatment base for chemical poisoning. Chinese J Indust Med 2009;22(4):313–5.

Song W, Qin C. Status of information consultation system for acute poisoning. J Clin Emerg 2002;3(5):205–7.

Wang S, Yan Jin Y, Nan Lang N, et al. Discussion on the construction of health emergency response capacity of poisoning treatment base. Chinese J Indust Med 2016;29(6):467–8.

Wu D, Hu D, Wu M. The structure and function of the Chinese disease prevention and control information system. Endemic Dis Bull 2007;22(2):65–7.

Xu L, Huo B, Huang W, et al. Establishment of the poison information system. J Hygiene Res 1994;23(II).

Yin Y, Jiang S, Cai J, et al. Brief introduction of information platform for emergency warning and treatment of sudden poisoning incidents. Chinese J Indust Med 2010;23(1):76–7.

Zhou P. Outline of advances in toxicology in China and brief discussion on toxicological research. Chinese J Pharmacol Toxicol 2016;30(12):1250–3.

Chapter 6.3

Taiwan

Chen-Chang Yang[a,b] and Jou-Fang Deng[b]
[a]*Institute of Environmental & Occupational Health Sciences, School of Medicine, National Yang Ming Chiao Tung University, Taipei, Taiwan,* [b]*Division of Clinical Toxicology & Occupational Medicine, Department of Medicine, Taipei Veterans General Hospital, Taipei, Taiwan*

Introduction

Acute poisonings, especially acute pesticide poisoning, used to be a major clinical as well as public health problem in Taiwan (Yang et al., 1996). However, there was neither formal clinical toxicology training nor a poison information service in Taiwan before 1985. The management of patients with acute poisoning primarily relied on emergency physicians and nephrologists who did not have specific training related to the treatment of acute poisonings. Moreover, online resources were generally lacking. Textbooks as well as other paper-based references were often unavailable to attending physicians who cared for acutely poisoned patients, which further complicated their prompt management. In response to the frequent occurrence of acute poisoning incidents in Taiwan, and in line with international trends, Taiwan's first national poison control center (PCC-Taiwan) was finally founded in July 1985. That event began the new era of clinical toxicology in Taiwan.

Poison control centers in Taiwan

Under the auspices of the Ministry of Health & Welfare (formerly known as the Department of Health) and the Taipei Veterans General Hospital (TVGH), PCC-Taiwan (http://www.pcc-vghtpe.tw/tc/index.asp) was founded by Dr. Jou-Fang Deng in July 1985. The center is located in the Division of Clinical Toxicology, Department of Medicine at TVGH and has been in full operation since January 1986 (Yang et al., 1996).

The goal of PCC-Taiwan is to provide prompt and relevant information on the first-aid, prompt diagnosis, and specific treatments (e.g., the use of antidotes or extracorporeal removal of toxicants) of various acute poisonings to both medical personnel and the general public. To achieve the above-mentioned goal, PCC-Taiwan adopted the Poisindex (Micromedex Inc.) database as its main reference library. PCC-Taiwan also established several

History of Modern Clinical Toxicology. https://doi.org/10.1016/B978-0-12-822218-8.00063-6

local databases that included various kinds of domestic toxicants such as pesticides, household products, and natural toxic substances including Chinese herbal medicines. PCC-Taiwan is staffed by a group of well-trained health professionals, including attending physicians (primarily internists), poison information specialists, and trained volunteers, to provide a 24-h telephone consultation service (Yang et al., 1996; Hung et al., 1998). All calls are answered by medical professionals with specific training in clinical toxicology. Information and treatment advice are offered to the public and health care professionals at no charge through the hotline (Telephone Number: #886-2-28717121).

PCC-Taiwan services

Currently, there are 6 physicians, 6 poison information specialists, and more than 10 trained senior medical student volunteers who work together at the PCC-Taiwan to provide 24-h daily telephone consultative services related to, but not exclusive of, the following subjects:

1. First-aid management and treatment of various pesticide poisonings.
2. Emergent management of accidental poisonings related to commonly used household chemicals such as disinfectants and cleaning agents.
3. Emergent management of accidental inhalation and ingestion of environmental pesticides or rodenticides.
4. Emergent treatment of bites and/or stings caused by venomous animals such as venomous snakes and wasp stings.
5. Prompt diagnosis and treatment of conventional drug abuse and new psychoactive substances (NPS) abuse.
6. Inquiries related to the pharmacological, toxicological and chemical properties of various drugs, Chinese herbal medicines and toxicants.
7. Treatment of acute and/or chronic health effects of exposure to numerous industrial chemicals.
8. Treatment and investigation of occupational injuries/diseases related to long-term exposure to specific chemicals.
9. Inquiries related to the range of toxicity and possible clinical symptoms of various poisonings.
10. Inquiries related to laboratory analyses of various acute poisonings such as new psychoactive substances (NPS)-related poisonings.
11. Treatment of animal poisonings.
12. Help in referring acutely poisoned patients to hospitals where advanced therapies (e.g., antidotes or intensive care) are more readily available.

Past poisoning outbreaks managed by PCC-Taiwan

In addition to providing online treatment information, interpretation of laboratory tests, and management options for acutely poisoned patients, PCC-Taiwan also serves as a training center for junior emergency physicians, clinical toxicologists, and poison information specialists in Taiwan as well as other Asian countries. By providing readily accessible service, timely advice and expertise in the treatment of numerous poisonings, PCC-Taiwan has earned an excellent reputation among patients, physicians and governmental agencies in Taiwan. More than that, PCC-Taiwan has also been functioning as a surveillance center to monitor any unusual poisonings. Through this channel, PCC-Taiwan has been involved in the investigation of many major poisoning outbreaks in Taiwan, such as a carbon tetrachloride-related poisoning in a color printing factory (1986), an epidemic of methamphetamine abuse (1990), a chlorine gas leakage-related exposure (1991 and 1992), a Chinese herbs-related podophyllotoxin (*Podophyllum pleianthum*) poisoning (1992), a mollusk-related tetrodotoxin poisoning (1995), a *Sauropus androgynus* poisoning (1995), a consumer terrorism (blackmail) related cyanide poisoning (2005), a fatal paramethoxymethamphetamine (PMMA) poisoning (2006), a leanness enhancing agents-related poisoning (2010), an ethylene chlorohydrin-related homicidal poisoning (2011), a work-related 1-bromopropane poisoning (2013), a thallium poisoning (2014), and many new psychoactive substance (NPS) poisonings (2016–2020).

Other poison control centers in Taiwan

Although PCC-Taiwan is the first and currently the only poison control center in Taiwan, three other poison control centers had been established in Taiwan in the past. All three centers were funded by the Ministry of Health and Welfare. The first of them was founded in 1995 and was located at Kaohsiung Medical University Hospital (KMUH), a tertiary medical center in Southern Taiwan. The center was finally closed in 2008 because it received a limited volume of telephone inquiries per year and most of the calls were either from KMUH or from other hospitals in Kaohsiung. The second and third poison control centers were located at Taichung Veterans General Hospital (a tertiary medical center in Central Taiwan) and Hualien Tzu-Chi Hospital (a tertiary medical center in Eastern Taiwan), respectively. Both centers were in full operation in 2004. Nevertheless, both centers were also closed in 2008 due to the same reason as the poison control center located at KMUH. After 2008, PCC-Taiwan became the only poison control center in Taiwan.

Poisoning data collection

Annually, PCC-Taiwan receives about 4000 (range 3000–5000) telephone inquiries. Collection of all poisoning exposure data is done by using a standardized data collection form. All reported cases are followed until they have a full recovery, die, have irreversible sequelae, or are lost to follow-up. At the end of follow-up, all medical charts are reviewed by a staff physician to decide whether the inquiry was indeed a poisoning case or not. The data of all poisoning cases are then entered into a computerized database for subsequent analysis. In the past three decades, PCC-Taiwan has collected data on nearly 150,000 cases. More than 20 papers have been published in international peer-reviewed journals by using the database. The first paper was published in 1996; it described the epidemiologic data of acute poisoning in Taiwan between 1985 and 1993 (Yang et al., 1996). Other studies have primarily analyzed the characteristics and risk factors of various acute poisonings in Taiwan (Chung et al., 1999; Chen et al., 2009; Lin et al., 2018), and evaluated the effectiveness of specific treatment modalities as well as antidotes (Yang and Deng, 2008; Doan et al., 2019).

Taiwan antidote network

The use of antidotes is one of the major treatment modalities of acute poisonings and is of critical importance in the management of specific poisonings such as methemoglobinemia and cyanide poisoning. In Taiwan, despite the establishment of a nationwide health insurance system in 1995 and easy access to healthcare facilities, the availability of certain antidotes, including methylene blue, cyanide antidotes, digoxin-specific antibody and physostigmine, was quite limited. In the mid-1990s, there were several cases presenting with severe methemoglobinemia after occupational chemical exposures. The workers later died due to the lack of timely treatment with methylene blue. To solve the problem of antidote unavailability and to have a better understanding of insufficient antidote stocking in Taiwan, a preliminary survey of all emergency departments in Taiwan was initiated in 1997 (Ong et al., 2000). Later on, the Center for Control and Administration of Specific Medical Antidotes in Emergencies (http://www.pcc-vghtpe.tw/antidote/) was established in 2000 at TVGH under the financial support of the Ministry of Health & Welfare. The purpose of the Center was to build a nationwide network of antidote stocking to relieve the difficulties faced by hospitals in Taiwan that did not have specific antidotes in toxicological emergencies. The Center also aimed to establish a comprehensive poisoning prevention system to respond to large-scale poisoning accidents.

Based on the findings of the preliminary survey (Ong et al., 2000), the National Antidote Stocking System identified antidotes of first priority that should be purchased and stocked in Taiwan. These antidotes were then collectively imported and distributed across selected hospitals (i.e., distribution sites) in Taiwan. Distribution sites were selected according to the probability of poisonings and suitability for stocking; and the antidotes were distributed according to their level of urgency of need in an emergency. The network consisted of one central control center, three main supply centers and approximately 60 antidote stocking hospitals. The distribution was completed in January 2001. Budgeting, procurement, and replenishment of antidotes were carried out each year according to the usage and expiration dates of the antidotes. A mechanism for the urgent allocation of antidotes in toxicological emergencies (such as chemical accidents) was also established. A website was created for sharing instantaneous information about antidote reserves, together with a reporting system for updates on stocking status, future distribution, data collection, and usage evaluation (Ong and Deng, 2012).

Both the purchase and distribution of antidotes are overseen by a committee that monitors and evaluates the utilization, effectiveness, and the demand for stocked antidotes. The control and supply centers also provide relevant information and emergent consultation services to all healthcare professionals who will use the antidotes. Moreover the antidote control center organizes and delivers educational and training programs to emergency physicians and nurses every year.

Clinical toxicology medical service

The first division of clinical toxicology was established by Dr. Jou-Fang Deng in January 1985 at TVGH. The staff of the division have worked closely with PCC-Taiwan in the last three decades to provide various medical services to all poisoned patients in Taiwan, especially those living in Northern Taiwan. To facilitate the diagnosis of patients with acute and/or chronic poisoning exposures, the division offers numerous toxicological analyses for conventional abuse substances as well as NPS, prescription drugs, Chinese herbal medicines, pesticides, heavy metals, and various chemicals. Currently the toxicology laboratory at TVGH is staffed by 12 medical technologists and/or research assistants and is equipped with various high-tech analytic instruments, including high performance liquid chromatography (HPLC), gas chromatography/mass spectrometry (GC/MS), liquid chromatography/tandem mass spectrometry (LC/MS-MS), quadrupole-time of flight (Q-TOF)/MS, GC/MS-MS, and inductively coupled plasma mass spectrometry (ICP-MS). In addition to routine analysis of the samples (blood, urine and hair) of poisoned patients, the toxicology laboratory has also been involved in the investigation of certain unusual poisoning outbreaks (Wu et al., 2012; Wang et al., 2015) and the identification of NPS-related acute poisonings leading to emergency department visits nationwide.

To offer better treatment of poisoned patients who need hospitalization, the division has 10 beds. Moreover, both an intensive care unit located in the emergency department and a medical intensive care unit in the hospital are available for patients with severe poisoning. Various extracorporeal removal modalities such as hemodialysis, hemoperfusion, and continuous veno-venous hemofiltration are also readily available to those in need. Extracorporeal Membrane Oxygenation (ECMO) is available as well for those patients with severe respiratory failure or cardiogenic shock.

The division was renamed as the Division of Clinical Toxicology & Occupational Medicine (https://wd.vghtpe.gov.tw/CT/Index.action) in November 2013 because all attending physicians of the division are also occupational medicine physicians and because the issue of occupational disease/injury diagnosis and prevention has become more important in the past two decades in Taiwan.

Currently, there are three full-time attending physicians and two adjunct attending physicians who are both licensed internists and occupational medicine physicians in the division. They provide outpatient medical services, emergency consultations, and inpatient care to poisoned patients who visit TVGH.

In addition to the Division of Clinical Toxicology & Occupational Medicine at TVGH, there are a few other divisions of clinical toxicology that also provide medical service to poisoned patients [e.g., Chang Gung Memorial Hospital (https://www1.cgmh.org.tw/intr/intr2/c31570/index.html) and China Medical University Hospital (https://www.cmuh.cmu.edu.tw/Department/Detail?depid=122)]. However, they do not offer the comprehensive toxicological analysis of toxicants or provide the same level of medical care of all aspects of acute poisoning as those provided by the Division of Clinical Toxicology & Occupational Medicine at TVGH.

Clinical toxicology training and education

According to the data collected by PCC-Taiwan as well as other statistics available in Taiwan, the number of both acute and severe human poisonings has been decreasing in recent years. Therefore, many healthcare professionals are becoming less familiar with acute poisonings that are infrequently seen in daily practice, such as venomous snakebites, wasp stings, pesticide poisonings, substance abuse, and plant/Chinese herbal medicine-related poisonings. With the specific goal of advancing knowledge and understanding of the diagnosis, treatment, and prevention of all forms of poisoning, PCC-Taiwan provides professional training and education to a wide variety of healthcare professionals in Taiwan. This includes a 1-month training module intended for junior emergency physicians, occupational medicine trainees, and rotating residents of the Department of Medicine of TVGH. PCC-Taiwan also provides 6–8 weeks training internships for pharmacists and public health students; 3–6 months training internships for foreign physicians; and 1–2 years training experiences for fellows of the Division of Clinical Toxicology & Occupational Medicine and medical student volunteers.

Education of the earlier-mentioned trainees is important as a means of disseminating higher standards of care for poisoned patients. These educational opportunities also create interest in this field among younger trainees who may later choose to obtain further training in clinical toxicology or pursue careers involving poison control centers. The main strength of the clinical toxicology training program at PCC-Taiwan is its vast number of cases collected over more than 35 years of operation. These invaluable data are available for retrospective analysis of the predictors and/or outcomes of various acute poisonings. The research findings are very important for both training and education in clinical toxicology. Another strength of the PCC-Taiwan is its laboratory facility that can provide a greater opportunity for the trainees to be immersed in the fascinating world of clinical toxicology.

Currently the major objectives of clinical toxicology training are as follows:

1. foster a better understanding of the principles and practice of clinical toxicology;
2. familiarize the trainee with the management of common and/or important poisonings in Taiwan;
3. familiarize the trainee with the management of common antidotes used in Taiwan;
4. familiarize the trainee with the laboratory procedures in clinical toxicology at PCC-Taiwan;
5. encourage research into all aspects of poisoning; and
6. facilitate the collection, exchange and dissemination of relevant information among individual members, poisons centers and organizations interested in clinical toxicology.

Proposed topics to be studied by the trainees of PCC-Taiwan include agrochemicals, animal envenomation, drug abuse, drug overdose, heavy metals, industrial materials, plants and herbal medicines, and other topics.

International collaboration

PCC-Taiwan has collaborated with many centers in Taiwan as well as foreign countries regarding training and research since its establishment in 1985. Junior medical doctors from many Asian countries, including Bangladesh, Chinese mainland, Hong Kong, India, Macao, Singapore, Thailand, and Vietnam have received training at PCC-Taiwan. Moreover, researchers from numerous countries such as Chinese mainland, Germany, Japan, Korea, the Philippines, Sweden, Thailand, and the United States have visited PCC-Taiwan. An international collaboration project on the diagnosis and management of snake envenomation is also ongoing between PCC-Taiwan and Cho Ray Hospital in Vietnam.

In addition to the receipt of training and the visits by foreign guests, the staff of PCC-Taiwan has also actively participated in international clinical toxicology conferences, including the North American Congress of Clinical Toxicology (NACCT), the scientific congress of European Association of Poisons Centres and Clinical Toxicologists (EAPCCT), the Asia Pacific Association of Medical Toxicology (APAMT), and the Asian Society of Toxicology (ASIATOX). Dr. Jou-Fang Deng and Dr. Chen-Chang Yang have also each served as the President of APAMT (https://www.apamt.org/board-members/).

Toxicology societies

Currently, there is no existing clinical/medical toxicology association in Taiwan. Therefore most clinical toxicologists join the Toxicology Society of Taiwan (TSTA) instead. The TSTA (https://twtoxicology.org.tw/) was founded in 1985 by a group of toxicologists led by Dr. Chen-Yuan Lee. TSTA was registered with the nation's Ministry of the Interior on June 20, 1987 (Satoh, 2015). Dr. Lee became the first president of TSTA and was succeeded by Dr. Jen-Kun Lin, Dr. Jou-Fang Deng, Dr. Tzuu-Huei Ueng, Dr. Tsung-Yun Liu, Dr. Huei Lee, Dr. Min-Liang Kuo, and Dr. Jaw-Jou Kang. The current president is Dr. Jih-Heng Li, and the Deputy President is Dr. Chen-Chang Yang.

TSTA is a member of both ASIATOX and International Union of Toxicology (IUTOX) and has actively participated in various scientific activities of both international associations. TSTA has also been the host organization of the 5th International Congress of ASIATOX held at the TVGH in 2009. In addition to ASIATOX, TSTA has regularly hosted the biennial cross-strait meetings between TSTA and Chinese Society of Toxicology (Satoh, 2015).

The Taiwan Environmental & Occupational Medical Association (TEOMA) is another medical association that enrolls quite a few clinical toxicologists in Taiwan (http://www.eoma.org.tw/). TEOMA was founded in 1992 by a group of occupational and environmental medicine experts. Dr. Jung-Deng Wang was the first president of TEOMA and was succeeded by Dr. Jou-Fang Deng, Dr. Yue-Leon Guo, Dr. Chi-Kung Ho, Dr. How-Ran Guo, Dr. Jiin-Chyuan John Luo, and Dr. Hung-Yi Chuang. The present president is Dr. Chen-Chang Yang. TEOMA is presently promoting the establishment of a "Clinical Toxicology" subspecialty under the specialty of Occupational Medicine. Hopefully, clinical toxicology will become a licensed subspecialty in Taiwan within 2–3 years. A clinical toxicology association is also expected to be founded after clinical toxicology becomes a formal subspecialty in Taiwan.

Future challenges

The development of clinical toxicology in Taiwan has spanned over 35 years. However, the number of well-trained clinical toxicologists remains relatively small in Taiwan. To expand the number of clinical toxicologists, more incentives and more financial support from the government are needed. The major challenges for PCC-Taiwan are its limited budget and human resources, versus its national role and position in serving all of the people of Taiwan. In recent years, PCC-Taiwan has asked for more funding support from the Taiwanese government so that a sufficient stock of antidotes in emergency care facilities can be assured. Moreover, the development and implementation of an artificial intelligence-assisted poison information service is also ongoing so that PCC-Taiwan can keep and even expand its current services without the need of extra human resources. Finally the inclusion of PCC-Taiwan into the Emergency Medical Care Act will help the center to have more sustainable funding support from the Taiwanese government.

References

Chen YJ, Wu ML, Deng JF, Yang CC. The epidemiology of glyophosate- surfactant herbicide poisoning in Taiwan, 1986-2007: a poison center study. Clin Toxicol 2009;47:670–7.

Chung K, Yang CC, Wu ML, Deng JF, Tsai WJ. Agricultural avermectins: an uncommon but potentially fatal cause of pesticide poisoning. Ann Emerg Med 1999;34:51–7.

Doan UV, Wu ML, Phua DH, Bomar YCC. Datura and Brugmansia plants related antimuscarinic toxicity: an analysis of poisoning cases reported to the Taiwan poison control center. Clin Toxicol 2019;59:246–53.

Hung DZ, Yang CC, Ong HC, et al. The present and future of poison control center in Taiwan. J Toxicol Sci 1998;23(Suppl 2):280–3.

Lin MS, Lin CC, Chen CY, Huang SY, Chou YH, Yang CC. Myocardial injury was associated with persistent and delayed neurological sequelae among patients with carbon monoxide poisoning in Taiwan. J Chin Med Assoc 2018;81:682–90.

Ong HC, Deng JF. Taiwan experience in the management of an antidote supply network. In: 11th Scientific Congress of Asia Pacific Association of Medical Toxicology (APAMT), Hong Kong; 2012.

Ong H, Yang CC, Deng JF. Inadequate stocking of antidotes in Taiwan: is it a serious problem? J Toxicol-Clin Toxicol 2000;38:21–8.

Satoh T. Toxicology in Asia - past, present, and future. Hum Exp Toxicol 2015;34:1291–6.

Wang TH, Wu ML, Wu YH, et al. Neurotoxicity associated with exposure to 1-bromopropane in golf-club cleansing workers. Clin Toxicol 2015;53:823–6.

Wu YH, Wu ML, Lin CC, Chu WL, Yang CC, Deng JF. Determination of caprolactam and 6-aminocaproic acid in human urine using hydrophilic interaction liquid chromatography-tandem mass spectrometry. J Chromatogr B Anal Technol Biomed Life Sci 2012;885-886:61–5.

Yang CC, Deng JF. Utility of flumazenil in zopiclone overdose. Clin Toxicol 2008;46:920–1.

Yang CC, Wu JF, Ong HC, et al. Taiwan National Poison Center: epidemiologic data 1985-1993. J Toxicol-Clin Toxicol 1996;34:651–63.

Chapter 6.4

The Philippines

Irma Reyes Makalinao[a,b] and Lynn Crisanta del Rosario Panganiban[a,b]

[a]*Department of Pharmacology and Toxicology, College of Medicine, University of the Philippines Manila,* [b]*University of the Philippines National Poison Management and Control Center, Philippine General Hospital, Manila, Philippines*

Origins of clinical toxicology

Creating toxicology as a distinct subspecialty of medicine in the Philippines is a journey worth revisiting. From a single individual who pioneered the field of toxicology in the Philippines in the 1960s by responding to poisoning referrals almost single-handedly and mentoring the first generation of toxicologists who became the pillars of the University of the Philippines (UP) National Poison Control and Information service, the field has since taken root. We pay tribute to Professor Emeritus Nelia P. Cortes-Maramba as the "Mother of Philippine Toxicology" and acknowledge the pioneers Kenneth Hartigan-Go, Lynn Crisanta R. Panganiban, Irma R. Makalinao, and Erle S. Castillo who advanced clinical toxicology as a medical specialty in the country.

On December 12, 1996, the only institutionalized clinical toxicology fellowship program in the Philippines, based in the University of the Philippines Manila, provided the impetus to create a professional organization called the Philippine Society of Clinical and Occupational Toxicology, founded in 1998. As a subspecialty of medicine, the entry fields for specialization in clinical toxicology were emergency medicine, family medicine, internal medicine, neurology, pediatrics, and psychiatry.

We have been expanding the horizon of toxicology not only as a professional discipline of medicine but also one that includes nursing and analytical toxicology.

To insure the sustainability of toxicology education in the Philippines, the UP College of Medicine, through the Department of Pharmacology and Toxicology, has included in the medical, nursing, and dental curriculum clinical toxicology lectures. Within the master's degree program there is a three-unit course in toxicology which includes regulatory and organ system toxicology.

Origins of poison control — Setting the stage

The practice of toxicology began in 1975 when a poison center was established at the Emergency Room Complex of the Philippine General Hospital (PGH),

History of Modern Clinical Toxicology. https://doi.org/10.1016/B978-0-12-822218-8.00062-4

the teaching hospital of the University of the Philippines Manila-College of Medicine (UPMCM). In a privileged communication with Prof. Maramba, she mentioned that this was made possible with the help of Dr. Mario Gutierrez who was then the head of the Department of Family Medicine and with the cooperation of the Department of Pediatrics. This development was in response to the rising incidence of poisoning caused by the indiscriminate use of pesticides. The center functioned as a treatment service focusing on the management of acute poisoning cases admitted in the hospital. In those years, documentation of poisoning cases was inadequate because of the lack of an effective system for poisoning information dissemination and data collection. In fact, the number of poisoning cases attended to from 1984 to 1989 only averaged 190 per year (Annual Reports, 1984–1989).

The misdiagnosis of cases resulted in under-reporting, probably due to limited avenues for formal training in toxicology. A learning activity was the monthly house-staff teaching hours for residents manning the emergency department, conducted by Professor Maramba, the only trained toxicologist in the country during that time.

The conditions mentioned earlier highlighted the need for setting up a national poison control center and its network of satellite centers to attend to poisoning-related matters not just in PGH but the whole country as well. Thus, in 1991, the Poisons Control and Information Service Network (NPCIS) project was implemented through the technical assistance from the World Health Organization-International Programme on Chemical Safety (WHO-IPCS), and grants from the International Development Research Centre (IDRC) and Gesselschaft fur Technische Zusammenarbeit (GTZ). At this time, the poison center was renamed as the National Poison Control and Information Service (NPCIS) with its own administrative and consultant staff based at the Philippine General Hospital. In 1992, a memorandum of agreement was entered into by the Department of Health (DOH) and the University of the Philippines Manila to formalize the network. With that set-up, NPCIS served as the central hub for all toxicology-related activities and coordinated country-wide activities with the DOH and other government agencies. These services included clinical treatment, poison information, analytical toxicology, teaching/training, research and development, toxicovigilance, linkages, and extension.

Organization and growth of NPCIS

The years covering 1991–2002 saw the growth of the NPCIS with strengthening of treatment and poison information services, including its laboratory capabilities. A team of doctors from NPCIS and different clinical departments of the PGH would go on a regular 24-h duty to attend to in-patient, out-patient, and telephone referrals. The NPCIS developed its own treatment algorithms for the management of poisoning cases (Maramba and Panganiban, 1998; Makalinao and Maramba, 1999) being used by hospital personnel as well as information monographs for health personnel in the field. Bedside toxicology tests and analytical toxicology procedures for common toxicants were developed and standardized. The growth of the NPCIS paved the way for the setting up of poison centers in different tertiary hospitals under the jurisdiction of the DOH.

Training

The NPCIS prioritized the development of its consultant staff to help them in the design and conduct of training programs. The clinical rotation and exposure to poison information provided by the Rocky Mountain Poison and Drug Center in 1993 through its Director, Dr. Richard C. Dart was incorporated in the blueprints of the 1996 clinical toxicology fellowship program and the training of specialists in poison information.

Notable among the NPCIS programs were the fellowship in clinical toxicology, the postgraduate course in toxicology administration and management, and the clinical toxicology rotation for resident physicians. To date, under the University of the Philippines National Poison Management and Control Center (UPNPMCC), residents from major hospitals in the Philippines continue to pursue elective rotations that started under NPCIS.

Data collection

Poisoning data collection was harmonized some time in 1997 through a WHO INTOX-INCHEM workshop. These poisoning data have been helpful in the issuance of health advisories on the accidental ingestion of yellow phosphorus from the deadly dancing firecracker "watusi" which was common during the Christmas season (Makalinao et al, 1993, Panganiban et al., 1993, Hartigan-Go and Pestano, 1995, Wallerstein, 1999). Other examples of advisories issued by the poison center have included methanol in alcoholic beverages, jatropha seed poisoning (Makalinao, 1993) and marine toxins (e.g., red tide) (Makalinao, 1997). The NPCIS also conducted research which assisted government agencies in policy formulation (Annual Report, 2004; UPNPMCC, 2020). Examples included restrictions on the use of mercury in artisanal gold-mining and severely toxic pesticides used in agricultural settings. Attention to hazards in the environment and the risks they pose to children is a particularly important consideration in crafting protective public health policies and legislation in the Philippines and everywhere (Makalinao, 2005).

Links to other resources

Linkages with national and international organizations were established, particularly with the DOH and the WHO, respectively. The NPCIS has maintained twinning arrangements with poison centers in the Western Pacific and European regions. NPCIS has offered short rotations and study visits by personnel from poison centers in Indonesia, Sri Lanka, Malaysia, and Mongolia. These linkages have been valuable because of the technical and financial support they have contributed to the growth of the unit. These linkages can be described as building on north–south and south–south cooperation in promoting toxicology as a distinct service and discipline (Annual Report, 2004).

Current UPNPMCC operations

In 2003 the NPCIS was recognized as a unit in the College of Medicine to concentrate on its national role under the leadership of Dr. Lynn Crisanta Panganiban (College Circular No. 2003-A32, 2003). Likewise, the PGH-Poison Control and Information Unit (PCIU) was created for the management of poisoning cases in the hospital with its first head, Dr. Irma Makalinao immediately followed by Dr. Erle Castillo (PGH Memorandum No. 2003-73, 2003). However, for the purpose of streamlining the toxicology-related activities, the UP Board of Regents in its 1192nd meeting held on January 27, 2005, approved the merging of the NPCIS and the PGH-PCIU (UP Board of Regents' Decision, 2005). The unit was named: University of the Philippines National Poison Management and Control Center (UPNPMCC). These developments over the past 15 years have highlighted the important role of UPNPMCC in the sustainable development of toxicology in the Philippines. It has exemplified leadership, excellence, and service to the Filipino people including some neighboring countries in Asia through work done with the World Health Organization.

Vision of the UPNPMCC

The vision of the UPNPMCC is "health advocates dedicated to the well-being of Filipinos through prevention and management of poisoning." It is committed "to protect the Filipino from poisoning through the promotion of chemical and pharmaceutical safety. The Center shall provide adequate training in toxicology and optimum management of poisoning cases." The UPNPMCC's objectives focus on the improvement of preventive and therapeutic management, education, information dissemination, and research.

Through the years, the UPNPMCC has been true to its calling. It has remained as a national focal point for the management of poisoning cases and training of health personnel (doctors, nurses, and laboratory analysts) for poison information and for clinical, occupational, and community work. It has been conducting research and health assessment activities on the health effects of chemical exposures. The UPNPMCC has provided technical advice to government agencies and legislative bodies in policy formulation and enhancement.

UPNPMCC has served a wider community as far as management of acute poisoning cases is concerned, as shown by the increasing number of telephone referrals (Fig. 6.4.1). And from 190 cases in the 1980s, the number of hospitalized in-patient cases attended to has grown to as high as 1509 in 2019 (Annual Reports, 2014–2019).

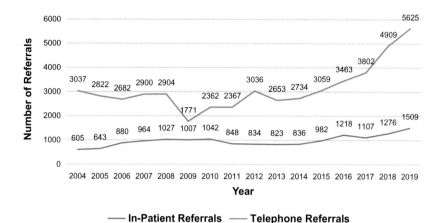

FIG. 6.4.1 Total number of poisoning referrals, National Poison Management and Control Center, UP—Philippine General Hospital, 2004–2019. *(Source: Annual Reports 2014–2019, Philippines: National Poison Management and Control Center, UP Philippine General Hospital, 2004–2019.)*

UPNPMCC has strengthened its toxicovigilance activities, partnering with both government and nongovernmental agencies. Notable is its campaign in the banning of cyanide in silver jewelry cleaning agents and mercury and lead in consumer products. It has been involved in chemical emergency preparedness and response particularly in the carbamate-contaminated cassava "maruya" cake poisoning incident (UPNPMCC, 2020). Other such incidents include bunker oil and elemental mercury spills (Calanog, 2006).

The valuable lesson that the UPNPMCC has gained through the years is the essential role of partnership and networking in sustaining the enterprise. Addressing the nation's toxicological issues has required teamwork, consisting of dedicated and committed professionals whose aim is one of keeping individuals and communities out of harm's way. The unique role of UPNPMCC in providing toxicology education across disciplines aligns with the vision of the UP system in shaping the minds that shape the future. This interdisciplinary approach to education is key in the sustainable development of poison centers across the country (Makalinao and Awang, 2005).

The toxicology training programs

Clinical toxicology

On the recommendation of the Dean of the UP College of Medicine and the Director of the Philippine General Hospital, the UP-Manila Chancellor signed and institutionalized the first ever and only clinical toxicology fellowship program in the Philippines on December 12, 1996. This decision subsequently underwent a process through the Training Coordinating Committee as presented by its first trainers: Professor Nelia P. Cortes-Maramba and Dr. Irma Makalinao, who became the first Program Director from 1997 to 2005. This action was immediately implemented on January 1, 1997. The 2-year program has consisted of a clinical rotation with house-staff teaching hours, weekly case conferences, in-patient and out-patient consults including telephone referral, and the clinical supervision of medical interns and residents rotating at the UPNPMCC. The second year has been dedicated to research and formal courses offered toward the Master of Science in Pharmacology degree. The master's degree program requires the inclusion of curricular content in basic toxicology and pharmacogenetics and additional electives to complete the required nine units of formal course work. In summary, the 2-year clinical toxicology program covers three major areas: training, research, and service. The major impact of this training program is shown by the fact that the alumni have become the heads in the DOH network of poison control centers (PCC) or poison control units (PCU) answering the need for trained specialists in Luzon (East Avenue Medical Center, Rizal Medical Center, Batangas Medical Center, Baguio General Hospital, Bicol Medical Center), Visayas (Eastern Visayas Regional Medical Center, Corazon Locsin Montelibano Memorial Regional Hospital), and Mindanao (Southern Philippines Medical Center, Northern Mindanao Medical Center, Zamboanga City Medical Center) regions of the Philippines.

Analytical toxicology training program

The analytical toxicology training program started in 1997 as a joint program of then UP National Poison Control and Information Service and the Department of Pharmacology of the UP College of Medicine. The primary aim was to have a composite team of toxicology-trained medical technologists or chemists mostly from the DOH hospitals. In recent years, this program has been offered to staff in both local government and private laboratories. The training includes lectures, hands-on laboratory work, attendance at weekly toxicology and laboratory conferences, and educational visits to selected government and private laboratories with analytical toxicology services. The participant is expected to have acquired basic knowledge and laboratory skills in analytical toxicology methodologies and procedures, knowledge of the basic principles of clinical toxicology and common causes of poisoning, and an appreciation of the importance of the ethical and medicolegal aspects of poisoning in the Philippines.

The hands-on laboratory work integrates basic knowledge in analytical toxicology through the performance of a range of methods, from colorimetric bedside toxicology to the use of more advanced techniques such as AAS, GC–MS/MS, and LC-MS/MS. To address developments in the fields of biosafety and biosecurity, these topics were introduced into the training package in 2018.

Toxicology training for nurses

In 2003, we graduated our first cohort of trainees in the toxicology training course for nurses jointly offered by the UP NPCIS and the PGH Poison Control Unit before the two entities were merged by the UP Board of Regents in 2005 to become the UPNPMCC. The initial trainees were emergency room nurses of government hospitals that were anticipated to have a need for trained medical and analytical toxicologists. The 3-month program includes formal lectures and in-house duties to answer telephone calls and assist in the management of poisoned patients under the supervision of toxicology consultants and fellows. Today, most of the graduates of the program form part of the network of DOH PCCs and PCUs working at the emergency departments or providing poison information. In October 2020, the Toxicology Nurses Association of the Philippines (TNAP) was officially registered in the Philippine Security and Exchange Commission with the aim of insuring relevant toxicology training in the nursing profession and to establish a standard of care among nurses in the management of poisoned patients.

The specialist in poison information

In 2018 the first formal training of the specialist in poison information was offered jointly by the UPNPMCC and certified by the Philippine Society of Clinical and Occupational Toxicology (PSCOT). The program included relevant lectures and hands-on training at the UPNPMCC. The trainee was evaluated as they handled telephone referrals, delivered case presentations, and joined rounds with the clinical team. At the end of the formal in-house training, a two part examination was given consisting of a written exam and a simulated telephone call. After passing the requirements set forth by UPNPMCC, the trainees returned to their sending institutions to answer telephone referrals under the supervision of their respective medical toxicologists. The individual trainee was asked to document the poison information calls in their respective hospitals for a period of 6 months. PSCOT, through its accreditation committee, administered both an oral and written examination for the purpose of certification. After 3 years, the certified specialist in poison information is required to take a re-certification examination.

National poison prevention week

On May 18, 2009, President Gloria Macapagal Arroyo signed Proclamation No. 1777, 2009 declaring the 4th week of June 2009 and every year thereafter as "National Poison Prevention Week (NPPW)" (Official Gazette, 2009). It cited the work of UPNPMCC in the management of toxicological problems in the country with the view that poisoning is preventable. The proclamation was made to address "the urgent need to increase the awareness on the preventive aspects of poisoning prevention at home, school, work and the general environment."

It has recognized the importance of education and information dissemination activities on poisoning prevention. NPPW is intended to provide valuable information to increase the awareness of the public and the working population (Go, 2018). The president's proclamation assigned the task to PSCOT and the DOH to plan and organize activities for the NPPW.

Current and future challenges and direction

The International Health Regulations Joint External Evaluation Mission report (WHO, 2005) referred to a network of 13 PCCs in the Philippines in varying stages of growth and development, strategically located in Luzon, Visayas, and Mindanao where chemical hazards have been identified. The report states:

"The capacities of the new PCCs need to be clarified and strengthened; not all will be designated as treatment centers—some will be information centers only. Currently, two are recognized as meeting WHO standards; increasing the number of the remaining PCCs that attain accreditation would enhance the quality of the national PCC network."

The following priorities for actions were recommended as pertaining to poison centers, namely:

1. Develop a national, integrated, multisectoral chemical incident preparedness, response, and recovery plan, incorporating an updated national chemical profile and hazard map.
2. Develop a national chemical security plan as described in the Philippines Chemical, Biological, Radiological, Nuclear (CBRN) National Action Plan.
3. Increase the number of PCC recognized as meeting WHO guidelines.
4. Develop a national, integrated, multisectoral chemical incident training and exercise program.

With the growing concern regarding chemical safety and security with recent examples, such as the massive explosion from ammonium nitrate in Beirut and the use of a chemical weapon like Novichok in 2020, the UPNPMCC sees its expanding role in chemical emergency preparedness, especially since the PGH has been the recipient of training and equipment on CBRN response and decontamination by the government of the United States. With 24-h availability all 365 days in a year, the UPNPMCC can provide timely advice in the event of a mass casualty chemical emergency.

The UPNPMCC with its long history and first ever institutionalized poison control center has served not only patients but also has created the continuity necessary for sustainability and growth. It accomplished this by creating the first ever toxicology training program whose impact can be seen by the graduates of the program who now serve as heads of poison centers in their respective areas of practice. The growth of training programs has also provided the path toward the professional societies that have emerged over time (such as the Philippine Society of Clinical and Occupational Toxicology and the Toxicology

Nurses Association of the Philippines). The multiplier effect is a testimony to the success of the training programs that espouse the vision of the UP in "shaping the minds that shape the future."

The history of the UP-based Poison Center is a story of humble beginnings whose foundation rests in the commitment of its pioneering pillars to serve the common good of the Filipino people and decrease mortality and morbidity from poisoning and to share best practices to our neighbors in the Association of Southeast Asian Nations (ASEAN) community. Anchoring the toxicology training programs to the UP has been a pivotal step in the right direction as it continues to sustain training and interest in the young medical students and nurses who will serve as the next generation of toxicologists. Future challenges include the sustained support to fund poison centers and accredit the different poison centers as they are being established.

We align ourselves with United Nations Sustainable Development Goal 3 (UN SDG 3) on insuring healthy lives and promoting the well-being for all at all ages (United Nations, 2020). Specifically, we recognize the important role of the PCC on strengthening the prevention and treatment of substance abuse, including narcotic drug abuse and harmful use of alcohol. Likewise, PCCs should work together to meet target 3.9 that "by 2030, substantially reduce the number of deaths and illnesses from hazardous chemicals and air, water, and soil pollution and contamination" (United Nations, 2020).

More than ever during the COVID-19 pandemic (UPNPMCC, 2020), we have seen a great potential for PCCs in public health emergencies and fulfilling UN SDG Goal 3D to "strengthen the capacity of all countries, in particular developing countries, for early warning, risk reduction and management of national and global health risks" (United Nations, 2020).

References

Annual Report. National Poison Management and Control and Information Service; 2004.

Annual Reports. Department of Family Medicine. UP Philippine General Hospital; 1984–1989.

Annual Reports. Philippines: National Poison Management and control Center, UP Philippine General Hospital; 2014–2019.

Calanog SS. Andrews mercury spill: Paranaque Philippines Region IX. February 16th, Accessed on 12/15/2020. https://response.epa.gov/site/site_profile.aspx?site_id=2291; 2006.

College Circular No. 2003-A32. Recognition of the National Poison Control and Information Service (NPCIS) as a Unit in the College of Medicine; 2003.

Go RGA. Zambo hospital to mark Poison Prevention Week with anti-drug campaign. Philippine News Agency; 2018. Accessed on 12/20/2020. https://www.pna.gov.ph/articles/1038293.

Hartigan-Go K, Pestano N. Watusi poisoning: a case report of yellow phosphorus ingestion. Philippine J Intern Med 1995;33(6):215–7.

Makalinao IR. A descriptive study on the clinical profile of jatropha seed poisoning. Vet Hum Toxicol 1993;35:4 [abstract 330].

Makalinao IR, Young P, Maramba NPC. The Clinical profile and treatment of Watusi poisoning in children. Vet Hum Toxicol 1993;35:4 [abstract].

Makalinao IR. Red tide poisoning: the Philippine experience. The Philippine J Microbiol Infect Dis 1997;26(1):S59.

Makalinao I. The environment as a determinant of children's environmental health: An emerging concern. Philippines: National Academy of Science and Technology; 2005.

Makalinao IR, Awang R. Poison control centers in developing countries and Asia's need for toxicology education. Toxicol Appl Pharmacol 2005;207(2 Suppl):716–21.

Makalinao IR, Maramba NPC. Watusi poisoning monograph: A comprehensive guide to human health effects, toxicity and treatment. Manila, Philippines: National Poison Control and Information Service; 1999.

Maramba NPC, Panganiban LRC. Algorithms of common poisoning: Part 1. 2nd ed. Manila Philippines National Poison Control and Information Service; 1998.

Official Gazette. Proclamation Number 1777 s. 2009. Declaring the 4th week of June 2009 and every year thereafter as "NATIONAL POISON PREVENTION WEEK". Accessed on 12/15/2020. https://www.officialgazette.gov.ph/2009/05/18/proclamation-no-1777-s-2009/; 2009.

Panganiban LCR, et al. Value of N-acetylcysteine in the management of Watusi-induced hepatotoxicity. Hum Vet Toxicol 1993;35:4 [abstract 127].

PGH Memorandum No. 2003-73. Creation of the PGH-Poison Control and Information Unit (PGH-PCIU); 2003.

United Nations. Sustainable Development Goals. Goal 3 - Ensure healthy lives and promote well-being for all at all ages. Accessed on 12/15/2020. https://www.un.org/sustainabledevelopment/health/; 2020.

University of the Philippines National Poison Management and Control Center (UPNPMCC). Training on the management of acute poisoning amidst the Covid-19 pandemic, December 10-11. Accessed on 12/15/2020 https://www.facebook.com/pages/National-Poison-Management-and-Control-Center/192954940751948?sk=timeline; 2020.

UP Board of Regents' Decision. 1192nd Meeting (January 27, 2005): Approval of the merging of the NPCIS and the PGH-PCIU and be named National Poison Management and Control Center. University of the Philippines Gazette; 2005. p. 12–3. 306 (1).

Wallerstein C. Christmas fireworks "sweets" kill hundreds of children. Brit Med J 1999;319:1222.

World Health Organization (WHO). Strengthening health security by implementing the international Health Regulations. Joint External Evaluations; 2005. Accessed on 12/15/2020. https://www.who.int/ihr/procedures/joint-external-evaluations/en/.

Chapter 6.5

Vietnam

Nguyen Trung Nguyen

Poison Control Center of Bach Mai Hospital, Hanoi, Vietnam

Clinical toxicology in Vietnam has developed in its own special way, mainly based on the clinical activities of individuals with toxicology expertise. This field has been afforded great opportunities and also challenges. Vietnam itself has been developing over time and now a large population exists.

Poison control in Vietnam: Origins and development

In the North of Vietnam

Origins

The Unit of Critical Care Toxicology was founded by Professor Vu Van Dinh in 1994, from the Department of Emergency and Intensive Care (A9 department) of Bach Mai Hospital. Bach Mai Hospital is a large teaching, tertiary care hospital in the North of Vietnam. The unit treated the most severely poisoned patients in critical condition sent to it from different provinces in the North and one part of the Central region of Vietnam. The physicians and nurses treating the poisoned patients were from the Department of Emergency and Intensive Care.

The Department of Clinical Toxicology was established from the Unit of Critical Care Toxicology on December 15, 1998 at Bach Mai Hospital. The Department had 10 beds and was directed by doctor Nguyen Thi Du. Notably the establishment of the Department of Clinical Toxicology as well as the poison control center was catalyzed by Dr. John Alan Haines who worked with the World Health Organization, visited the hospital, and consulted with the Ministry of Health of Vietnam.

Toxicology laboratory tests were performed within the campus of the department and included thin layer chromatography tests for common pesticides (i.e., organophosphate, carbamate, and organochlorine), opiates, phenobarbital, diazepam, aconitine, strychnine, belladonna, and gelsemium alkaloids.

The most common poisoning agents seen by staff in the Department of Clinical Toxicology included organophosphates, carbamates, sodium fluoroacetate/fluoroacetamide, snakebite, phenobarbital, diazepam, and heroin.

History of Modern Clinical Toxicology. https://doi.org/10.1016/B978-0-12-822218-8.00039-9

The physicians and nurses treating these patients were from the Department of Emergency and Intensive Care. The death rate of poisoned patients treated at the department was reduced after its establishment: from 8.5% in 1998 to approximately 2% in 1999 (source: poison control center database, unpublished).

Regulation

The Poison Control Center of Bach Mai Hospital was set up by the Ministry of Health on September 17, 2003. It was based within the Department of Clinical Toxicology and is now considered the national poison control center. The poison control center has been working under the guidance set forth by the Regulation of Emergency, Intensive Care, and Clinical Toxicology promulgated by the Ministry of Health.

The poison control center has also been working with the Training Department of Bach Mai Hospital and collaborates with medical colleges (particularly the Faculty of Intensive Care, Emergency Medicine and Clinical Toxicology of Hanoi Medical University), and the Vietnam Association of Emergency, Intensive Care and Clinical Toxicology. These agencies assist the poison control center in implementing its assigned functions. They also assist the center in promoting poison control throughout the country (details are presented later). The establishment and development of expertise in clinical toxicology in the North of Vietnam had a lot of technical and training support from international colleagues and institutions including Thailand (Ramathibodi Poison Center), the United States (Rocky Mountain Poison and Drug Center), and Taiwan (National Poison Control Center).

In 2008 the Ministry of Health issued a regulation regarding intensive care, emergency medicine and poison control. This regulation included explicit guidance concerning the organization, functions, and staffing of poison control centers and departments of clinical toxicology. The regulation also required all provincial hospitals to have their own departments of intensive care and clinical toxicology.

Vietnam Military Medical University

The Faculty of Toxicology and Radiation of Vietnam Military Medical University has operated since 1959 with functions of research, training, and education in toxicology and radiation in the army. A poison control center was established by the University in 2000. The activities of this center focused on research, training, and education in army poison control. The center also conducted important research and training in poison management and the prevention of poisoning from natural toxins, especially in the Northern mountainous provinces of Vietnam. The poison control center and the Faculty of Toxicology and Radiation were merged into the Center for Training and Research in Toxicology and Radiation in 2017.

In the South of Vietnam

Cho Ray Hospital

Clinical toxicology has been carried out for many years at Cho Ray Hospital which has followed the model of and operates similarly to the Clinical Toxicology Unit in Bach Mai Hospital. The most severely poisoned patients are treated at the Department of Emergency Medicine and Intensive Care Unit of the hospital. They are often transferred there from different provinces in the South. Recently, a unit of clinical toxicology was set-up and has been working within the Department of Tropical Diseases of the hospital. The unit has received great support from the National Poison Control Center of Taiwan in terms of training.

Cho Ray Hospital also has its own Center of Training and Education to carry out training programs for other healthcare facilities in the South. Its staff work closely with the Faculty of Intensive Care, Emergency Medicine and Clinical Toxicology of the University of Medicine and Pharmacy at Ho Chi Minh City.

Current clinical toxicology network operations

Poison Control Center

There is only one poison control center (the Poison Control Center of Bach Mai Hospital) in Vietnam and it is composed of a Clinical Toxicology Unit, Poison Information Unit and Toxicology Laboratory Unit. The poison control center has 52 staff members of which 8 are physicians and 35 are nurses. It has developed many recommendations for the prevention and management of poisonings based on their own clinical experiences. These recommendations are available to the public.

Clinical toxicology unit

The Department of Clinical Toxicology is also a poison treatment center with 50 beds including 12 intensive care beds. The physicians in the department are trained in emergency medicine, intensive care, and clinical toxicology. The clinical staff is capable of performing extracorporeal procedures (e.g., hemodialysis, continuous renal replacement therapies, plasma exchange, and hemoperfusion).

The number of poisoned patients treated at the Bach Mai Hospital has steadily increased and reached 4000 cases in 2019. The most common admission diagnoses were pesticide poisonings, drug overdoses, snakebites, alcohol and drug abuse. Patients were treated according to our protocols of the poison control center.

Poison information unit

The poison information unit is housed in one room and has a library. It is staffed by one assistant and one physician from the Department of Clinical Toxicology.

The unit's activities include patient data collection, answering certain public telephone inquiries, and providing toxicology consultations to physicians within Bach Mai Hospital and outside hospitals.

Toxicology laboratory unit

The toxicology laboratory unit is located within the poison control center and offers 24 h a day and 7 days a week service. It is staffed by five chemists with bachelor or graduate degrees. Our laboratory testing uses methods that include high performance liquid chromatography, gas chromatography, an ELISA system for snake venom analysis, a system for thin layer chromatography (TLC), quick tests for drug abuse, an ammonia analyzer, a blood gas analyzer, and an osmolarity analyzer.

Quantitative testing in our laboratory includes serum acetaminophen, phenobarbital, paraquat, ethanol, and methanol. Qualitative testing by TLC is available for a wide range of agents including pharmaceutical products, pesticides, and alkaloids. Tests unavailable on-site (e.g., heavy metals) are sent to an outside laboratory.

Toxicovigilance and pharmacovigilance

Notably, toxicovigilance and pharmacovigilance tasks are carried out and the data is monitored actively by the poison control center. From the cases of poisoning either treated at the center or consulted on from other hospitals, workers in the poison control center identify trends in either the risks or the problems of poisoning involved. Poison control center leaders can use this data to make suggestions or recommendations in official documents for the authorities responsible for public health agencies, other stakeholders (both individuals and organizations) and the general public. Appropriate measures are recommended to stop/avoid/minimize the poisoning. Many unsafe pharmaceutical and food products and unsafe working conditions have thereby been identified, addressed, and resolved.

Public education

One of the most dominant activities of the poison control center is public education. Without funding, the center cooperates actively with the Department of Social Affairs and Public Communication of Bach Mai Hospital and all media, including television outlets and newspapers. A huge number of articles and news relating to notifications, information, and recommendations from the poison control center have been posted. It has been estimated that every 2 days there is one article or news item mentioning new information from the poison control center. The awareness of not only the general public but also many leaders and public officials regarding poisoning-related issues may thereby be enhanced.

Training

The Ministry of Health issued a regulation for large hospitals including Bach Mai Hospital to support provincial hospitals and other equivalent hospitals in the North of Vietnam in terms of technical issues via training and education programs. The management of poisoning is one of the selected topics. The poison control center has sponsored many training courses, teaching activities, continuous medical education programs, and field visits to almost all provinces. The training can be at local hospitals or at the poison control center. All of these activities are organized in collaboration with the training center of the hospital.

The poison control center has been a busy practicing facility for training institutions, especially Hanoi Medical University and the Nursing School of Bach Mai Hospital for medical students, nursing students, and postgraduates. Clinical toxicology is one of three modules for postgraduate training (i.e., emergency medicine, intensive care, and clinical toxicology). Physicians and nurses of the center are also regular lecturers or co-lecturers at those training institutions.

There are annually approximately 800 learners practicing or rotating at the poison control center. The poison control center also sponsors coursework in clinical toxicology for professionals from other countries. For example, 26 senior doctors from India trained in Vietnam in a 1 month course on the diagnosis and treatment of acute poisonings in 2009, funded and organized by the World Health Organization.

Emergency response

The poison control center has organized an emergency response team. Together with staff from other departments of Bach Mai Hospital, they are sent to the site of a poisoning incident/outbreak. The team may also be sent to help manage complicated cases which exceed the competency of local resources. The team participates or helps to resolve the situation/cases and find the causes of the problems.

The poison control center is also consulted as an advisory agency by the Ministry of Health and other responsible public health agencies about policies and guidelines. The poison control center assists in the resolution of complicated issues related to toxicology expertise and poison control.

Clinical toxicology at Cho Ray Hospital

The Unit of Critical Care Toxicology (in the Intensive Care Department) and Unit of Clinical Toxicology (in the Department of Tropical Disease) of Cho Ray Hospital treat a volume of poisoned patients equivalent to that treated at the Poison Control Center of Bach Mai Hospital. However, there is currently no toxicology laboratory unit or poison information service at Cho Ray Hospital.

Training in clinical toxicology is also carried out by the Center for Training and Education of Cho Ray Hospital, assisted by the faculties of emergency medicine, intensive care, and clinical toxicology of the University of Medicine and Pharmacy at Ho Chi Minh City. The methods, curriculum, and mechanisms of training here are similar to those applied by the Poison Control Center of Bach Mai Hospital.

Provincial hospitals in Vietnam

There are 63 provinces in Vietnam. All of the provincial hospitals with departments of intensive care and clinical toxicology have postgraduate doctors trained at the Poison Control Center of Bach Mai Hospital or at the Intensive Care Unit of Cho Ray Hospital. Poisoned patients are treated by these departments of intensive care and clinical toxicology. If the conditions of the patients are complicated and exceed the ability of the hospitals, they can be transferred to larger or tertiary hospitals. There are frequent exchanges of information and consultation between these two levels of healthcare facilities.

Association of Emergency Medicine, Intensive Care and Clinical Toxicology

Members of the Vietnam Association of Emergency Medicine, Intensive Care, and Clinical Toxicology are doctors working in the field of emergency medicine, intensive care and clinical toxicology in provincial hospitals, district hospitals, tertiary hospitals and departments of emergency medicine and intensive care of private hospitals. There are annual scientific meetings or workshops sponsored by the Association. At least one session of the program at each meeting is devoted to clinical toxicology. There are also Association branches in Hanoi and Ho Chi Minh City with active participation by Association members in the North and the South, respectively.

Financial issues

The poison control center and the departments of clinical toxicology are both contained within large, public hospitals. There is a trend in the policy that all the large public hospitals, from provincial hospitals to higher level tertiary care hospitals, have to operate under a financially self-sustaining mechanism. Leaders at Bach Mai Hospital have been working under the financial constraints of this self-sustaining expectation; no source of funding from the government exists. The hospital therefore has had to invest in those services that can earn money rather than free services like poison information or public education. Public healthcare insurance covers all diagnostic and treatment costs for a small number of patients; it can only pay up to 80% for a majority of patients. Charity activities for poor patients are organized; there are calls for financial support from public and business sectors to help severely poisoned patients with excessive treatment costs.

Without funding from the government, the poison control center cannot maintain its work load and function adequately. The funding from international agencies and programs is less accessible when the country becomes designated by WHO as a "low middle income country." The Poison Control Center of Bach Mai Hospital has to manage its budget on the income stream from clinical services at the center to pay the salary of the staff.

Future challenges

The income of the poison control center generated from the clinical practice is very low, not enough to pay for the salary of staff or to make the center self-sustaining financially. Meanwhile, they have to do work including the provision of poison information to health professionals and the general public without payment. The number of staff, especially physicians, is decreasing. The poison control center has thus been facing difficulties in maintaining its operations. The financial self-sustaining mechanism is inappropriate for the development of poison control. Government funding in this area is mandatory.

Conclusion

The clinical toxicology network offers distinct advantages for training, education, and research in clinical toxicology. There are increasing demands for toxicology-related clinical services in Vietnam. The population has grown to more than 97.3 million people (Google, 2020) and the economy has been developing. The operation of the poison control center of Bach Mai Hospital, the only poison control center in Vietnam currently, shows that there needs to be two additional poison control centers: one each in the Central region and the South of the country. The network of three poison control centers working together is the best model to deliver these services.

Reference

Google. Population of Vietnam 2020. Accessed on November 7, 2020. https://www.google.com/ search?source=hp&ei=goGmX9WLHMO7ggefjKmoDw&q=population+of+vietnam+2020 &oq=Population+of+Vietnam&gs_lcp=CgZwc3ktYWIQARgBMggIABCxAxDJAzICCA- AyAggAMgIIADICCAAyAggAMgIIADICCAAyAggAMgIIADoICAAQsQMQgwE6Aggu OgUIABCxAzoLCC4QsQMQxwEQowI6DgguELEDEMcBEKMCEJMCOgUILhCxAzoL- CAAQsQMQgwEQyQM6BQgAEMkDUJkHWN0tYNNCaABwAHgBgAG7AYgBnAmSAQ QyMC4xmAEAoAEBqgEHZ3dzLXdpeg&sclient=psy-ab.

Chapter 6.6

Thailand

Winai Wananukul[a,b] and Charuwan Sriapha[a]

[a]*Ramathibodi Poison Center, Faculty of Medicine Ramathibodi Hospital, Mahidol University, Bangkok, Thailand,* [b]*Department of Medicine, Faculty of Medicine Ramathibodi Hospital, Mahidol University, Bangkok, Thailand*

Introduction

Thailand, during 1980–1990, was in the period of transforming from an agricultural to an industrial country. Many chemicals were used routinely in agriculture and in industry, as well as in the household. Because of insufficient control and inadequate knowledge among the users, the inappropriate use of the chemicals frequently happened. According to one report from the Thai Ministry of Public Health during the period 1990–1995, the incidence of poisoning in the country was 30 per 100,000 population, with 300 deaths per year (Kaojarern, 1998). At Ramathibodi Hospital, a university hospital in Bangkok, there were 200 poisoned in-patients per year in the medical wards, accounting for 4.1% of all hospitalizations. Meanwhile the average number of nonadmitted poisoning cases was estimated to be 4000 per year (Kaojarern, 1998). It was found that poisoning was usually under-reported. Among poisoning cases, pesticide poisoning was most commonly observed. There were 289 deaths recorded as outcomes of 4046 pesticide poisoning cases, representing a 7.1% mortality rate in 1985 (Jeyaratnam, 1990). The cases were more common in hospitals outside of the Bangkok metropolitan area; notably, there were no clinical toxicologists outside the capital.

Origins of Thai clinical toxicology

Before a poison center was set up in Thailand, there were a small number of physicians who were interested in toxicology and partially worked as clinical toxicologists. They were scattered and in many fields of medicine, such as internal medicine, pediatrics, occupational medicine, preventive medicine, and forensic medicine. They had specific toxicology-related topics in which they were interested, according to their main specialties, such as toxicology, occupation-related poisoning, or laboratory analysis.

When the Faculty of Medicine at Ramathibodi Hospital was established in 1969, there was a Division of Industrial Medicine in the Department of Medicine.

History of Modern Clinical Toxicology. https://doi.org/10.1016/B978-0-12-822218-8.00040-5

The functions within the Division of Industrial Medicine included teaching and providing services in occupational medicine and clinical toxicology. The Division's name was changed to that of Clinical Toxicology in 1972 when Dr. Polwat Jennawasin, followed by Dr. Sming Kaojarern, finished their training in clinical pharmacology and toxicology in the U.S. The Division changed its name again to the Division of Clinical Pharmacology and Toxicology in 1984. Teaching of clinical toxicology and the provision of consultative services were formally conducted starting in 1984. Unfortunately, Dr. Jennawasin passed away in an accident in that same year.

During 1992–1995, there were three internal medicine physicians who had also trained in clinical pharmacology and toxicology in the United States. By 1995, there were only four clinical toxicologists in the three teaching hospitals; two were at Ramathibodi Hospital. Apart from the clinical services, the toxicological laboratory in the Department of Pathology, Faculty of Medicine Ramathibodi Hospital was also actively developed. It was operated to conduct toxicological testing nationwide. The clinical toxicology faculty had an advanced degree of expertise and were well-integrated into the Division at that time.

Origins of Ramathibodi Poison Center

Most physicians had insufficient knowledge regarding diagnosis and management of poisoning because of a limited opportunity to learn clinical toxicology during their medical school years. There were also limited resources for physicians to search for reliable information related to toxic chemicals and poisoning during that time. As a result of these factors, poisoning cases were inevitably poorly managed. The International Programme of Chemical Safety (IPCS), World Health Organization (WHO) declared that a poison center would be a specialized unit to help health personnel in diagnosis, treatment and prevention of poisoning. IPCS promoted and encouraged all country members to set up poison centers for this purpose.

In Thailand, the Faculty of Medicine Ramathibodi Hospital was found to be the most suitable group to set up a poison center for the country. At the same time, there was a need for clinical toxicology consultation nationwide. Additionally, with the strong support of Professor Atthasit Vejjajiva (who was Dean of the Faculty at the time), Professor Sming Kaojarern proposed to set up a poison center under the faculty in 1991. Human resources and facilities were gradually organized.

The Ramathibodi Poison Center (RPC) was formally opened for operations in August 1996. There were two clinical toxicologists, two information scientists, and one clerical staff. An in-house clinical toxicology training course was initiated. Multidisciplinary medical personnel including nurses from the emergency department, intensive care unit, and medicine ward, and pharmacists have all been trained as part-time specialists in poison information (SPI). Meanwhile, international databases such as the Clinical Information System, Drug Information Source, Physician Desk's reference, Toxline, Chem-Bank, and OSH-ROM were prepared for use as the poison information resources.

Since its beginning in 1996, RPC has formally provided its services around the clock, 24 h daily throughout the year (Kaojarern, 1998; Wananukul et al., 2007). RPC is integrated with several departments including internal medicine, emergency medicine, pediatrics, and pathology. Its services include information and consultation services, clinical services, and laboratory services. These information and consultation services serve health care professionals nationwide free of charge. Initially, the center consisted simply of a telephone and a designated SPI to answer the telephone. The SPIs were continuously trained to give information addressing all types of inquiries. They worked under the supervision of clinical toxicologists, especially for complicated or uncertain cases (Wananukul et al., 2007). However, data collection was fragmented and recorded on non-standardized paper forms.

In 1998, the poison center started to pursue follow-up calls for those poisoning cases on which it had been consulted. The objectives were to verify the cases and exchange more information between the center and frontline health care teams who were treating the patients. At the same time, the poison center developed its data management system with digitalized forms by the harmonization of terms and data collection with the IPCS INTOX program and American Association of Poison Control Centers' Toxic Exposure Surveillance System. The provision of timely and practical information to physicians and health personnel increased the center's recognition.

In 2000, three in-house local databases were created to identify chemical substances and venomous animals. These covered registered pesticide products, registered household products, and venomous snakes in Thailand. In addition, specialists in related areas such as botany, mycology, entomology, and zoology, were invited to be advisors to the center. Meanwhile, other activities progressively expanded, including the training workshop for healthcare providers in rural areas and new initiatives in cooperation with other health organizations, particularly the National Health Security Office (NHSO). With funding from NHSO to enhance the accessibility of the center, the service system was upgraded to a call center system in 2005. The number of calls subsequently increased annually from 409 calls the year of its inception to 16,883 calls recorded in 2011. A nationwide four-digit hotline number (i.e., 1367) was introduced in 2012 to improve the accessibility of the communication system.

Current RPC operations

The center now uses a modern call center system integrated with messaging apps for poison information service. It clearly enhances the precision and efficiency of the service. There are now 4 clinical toxicologists, 5 full-time SPIs, 1 full-time laboratory scientist, 1 clerical staff, and 25 part-time SPIs who work at the center. The RPC currently manages over 24,000 calls each year.

During the past several years, the data collection system has been standardized to an advanced digital format, that is, the RPC Toxic Exposure Surveillance System. Its dataset holds enormous potential for broadening the scope of research on human toxicology; the collected data are a resource for conducting research studies. In 2015, the center was officially announced as one of the Centers of Excellence of the faculty (NHSO, 2020). The center was also designated as a WHO Collaboration Center for Poison Control and Prevention in 2018 (WHO, 2018).

The fields of interest for faculty affiliated with RPC include pesticide poisoning, heavy metal poisoning, snake bite, natural toxins, substance abuse, pharmaceutical products, and the poisoning management system itself. The center also works with several agencies to solve problems related to its function, such as the Office of Narcotic Control Board, NHSO, and Ministry of Public Health.

Siriraj Poison Center

In 2006, the Faculty of Medicine at Siriraj Hospital, which is affiliated with Mahidol University in Bangkok, set up the second poison center: the Siriraj Poison Center. The poison center originally was a toxicological laboratory service. It started as a toxicological laboratory, along with a drug information unit operated by hospital pharmacists and a clinical service staffed by toxicologist clinicians. It subsequently developed over time into a formal poison center as defined by the previously mentioned IPCS guideline for poison control (Sirisamut, 2008). The strengths of the Siriraj Poison Center include its simulation training, clinical expertise in pediatric and adolescent toxicology, and its ongoing research efforts related to acetaminophen poisoning, recreational drugs, and edible insect safety.

Thai Society of Clinical Toxicology

The field of clinical toxicology in Thailand has grown enormously since the development of the Ramathibodi Poison Center. The RPC holds an "Inter-Hospital Tox Conference" monthly as an educational activity for staff and residents in rotations. In 2003, an emergency medicine residency training program was established there, with clinical toxicology as one of the selective subjects for the residents. These training opportunities have added to the visibility of clinical toxicology as a medical specialty in Thailand.

In 2006, the Thai Society of Clinical Toxicology was established. It hosted the 6th Scientific Congress of Asia Pacific Association of Medical Toxicology (APAMT) in 2007. Several activities, especially those involving education, have been run under the society. With the cooperation of the Thai Society of

Toxicology, the Thai Society of Clinical Toxicology, the Thai Environmental Mutagen Society and other alliances, the National Conference in Toxicology has been held annually since 2008. It is a platform for all branches of toxicology to meet and share their knowledge. After the National Antidote Project was initiated in 2010, there were annual workshops held in all four regions of Thailand. More than 1200 physicians, nurses, and pharmacists attended these workshops. All of these have been the major drivers of the development and recognition of clinical toxicology in Thailand to be one of the prominent disciplines of medicine.

Education and training

The need for trained clinical toxicologists was expanding in Thailand, as well as the need to increase medical staffing in the poison centers to accommodate the increasing numbers of clinical cases. To meet these needs, a fellowship training program in clinical toxicology and pharmacology was approved by the Medical Council of Thailand in 2011. The training curriculum is now sponsored and overseen by The Royal College of Physicians of Thailand (RCPT). Physicians who have earned a diploma from the Thai Board of Internal Medicine or Emergency Medicine are eligible for the training program. There are two programs: one each in the Ramathibodi and Siriraj Poison Centers. Over the years, the number of clinical toxicologists has gradually increased, as well as various aspects of research work in this field.

The challenges of poison centers

The major challenges facing the Thai poison centers in the future are financial support and human resources (Kaojarern, 1998). Though the services of both poison centers are available to all health facilities and the public nationwide, the operating budgets are totally dependent on the Faculties. There is no income from their main services. Both poison centers have never received any financial support from Ministry of Public Health. NHSO provided support to RPC for improving hardware for the services, but not on a regular basis to sustain their operations. The centers will need in the future to create income streams from other activities. However, at present such alternative sources of income are not enough to compensate the expense.

Because there is no specific and comprehensive national training program for SPIs, the poison centers have developed their own in-house training course for them. These SPIs are also required to take continuing education courses to maintain their expertise.

Human poisoning in Thailand

According to analyses of data from the poison center surveillance system, the common human poison exposures in Thailand are pesticides, pharmaceutical products, and household products (Wananukul et al., 2007; Saoraya and

Inboriboon, 2013). Pesticide poisoning has been not only the most common but also the cause of the highest mortality rates.

According to circumstances of poison exposure, there are two high-risk groups of poisoned patients. The first group is children aged 0–6 years. The other is teenagers and young adults (those who are 20–29 years old). Accidental exposure is the circumstance seen in the majority of poisonings occurring in the children but intentional self-harm is the most common in teenagers and young adults (Wananukul et al., 2007).

Venomous snake bite is an important natural toxin. Specific monovalent and polyvalent anti-venoms are produced locally by Queen Saovapha Memorial Institute. With accessible anti-venom and available guidelines as well as consultation from the poison center, the mortality rate due to snake bite is relatively low. Poisonous mushrooms, tetrodotoxin, and cyanogenic glycoside poisoning are all causes of seasonal poisoning in Thailand (Swaddiwudhipong et al., 1989). An event of mass botulism from eating pickled bamboo shoots in 2006 was the most challenging toxicological disaster in Thailand (CDC, 2006). Of 209 patients, 119 were hospitalized and 42 required intubation and respiratory support. With the collaboration of national and international experts, all patients finally recovered. There was no mortality resulting from this incident.

Poison center activities

In addition to providing its information and consultation services, the poison centers have identified other needs related to poisoning. Some of the activities are as follows:

1. Training workshop in pesticide poisoning for health personnel in rural areas

According to data from RPC, pesticide poisoning has been the most common type of poisoning seen in adults and causes the highest mortality rate. Unfortunately, most of the cases occur in the rural areas of Thailand where health personnel are lacking in the competencies necessary to deal with these serious cases. RPC arranged a 1–2 day workshop on pesticide poisoning in the rural areas. The objective was to educate health personnel in the diagnosis and proper management of pesticide exposures, so that poisoned patients would receive appropriate medical management at the earliest time possible.

2. The Thai National Antidote Project

One of the major challenges in the treatment of poisoned patients in Thailand is the lack of several antidotes. Though the knowledge to diagnose and treat the patients may exist, a lack of the specific antidote compromises the treatment outcome. Therefore a project called "Nationwide Access to Antidote" was set up in 2010 (Suchonwanich and Wananukul, 2018). There are several paradigm shifts and innovations associated with this project. It is a collaborative work among several agencies in Thailand and it receives its budget from the NHSO (2017).

The main concept in the project is central management, with the sharing of resources and networking. The essential but unavailable antidotes are identified. To solve their shortage, local production of these antidotes is encouraged. For some antidotes which are not produced locally, the Government Pharmaceutical Organization is responsible for search and procurement. All antidotes procured in the program belong to NHSO. Public hospitals at all levels, from university hospitals to regional, provincial and community hospitals, are invited to be the sites for the stocking of antidotes. The drugs are distributed according to the urgency of their need, availability and cost. Educational and training activities and materials are provided to health care personnel at all levels.

An online capacity to search for antidotes was developed, assisted by real-time stocking data using a global positioning system (GPS). The stock was maintained by vendor management inventory. Poison centers play important roles in verifying, supervising and following the patients who have received one of the antidotes. In this way, patients are able to gain access to the antidotes, as well as anti-venoms, quickly and sufficiently. The project is also cost-effective and saves the total budget (Suchonwanich and Wananukul, 2018). The Thai National Antidote Project has been able to demonstrate a reduction of the mortality rate (Srisuma et al., 2018) and has relied on the national budget for purchasing the drugs. A new initiative, called the "Initiative for Coordinated Antidotes Procurement in the South-East Asia region (iCAPS)," which was developed from this project, was established by WHO in 2019 to cover the region (WHO, 2019).

International collaboration

The institutional collaboration between Thai toxicologists within the country and those internationally is mainly facilitated by WHO and APAMT. APAMT is an important platform for clinical toxicologists in the region to meet and exchange their experience. The Thai toxicologists and poison centers have collaborative research projects and other initiatives with others in the region and globally. Projects with colleagues in both the Taiwan National Poison Center and Hong Kong Poison Center are examples of this good collaboration.

The poison centers have been hosting international toxicology elective rotations for foreign medical students, physicians, and toxicology fellows. To experience toxicology management in the Thai context, the visitors participate in academic activities, table rounds, bedside consultations, and clinics under the supervision of the Thai staff. The visiting students or fellows also have optional experiences, such as visits to regional hospitals, community hospitals, or a snake farm. Some of the visitors have conducted research collaborations as well.

To expand the perspectives of Thai toxicology fellows, the centers have invited foreign speakers or arranged video conferences with poison centers in other countries. Thai fellows-in-training also have opportunities to visit poison centers in other countries such as Taiwan or United States as part of their elective rotations. The objectives of such international electives are to gain experiences in different settings and paradigms and to network with experts in clinical toxicology to set up any future collaborations.

Conclusion

Clinical toxicology in Thailand is relatively new and small, but is now expanding. Poison centers in Thailand are located in the medical schools and provide 24/7 information and consultation services. Beside services, they provide teaching, training, conducting research, and work systems which are related to country's toxicological problems. The major challenges are budget and human resources. Poison centers have developed robust roles and they have proven their value for the country.

References

Centers for Disease Control and Prevention (CDC). Botulism from home-canned bamboo shoots-Nan Province, Thailand, March 2006. MMWR Morb Mortal Wkly Rep 2006;55(14):389–92.

Jeyaratnam J. Acute pesticide poisoning: a major global health problem. World Health Stat Q 1990;43:139–44.

Kaojarern S. Recent situation of the poison center in Thailand. J Toxicol Sci 1998;23(Suppl 2):287–91.

National Health Security Office (NHSO). NHSO Annual Report Fiscal Year 2017. Bangkok, Thailand: National Health Security Office; 2017, p. 51–2. Available from: http://eng.nhso.go.th/assets/portals/1/files/annual_report/Annual-Report-NHSO-2017-Eng(1).pdf. Accessed 7 April 2021.

National Health Security Office (NHSO). Ramathibodi Poison Center's role as a great pillar in the fight against poison. National Health Security Office; 2020. (updated 28 January 2020; accessed 30 April 2020). Available from: https://eng.nhso.go.th/view/1/DescriptionNews/Ramathibodi-Poison-Centers-role-as-a-great-pillar-in-the-fight-against-poisons/62/EN-US. Accessed 7 April 2021.

Saoraya J, Inboriboon PC. Acute poisoning surveillance in Thailand: the current state of affairs and a vision for the future. ISRN Emergency Med 2013;1–9.

Sirisamut T. Siriraj poison control center: an analysis of a 2-year cooperation. Thai Pharm Health Sci J 2008;3:405–10.

Srisuma S, Pradoo A, Rittilert A, Wongvisavakorn S, Tongpoo A, Sriapha C, et al. Cyanide poisoning in Thailand before and after establishment of the National Antidote Project. Clin Toxicol (Phila) 2018;56(4):285–93.

Suchonwanich N, Wananukul W. Improving access to antidotes and antivenoms, Thailand. Bull World Health Organ 2018;96(12):853–7.

Swaddiwudhipong W, Kunasol P, Sangwanloy O, Srisomporn D. Foodborne disease outbreaks of chemical etiology in Thailand, 1981-1987. Southeast Asian J Trop Med Public Health 1989;20(1):125–32.

Wananukul W, Sriapha C, Tongpoo A, Sadabthammarak U, Wongvisawakorn S, Kaojarern S. Human poisoning in Thailand: the Ramathibodi poison Center's experience (2001-2004). Clin Toxicol (Phila) 2007;45(5):582–8.

World Health Organization (WHO). WHO Collaborating Centres Global database: WHO Collaborating Centre for the Prevention and Control of Poisoning, 2018. Available from: https://apps.who.int/whocc/List.aspx?A3urjfLCtPUcfza890bjdA==. Accessed 7 April 2021.

World Health Organization (WHO). Improving access through inter-country collaboration in procurement. In Access to medical products in the South-East Asia Region, 2019: Review of progress. New Delhi, India: World Health Organization, South-East Asia Region; 2019. p. 18–9.

Chapter 6.7

South Korea

Hyung-Keun Roh
Past President, The Korean Society of Clinical Toxicology

Governmental projects for poison information

After the turbulent time of the 1950s following the Korean War, regulatory policies addressing toxic substances began with the *Law for Poison and Hazardous Materials*, which was legislated in 1963. This law aimed to prevent accidental poisoning and became a base for regulating the production, transport, sales and manufacture of toxic substances (Jung and Ma, 2016). In the 1980s, industrial development in Korea entailed a massive increase in the use of synthetic chemicals. After the *Toxic Chemicals Control Act* was established in 1991, the control of toxic substances was accelerated (Yoon et al., 2014). Korea's joining the Organization for Economic Cooperation and Development in 1996 reinforced compliance with the international regulations concerning the control and management of toxic chemicals (Moon and Kim, 2014).

Some government ministries started to make their own databases for toxic substance information. There have been three major databases: from the Ministry of Environment, the Ministry of Employment and Labor, and the Ministry of Food and Drug Safety (Ju, 2006). In preparation in anticipation of any future accident, the National Institute of Environmental Research (affiliated with the Ministry of Environment) made a chemicals information system including hazardous chemical substances (i.e., those substances subject to intensive control). The Occupational Safety & Health Research Institute of the Ministry of Employment and Labor also operated an information search system for chemical substances and material safety data sheets. The National Institute of Food and Drug Safety Evaluation (NIFDS) under the Ministry of Food and Drug Safety made the Toxicity Information Service System (Tox-Info; https://www.nifds.go.kr/toxinfo) to provide both the public and medical professionals with information on toxic substances and acute poisoning.

All of these information systems covered a wide range of toxicology, but they included little in the way of clinical contents, except for the clinical information on acute poisoning provided by Tox-Info, which was added in 2007.

History of Modern Clinical Toxicology. https://doi.org/10.1016/B978-0-12-822218-8.00001-6

The Asan Medical Center in Seoul set up a poison information service system supported by Ministry of Health and Welfare from 2004 to 2012, but the system was not fully activated.

Private activities on poison control

Soon Chun Hyang University Hospital

In 1991, Soon Chun Hyang University Hospital established a research center for pesticide poisoning in Chunan where there was a large agricultural population. Pesticide poisoning was common in the rural area at that time, so that the research center was able to conduct a large number of studies related to the diagnosis and treatment for pesticide poisoning. The high incidence of acute paraquat poisoning there enabled them to collect a great number of cases, and their research was very active, especially investigations of paraquat poisoning (Hong et al., 2014). They also provided online consultation services for the public and for the victims of pesticide poisoning.

Inha University Hospital

Inha University Hospital, located in Incheon, operated a poison center from 1996 to 2007, managing acutely intoxicated patients. The center covered a wide range of acute poisoning, and several departments, including internal medicine and emergency medicine, took part in the activities of the center. Considering the large proportion of patients with intentional poisonings seeking the hospital's services, psychiatric consultation and treatment services were actively introduced for the cases involving a suicide attempt. A small-scale toxicology laboratory was set up to analyze the patients' samples for diagnosis, and the service was expanded to respond to the requests of other area hospitals. The samples were analyzed immediately in an emergency when needed. An information service to the public was limited due to a shortage of manpower but a consultation service for acute intoxication was possible at the request of physicians from other hospitals. Although this center was private and there was no support by the government, it covered the major functions of a poison center, such as treatment, an information service, and toxicological analyses. The center suggested a model for the type of regional poison center that the government should establish in the future.

The Korean Society of Clinical Toxicology

Acute poisoning with toxic substances commonly occurred in Korea, and the incidence of severe cases and mortality rates was high. But Korean academic research in this field was not as active as that in Western countries. Many physicians and other experts involved in the management of acute poisoning recognized the need for more academic exchanges in clinical toxicology. They were gathered from various fields, such as emergency medicine, internal medicine, pediatrics, psychiatry, industrial medicine and forensic science, and together, they inaugurated the Korean Society of Clinical Toxicology (KSCT) in 2003.

Korean Society of Clinical Toxicology meetings

The KSCT has been active in discussing an extensive range of issues in clinical toxicology, not only with the clinicians experienced in acute poisoning cases but also with other specialists invited from inside and outside of the country. In addition to academic discussions, some safety guidelines for the management of hazardous materials were also developed. Professional opinions regarding public toxicological issues were also provided. Through annual conferences and small meetings, subjects of acute poisoning commonly encountered in emergency rooms were preferentially discussed; poisoning topics specific to Korea were included.

Korean Society of Clinical Toxicology meeting topics

Acute poisoning cases in Korea were characterized as more intentional than accidental (Kim et al., 2015), and the incidence of severe cases was relatively high. Topics related to pesticide poisoning were common in the conferences, especially those topics related to paraquat and organophosphate poisoning due to their severity and high mortality rates (Cha et al., 2014). Caustic ingestion, acute poisoning in industry, plant toxins like mushrooms and herbal products, animal toxins including tetrodotoxin and snake venom, household chemicals, and heavy metals were also important subjects. The toxicological laboratory service's ability to identify causative toxic substances, which was of interest to all members, was often discussed. The high incidence of suicide attempts by acute poisoning in Korea made clinical toxicologists work together with psychiatrists through these conferences. For understanding the current poisoning status and managing the data, it was also frequently discussed how a toxicology surveillance system would be set up. In 2017, the KSCT started annual training courses to educate young physicians, nurses, paramedics, and emergency medical technicians involved in managing acutely intoxicated patients.

Korean Society of Clinical Toxicology's role in disaster preparedness

Related to national security, the KSCT took a leading role in providing scientific suggestions for preparedness in the event of chemical disasters or terrorism, although it is not an official arm of the Korean government. KSCT experts and representatives from Ministry of Health and Welfare, Ministry of Environment, Ministry of Labor, Ministry of Defense, National Police Agency, and National Fire Agency were all invited to KSCT symposiums to discuss how to prepare for such an emergency through close collaborations between governmental offices and a number of private hospitals.

Journal of the Korean Society of Clinical Toxicology

The *Journal of the Korean Society of Clinical Toxicology* was first published in 2003 when the KSCT was inaugurated. This journal has been issued twice each year as an academic journal registered in the National Research Foundation of Korea, and it has become a main journal in the field of clinical toxicology in Korea.

Pesticide research project

Between 2005 and 2007, when pesticide poisonings were common in agricultural areas, the Korean Rural Development Administration, together with experts in clinical toxicology mainly from the KSCT, carried out a research project called "Establishment of a Pesticide Control System." Surveillance of acute pesticide poisoning, guidelines for its diagnosis and treatment, an information system for pesticide poisoning prophylaxis and emergency management, and the monitoring of chronic pesticide poisoning in rural areas were all prospectively studied (Roh et al., 2008).

Thirty-eight hospitals nationwide participated in this project, and the pesticide poisoning data were collected and analyzed (Lee et al., 2007). The project offered practical diagnostic methods and treatment guidelines, especially on paraquat and organophosphate poisoning. These two pesticide categories showed high mortality rates; poisonings with these products commonly produced life-threatening conditions. Data on about 1900 items produced by the pesticide manufacturers were collected and computerized so that the data were able to be used for confirming the constituents of pesticides when treating a victim of acute intoxication. Clinical data collected from the farmers who were chronically exposed to pesticides were analyzed to suggest criteria needed for early detection of chronic pesticide poisoning (Roh et al., 2008).

Poison information database system

A poisoning emergency needs immediate treatment; it is important for patient management to identify the causative toxic substance and quickly obtain its information. While the toxic substance information in English was generally easy to access, similar information in Korean was very limited. Furthermore, the toxicity information suitable to and useful for treating a Korean patient was difficult to find, especially for animal and plant toxins. Such information should be described using Korean terms. Thus the NIFDS conducted a poison information system project between 2007 and 2016. A writing staff of about 15 experts drawn mainly from the scientific committee of the KSCT compiled the clinical information on 50–60 toxic substances every year. The table of contents for the paper on each substance consisted of an introduction, the toxicokinetics/toxicodynamics, clinical manifestations, diagnosis, treatment, and others. These papers were written according to the style of a review paper, with the inclusion of references.

The information gathered about the substance in each paper was summarized in two pages to give a quick overview for use in an emergency (Roh, 2008).

It was doubtful in the beginning whether such a compilation involving a small number of substances would be helpful for physicians managing an acute poisoning because the number of toxins is usually thought to be countless. The writing started with the substances that were known to have high incidences of occurrence in Korea, through previous studies on the frequencies of various acute poisonings in the country. The toxic substances included in these papers increased in number annually; by 2014, 470 substances had been reviewed. One study retrospectively reviewed the medical records of the acutely intoxicated patients who had visited 20 different emergency departments in one short year. A total of 10,887 cases of intoxication among 8145 patients was collected. The coverage rates of the poison information database for both the number of poisoning cases and the kinds of toxic substances were calculated. The 470 substances registered in the database covered 89% of the identified cases related to acute poisoning, although the same substances only covered 45% of the identified toxic substances (Kim et al., 2016). This study revealed that the poison information database covered a large proportion of the real poisoning cases in Korea and would have been helpful for the physicians in an emergency.

Antidote project

While some of the commonly used antidotes were reserved by most hospitals, many of the uncommon antidotes that were clinically important but rarely used were not stocked even in the large university hospitals. Even if hospitals stocked expensive antidotes for use in rare emergency cases, there was no guarantee that they would be needed before their expiration dates. Thus, hospital pharmacies became more passive for purchasing such expensive items to cut their losses. Considering the relative lack of experts in clinical toxicology in Korea, the hospitals did not expect that someone would actively advocate for the routine stocking of antidotes. When pharmaceutical manufacturers did not produce or import a specific antidote, no hospitals were able to purchase it at all.

In 1999, the Korea Orphan and Essential Drug Center was launched. This center started to import some antidotes which were difficult for individual hospitals to purchase. However, the center had no system to quickly deliver the antidotes to the hospitals in an emergency, so the antidote utilization was restricted and not successful. To stock the antidotes internationally recommended for emergencies but not produced in Korea, it was necessary to have an antidote supply system supported by a relevant governmental office. It was also suggested that if the governmental office could reliably inventory the antidotes possessed in each local hospital and manage their dates of expiration through a system of antidotes exchange among the hospitals, then the antidotes would be always available to all the hospitals (Roh, 2013).

Based on the experience of a pilot program for antidotes stocking and distribution conducted by the Seoul Asan Hospital between 2010 and 2012 (Park et al., 2013), the National Emergency Medical Center (NEMC) started an antidotes managing system in 2016. Twenty "base hospitals" were designated nationwide for antidote stocking. Since then, antidotes have been rapidly supplied by private ambulance service to any hospital close to the base hospitals in a time of need (NEMC, 2019a).

Laboratory services for toxic substances

Toxicology laboratories to confirm the causative substances of acute poisoning were sometimes needed to treat a patient with acute poisoning. However, in most of the hospitals that frequently managed poisoned patients, it was difficult to set up the necessary analyzing equipment. Although commercial laboratory services were available for identifying the toxic materials, their services were not always available in an emergency. Also, it took time to get the results, so that they were not widely utilized, except for confirming the toxic materials that had been involved after the event.

Through some pilot projects to establish an analytical laboratory service, the NEMC was able to support a new system to analyze toxic substances. Since 2019, two university hospitals and four branch institutes of the National Forensic Service have been designated to run the regional laboratories needed to cover the whole country (NEMC, 2019b). The opportunity to use the toxicology laboratory has increased by this system in which any hospital can send patients' samples to the laboratory for analysis. However, the emergency analyses are only available in the two university hospitals. The clinical information accompanying the samples is sometimes not well-informed; thus, proper medical interpretation of the results is not always possible. New strategies should be considered.

Future challenges

Poison control activities in Korea have been gradually and partially developed by members of the KSCT as the need arose. Korean clinical toxicologists and other experts have tried to build a national network of regional poison centers which would integrate the important core functions, considering the considerable distance for some patients to be immediately reached in an emergency. To achieve this goal, cooperation between the academic institutions and the relevant governmental offices should be deliberated in detail.

Clinical toxicology is not yet acknowledged as a separate professional discipline in Korea, and adequately trained physicians in this field are still limited. Therefore the educational curriculum in medical schools should be set up to strengthen the understanding of poison control, and in the future, programs will need to be developed to train a workforce and foster the careers of specialists in clinical toxicology.

References

Cha ES, Khang YH, Lee WJ. Mortality from and incidence of pesticide poisoning in South Korea: findings from national death and health utilization data between 2006 and 2010. PLoS One 2014;9(4):1–8.

Hong SY, Lee JS, Sun IO, Lee KY, Gil HW. Prediction of patient survival in cases of acute paraquat poisoning. PLoS One 2014;9(11):1–7.

Ju IJ. Interministrial Cooperation Program for Toxic Chemical Management. Natl. R&D Rep; 2006.

Jung HK, Ma JK. A study on legal systems and politics to control chemicals. Adm Law J 2016;44:191–222.

Kim KH, Choi JW, Park M, Kim MS, Lee ES. A nationwide study of patients hospitalised for poisoning in Korea based on Korea National Hospital Discharge in-Depth Injury Survey data from 2005 to 2009. BMJ Open 2015;5(11):1–9.

Kim SJ, Chung SP, Gil HW, Choi SC, Kim H, Kang C, Kim HJ, Park JS, Lee KW, Cho J, Yoon JC, Cho S, Choe MSP, Hwang TS, Hong DY, Lim H, Kim YW, Kim SW, Kang H, Kim WJ. The poisoning information database covers a large proportion of real poisoning cases in Korea. J Korean Med Sci 2016;31(7):1037–41.

Lee MJ, Kwon WY, Park JS, Eo EK, Oh BJ, Lee SW, Suh JH, Roh HK. Clinical characteristics of acute pure organophosphate compounds poisoning - 38 multi-centers survey in South Korea. J Korean Soc Clin Toxicol 2007;5(1):1–11.

Moon SG, Kim KH. Regulatory policies of toxic chemical substances in Korea: examining toxic substances registration and evaluation act. EWHA Law J 2014;19(2):249–78.

NEMC. Emergency medical service guidelines for stocking and distribution of antidotes. NEMC Guidel 2019a;4–6.

NEMC. Emergency medical service guidelines for toxicological analyses. NEMC Guidel 2019b;7–10.

Park SY, Oh BJ, Sohn CH, Jeong RB, Lim KS, Kim W, Ryoo SM. The experiences of the emergency antidote stock and delivery service by the Korean Poison Information Center. J Korean Soc Clin Toxicol 2013;11(1):9–18.

Roh HK. Establishment of poison information system. Seoul: Natl. R&D Rep; 2008.

Roh HK. Need for stocking of emergency antidotes. J Korean Med Assoc 2013;56(12):1054–6.

Roh HK, Lim KS, Hong SY. Establishment of management systems for pesticide poisoning. Suwon: Natl. R&D Rep; 2008.

Yoon CS, Ham SH, Park JH, Kim SJ, Lee SA, Lee KS, Park DG. Comparison between the chemical management contents of laws pertaining to the Ministry of Environment and the Ministry of the Employment and Labor. Korean J Environ Heal Sci 2014;40(5):331–45.

Index

Note: Page numbers followed by *f* indicate figures, *t* indicate tables, and *b* indicate boxes.

Printed in the United States
by Baker & Taylor Publisher Services